LEARNING INTERVENTIONAL RADIOLOGY

T0127754

Edited by:

JUSTIN SHAFA, MD
Radiology Resident
Jacobi Medical Center
Albert Einstein College of Medicine
Bronx, New York

STEPHEN T. KEE, MD, FSIR
Professor of Radiology
Ronald Reagan UCLA Medical Center
Los Angeles, California

ELSEVIER

ELSEVIER

1600 John F. Kennedy Blvd.
Ste 1600
Philadelphia, PA 19103-2899

LEARNING INTERVENTIONAL RADIOLOGY, FIRST EDITION

ISBN: 978-0-323-47879-3

Copyright © 2020 by Elsevier, Inc. All rights reserved.

No part of this publication may be reproduced or transmitted in any form or by any means, electronic or mechanical, including photocopying, recording, or any information storage and retrieval system, without permission in writing from the publisher. Details on how to seek permission, further information about the Publisher's permissions policies and our arrangements with organizations such as the Copyright Clearance Center and the Copyright Licensing Agency, can be found at our website: www.elsevier.com/permissions.

This book and the individual contributions contained in it are protected under copyright by the Publisher (other than as may be noted herein).

Notice

Practitioners and researchers must always rely on their own experience and knowledge in evaluating and using any information, methods, compounds or experiments described herein. Because of rapid advances in the medical sciences, in particular, independent verification of diagnoses and drug dosages should be made. To the fullest extent of the law, no responsibility is assumed by Elsevier, authors, editors or contributors for any injury and/or damage to persons or property as a matter of products liability, negligence or otherwise, or from any use or operation of any methods, products, instructions, or ideas contained in the material herein.

Library of Congress Control Number: 2019935103

Content Strategist: Marybeth Thiel
Content Development Specialist: Marybeth Thiel
Publishing Services Manager: Shereen Jameel
Project Manager: Radhika Sivalingam
Designer: Bridget Hoette

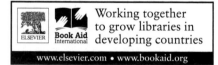

Printed in United States of America.
Last digit is the print number: 9 8 7 6 5 4 3 2

LEARNING INTERVENTIONAL RADIOLOGY

CONTENTS

CONTRIBUTORS

Lourdes Alanis, MD, MPH
Radiology Resident
Cooper University Health Care
Camden, NJ

Ronald S. Arellano, MD
Associate Professor of Radiology
Massachusetts General Hospital
Harvard Medical School
Boston, MA

Christopher R. Bailey, MD
Radiology Resident
The Johns Hopkins Hospital
Baltimore, MD

David H. Ballard, MD
Radiology Resident/T32 Research Fellow
Mallinckrodt Institute of Radiology
Washington University School of Medicine
St. Louis, MO

Adam M. Berry, DO
Interventional Radiology Resident
University of Arkansas for Medical Sciences
Little Rock, AR

Stuart E. Braverman, MD
Interventional Radiologist
Santa Barbara Cottage Hospital
Santa Barbara, CA

Peter R. Bream, Jr., MD, FSIR
Professor of Radiology
University of North Carolina at Chapel Hill
Chapel Hill, NC

Andrew M. Brod, MD
Resident Physician
University of Florida
Gainesville, FL

Jeffrey A. Brown, MD
Interventional Radiology Fellow
Yale University
New Haven, CT

Charles T. Burke, MD
Professor of Radiology, Vice Chair of
    Interventional Services, and Division
    Chief of Vascular-Interventional
    Radiology
University of North Carolina at Chapel Hill
Chapel Hill, NC

Jeffrey S. Carpenter, MD
Professor of Neurology, Neurosurgery, and
    Radiology
West Virginia University
Morgantown, WV

Rajat Chand, MD
Radiology Resident
John H. Stroger, Jr. Hospital of Cook
    County
Chicago, IL

Philip Yue-Cheng Cheung, MD, MEng
Interventional Radiology Resident
Stanford University Medical Center
Stanford, CA

Jason Chiang, MD, PhD
Radiology Resident
UCLA Medical Center
Los Angeles, CA

Clayton W. Commander, MD, PhD
Radiology Resident
University of North Carolina
Chapel Hill, NC

**Bairbre L. Connolly, MB, FFRRCSI,
FRCP(C)**
Centre of Image Guided Therapy
Department of Diagnostic Imaging
The Hospital for Sick Children
Toronto, Canada;
Associate Professor, Department of Medical
    Imaging
University of Toronto
Toronto, Canada

Nathan A. Cornish, DO
Radiology Resident
Maimonides Medical Center
Brooklyn, NY

Alexander A. Covington, MD, MBA
Interventional Radiology Fellow
University of New Mexico Health Sciences
    Center
Albuquerque, NM

**Horacio R.V. D'Agostino, MD, FACR,
FSIR**
Professor of Radiology, Surgery, and
    Anesthesiology
Chairman of the Department of Radiology
LSU Health - Shreveport
Shreveport, LA

Daniel M. DePietro, MD
Resident, Interventional Radiology
Hospital of the University of Pennsylvania
Philadelphia, PA

Kavi K. Devulapalli, MD, MPH
Interventional Radiologist
Duke Regional Hospital
Durham, NC

Gustavo A. Elias, MD
Interventional Radiology Fellow
Yale University
New Haven, CT

Alicia L. Eubanks, MD
General Surgery Resident
University of Virginia
Charlottesville, VA

Anthony Febles, MD
Assistant Professor of Radiology
Zucker School of Medicine at
    Hofstra/Northwell
Hempstead, NY

**Aaron M. Fischman, MD, FSIR
FCIRSE**
Associate Professor of Radiology and
    Surgery
Icahn School of Medicine at Mount Sinai
New York, NY

Sarah T. Flanagan, MD, MPA
Radiology Resident
LSU Health - Shreveport
Shreveport, LA

Jacob W. Fleming, MD
Interventional Radiology Resident
University of Texas Southwestern Medical
    Center
Dallas, TX

Daniel E. Fuguet, MD
Radiology Resident
St. Joseph Mercy Oakland
Pontiac, MI

Ron C. Gaba, MD
Associate Professor of Radiology and
    Pathology
Vice Chair for Research, Department of
    Radiology
University of Illinois Health
Chicago, IL

Vincent Gallo, MD
Interventional Radiologist
Holy Name Medical Center
Teaneck, NJ

Judy W. Gichoya, MD, MS
Radiology Resident
Indiana University
Indianapolis, IN

Makida T. Hailemariam, MD
Radiology Resident
Michigan State University
Southfield, MI

Monte L. Harvill, MD
Chief of Vascular and Interventional
    Radiology
Harper University Hospital
Wayne State University SOM
Detroit, MI

Nauman Hashmani, MBBS
Resident Physician
Hashmanis Hospital
Karachi, Pakistan

Junjian Huang, MD
Radiology Resident
Pennsylvania Hospital, University of
    Pennsylvania Health System
Philadelphia, PA

Ari J. Isaacson, MD
Assistant Professor of Vascular -
    Interventional Radiology
University of North Carolina
Chapel Hill, NC

Stephen T. Kee, MD, FSIR
Professor of Radiology
Ronald Reagan UCLA Medical Center
Los Angeles, California

Joanna Kee-Sampson, MD
Assistant Professor of Radiology
University of Florida - Jacksonville
Jacksonville, FL

Frederick S. Keller, MD
Cook Professor, Charles Dotter Department
    of Interventional Radiology
Oregon Health & Sciences University
Portland, OR

Andrew Kesselman, MD
Assistant Professor of Interventional
    Radiology
Weill Cornell Medicine
New York

Akhil Khetarpal, MD
Interventional Radiology Fellow
Medical College of Wisconsin
Milwaukee, WI

Ryan M. Kiefer, MD
Interventional Radiology Resident
Hospital of the University of Pennsylvania
Philadelphia, PA

Eric C. Kim, MD, MS
Radiology Resident
University of Chicago
Chicago, IL

Jeremy I. Kim, MD
Radiology Resident
University of North Carolina
Chapel Hill, NC

Eric C. King, MS, MD
Radiology Resident
Kaiser Permanente Los Angeles Medical
    Center
Los Angeles, CA

Maureen P. Kohi, MD, FSIR
Associate Professor of Clinical Radiology
    and Chief of Interventional Radiology
University of California, San Francisco
San Francisco, CA

Marcin K. Kolber, MD
Assistant Professor of Interventional
    Radiology
UT Southwestern Medical Center
Dallas, TX

Nathan Kwok, MD
Radiology Resident
University of Utah
Salt Lake City, UT

Cuong (Ken) Lam, MD, MBA
Vascular and Interventional Physician
Kaiser Permanente Vascular and
    Interventional Specialists,
    Los Angeles
Los Angeles, CA

**Edward Wolfgang Lee, MD,
PhD, FSIR**
Associate Professor of Radiology and
    Surgery
Director of Research
UCLA Medical Center
Los Angeles, CA

Luke A. Lennard, MD
Abdominal Imaging Fellow
University of Alabama at Birmingham
Birmingham, AL

Paul B. Lewis, MD
Clinical Assistant Professor of Vascular and
    Interventional Radiology
University of Pittsburgh Medical Center
    (UPMC)
Pittsburgh, PA

Millie Liao, DO, MS
Interventional Radiology Resident
Loma Linda University
Loma Linda, CA

Viky S. Loescher, MD
Radiology Resident
Mount Sinai Medical Center
Miami Beach, FL

Mohammed F. Loya, MD
Radiology Resident
Nassau University Medical Center
East Meadow, NY

Mina S. Makary, MD
Assistant Professor
Division of Vascular and Interventional
    Radiology
Department of Radiology
The Ohio State University Wexner
    Medical Center
Columbus, OH

Larry E. Mathias, III, DO, MBA
Radiology Resident
Baylor Scott and White/Texas A&M
Temple, TX

Kimberly C. McFarland, MD
Interventional Radiology Fellow
SUNY Downstate Medical Center/Kings
    County Hospital
Brooklyn, NY

Justin P. McWilliams, MD
Associate Professor of Radiology
UCLA Medical Center
Los Angeles, CA

John M. Moriarty, MD, FSIR
Associate Professor of Radiology and
    Medicine
UCLA Medical Center
Los Angeles, CA

James J. Morrison, MD, MBI
Assistant Professor of Radiology
Advanced Radiology Services, Michigan
    State University
Grand Rapids, MI

Pranav Moudgil, MD
Resident Physician
Oakland University William Beaumont
    SOM
Beaumont Health System
Royal Oak, MI

Marwan H. Moussa, MD
Interventional Radiology Fellow
Beth Israel Deaconess Medical Center
Boston, MA

Daniel C. Murph, MD
Radiologist
IU Health University Hospital
Indianapolis, IN

Brittany K. Nagy, MD
Interventional Radiologist
Lake Vascular Institute at Lake Medical
    Imaging
Leesburg, FL

Andrew S. Niekamp, MD
Interventional Radiology Fellow
Miami Cardiac and Vascular Institute
Miami, FL

Myles Nightingale, MD
General Surgery Resident
Temple University Hospital
Philadelphia, PA

Muhammad Umer Nisar, MD
Resident Physician
University of Pittsburgh Medical Center
Pittsburgh, PA

Emily R. Ochmanek, DO
Interventional Radiology Fellow
University of Colorado School of
    Medicine
Aurora, CO

Brandon P. Olivieri, MD, RPVI
Interventional Radiologist
Department of Vascular & Interventional
    Radiology, @SOBE_Vascular
Mount Sinai Medical Center
Miami Beach, FL

Shivang S. Patel, DO, MS
Radiology Resident
Saint Barnabas Medical Center
Livingston, NJ

Keith Pereira, MD, DABR
Assistant Professor
Division of Vascular and Interventional
    Radiology
Saint Louis University
St. Louis, MO

David A. Petrov, MD
Radiology Resident
Allegheny Health Network
Pittsburgh, PA

Thomas Powierza, MD
Radiology Resident
Baptist Memorial Healthcare
Memphis, TN

Uma R. Prasad, MD
Associate Professor of Radiology
Director of Non-Vascular Interventions
    and Ultrasound
VCU Health System
Richmond, VA

Poyan Rafiei, MD
Vascular and Interventional Radiologist
Radiology Partners Gulf Coast
Houston, TX

Driss Raissi, MD
Assistant Professor of Radiology, Medicine
    and OB/GYN
University of Kentucky
Lexington, KY

Bipin Rajendran, MD
Interventional Radiology Fellow
Massachusetts General Hospital
Boston, MA

Priyanka Ramesh, MBBS
General Surgery Resident
Patel Hospital
Karachi, Pakistan

Hunaid Nasir Rana, MD
Resident Physician
LSU Health Sciences Center
Baton Rouge, LA

Fareed R. Riyaz, MD
Interventional Radiology Fellow
Massachusetts General Hospital
Boston, MA

Jeffrey H. Savin, MD
Radiology Resident
Beaumont Health/Oakland University
    William Beaumont School of Medicine
Royal Oak, MI

Michael A. Savin, MD, FSIR
Associate Professor of Diagnostic and
    Interventional Radiology
Beaumont Health/Oakland University
    William Beaumont School of Medicine
Royal Oak, MI

Stephen Seedial, MD
Interventional Radiology Fellow
Northwestern Memorial Hospital
Chicago, IL

Kimberly D. Seifert, MD, MS
Radiology Resident
Yale University School of Medicine
New Haven, CT

Justin Shafa, MD
Radiology Resident
Jacobi Medical Center
Albert Einstein College of Medicine
Bronx, NY

Salman S. Shah, MD
Chief, Division of Vascular and
    Interventional Radiology
Nassau University Medical Center/
    NuHealth
East Meadow, NY

Pratik A. Shukla, MD
Assistant Professor
Division of Interventional Radiology
Department of Radiology
Rutgers New Jersey Medical School
Newark, NJ

Andrew Sideris, MD
Interventional Radiology Resident
New York-Presbyterian
    Hospital/Columbia University
    Medical Center
New York

Nadia V. Silva, MD
Resident Physician
University of Texas Health at San Antonio
San Antonio, TX

Manu K. Singh, MD
Staff Interventional Radiologist
Santa Barbara Cottage Hospital
Santa Barbara, CA

Sara E. Smolinski-Zhao, MD
Assistant Professor of Radiology
University of Michigan
Ann Arbor, MI

Jared T. Sokol, BA
Medical Student
University of Chicago Pritzker School of
    Medicine
Chicago, IL

Eric vanSonnenberg, MD
Clinical Professor of Radiology
University of Arizona College of Medicine
    Phoenix
Phoenix, AZ;
Visiting Professor of Medicine and Clinical
    Professor of Radiology
UCLA Medical Center
Los Angeles, CA

Tameem M. Souman, MD, MPH
Vascular and Interventional Radiology
    Attending
Mt. Sinai Health System
Chicago, IL

Malcolm K. Sydnor, MD
Division Chair of Vascular and
    Interventional Radiology
VCU Health
Richmond, VA

Thaddeus F. Sze, MD
Vascular and Interventional Radiologist
Santa Fe Imaging
Santa Fe, NM

David M. Tabriz, MD, RPVI
Assistant Professor of Radiology
Rush University Medical Center
Chicago, IL

Chad Thompson, MD
Interventional Radiologist
Integris Baptist Medical Center
Oklahoma City, OK

Samuel K. Toland, MB, BCh, BAO
Resident Physician
Mater Misericordiae University Hospital
Dublin, Ireland

Scott O. Trerotola, MD
Associate Chair and Chief of
    Interventional Radiology
Vice Chair for Quality, Department of
    Radiology
Perelman School of Medicine at the
    University of Pennsylvania
Philadelphia, PA

Ryan Trojan, MD
Vascular and Interventional Radiologist
INTEGRIS Baptist Medical Center
Oklahoma City, OK

Muhammad Umair, MB, BS
Radiology Resident
Northwestern University, Feinberg School of
    Medicine
Chicago, IL

Laurie M. Vance, MD
Diagnostic Radiologist
Henry Ford Health System
Detroit, MI

Eric M. Walser, MD
Professor and Chair, Radiology
Department of Radiology
The University of Texas Medical Branch
Galveston, TX

James P. Walsh, MD
Assistant Clinical Professor of Radiology
SUNY Downstate
Brooklyn, NY

Jennifer Wan, MD
Vascular and Interventional Radiologist
Mills-Peninsula Medical Center
Sutter Health
Burlingame, CA

Shantanu Warhadpande, MD
Radiology Resident
University of Pittsburgh Medical Center
Pittsburgh, PA

Clifford R. Weiss, MD, FSIR, FCIRSE
Associate Professor of Radiology, Surgery
    and Biomedical Engineering
Interventional Radiology Center
Department of Radiology
The Johns Hopkins Hospital
Baltimore, MD

Kevin T. Williams, MD
Associate Professor of Radiology
University of New Mexico
Albuquerque, NM

Thaddeus M. Yablonsky, MD
Chief of Interventional Radiology
Morristown Medical Center
Morristown, NJ;
Clinical Assistant Professor of Radiology
Sidney Kimmel Medical College of Thomas
    Jefferson University
Philadelphia, PA

Timothy E. Yates, MD, DABR, RPVI
Interventional Radiologist
Associate Diagnostic Radiology Program
    Director
Mount Sinai Medical Center
Miami Beach, FL

Zachary Zhang, MD
Interventional Radiology Fellow
Brigham and Women's Hospital/Harvard
    Medical School
Boston, MA

To Noah, my first nephew—dream big!

—Justin Shafa

Dedicated to the hard-working staff in Interventional Radiology
at UCLA Health—you made it all possible.

—Stephen Kee

First proposed as a concept by the preeminent interventionalist Charles Dotter in 1963, interventional radiology (IR) is a relatively new field in medicine that is growing exponentially in its role in patient care. To define all that the field encompasses, it was Dr. Dotter himself who so eloquently said: "If a plumber can do it to pipes; we can do it to blood vessels." Not so barbaric in practice, the genius of the statement is immediately evident—blood vessels traverse the entirety of the human body, and, as such, a catheter can theoretically be directed anywhere in the body via these vascular networks. From these humble beginnings, the discipline has since flourished throughout the world. That initial meeting of the Society of Cardiovascular Radiology, held in 1973, included less than 100 members; in 2018, the Society of Interventional Radiology (SIR) had more than 7,000 members in the United States alone.

By far the most rapid growth in membership in the past few years has been in the number of medical students and residents. With modern high-definition imaging at hand, the minimally invasive nature of our techniques results in excellent initial outcomes and dramatically reduced recovery times for patients, which appeals directly to the imagination of young, tech-savvy, forward-thinking trainees.

Interventional radiology is all encompassing—it's pediatrics to geriatrics, head-to-toe, and one must maintain a basic knowledge of all aspects of health care. I truly believe that. Barely a day has passed in the 20 plus years since I started my IR fellowship with Michael Dake at Stanford University that I have not had to think back to my basic medical training to better understand a disease concept, or to my anatomy classes in Dublin many years ago, as I arranged the steps of a procedure in my mind.

Interventional radiology may not always be fun, but it is never boring. Even the most trivial, routine procedure can become an entertaining challenge when an unexpected anatomic variant is encountered or a previously unentertained diagnosis suddenly presents itself.

The diversity and breadth of interventional radiology result in difficulties in training. Traditional IR fellowships have consisted of a single year of apprenticeship at the end of 4 years of diagnostic radiology residency, during which the trainees only receive 12 weeks of IR exposure. This is simply not enough time for these individuals to absorb an IR curriculum, become adept at basic and some advanced procedures, remind themselves how to perform basic patient assessment, obtain experience in a clinic setting, and develop some understanding of the management of complex ICU or/ and trauma cases. The society has successfully undertaken the development of an IR residency, encompassing multiple entry methods, resulting in at least 24 months of IR training. This major step forward comes into effect beginning July 1, 2020.

This book was written in an attempt to assist trainees with this novel curriculum and provide a basic and advanced understanding of the types of conditions encountered by medical students and residents on an IR rotation. Thanks to Justin, the contents cover a very broad range of diseases and procedures. Hopefully physicians from other specialties can use this to learn more about what assistance they can obtain from their interventionalists colleagues. This may not be the only text required, but it provides an essential basis and will provide an in-depth resource for physicians hungry for more information.

- Stephen Kee

ACKNOWLEDGMENT

We would like to extend many thanks to all of the medical students, residents, fellows, and attendings whose valued contributions made this publication possible.

History of Interventional Radiology

Andrew M. Brod, Marwan H. Moussa, Driss Raissi

This opening chapter aims to introduce the pioneers who conceived the concept of interventional radiology (IR) and developed the field to its current form. Whether it is Dotter's innovative brilliance or Baum's visionary approach to sharing new technologies, these minds were paramount in laying the groundwork for the field. No less important, the intimate relation between translational research and the innovative nature of IR is a dominant trait in the conception and development of IR. This chapter is by no means a comprehensive presentation of the exciting history of IR. However, it is an attempt to shed some light on some of the forefathers of this growing field and their pivotal landmarks, which have positioned IR to be on the cutting edge of contemporary medicine.

EGAS MONIZ—CEREBRAL ANGIOGRAPHY

- *Moniz pioneered cerebral angiography and developed Thorotrast.*
- *He won the Nobel Prize in Physiology or Medicine for developing lobotomy.*

Egas Moniz was born in 1874 in Avanca, Portugal to an aristocratic family. Moniz attended medical school at the University of Coimbra in Portugal and later traveled to France, where he trained in neurology and psychiatry with some of the most renowned French authorities in those specialties.

Cerebral angiography stands as Moniz's seminal contribution to medicine. Convinced that radiographic visualization of the cerebral vasculature would yield more accurate localization of brain tumors, he set out with his neurosurgical collaborators, Drs. Lima and Dias, to develop a technique that would fulfill this function. Numerous in vitro and cadaveric studies established potential intravenous contrast agents and the normal radiographic anatomy of the internal carotid artery.

In the early animal and cadaver studies, strontium bromide was discarded in favor of sodium iodide after four failed attempts and the death of one patient. The first satisfactory examination was that of their ninth patient, a 20-year-old man whose films showed displacement of intracranial vessels secondary to a pituitary tumor. The technique was further optimized by roentgenologist Jose Pereira Caldas, who devised a "radio carousel" that allowed for the rapid sequential exposure of six films to capture the arterial, capillary, and venous phases of cerebral blood flow. By 1934, Moniz and his collaborators had described his group's experience in an impressive series of cases studies.

In an effort to improve his angiographic technique, Moniz developed Thorotrast (thorium dioxide), a contrast agent with less immediate side effects and higher image resolution. However, Thorotrast, an alpha emitter, fell out of use due to an increased risk of malignancy after a single use. Moniz is perhaps best known for his work on frontal lobotomy for the treatment of refractory neuropsychiatric disorders. For this, he received the 1949 Nobel Prize in Physiology or Medicine.

SVEN IVAR SELDINGER—SELDINGER TECHNIQUE

- *Seldinger developed the Seldinger technique for simple percutaneous arterial access and catheterization.*
- *He pioneered percutaneous transhepatic cholangiography.*

Sven Ivar Seldinger was born in Mora, Sweden on April 19, 1921. He came from a long line of gifted mechanics who ran the Mora Mechanical Workshop and were said to be "technical geniuses." He is credited with the development of the technique that bears his name, which has been called the "single technical contribution [that] has impacted the development of angiography, and consequently the realization of interventional radiology."

Prior to Seldinger's breakthrough, numerous well-respected authorities had developed multiple techniques to catheterize arteries and perform angiography. They were all plagued with risky approaches—such as direct catheterization of the aorta or surgical cutdowns—that were deemed unpopular and difficult to adopt. Catheters also had a short reach beyond the needle tip, making the opacification of deep visceral arteries an uncharted territory. The potential in angiography was great, but a less invasive method of catheter placement was required.

In 1952, Seldinger, then a young radiology resident, conceived of his technique and later demonstrated in phantom models how it could be utilized to reach all arteries of the body. Seldinger best describes the moment when he had his epiphany the following is a quotation from "A Leaf out of the History of Angiography" (In: Pioneers in Angiography, M.E. Silvestre, F. Abecasis, J.A. Veiga-Pires eds. Elseviers Science Publishers [Biomedical Division], 1987), "After an unsuccessful attempt...I found myself disappointed and sad, with three objects in my hand—a needle, a wire and a catheter—and in a split second I realized in what sequence I should use them: Needle in—wire in—needle off—catheter on wire—catheter in—catheter advance—wire off." Although revolutionary, the idea was described by Seldinger's department chair as too simple to constitute the basis for his thesis. This sent Seldinger off to develop yet another technique, percutaneous transhepatic cholangiography. Seldinger published his method in 1953, ushering angiography into a new era. He also described and wrote about catheterization of the spleen and liver, pressure readings in the portal vein in pathologic conditions and after administration of various chemical compounds, percutaneous transhepatic cholangiography, pancreatic diagnostics, and vascular anomalies in the extremities, thus cementing his place in the history of IR.

CHARLES DOTTER—INTERVENTIONAL RADIOLOGY

- *Dotter was the youngest American radiology department chair at the age of 32.*

- *He conceived the idea of IR in 1963 and treated his first patient by percutaneous transluminal dilatation in 1964.*

Born in Boston in 1920, a young Charles Dotter was quite inquisitive, always trying to disassemble any machine that came his way. That interest and derived satisfaction were most likely an earlier manifestation of Dotter's famous conceptual trademark, the crossed pipe and wrench. At the age of 32, Dotter was named chairman of the Department of Radiology at Oregon Health Sciences University, a position he held for 33 years until his death.

Dotter first discussed what would become the foundation of IR at the Czechoslovak Radiologic Congress held in Karlovy Vary, Czechoslovakia in 1963. In his closing remarks, he envisioned the future of the field: "The angiographic catheter can be more than a tool for passive means for diagnostic observation; used with imagination it can become an important surgical instrument." In 1964, Dotter was presented with his first opportunity to perform transluminal vascular dilatation on Laura Shaw, an 82-year-old woman who was referred to Dotter by Dr. William Krippaehne for an angiogram. She had previously refused recommended amputation of her left foot due to gangrenous toes and a nonhealing ulcer. The short segmental stenosis of the superficial femoral artery was easily and quickly dilated by Dotter's experimental percutaneous dilating catheters. Angiograms performed 3 weeks after the intervention demonstrated persistent patency of the vessels (Fig. 1.1). In fact, Shaw lived for another 3 years until she succumbed to congestive heart failure. She is famous for having said, while on her deathbed, "[I'm] still walking on my own two feet."

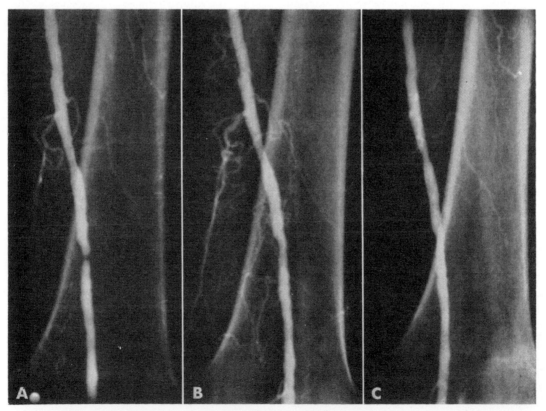

Fig. 1.1 Angiograms of Dotter's First Catheter Patient, Laura Shaw. (A) Before transluminal dilation of the left superficial femoral artery. (B) Immediately after dilation. (C) Three weeks after the procedure. (From Dotter CT, Judkins MP. Transluminal treatment of arteriosclerotic obstruction. Description of a new technic and a preliminary report of its application. *Circulation.* 1964;30:654–670, Fig. 1.)

Acceptance of this radical technique was anything but swift. In the year following Ms. Shaw's successful procedure, Dotter and his colleagues reported the results of 113 procedures in 74 patients with iliofemoral obstruction. In the famous case of "visualize but do not try to fix," Dotter obliged and imaged the diseased superficial femoral artery without intervention as requested. As a cunning clinician, however, Dotter recognized a second lesion in the deep femoral artery and seized the opportunity to dilate it. To Dotter's delight, the patient was spared amputation even after failure of the open surgical repair of the superficial femoral artery thanks to the left profunda he had repaired through angioplasty (Fig. 1.2) (see video at https://www.youtube.com/watch?v=LsaS5vhqhiQ). In addition to his pioneering angioplasty work, Dotter's further contributions to the field include the use of streptokinase in the treatment of thromboembolic disease; embolization in the treatment of acute gastrointestinal bleeding; transluminal extraction of catheter and guidewire fragments; and the transjugular approach to the hepatic, biliary, and portal circulation. Dotter exhibited a unique display of physical and mental resilience. Despite two bouts with Hodgkin lymphoma and two open heart surgeries for coronary artery stenosis, he continued to work until his death. He would schedule his own radiotherapy around his patients' appointments such that patient care never took a back seat to his own. Dotter possessed a larger-than-life personality. Cunning and aggressive in his pursuit, Dotter paved the way for the interventional radiologist to rise. He was not daunted by skeptics or by their ridicule, truly earning the nickname *Crazy Charlie*.

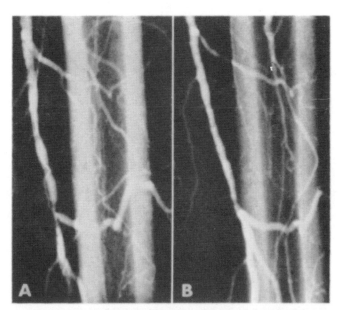

Fig. 1.2 Angiograms of the "Do not try to fix" patient, showing significant narrowing of the left profunda. (A) before and (B) after transluminal dilation. Dotter's intervention spared this patient's limb since the surgical repair of his superficial femoral artery had failed. (From Dotter CT, Judkins MP. Transluminal treatment of arteriosclerotic obstruction. Description of a new technic and a preliminary report of its application. *Circulation.* 1964;30:654–670, Fig. 4.)

ANDREAS GRÜNTZIG—BALLOON ANGIOPLASTY

- *Grüntzig further developed balloon angioplasty, giving rise to the dawn of percutaneous transluminal coronary angioplasty (PTCA).*

Andreas Grüntzig was born on June 25, 1939, in Dresden, Germany. As a medical student, he was mentored by Dr. Schettler, one of Germany's foremost atherosclerosis experts. After his internship, Grüntzig secured a postdoctoral research fellowship in London that included training in public health and statistics. It would leave an everlasting imprint on his view of atherosclerosis. After spending 3 years studying and publishing papers about atherosclerosis and its risk factors, Grüntzig decided to embark on a career in clinical medicine.

In 1969 he joined the Angiologische Klinik, a hospital specializing in vascular medicine, as a clinical fellow. During his training he would have the opportunity to meet Dr. Eberhard Zeitler, a radiologist who introduced him to "Dottering," the word for angioplasty at the time.

In 1973, collaborating with Dr. Heinrich Hopff, a retired professor of chemistry, Grüntzig succeeded in crafting a balloon catheter. He performed his first balloon angioplasty in 1974 on a 74-year-old man with severe claudication. The femoral artery was successfully dilated, and the patient became symptom-free. Emboldened, Grüntzig went on to make custom designs and to craft balloon catheters in his kitchen for each individual patient based on preprocedural angiograms. After his success with peripheral arteries, Grüntzig shifted his attention to the coronary arteries, experimenting with smaller balloon catheters on dogs and human cadaveric coronary arteries.

In 1977, Grüntzig submitted his thesis, titled "Percutaneous Transluminal Recanalization," and patented the balloon catheter concept. He then performed the first successful renal artery balloon angioplasty. In September of that year, Grüntzig was presented with an ideal opportunity to validate his principle, a 38-year-old male with isolated stenosis of the proximal left anterior descending artery. With support and backup in the operating theater from Dr. Åke Senning, a cardiothoracic surgeon credited with inventing and implanting the first-ever cardiac pacemaker, Grüntzig proceeded with and successfully performed the first successful coronary angioplasty (see video at https://med.emory.edu/gamechangers/researchers/gruentzig/interview.html).

JOSEF RÖSCH—CREATOR OF THE TRANSJUGULAR INTRAHEPATIC PORTOSYSTEMIC SHUNT

- *Rösch pioneered both the transhepatic intrajugular portosystemic shunt (TIPS) procedure and the use of embolization for controlling acute gastrointestinal bleeding.*

Josef Rösch was born in Pilsen, Czechoslovakia in 1925. Dotter and Rösch were lifelong friends and collaborators, having met at the Czechoslovak Radiologic Congress where Dotter gave his famous lecture on angiography in 1963. Dotter offered Rösch a 1-year fellowship at Oregon Medical School (now Oregon Health & Science University, or OSHU), which he pursued in 1967, followed by an additional fellowship at the University of California Los Angeles (UCLA), where he developed the TIPS technique. He is credited with numerous advances in the field of IR. A prolific physician-scientist, he authored or coauthored 495 articles and book chapters, the most meaningful of which covered the TIPS procedure and the use of embolization for controlling acute gastrointestinal bleeding.

CESARE GIANTURCO—COILS AND STENTS

- *Gianturco described percutaneous cardiac catheterization, vena cava filters, and the stenting of vessels.*
- *He initiated the use of steel coils for vascular occlusion.*

Cesare Gianturco was born in Naples, Italy, in 1905. He is credited with the technique of percutaneous deployment of steel coils for vascular occlusion, which he first presented in 1975. He additionally described the stenting of aortic dissections, stenting across biliary constrictions, and the potential applications of stenting in the tracheobronchial tree. Transcatheter intraarterial infusion of chemotherapy, intraarterial coronary drug therapy, and the vena cava filter are also among his innovations. In 1985, he introduced the Gianturco Z stent to relieve obstructions of large veins. Gianturco was hailed by his family as a loving and devout father, by his colleagues as an exceptional teacher and scientist, and by the medical community as a giant. None summarized it more eloquently than Dr. R. David Fisher's memorial of Gianturco and his impact on the field of interventional cardiology: "In every corner beneath the polished surface are found the contributions of Dr. Gianturco."

ANDERS LUNDERQUIST—PANCREATIC VENOUS SAMPLING

- *Lunderquist capitalized on unintentional findings that led to pancreatic venous sampling and transhepatic variceal embolization techniques.*

Anders Lunderquist was born on July 17, 1925 in Lycksele, Sweden. He visited Dotter at Oregon Medical School in 1969 to learn angioplastic techniques, and he continued to be in close contact with Dotter and other American colleagues for the remainder of his career. Lunderquist had a keen eye for serendipitous findings that could lead to new techniques in IR. He passionately told of having accidentally accessed a portal vein branch while performing a biliary drainage. Instead of retracting his needle, he catheterized the portal venous system, which later led to his development of transhepatic variceal embolization in 1974. Lunderquist is also credited with having developed pancreatic venous sampling, which he stumbled upon during a transumbilical catheterization of the portal vein in a study of hepatic tumors.

KURT AMPLATZ—INVENTOR OF THE SEPTAL OCCLUDER

- *The septal occluder revolutionized the treatment of septal defects and became the standard of care.*

Kurt Amplatz was born in 1924 in Weistrach, Austria. Following a residency in Detroit, he joined the University of Minnesota School of Medicine as an attending radiologist in 1957. At that time Minnesota was a powerhouse and pioneer in open-heart surgery. Dr. Walton Lillehei had performed the first open-heart operation in 1954, and Dr. Richard DeWall had pioneered the heart-lung machine.

Like that of many of the founding fathers of IR, Amplatz's career is decorated with many publications. His name is associated with 7 textbooks, 68 textbook chapters, and more than 1000 scientific presentations at national and international scientific meetings. His landmark innovation, the Amplatzer Septal Occluder, has spared over 30,000 patients from having open-heart surgeries. Today, the Amplatz name is ubiquitous in the angiography suite (Amplatz plug, Amplatz gooseneck snares, Amplatz catheters, etc.) because of his dedication to innovation.

JOHN DOPPMAN—SPINAL VASCULAR INTERVENTION

- *Doppman performed the first percutaneous AVM embolization and was a leader in endocrine interventions.*

John Leo Doppman was born on June 14, 1928 in Springfield, Massachusetts. An ardent subscriber to the Latin proverb *litera scripta manet* ("written letters remain"), Dr. Doppman had a prolific publishing career, totaling 516 scientific articles and 38 textbook chapters. His passion for writing and research was enhanced by the growing field of radiologic endocrinology, in which there were not many publications at the time.

Through his foundational fluency and endless radiologic and angiographic talents, Dr. Doppman was the first physician to conduct percutaneous arteriovenous malformation embolization in 1968; this ultimately led to his textbook on the subject of spinal cord blood supply. In the 1970s, Dr. Doppman shifted gears and began focusing on the diagnosis, lateralization, and embolization of endocrine adenomas. He and his team focused in on adrenal vein sampling in the diagnosis of aldosteronomas vis-à-vis bilateral adrenal hyperplasia. In the 1980s, he was the first to describe bilateral inferior petrosal sinus sampling, which is now the mainstay technique used to diagnose and lateralize Cushing disease. In the 1990s, Dr. Doppman switched his focus to the pancreas and developed techniques to find and diagnose gastrinomas, insulinomas, and other islet cell tumors.

JULIO PALMAZ—CORONARY STENT

- *Palmaz invented the balloon-expandable mesh stent used in coronary angioplasty and revolutionized cardiovascular medicine.*

Born on December 13, 1945, in La Plata, Argentina, Julio Palmaz had a deep interest in mechanics from a young age. After completing medical school and internship in Argentina, he moved to California for radiology residency in 1977. In 1978, Palmas met Andreas Grüntzig at a conference in New Orleans. After this meeting, Palmaz used his mechanical mind to marry the Dotter (metal spring) and Grüntzig (balloon dilation) techniques of angioplasty, ultimately leading to his development of a balloon-expandable mesh stent.

Despite resistance to change and repeated failure, Palmaz eventually achieved approval from the US Food and Drug Administration for use of his stent in peripheral arteries in 1991 and in coronary arteries in 1994. By 1998, the Palmaz-Schatz stent was used in over 80% of percutaneous coronary angioplasties, and approximately a million of these stents are deployed annually worldwide (see a Dr. Julio Palmaz tribute film at https://www.youtube.com/watch?v=87tVZbxKaaY).

IRVIN F. HAWKINS

- *Hawkins developed carbon dioxide digital subtraction angiography.*

Irvin F. Hawkins was born in Baltimore, Maryland in 1936. His major contribution to the field of IR was his development of carbon dioxide digital subtraction angiography as an alternative to iodinated contrast. The initial development of this technique came serendipitously when Dr. Hawkins inadvertently injected a patient with 70 mL of room air instead of iodinated contrast. Fortuitously, a full range of images was obtained, and even better, the patient suffered no adverse effects. Over the coming decades—with advances in technology, the increasing sophistication of digital subtraction imaging, and reliable sourcing of gaseous carbon dioxide—the technique was further refined through animal studies.

Throughout Dr. Hawkins's career, he pioneered advances in IR with a focus on patient safety. He was one of the first to adopt smaller-bore catheters, which eventually paved the way for microvascular techniques. He also introduced blunt needles for carotid access, coaxial guide needle systems, and the microneedle TIPS set, all in the name of reducing potential complications.

WILLIAM COOK—FIRST SUPPLIER OF INTERVENTIONAL RADIOLOGY INSTRUMENTATION

- *Cook founded Cook, Inc., by manufacturing wires and catheters in his spare bedroom; over time, this little business grew to be the largest family-owned medical device manufacturer in the world.*

As interventional techniques became the standard of care, the need for mass-produced, high-quality instruments and material became apparent. Enter Bill Cook.

William A. "Bill" Cook was born on January 27, 1931 in Mattoon, Illinois. He grew up aspiring to be a physician and later went on to pursue a degree in biology at Northwestern University. After graduating in 1953, he planned to go to medical school but was instead drafted into the US Army, where he served as an anesthesia technician. In this role, for 2 years, he taught the physics of anesthesia to army anesthesiologists. Thereafter, instead of continuing to provide direct medical care, Cook began his business career.

Cook, Inc., was officially founded in 1963. Bill and his wife, Gayle, began manufacturing guidewires, catheters, and needles in the spare bedroom of their Bloomington, Indiana, apartment. That same year, at a meeting of the Radiological Society of North America, Cook first met Charles Dotter. As the story goes, there was a "short, muscular, bald man with darting eyes" lurking around the Cook booth. When Cook asked if he needed anything, the bald man left. At the end of the day, the bald man returned to the booth and asked Cook if he could borrow his blowtorch and some Teflon tubing. Without backup equipment or knowledge of the requestor, Cook obliged. When he later asked for the mystery man's name, he replied "Charles Dotter." The next day, Dotter returned with 10 perfectly constructed Teflon catheters, and Cook, the natural businessman, sold each for $10. Not long after this, Dotter invited Cook to Portland, Oregon, where he gave Cook diagrams of the catheters required to perform the first-ever percutaneous transluminal angioplasty.

After his successful partnership with Dotter, Cook also partnered with some of the other founding fathers of IR, including Andreas Grüntzig and Cesare Gianturco. Cook's attention to detail and drive to create reliable products led to the rise of Cook, Inc., to become the largest family-owned medical device supplier in the world. Without the tools supplied by Cook, Inc., physicians in the field of angiography would not be able to do their work.

JOHN ABELE—DRIVER OF THE INDUSTRY

- *Abele founded Boston Scientific in 1979.*

While John Abele made his name in medical device manufacturing, his main goal was to drive collaboration among as many people as he could in order to encourage the advancement of what was then known as "less invasive surgery." Upon graduating from Amherst College in 1959, Abele began working for Advanced Instruments, a company that specialized in cutting-edge laboratory equipment such as osmometers and flame photometers. At the time, these were novel and disruptive technologies, and Abele spent much of his time trying to change the minds of skeptical established scientists and persuade them of the need for these tools. Thanks to his natural salesman's skills as well as his scientific acumen, he was able to accrue a sizable client base.

In 1965 Abele allied himself with many of the premier cardiac surgeons of the time in order to adopt standards for medical instrumentation in the operating room. From there, Abele was hooked on novel technologies and the development of new tools for practicing clinicians. Abele joined Medi-Tech, a development company, in 1969. One of their premier products at that time was a steerable multilumen catheter that would soon provide a stepping stone for the next chapter in Abele's career. It was then that Andres Grüntzig contacted Medi-Tech about their steerable catheter, and Abele not only sent him some samples but also traveled to Zürich to watch Grüntzig at work. This relationship was fruitful for both parties, as Abele later introduced Grüntzig to the cardiologist Richard Myler, with whom Grüntzig would work to perform the first human coronary angioplasty.

In 1979, Abele and a partner formed Boston Scientific. Early on, the company was focused on producing angioplasty and valvuloplasty balloons. After the work of Julio Palmaz set the table for balloon-expandable stents, later advances included paclitaxel-eluting coronary stents. In 2002, Boston Scientific went public in order to generate the revenue needed to make a series of business acquisitions that would further entrench the company within the field of IR. Among those business purchases was that of SciMed, which at the time was the market's leading manufacturer of catheters.

STANLEY BAUM—THE FOUNDER OF INTERVENTIONAL RADIOLOGY'S FIRST PROFESSIONAL SOCIETY

- *Baum founded the Society of Cardiovascular Radiology, which later became the Society of Interventional Radiology.*

Stanley Baum completed his residency in radiology at the University of Pennsylvania. Merging his interests in both radiology and the cardiovascular system, he then went to the Stanford University where he completed a fellowship in cardiovascular radiology in 1962. Although most of his focus and time were on cardiovascular radiology, Baum expanded his scope to include acute gastrointestinal bleeds. He and Dr. Moreye Nusbaum, his surgical colleague, described the role of angiography in the diagnosis of acute bleeds with extravasation rates as low as 0.5 mL/min. After a successful experimental series in dogs, human trials in the late 1960s elucidated the use of selective arterial infusion of vasoconstrictors to slow or stop these bleeds intravascularly. This use of "emergency angiography" was the standard of care prior to the wide adoption of endoscopy.

In 1973 Baum founded the Society of Cardiovascular Radiology (SCR) and became its first president. The main goals of the society were to increase communication among practitioners in the field, spur innovation and development to improve patient care and outcomes, and advance the training and scientific research conducted in cardiovascular radiology and IR. Moreover, membership was limited to the most active individuals in cardiovascular radiology, especially those keen on developing new investigative techniques. After several name changes throughout the years, the Society of Cardiovascular Radiology became known as the Society of Interventional Radiology, the major professional society for interventional radiologists.

SOCIETY OF CARDIOVASCULAR AND INTERVENTIONAL RADIOLOGY— A PLACE TO CALL HOME

- *This society was founded in 1973 by small group of innovative radiologists.*
- *It championed the creation of IR-specific residency programs.*

As discussed earlier, it was through the work of Stanley Baum in 1973 that the first professional society in IR was founded. Its goal, like that of any other professional society in medicine, was to provide a place where active members could discuss new techniques, fields of research, therapies, and technologies. Moreover, the society established a governing body to ensure that the interventions and trials being conducted were of high quality and to otherwise promote excellent standards of care.

The first formal meeting of the SCR, attended by 24 radiologists, took place in 1975 in Key Largo, Florida. As the pioneers in the field continued to innovate and expand their practices, the SCR felt the need to change its name to reflect the increasing use of therapeutic interventions. Thus, in 1983, the Society of Cardiovascular and Interventional Radiology (SCVIR) was born. In 1989, the society became associated with the journal *Radiology* and released a special volume that included articles, reviews, and news items specifically related to cardiovascular medicine and IR. In 1990, the *Journal of Vascular and Interventional Radiology* (JVIR) was launched as the society's own journal. The 1990s were a decade of growth for the SCVIR. Political activism became important to the group, as demonstrated by the formation of the Interventional Radiology Political Action Committee (IRPAC). Ensuring a steady stream of interventionalists, the society remained active in the fellowship match program. Most significantly, SCVIR began talks with the American Board of Radiology to seek formal designation as a subspecialty of radiology. Gains in appropriate billing codes, standards of practice, and quality guidelines were also established in the decade that laid the foundation for future growth of the discipline.

In 2002, the society changed its name once again to reflect the growing role of IR. Now it was no longer limited to the cardiovascular system. The new name, the Society of Interventional Radiology (SIR), encompassed just that. A subsection of the SIR was formed in 2009 to capture medical students and residents interested in pursuing IR. The resident, fellows, and students' section of the SIR (rfs.sirweb.org) offers like-minded trainees a forum within which they can come together to discuss the future of the field.

Over the past decade, the SIR has been very active in solidifying the future of IR. In 2012, it lobbied the American Board of Medical Specialties to recognize IR as a primary specialty. In 2013, the American Board of Radiology announced that IR physicians would be certified in both diagnostic radiology and IR. Also in 2013, the Accreditation Council for Graduate Medical Education approved the formation of direct IR residency programs, which for the first time gave graduating medical students an opportunity to match directly into the field, which happened for the first time in 2017.

🏠 TAKE-HOME POINTS

Milestone Procedures in the History of Interventional Radiology

Year	Procedure	Physician
1963	Angiographic diagnosis of acute gastrointestinal bleeds	Baum, Nusbaum
1964	Transluminal angioplasty	Dotter
1966	Embolization of endocrine tumors and spinal cord AVMs	Doppman
1967	Judkins technique of coronary angiography	Judkins
1967	Selective vasoconstriction for controlling gastrointestinal bleeds	Baum, Nusbaum
1969	Percutaneous stent placement	Dotter
1970	Percutaneous removal of biliary stones	Fennessey, Kawai, Classen, Burhenne
1970	Selective embolization for controlling gastrointestinal bleeds	Rosch
1972	Catheter-directed thrombolysis	Dotter
1972	Embolization for pelvic trauma	Margolies
1974	Transhepatic variceal embolization	Lunderquist
1975	Vascular occlusive coils	Gianturco
1975	Percutaneous nephrolithotomy	Frenstrom
1975–1985	Percutaneous extraction of gallstones	Wiechel, Dotter, Rosch, Kerlan
1977	Embolization of pulmonary AVMs and varicoceles	Porstmann (AVM), Lima (varicocele)
1977	Bland embolization and chemoembolization of hepatocellular cancer	Doyon, Yamada, Freidman, Misra, Wheeler
1982	Transjugular intrahepatic portosystemic shunt	Richter
1983	Balloon-expandable stent	Palmaz
1985	Self-expandable stent	Wallsten
1989	Biliary stents	Irving, Lunderquist, Roche, Coons
1990	Y-90 embolization of solid tumors	Shapiro, Andrews
1990	Uterine artery embolization	Ravina, McLucas, Goodwin
1990	Abdominal aortic stent grafts	Parodi
1991	Balloon-occluded retrograde transvenous obliteration of gastric varices	Kanagawa
1992	Radiofrequency ablation of liver tumors	Buscarini and Rossi
1999	Percutaneous delivery of islet cells to liver for transplantation	Sutherland, Shapiro

AVMs, Arteriovenous malformations.

REVIEW QUESTIONS

1. Sven Ivar Seldinger is best known as a founding father of interventional radiology for having introduced
   a. an injectable contrast agent.
   b. stents.
   c. the vascular access technique.
   d. balloon angioplasty.
2. Julio Palmaz is best known as a founding father of interventional radiology for having introduced
   a. digital subtraction angiography.
   b. balloon-expandable stents.
   c. stents.
   d. an injectable contrast agent.
3. Andreas Grüntzig is best known as a founding father of interventional radiology for developing the
   a. balloon-expandable stent.
   b. an injectable contrast agent.
   c. the vascular access technique.
   d. balloon angioplasty.
4. Irvin Hawkins is best known as a founding father of interventional radiology for having introduced
   a. digital subtraction angiography.
   b. injectable contrast agents.
   c. stents.
   d. the vascular access technique.
5. Egas Moniz is best known as a founding father of interventional radiology for introducing
   a. digital subtraction angiography.
   b. balloon-expandable stents.
   c. the vascular access technique.
   d. injectable contrast agents.

SUGGESTED READINGS

Baum RA, Baum S. Interventional radiology: a half century of innovation. *Radiology*. 2014;273(2 suppl):S75–S91.

Rösch J, Keller FS, Kaufman JA. The birth, early years, and future of interventional radiology. *J Vasc Interv Radiol*. 2003;14 (7):841–853.

Murphy TP, Soares GM. The evolution of interventional radiology. *Semin Intervent Radiol*. 2005;22(1):6–9.

Basics of Interventional Radiology

Brandon P. Olivieri, David M. Tabriz, Fareed R. Riyaz, Adam M. Berry,
Stephen T. Kee

PREOPERATIVE BASICS

This section reviews general preoperative considerations for Interventional Radiology (IR) procedures, assuming that a **history**, **physical**, and thorough **evaluation** have been conducted and that an appropriate procedural **indication** has been confirmed (specific procedural indications/contraindications and other unique considerations are reviewed in the respective procedural sections that follow).

Informed Consent

- Informed consent for both the procedure and appropriate level of sedation need to be obtained in non-life-threatening scenarios. At a minimum, discussion with the patient or patient surrogate should include:
  - Reason for and method of the procedure/treatment
  - Benefits, risks, and potential complications of the procedure/treatment
  - Risks and prognosis if the procedure/treatment is refused
  - Reasonable alternative procedure/treatment(s) and their risks/benefits
- Further guidelines for informed consent are detailed in the *ACR-SIR Practice Parameter on Informed Consent for Image Guided Procedures.*

Review of Medications and Allergies

- Any patient medication, primarily anticoagulation medications, and known allergies, particularly any adverse reactions to iodinated contrast, should be reviewed prior to any image-guided procedures.

Approach to Anticoagulant Drugs

- Estimate thromboembolic risk—those with atrial fibrillation, prosthetic heart valves, or recent venous thromboembolism (VTE) are at greatest risk—and delay surgery when possible in patients with a transiently increased risk.
  - CHA_2DS_2-VASc score
    - One point for each of the following: history of congestive heart failure, hypertension, diabetes, vascular disease, age greater than 65, and female gender

- Two points for each of the following: age greater than 75 or previous stroke
  - In general, no therapy is recommended for those with a score of 0; aspirin or oral anticoagulation should be considered for a score of 1; oral anticoagulation is recommended for a score of 2.
- Estimate bleeding risk.
  - HAS-BLED scores ≥ 3 confer increased risk:
    - One point for each of the following: **H**ypertension, **A**bnormal renal or liver function, **S**troke, **B**leeding tendency, **L**abile INRs, **E**lderly, antiplatelet **D**rugs, and alcohol.
- Determine the timing of anticoagulation interruption
  - Based on the RE-LY trial, a randomized trial of 18,000 patients comparing dabigatran and warfarin (Tables 2.1 and 2.2)
- Determine whether to use bridging anticoagulation
  - Typically not done, as it increases bleeding risk without reducing rate of VTE, but it may benefit patients on warfarin with high VTE risk.

Laboratory Evaluation

- **Renal function:** renal function assessment is warranted prior to procedures requiring contrast.
  - **Blood urea nitrogen (BUN):** increased values may indicate renal failure or conditions resulting in increased urea production (e.g., steroid use, fever, burns, dehydration).
  - **Creatinine/creatinine clearance (Cr/CrCL):** increased creatinine and, more accurately, decreased CrCL indicate renal insufficiency.
- **Hemostasis**
  - Hemostasis consists of the tissue factor (TF; formerly "extrinsic") and activation (formerly "intrinsic") pathways, which converge onto a common clotting cascade pathway.
  - Common laboratory tests used to measure hemostasis include:
    - **Prothrombin time (PT)/international normalized ratio (INR):** evaluates vitamin K–dependent clotting factors (II, VII, IX, X), TF, and common pathways.

- **Platelet count:** number is predictive of clotting propensity; however, various comorbid conditions (e.g., liver failure) alter platelet adhesion capability.
- **Activated partial thromboplastin time (aPTT):** evaluates contact activation and common pathways

- **Fibrin:** activated from fibrinogen, fibrin organizes initial clot and scaffolds platelets.
- In settings of trauma, transplant, and hepatic failure, **thromboelastography (TEG)** is a dynamic laboratory exam that determines specific deficits within the

TABLE 2.1	**RE-LY Trial**					
Drug	**Method of Action**	**Relevant Labs**	**Discontinuing**	**Restarting**	**Reversal Agents**
Warfarin (Coumadin)	Blocks vitamin K–dependent steps in the clotting cascade, specifically synthesis of factors II, VII, IX, and X	PT/INR	5–6 days before surgery, depending on INR (over or under 3). On the day before surgery, if INR > 1.5, administer low-dose oral vitamin K (this timing is based on half-life, which is 36–42 h)	If withheld for 5 days and restarted 12 h postop, INR will have been subtherapeutic for 8 days. Consider bridging therapy (LMW heparin) for high-risk patients.	Semiurgent: IV vitamin K Immediate: FFP
Dabigatran (Pradaxa)	Direct thrombin inhibitor, blocking conversion of fibrinogen to fibrin	aPTT	2–5 days, depending on creatinine clearance (O/U 50)	Delay for 2–3 days postop due to rapid onset of action.	None
Rivaroxaban (Xarelto) and apixaban (Eliquis)	Direct factor Xa inhibitor, blocking conversion of prothrombin to thrombin	Antifactor Xa	1–2 days preop	Delay for 2–3 days postop due to rapid onset of action.	In development
Aspirin	Irreversibly inhibits COX-1, along the prostaglandin synthesis pathway	Platelet count			
Clopidogrel (Plavix)	Inhibits platelet aggregation by inhibiting GPIIb/IIIa complex	Platelet count	See Table 2.2		

INR, International normalized ratio; *PT*, prothrombin time; *PTT*, partial thromboplastin time.

TABLE 2.2	**Aspirin and Clopidogrel (Plavix) Risk Levels**		
Bleeding Risk	**CARDIAC RISK LEVEL**		
	Low	**Intermediate**	**High**
Low	Maintain aspirin and/or Plavix	Elective/urgent surgery: proceed with surgery, maintaining the patient on aspirin and/or Plavix	Elective surgery: postpone Urgent surgery: perform with the patient on aspirin and/or Plavix
Intermediate	Maintain aspirin and/or Plavix	Elective surgery: balance versus risk discussion Urgent surgery: perform with the patient on aspirin and/or Plavix	Elective surgery: postpone Urgent surgery: perform with the patient on aspirin and/or Plavix
High	Stop aspirin and/or Plavix, if necessary, 5 days before surgery, and restart within 24 h of surgery.	Elective surgery: postpone Urgent surgery: perform Continue the patient on aspirin Stop Plavix, if possible, 5 days before surgery, and restart within 24 h after surgery	Elective surgery: postpone Urgent surgery: perform Continue the patient on aspirin Stop Plavix 5 days before surgery but consider substituting with intravenous tirofiban (Aggrastat) or eptifibatide (Integrilin) in the days before the operation

coagulation cascade and guides targeted replacement with fresh frozen plasma, cryoprecipitate, platelets, or specific medications.

- The *SIR Standards of Practice Consensus Guidelines for Periprocedural Management of Coagulation Status and Hemostasis Risk in Percutaneous Image-Guided Interventions and Addendum of Newer Anticoagulants to the SIR Consensus Guideline* offers guidelines for coagulation parameters based on procedure invasiveness (Table 2.3).

Sedation Plan

- Evaluation of the appropriate sedation requirements (no sedation, local anesthesia, minimal sedation, moderate sedation, deep sedation, or general anesthesia) based on patient safety and procedural complexity
- Moderate sedation is discussed later in this chapter.

Antibiotic Prophylaxis

- The Society of Interventional Radiology *Practice Guideline for Adult Antibiotic Prophylaxis during Vascular and Interventional Radiology Procedures* classifies procedures (Table 2.4).

- Antibiotic prophylaxis is generally recommended for any procedure not considered clean. The choice of antibiotic depends on the expected bacterial flora encountered. Common choices include:
  - 1 g cefazolin (Ancef) IV
  - 1 g vancomycin IV
  - 900 mg clindamycin IV

Radiation and Magnetic Resonance Safety

- For image-guided procedures associated with high levels of radiation, explanation and probability of deterministic injury (e.g., skin burn) should be discussed with the patient as part of the consent process.

GENERAL POSTOPERATIVE MANAGEMENT

Basic Postoperative Orders

- A mnemonic for postoperative orders is "**ADC VANDALISM**":
  A—Admit to (e.g., ICU, general surgical floor, general medical floor)
  D—Diagnosis
  C—Condition
  V—Vital signs (e.g., q4h, q shift)

TABLE 2.3 Coagulation Parameters Based on Procedure Invasiveness

Category 1	Category 2	Category 3
Procedure		
Nontunneled venous catheter	Angiography (arterial intervention with access size up to 7 Fr)	TIPS
Dialysis access interventions	Venous interventions	Renal biopsy
Central line removal	Chemoembolization/radioembolization	Radiofrequency ablation
IVC filter placement	Spinal procedures (vertebroplasty, kyphoplasty, lumbar puncture, epidural injection, facet block)	Nephrostomy tube placement
Venography	Uterine artery embolization	Biliary interventions (with new tract formation)
Catheter exchanges (biliary, nephrostomy, abscess drainage catheter)	Transjugular liver biopsy	
Thoracentesis	Tunneled venous catheter	
Paracentesis	Subcutaneous port device placement	
Thyroid biopsy	Abscess drainage	
Joint aspiration/injection	Biopsy (excluding superficial and renal)	
Superficial aspiration, drainage, and/or biopsy (excluding intrathoracic or intraabdominal sites)	Percutaneous cholecystostomy	
	Enteric tube placement	
Tests		
Recommended: INR, aPTT	Recommended: INR, aPTT, platelet count	Recommended: INR, aPTT, platelet count
Not recommended: platelet count, hematocrit	Not recommended: hematocrit	Not recommended: hematocrit
Thresholds		
INR: correct to ≤2.0	INR: correct to ≤1.5	INR: correct to ≤1.5
Transfuse if platelets ≤50,000/μL	Transfuse if platelets ≤50,000/μL	Transfuse if platelets ≤50,000/μL
aPTT: no consensus	aPTT: trend toward correcting for values ≥1.5 × control	aPTT: correct so that value is ≤1.5 × control

INR, International normalized ratio; *PTT*, partial thromboplastin time.

TABLE 2.4   Interventional Radiology Procedure Classifications

Procedure Classification	Description	Example
Clean	No entry into the GI, GU, or respiratory tracts No inflammation evident No break in aseptic technique	Diagnostic angiogram
Clean-contaminated	Entry into the GI or GU tract No inflammation evident No break in aseptic technique	PCN with sterile urine
Contaminated	Entry of inflamed/colonized GI or GU tract without frank pus Major break in aseptic technique	PCN with pyelonephritis
Dirty	Entry of infected purulent site	Abscess drainage

A—Allergies

N—Specific nursing orders (e.g., strict I/O, drainage catheter flush duration)

D—Diet

A—Activity (e.g., strict bedrest with head of bed elevated for 2 hours)

L—Labs

I—IVF (type and rate)

S—Studies (imaging)

M—Medications

Brief Operative Note

- Typically includes patient name, identifier, date of birth, date of procedure, operator(s), procedure(s), preprocedure diagnosis, postprocedure diagnosis, medications given, amount of contrast given, estimated blood loss, complications (Box 2.1), findings, fluoroscopy time, air kerma (mGy), DAP (mGy.cm^2).

VASCULAR ACCESS: THE SELDINGER TECHNIQUE

- The Seldinger technique was introduced in 1953 as an improved method of vascular access.
- Percutaneous needle puncture for angiography was an established procedure prior to the introduction of the Seldinger technique.
  - However, these previous methods required the puncture of a vessel with a large-bore needle through which a narrower-bore catheter was threaded, restricting the use of these methods to relatively large vessels.
  - These methods created relatively large defects in the vessel wall, increasing the risk of hemorrhage and vessel wall damage.
- With the Seldinger technique, the vessel is accessed with a percutaneous needle, a flexible metal **guidewire is introduced through the needle lumen and into the vessel**, the percutaneous needle is removed from the vessel over the guidewire, and a flexible catheter is subsequently threaded over the guidewire and into the vessel.
- Advantage of this technique is that **much smaller percutaneous needles can be used** since the whole catheter need not be threaded through the percutaneous needle.

- This allowed **smaller vessels to be accessed** with **lower risks of complication** than previous methods.

Basic Steps of Vascular Access

- **Ultrasound** the expected site of vascular access (e.g., the neck for internal jugular vein access, the groin for femoral artery access). Evaluate for stenosis, clot, or any other potential complicator to obtaining access.
- **Sterilize** the site of entry with an iodinated or chlorhexidine prep, and **sterilely drape** the patient.
- **Numb the subcutaneous tissues** at the site of entry:
  - Use 1% to 2% lidocaine (without epinephrine). Consider adding 1 mL of sodium bicarbonate to 9 mL of lidocaine to minimize the burning sensation of the lidocaine.
  - Create a small, superficial skin wheal of lidocaine at the site of access with a 25-gauge needle.
  - Avoid entering the vessel wall/lumen or injecting lidocaine into either of these structures.
- Create a superficial skin incision at the anesthetized site with a **No. 11 scalpel blade**.
- Use curved mosquito **forceps** or other similar tools to dissect apart the subcutaneous tissues at the incision site. Avoid overdissection at this point, as this will make closure more difficult at the end of the procedure.

BOX 2.1   Society of Interventional Radiology Classification of Procedural Complications

Minor Complications
- Require no therapy and of no consequence
- Require nominal therapy but of no consequence; includes overnight admission for observation only

Major Complications
- Require therapy, minor hospitalization (<48 h)
- Require major therapy, unplanned increase in level of care, prolonged hospitalization (>48 h)
- Permanent adverse sequelae
- Death

From Sacks D, McClenny TE, Cardella JF, Lewis CA. Society of Interventional Radiology clinical practice guidelines. *J Vasc Interv Radiol.* 2003;14(9 Pt 2):S199–S202, Table 2.

- **Primary access** with access needle
  - Enter the subcutaneous tissues at the site of skin incision with the needle:
    - Visualize the vessel to be accessed with ultrasound at the site of your skin incision.
    - Angle the needle parallel to the vascular structure to be entered, at approximately 40 degrees with respect to the skin.
      - 18- or 21-gauge needles are generally used.
      - Grasp the needle with your thumb and index finger, placing the remaining fingers on the patient in order to stabilize your hand.
    - Advance the needle into the skin incision. Continuously visualize the tip of your needle under ultrasound as you advance.
  - Enter the vessel:
    - If possible, access only the near wall of the vessel, and land the tip of your needle within the vessel lumen (i.e., **a single-wall entry**), especially if the patient has abnormal clotting parameters or if prevention of puncture-site bleeding is preferred.
      - However, this is not always possible, and sometimes going through and through the vessel is necessary (i.e., **a double-wall entry**).
    - Upon entering the vessel lumen, one will often get blood return through the external aspect of the needle. However, if the intravascular pressure is low, this may not be the case.
      - In situations where one is fairly confident that one is within the vessel lumen but is getting no blood return, a syringe can be carefully attached to the needle, and blood can be aspirated.
      - If blood does not aspirate back, it may be necessary to attempt to re-access the vessel.
    - Once the vessel has been accessed, the needle can be "flattened out" and made more parallel with the skin surface in order to improve the angle of the needle within the vessel.
- Introducing the **guidewire**
  - Once the vessel has been accessed, a guidewire is then threaded through the needle **into the vessel lumen**.
  - The guidewire should slide smoothly into the vessel lumen. If it does not, this suggests that the guidewire is within the patient's soft tissues rather than the vessel lumen.
    - One method of troubleshooting at this point is to use fluoroscopy to see if the guidewire seems to "ball up" in the skin, suggesting that it is indeed in the patient's subcutaneous tissues or if it elongates appropriately and takes the expected course of a vascular structure.
    - If the guidewire "balls up," it will likely be necessary to reaccess the vessel completely.
  - Once a significant portion of the guidewire has been advanced into the vessel to give yourself "purchase," the needle can be removed over the guidewire.
- Introducing **devices** over the guidewire

- Various sheaths, dilators, or other equipment/devices can be passed over the guidewire and into the vessel lumen.
  - In the original technique described by Seldinger in 1953, a catheter was introduced at this point over the guidewire and into the vessel lumen.
  - In the **modified Seldinger technique** (Fig. 2.1)—a more modern variation on the original—a combination device consisting of a sheath and dilator is introduced into the vessel lumen, after which the dilator is unscrewed from the sheath and removed, while the sheath is left in place.
- Depending on the procedure, multiple devices can now be threaded over the guidewire:

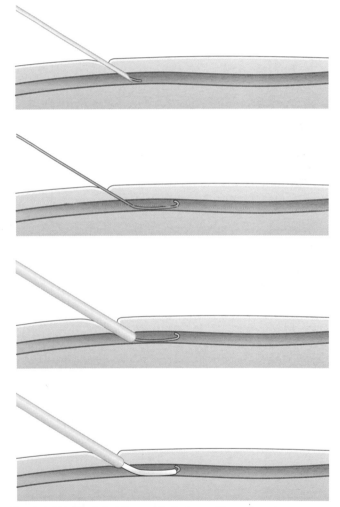

Fig. 2.1 Modified Seldinger Technique. Illustration demonstrates the technique of vascular access. *Top to bottom*: A hollow needle is used to puncture the anterior wall of the vessel, and a guidewire is inserted through the needle once the intravascular location of the needle is confirmed by visualization of blood dripping at the hub of the needle. Next, the wire is fixed, and the needle is removed. During this step, firm pressure is applied over the puncture site to avoid hematoma formation. Then, a sheath is introduced over the wire. Finally, the selected catheter is introduced through the sheath to enter the vessel of interest. (Reused with permission from Hedgire SS, Kalva SP. Catheter Angiography [Vascular] in Problem Solving in Cardiovascular Imaging by Abbara S and Kalva SP, 2012, 155–162, Fig. 9.1. Elsevier, Philadelphia)

- For example, to place a **central venous catheter**, serial dilation of the subcutaneous tissues is performed over the guidewire with dilators of increasing size, followed by placement of the catheter into the vessel.
  - Or, to perform an **angiography**, a catheter can be threaded over the guidewire to the desired endpoint, followed by removal of the guidewire and injection.
- The Seldinger technique and its modification, with its placement of the guidewire into the vessel lumen as a "track" for other medical devices to follow over, forms the basis of vascular access and is the technique that has allowed our field to grow.

CONTRAST

Contrast Media Used in the IR Suite

- Ionic agents are first generation and are not commonly used, due to their high osmolality and subsequent increased risk of side effects/adverse reactions.
- Nonionic agents have been developed, including:
  - Low-osmolal formulations like **Isovue** (iopamidol) and **Omnipaque** (iohexol)
    - Keep in mind that low-osmolal agents have nearly twice the osmolality of serum and have a greater osmolality than iso-osmolal agents.
    - Only Omnipaque is indicated to use intrathecally.
  - Iso-osmolal (relative to serum osmolality ∼290 mosmol/kg) formulations like **Visipaque** (iodixanol)
    - Prolonged fasting or use of laxatives in the pediatric population is a contraindication to using Visipaque.

 CLINICAL POINT

Osmolality has the strongest association with side effects and adverse reactions related to contrast use. Therefore, an iso-osmolal agent has the best safety profile.

CLINICAL POINT

Warming iodinated contrast agents to body temperature decreases viscosity and in turn reduces the necessary injection pressure.

Precautions

- Iodinated contrast agents decrease the uptake of radioactive iodine-131 by the thyroid for 3 weeks. Therefore, alternatives should be discussed for patients undergoing iodine-131 therapy or those who may require iodine-131 within 3 weeks of iodinated contrast administration.
- Patients taking Glucophage or Glucophage XR (metformin) who develop acute kidney injury/contrast-induced nephropathy (AKI/CIN) are at risk for developing lactic acidosis. Therefore, the FDA recommends the temporary

discontinuation of metformin prior to or at the time of contrast injection in the following situations:
  - Patients receiving intraarterial iodinated contrast
  - Patients receiving intravenous iodinated contrast media with an estimated glomerular filtration rate (eGFR) between 30 and 60 mL/min/1.73 m^2
  - Patients with a history of liver disease, alcoholism, or heart failure
- Metformin is to be withheld for 48 hours after contrast administration and only reinstituted after confirmation of stable and appropriate eGFR values.

Adverse Reactions

- Adverse reactions to contrast use may be more common in patients with a history of asthma, allergies, cardiovascular disease, congestive heart failure (CHF), beta-blocker usage, renal insufficiency, thyroid disease, myasthenia gravis, or diabetes.
- Beta-blocker therapy
  - May lower the threshold for contrast reactions
  - May lead to more severe contrast reactions
  - May decrease the response to epinephrine in the treatment of anaphylactic reactions
- Renal insufficiency
  - Increased risk of postcontrast acute kidney injury (PC-AKI) and CIN
  - There are no standard criteria for diagnosis. However, the Acute Kidney Injury Network is a consensus group and has attempted to standardize the diagnosis of AKI as any of the following occurring within 48 hours of iodinated contrast administration:
    - Absolute serum creatinine increase of 0.3 mg/dL
    - Percentage increase of serum creatinine ≥50%
    - Urine output reduced to ≤0.5 mL/kg/h for at least 6 hours
  - When CrCL is used to calculate GFR, a normal serum creatinine is maintained until the GFR is decreased by ∼50%.
- Risk factors
  - The most important risk factor is preexisting renal insufficiency (eGFR <60 mL/1.73 m^2), especially in diabetics.
  - Other risk factors include dehydration, diabetes, cardiovascular disease leading to decreased renal perfusion, and large volumes of contrast or multiple contrast studies within 24 to 48 hours.
- Prevention
  - Select an alternate contrast agent such as CO_2.
  - IV volume expansion with isotonic fluids prior to and following the completion of the procedure
  - Studies on the efficacy of sodium bicarbonate and N-acetylcysteine are conflicting.

CLINICAL POINT

Cystatin C is an endogenous compound produced by nucleated cells. It has proven to be more sensitive at estimating small changes in GFR. Currently, equations using values for both creatinine and cystatin C are accepted as the most accurate estimation of GFR.

- Allergies
  - Risk factors
    - Previous reaction to contrast media
    - Any known allergic diathesis
      - Highest risk in those with multiple allergies/severe reactions
      - There is no evidence supporting seafood and/or shellfish allergies to a potential subsequent allergic reaction to iodinated contrast media.
  - Manifestations
    - Mild—urticaria and pruritis, often self-limited
    - Moderate—urticaria and pruritis, requiring medical management
    - Severe—anaphylactic shock (hypotension and tachycardia), diffuse edema, hypotension, laryngeal edema, bronchospasm, hypoxia, all of which are life threatening and require immediate medical management.
  - Prevention
    - Patients with a history of or at an increased risk of allergic reaction can be offered premedication.
    - Pediatric regimen:
      - Prednisone 0.5 mg/kg (max dose 50 mg) PO at 13, 7, and 1 hour prior to the procedure
      - Diphenhydramine 1.25 mg/kg (max dose 50 mg) PO, IV, or IM 1 hour prior to the procedure
    - Adult regimen:
      - Prednisone 50 mg PO at 13, 7, and 1 hour prior to the procedure
      - Diphenhydramine 50 mg PO, IV, or IM 1 hour prior to the procedure

Carbon Dioxide

- Physical properties
  - Carbon dioxide (CO_2) is highly soluble and a rapidly absorbed molecule with low viscosity.
  - The buoyancy of CO_2 permits it to act as a negative contrast agent by displacing blood when injected intravascularly.
  - Image acquisition is obtained through digital subtraction angiography (DSA).
- Advantages over iodinated contrast agents:
  - No risk of allergic reaction, hepatotoxicity, or nephrotoxicity
    - Therefore, it is the preferred agent during renal arteriography.
  - Useful for complex cases or those requiring large volumes of contrast, as there is no dose limitation. CO_2 is dissolved and rapidly exhaled with complete dissolution within approximately 2 minutes.
  - The low viscosity and compressibility of CO_2 makes it particularly useful during TIPS procedure. It allows for the visualization of the portal system following wedge hepatic venography.
  - Increases visualization of collateral vessels because, unlike iodinated agents, CO_2 does not mix with blood and therefore does not become dilute in collateral circulation. It increases sensitivity in detecting small arterial bleeds.

- Indications for use:
  - Arteriography of the lower extremities and abdomen (below the diaphragm)
  - Venography
  - Alternative for patients with allergy to iodinated contrast agents
  - Alternative for patients with decreased renal function who are not on dialysis
  - Patients requiring I-131 radiotherapy
- Contraindications
  - No absolute contraindications
  - Relative contraindications include:
    - Use in the thoracic aorta, coronary arteries, and cerebral circulation (including brachiocephalic trunk)
    - Use in patients with cardiac septal defects (potential for right-to-left shunt) or pulmonary AVMs due to risk of air emboli
    - Patients with pulmonary hypertension or insufficiency due to possibility of CO_2 increasing pulmonary artery pressure
- Adverse reactions
  - Pain from explosive delivery of pressurized CO_2
  - Gas emboli from air contamination
    - Spinal, coronary, or cerebral arteries are at risk when used for arteriography above the diaphragm
    - Tissue ischemia
    - Pancreatitis
  - "Vapor lock" phenomenon from air contamination or excessively large volumes of CO_2 can lead to:
    - Hypotension when occurring in the pulmonary artery
    - Visceral ischemia when occurring in an aortic aneurysm

> ## CLINICAL POINT
>
> Catheters should never be connected directly to the source of CO_2, as they contain significant volumes of the gas at high pressure.

- Methods and systems for CO_2 delivery
  - Source of CO_2 should be laboratory grade with a concentration of 99.99%.
  - Handheld syringe method
    - Fill syringe directly from the source.
    - Quickly open and close the three-way stopcock to allow the pressure within the syringe to reduce to atmospheric pressure and avoid explosive delivery.
    - Improper technique to fill syringe or incomplete closure of the stopcock that allows air to replace CO_2 gas can lead to air contamination.
  - Plastic bag system
    - Purchased as a custom waste bag and contrast delivery system used off-label for CO_2 administration
    - A plastic bag is connected to the CO_2 source and filled with CO_2 through tubing with a microfilter and stopcock. The bag is filled a total of three times, completely purging the bag each time to ensure complete removal of air.

- Improper technique to fill the bag, loose connections, and improper use of stopcocks can lead to air contamination.
- CO_2mmander with AngiAssist—the **only FDA-approved medical CO_2 delivery system**
  - CO_2mmander is a small, portable, CO_2 source system that uses disposable CO_2 cartridges. AngiAssist is a delivery system that connects to the CO_2mmander source.
  - Kit consists of single piece of tubing with an end that connects to the CO_2mmander (port 1), a "reservoir" syringe (port 2), an "injection" syringe (port 3), and an end that connects to an angiographic catheter (port 4); additionally, a K valve is included that is used to direct the flow of CO_2 through the system.
    - The "reservoir" syringe connected to port 2 is used to draw CO_2 from the CO_2mmander source. The "injection" syringe connected to port 3 is filled with the desired volume of CO_2 to be injected. A turn of the K valve to the catheter directs flow through the system.
  - Advantages over other delivery options:
    - FDA approved
    - Kit comes preassembled as a closed system (does not utilize stopcocks) and does not require the use of reservoir bags. Thereby, the risk of air contamination is significantly decreased.

SEDATION

Principles of Sedation for the Interventional Radiology Patient

- An appropriately credentialed staff member who can administer narcotics and other medications should be available to monitor the patient during and after the procedure.
- Continuous monitoring of vital signs including heart rate (HR) and rhythm via electrocardiogram, oxygen saturation, and intermittent blood pressures should be performed in all patients prior to and throughout the duration of procedural sedation.
  - Pulse oximetry and blood pressure should be monitored in an extremity that is not undergoing an intervention.
  - Nasal cannula should be in place prior to administration of medications in order to prevent the delay of resuscitative efforts, should they become necessary.
- PACs or PVCs may be observed on EKG and serve as an indication that a guidewire or catheter is within one of the heart chambers and should be repositioned.

Moderate Sedation

- The objective is to ensure that the patient has obtained an acceptable level of comfort without the loss of spontaneous respirations or the ability to respond to physical or verbal stimuli in order to facilitate in the safe completion of the procedure.

- Contraindications
  - No absolute contraindications
  - Relative contraindications include:
    - American Society of Anesthesiologists (ASA) class III or higher
    - Airway abnormalities
    - Increased risk of aspiration (i.e., bowel obstruction)
    - Extremes of age
    - Altered mental status
- Complications
  - Respiratory complications (most common, with significant compromise in <1%), vomiting and aspiration, and cardiovascular instability
    - Guidelines from the American Society of Anesthesiologists recommend a minimum of 2 hours NPO status following a clear liquid diet or 6 hours NPO following a solid diet prior to being sedated.

Agents for Adults: Combination of Analgesics and Anxiolytics/Sedatives

- Analgesic
  - Fentanyl, an opioid; it is short acting (duration of 30–60 minutes), metabolized by the liver, and excreted in urine.
  - Dosing
    - 0.5 to 1 mcg/kg IV
    - Repeat 0.5 mcg/kg IV q2min to desired effect
  - Risk of respiratory depression and hypotension, potentiated by the coadministration of sedatives like Versed
- Anxiolytics/sedatives
  - Versed (midazolam), a benzodiazepine; it is short acting (duration of 10–40 minutes), metabolized by the liver, and excreted in urine
  - Dosing
    - 0.25 to 1 mg IV pushed over 1 to 2 minutes
    - Repeat q2–5min to desired effect
  - Risk of respiratory depression, potentiated by coadministration with opioids
  - Amnestic effect is beneficial.

Pediatric Agents

- Ketamine, a phencyclidine derivative; it is short acting (duration of 15–30 minutes), metabolized by the liver, and excreted in urine.
- Ketamine is a dissociative sedative that offers both an analgesic and sedative effect.
  - More effective and poses a decreased risk for respiratory depression in comparison to fentanyl and midazolam/propofol combination.
- Contraindications
  - Absolute
    - Known or suspected psychosis
    - Age <3 months old
  - Relative
    - Active pulmonary infections, cardiac or thyroid disease, increased intracranial pressure, porphyria, or glaucoma
    - Age <12 months old

- Dosing
  - 1 to 1.5 mg/kg IV
  - Repeat 0.5 to 1 mg/kg IV q10min to desired effect
- Side effects
  - Vomiting is a commonly encountered side effect. Prevent with Zofran (ondansetron) 0.15 mg/kg.
  - Laryngospasm and respiratory depression are rare and can typically be managed with basic airway support measures.
  - Increased salivation, most commonly seen in infants. Manage with suction and, if necessary, glycopyrrolate or atropine.
  - Emergence phenomenon

Reversing Sedation

- Required to overcome moderate sedation that has resulted in respiratory depression unable to be overcome by supplemental O_2 or stimulation.

Opioid Reversal

- Goal is to restore adequate ventilation.
- Naloxone
  - Partial reversal: 0.1 to 0.2 mg IV q2–3min PRN
  - Full reversal: 0.4 to 2 mg IV q2–3min PRN
- Monitoring should continue for at least 1 hour s/p administration of naloxone, as the reversal agent may be cleared more rapidly than the opioid, leading to resedation.
- Considerations
  - Withdrawal symptoms and/or painful episodes may be precipitated in opioid-dependent patients.
  - Use caution in the elderly and those with cardiovascular disease, as naloxone causes the release of catecholamines that could lead to cardiovascular complications.

Benzodiazepine Reversal

- Flumazenil
  - Adults
    - 0.2 mg IV q1min × 1–5 doses to desired effect
    - Can be repeated q20min to a maximum dose of 1 mg per 20 minute interval.
  - Pediatrics
    - 0.01 mg/kg IV q1min × 1–5 doses to desired effect (maximum single dose of 0.2 mg)
    - Can be repeated q20min to a maximum dose of 1 mg per 20 minute interval.
  - Monitoring should continue for at least 1 hour s/p administration of flumazenil, as the reversal agent may be cleared more rapidly than midazolam, leading to resedation.
  - Maximum effect of a dose is observed at 6 to 10 minutes post administration.
  - Flumazenil has not been proven to consistently reverse respiratory depression, and its application is mostly limited to those with chronic exposure to benzodiazepines.

- Contraindications/precautions
  - Use care in patients with seizure disorder or those taking high-dose tricyclic antidepressants or carbamazepine due to the risk of precipitating seizures.
  - Use care in patients with a history of chronic benzodiazepine use due to the risk of precipitating withdrawal symptoms that include seizure and death.

Ketamine Reversal

- There is no agent for ketamine reversal. Supportive measures and standard care should be given for any adverse reactions.

TOOLS

Wires

- Function as a rail for safe passage of catheters and sheaths, preventing injury to vessel walls (Table 2.5)
- Guidewire characteristics:
  - *Trackability* is the ease with which a wire is able to follow a tortuous course.
  - *Malleability* is the ability of a wire to attain and keep shape.
  - *Flexibility* describes the ability of a wire to bend around areas of external pressure.
  - *Stiffness* describes the strength of a wire.
  - *Torquability* is the ability to transmit rotational force from the proximal tip (operator's hand) to the distal tip.
  - *Tactile feedback* describes how much of the wire tip's interaction with the surrounding environment is transmitted back to the operator's hands.

Basic Guidewire Design

- Core diameter
  - 0.014, 0.018, and 0.035 inch are the most widely used options
  - Strength of wire is related to wire radius
    - The larger the diameter, the stiffer the rail
    - The smaller the diameter, the greater the flexibility
  - Knowledge of unique wire attributes is crucial to address the task at hand as choice of wire is often determined by compatibility with accessory devices.
    - Most atherectomy systems require 0.014 wires
- Core material
  - Stainless steel
    - Rigidity provides good support rail with good torquability
  - High-tensile-strength stainless steel
    - More rigid than the above, with even greater torquability
  - Nitinol
    - Kink-resistant and increased flexibility that is able to navigate around stenoses, acutely angled vessels, and/or otherwise tortuous vessels

TABLE 2.5   Frequently Used Wires

Wire Name	Features	Common Uses
Bentson Wire (Cook Medical, Bloomington, IN)	• Long, soft, floppy distal tip with long transition to stiffer shaft	• Floppy tip makes great for initial access wire • Long taper is helpful for passing through long, difficult curves (such as aortic bifurcation)
Wholey wire (Covidien, Mansfield, MA)	• Atraumatic tip • Shapeable tip • Gradual transition from floppy tip to stiffer shaft • High torquability	• Great for initial access • Atraumatic tip allows for safe passage through stenotic vessels • High torquability allows for precise manipulation
GLIDEWIRE Wire (Terumo, Somerset, NJ)	• Has an elastic nitinol core surrounded by polyurethane with hydrophilic outer coating • Comes in standard and stiff varieties	• Hydrophilic coating allows for traversing tight stenoses and occlusions • Resistant to kinking • NOTE: Low tactile feedback results in increased risk of vessel perforations and dissections
AMPLATZ Wire (Boston Scientific, Marlborough, MA)	• Thicker core wrapped with flat steel band creates a stiffer wire relative to outer diameter	• Provides stiff rail for advancing sheath over angled or tortuous aortic bifurcations

- Hybrid—nitinol tip and stainless steel shaft
  - Flexibility of the tip allows for improved navigation around lesions
  - Strong shaft gives increased torquability to the wire tip and increases rail support for device delivery
- Tip design
  - Penetration power = Tip stiffness/Area of the tip
    - Penetration power determines the ability of the tip to push through plaque
  - If core extends to tip of wire:
    - Increased tactile feedback, strength, and torquability
    - More likely to injure a vessel
  - If core does not extend to tip of wire:
    - Increased malleability and flexibility
    - Less likely to injure vessel
- Taper
  - Determines the transition of stiffness along the length of the wire from the flexible tip to the stiffer proximal end
  - Gradual taper:
    - Improved trackability (i.e., easier to track wire up and over aortic arch into contralateral limb)
    - Less support and penetration power
  - Abrupt taper:
    - Good support and penetration power
    - Less trackability
- Coatings
  - Polymer or plastic coatings enhance lubricity, which increases trackability and decreases tactile feedback
- Wire length
  - Longer wire confers less torquability

Catheters

- Two main types: nonselective (flush) and selective catheters (Table 2.6)
  - Nonselective catheters are used to inject contrast into medium- and large-sized vessels and have both side holes and an end hole.
  - Side holes are commonly used for pump injection.
  - End holes are commonly used for hand injection.
- Selective catheters can be shaped to a wide variety of angles to allow for the direct catheterization of vessels.
- Available in a variety of shapes, sizes, and materials, depending on use
- Three important values in catheter size: total length, outer diameter, and inner diameter
  - Catheters are sized in French (Fr)—1 Fr = 0.33 mm.

ANGIOPLASTY

Angioplasty Balloons

- Technical specifications
  - *Nominal pressure* is the pressure at which the balloon reaches its labeled diameter.
  - *Rated burst pressure* is the pressure at which 99.9% of balloons will not burst with 95% confidence.
  - *Compliance* is change in balloon diameter as a function of inflation pressure.
    - The majority of angioplasty balloons are noncompliant, meaning they maintain a fixed diameter despite increasing pressure.
- Balloons achieve luminal gain via controlled iatrogenic vessel wall injury by causing:
  - Longitudinal and radial plaque redistribution
  - Arterial expansion
  - Plaque rupture
  - Disruption of vessel media
- Complications
  - Early:
    - Flow-limiting dissection
    - Elastic recoil
    - Vessel rupture

TABLE 2.6   Frequently Used Catheters

Catheter Type	Features	Common Uses
Pigtail catheter (nonselective)	End hole and multiple side holes extending down to the distal 1–2 cm of the shaft Pigtail loop measures approximately 15 mm across	Side holes allow for homogeneous contrast bolus Pigtail curve minimizes catheterization of small branch vessels
Straight catheter (nonselective)	End hole and multiple side holes on a straight shaft	Used in vessels that are too small to form pigtail in but still have a reasonable rapid flow (i.e., iliac)
Cobra (selective)	"Shepherd's crook" curve at distal end of catheter Comes in three sizes of curve (C1–C3), with each curve progressively widening	Invaluable catheter for visceral and peripheral vessel selection Does not need to be formed Used for accurate selection of desired branching vessels
Berenstein (selective)	Angled tip catheter No side holes End hole only	Best when catheterizing forward-facing vessels One of the simplest catheters to use Very good at selective catheterization

- Late:
  - Vessel wall trauma leading to late lumen loss by neointimal hyperplasia, as caused by thrombogenic, vasoactive, and mitogenic factors, and fibroblast proliferation.

Drug-Coated Balloons

- Balloons are coated with paclitaxel, which interferes with microtubule dynamics preventing mitosis, inhibiting smooth muscle cell proliferation, and preventing restenosis via neointimal hyperplasia. To be effective, the drug must:
  - Arrive intact to the lesion site
    - Potential to be washed off of the balloon prior to target application during device handling
  - Be efficiently transferred from the balloon to the vessel wall
    - Determined by coating technique
      - Crystalline coatings have greater biological efficacy.
      - Amorphous coatings have better uniformity of application and less particulate formation.
    - Dependent on inflation time
      - Typically, between 95% and 100% of the drug is released after the balloon has been inflated for 3 minutes.
  - Be retained in vessel wall for a sufficient period of time.
    - Drug is deposited in the vessel wall, which serves as a reservoir for elution into close adjacent arterial segments, as well as deeper into the arterial wall.
    - Drug tissue levels are potentially detectable for up to 180 days.
- See Table 2.7 for frequently used balloons, and see Table 2.8 for supplemental information.

Important Clinical Trials

IN.PACT SFA Randomized Trial

- Patients with SFA and/or popliteal artery lesions were randomly assigned to either a plain balloon angioplasty (PTA) or drug-coated balloon (DCB) group. The IN.PACT Admiral Drug Coated Balloon (Medtronic, Minneapolis, MN) was used.
- Primary endpoint: primary patency (freedom from restenosis or clinically driven target lesion revascularization [TLR])
  - 12-month primary patency: DCB (82.2%) versus PTA (52.4%); $P < .001$
  - 24-month primary patency: DCB (78.9%) versus PTA (50.1%); $P < .001$
  - 12-month clinically driven TLR: DCB (2.4%) versus PTA (20.6%); $P < .001$
  - 24-month clinically driven TLR: DCB (9.1%) versus PTA (28.3%); $P < .001$

LEVANT

- Patients with femoropopliteal stenosis with claudication or rest pain were randomly assigned to the plain balloon angioplasty (PTA) group or Lutonix Drug-Coated Balloon (Bard Peripheral Vascular, Tempe, AZ) group.
- Primary endpoint: primary patency (binary patency and freedom from TLR)
  - 12-month primary patency: DCB (65.2%) versus PTA (52.6%); $P = .02$
  - 24-month primary patency: DCB (58.6%) versus PTA (53%); $P = .05$

▶▶ CLINICAL POINT

Based on these trials, femoropopliteal lesions treated with DCBs may have better primary patency compared with plain balloon angioplasty up to 2 years post procedure.

STENTS

Bare Stents

- Stents achieve luminal gain via rigid scaffolding that displaces plaque out of the lumen by exerting chronic outward radial force (Table 2.9).
- Complications
  - Late lumen loss via in-stent restenosis (ISR)

TABLE 2.7   Frequently Used Balloons

Balloon Type	Sample Brand Names	Features	Common Uses
Plain angioplasty balloons (POBAs)	Ultraverse PTA Dilatation Catheter (Bard Peripheral Vascular, Tempe, AZ) Evercross PTA Balloon Catheter (eV3 Endovascular Inc., Plymouth, MN) Charger Balloon Dilatation Catheter (Boston Scientific, Marlborough, MA)	Angioplasty balloons come with a variety of features and benefits, including compliant and semicompliant systems, low-profile systems, increased trackability, increased pushability, and radiopaque markers to increase visualization and reduce fluoroscopy time	Prepping vessels prior to DCB angioplasty or stenting Further postdilating following atherectomy Postdilatation of stents
Focal force balloons	VascuTrak PTA Dilatation Catheter (Bard Peripheral Vascular, Tempe, AZ)	Wire at external surface of balloon delivers focused force for eccentric delivery of radial force, allowing lower inflation pressures	Primary therapy in "no-stent" zones (CFA, popliteal) Resistant and highly calcified lesions Further postdilate following atherectomy Vessel prepping prior to DCB
Plaque-modifying balloons	Chocolate PTA Balloon Catheter (manufactured by TriReme Medical, LLC, Pleasanton, CA; distributed by Cordis Corporation, Bridgewater, NJ)	Nitinol-constraint creates alternating constrained pillows and grooves that facilitate uniform distribution of angioplasty forces in order to minimize vessel wall trauma and reduce dissection rates	Primary therapy in "no-stent" zones (CFA, popliteal) Resistant and highly calcified lesions Further postdilate following atherectomy Vessel prepping prior to DCB
Scoring balloons	AngioSculpt Scoring Balloon (Spectranetics Corporation, Colorado Springs, CO)	External helical nitinol scoring struts secure balloon in place during angioplasty to preven slippage during inflation and allow increased outward radial force delivery in order to reduce vessel wall trauma and therefore limit dissection rates	Can be used as primary angioplasty balloon Resistant and highly calcified lesions Further postdilate following atherectomy Vessel prepping prior to DCB
Drug-coated balloons (DCBs)	IN.PACT Admiral Drug Coated Balloon (Medtronic, Minneapolis, MN) Lutonix Drug Coated Balloon (Bard Peripheral Vascular, Tempe, AZ)	Balloon coated in paclitaxel with different combinations of carriers + excipients Paclitaxel interferes with microtubule dynamics, preventing neointimal hyperplasia	Prevents restenosis of treated lesions Can be used as primary therapy for lesions with stent-like results without leaving behind foreign body Effects are affected by a number of different characteristics that vary based on balloon type, but drug can last up to 180 days in the arterial wall

TABLE 2.8   Supplemental Information on Angioplasty Balloons

Trade Name	Balloon Type	Diameter	Length	Cost	NP	RBP	Wire
Ultraverse (Bard)	Standard pressure	3–12 mm	20–300 mm	$80–85	6–8 atm	9–21 atm	.035
Dorado (Bard)	Standard pressure	3–10 mm	20–200 mm	$160–170	8 atm	20–24 atm	.035
Atlas (Bard)	Standard pressure	12–26 mm	20–60 mm	$260–465	4–7 atm	12–18 atm	.035
Mustang (Boston Scientific)	Standard pressure	3–12 mm	12–200 mm	$370–380	8–10 atm	14–24 atm	.035
Conquest (Bard)	High pressure	5–12 mm	20–80 mm	$150–155	6–8 atm	20–30 atm	.035
Peripheral Cutting (Boston Scientific)	Cutting	2–8 mm	15–20 mm	$820–830	4–6 atm	8–12 atm	.014–.018

TABLE 2.9	Frequently Used Stents	
Stent Type	**Sample Brand Names**	**Features and Uses**
Bare metal stents (BMSs)	LifeStent (Bard Peripheral Vascular, Tempe, AZ)	Must use self-expanding stents to resist compressive/crushing forces in the limbs Different BMS have different characteristics, with some with higher levels of flexibility
Vasculomimetic	Supera Peripheral Stent System (Abbott Vascular, Abbott Park, IL)	Interwoven nitinol design withstands compression with little radial outward force Because of this design, must prepare the vessel with balloon larger than or equal to the stent diameter to attain maximal stent diameter Mimics natural structure and anatomic movement of vessel, reducing chances of stent fracture Useful for areas prone to compression and torsional forces Useful in treating de novo lesions or restenotic or occlusive femoropopliteal lesions
Endoprosthesis	GORE Viahbahn Endoprosthesis (W.L. Gore & Associates, Inc., Flagstaff, AZ)	Flexible stent-graft constructed with ePTFE liner with heparin-bonded surface attached to external nitinol stent Used to effectively create endoluminal bypass Useful for relining stents that have closed down or developed in-stent restenosis Useful for covering fractured stents Useful for sealing off arterial ruptures or excluding pseudoaneurysms from circulation
Drug-eluting stents (DESs)	Zilver PTX Drug-eluting Peripheral Stent (Cook Medical, Bloomington, IN)	Paclitaxel elutes from stent into vessel wall within 72 h Remains in vessel wall for up to 56 days Inhibits neointimal hyperplasia

- Stent placement inhibits normal arterial movement, resulting in damage due to dynamic stresses of compression, flexion, and torsion
- In addition, radial outward force causes chronic inflammation. Lastly, the stent incites a foreign body reaction.
- Fractures
  - Stents are subject to fracture over time, especially in areas of high torsional or compressive forces (common femoral artery (CFA), proximal superficial femoral artery (SFA), popliteal artery).
- Limits potential for future surgical bypass/revascularization by covering potential targets

Drug-Eluting Stents
- ISR rates differ between devices (bare nitinol stents vs. sirolimus-covered stents vs. paclitaxel-covered stents) and location of treated artery
- The 2006 SIROCCO trial compared bare nitinol to sirolimus-covered stents for SFA lesions:
  - Results were initially encouraging, but benefit was lost after 18 months.
    - Bare nitinol stents had a 21.1% ISR rate.
    - Sirolimus-covered stents had a 22.9% ISR.
- The ZILVER PTX randomized controlled trial showed 5-year primary patency of SFA lesions as:
  - 66.4% for those treated with the ZILVER PTX drug-eluting stent
  - 43.4% for those treated with balloon angioplasty or bare metal stent

ATHERECTOMY
- Used as an alternative or adjunct to angioplasty and/or stenting
- Instead of displacing plaque radially and longitudinally along the vessel wall to achieve luminal gain, as is done in angioplasty and stenting, atherectomy devices physically remove plaque from the artery.

> ### ⏩ CLINICAL POINT
> Many device manufacturers mandate the use of an embolic protection device in the artery distal to the atherectomy site to catch any potential atheroembolism.

Types of Atherectomies
- Laser atherectomy
  - Example: excimer laser (Spectranetics; Colorado Springs, CO)
  - Mechanism: uses pulsed UV light to photo-ablate plaque, penetrating the atheroma and vaporizing plaque through thermokinetic interactions
  - Specific uses
    - ISR
    - Recanalization of native arteries in the setting of occluded bypass grafts
    - Total occlusions that remain crossable by guidewire
    - Lesions that cannot be traversed by guidewire
    - See Box 2.2.

> **BOX 2.2   EXCITE In-Stent Restenosis Trial: EXCimer Laser for Treatment of FemoropopliTEal In-Stent Restenosis**
>
> Patients with claudication (Rutherford class 1 through 4) and in-stent restenosis of previously placed femoropopliteal bare metal stents were randomized to receive either angioplasty alone (PTA) or both excimer laser atherectomy and angioplasty (ELA + PTA)
> - Primary efficacy endpoint: freedom from lesion recurrence at 6-month follow-up
> - No lesion recurrence at 6-month follow-up:
>   - 73.5% in the ELA + PTA group
>   - 51.8% in the PTA group
> - Study enrollment was stopped at 250 patients due to early efficacy in the ELA + PTA group
> - ELA + PTA associated with 52% reduction in lesion recurrence

> **BOX 2.3   DAART: Directional Atherectomy and Anti-Restenotic Treatment**
>
> - Placing permanent stents has repercussions, and in general, practitioners prefer to not to leave objects behind.
> - While drug-coated balloon technology has demonstrated improved outcomes compared with conventional angioplasty, it has limitations in heavily calcified lesions where there is thought to be reduced drug uptake.
>   - A treatment option known as DAART, where plaque is first removed by atherectomy followed by drug delivery using a paclitaxel-coated balloon, was studied in the DEFINITIVE AR trial. The trial demonstrated higher patency rates in lesions treated with the combination of directional atherectomy and DCB compared with those treated with DCB alone.
>   - In the DAART group, more plaque removed from the vessel (<30% residual stenosis) prior to DCB treatment was associated with higher primary patency rates than when less plaque was removed (>30% residual stenosis).

DCB, Drug-coated balloon.

- Orbital atherectomy
  - Example: Diamondback Orbital Atherectomy System (Cardiovascular Systems, Inc.; St. Paul, MN)
  - Mechanism: abrasive diamond-coated rotating crown creates an ablative surface that selectively targets rigid, diseased tissue (healthy tissue flexes away). Greater rotational speeds create larger luminal sizes.
  - Specific uses
    - 360-degree plaque removal effective for circumferential calcified plaque
- Directional atherectomy
  - Example: TurboHawk plaque-excision system (Covidien; Mansfield, MA)
  - Mechanism: directional series of cutters at the end of the catheter are positioned at area of highest plaque burden to chip away at the plaque, which is then collected in the catheter's nose cone and removed from the body

- Can serve as standalone therapy for difficult areas where stenting is not desired (i.e., adjacent to the CFA or in the popliteal artery)
- See Box 2.3.
- Rotational atherectomy
  - Example: JetStream Atherectomy System (Boston Scientific; Marlborough, MA)
  - Mechanism: uses rotating series of blades at the end of the catheter to debulk plaque circumferentially with simultaneous aspiration to reduce the chance of distal embolization
  - Lesion debulking with the JetStream device has been shown to improve the patency rates of heavily calcified lesions that are subsequently treated with DCBs.

> ## 🏠 TAKE-HOME POINTS
>
> - Informed consent should cover both the procedure and the sedation type, including (1) reason for the procedure; (2) method of the procedure; (3) benefits, risks, and potential complications of the procedure; (4) risks if the procedure is refused; and (5) alternatives to the procedure.
> - Holding aspirin and Plavix prior to a procedure should be a decision weighing cardiac risk versus bleeding risk.
> - Acute kidney injury after contrast administration is manifested by an increase in serum creatinine of 0.3 mg/dL or more, a percentage increase of serum creatinine of 50% or more, or a decrease in urine output to less than 0.5 mL/kg/h.
> - Patients with a history of contrast allergies should be premedicated with an appropriate regimen, such as:
>   - Prednisone 50 mg PO at 13, 7, and 1 hour prior to the procedure
>   - Diphenhydramine 50 mg PO, IV, or IM 1 hour prior to the procedure
> - Most common "cocktail" for conscious sedation is a combination of fentanyl, an analgesic, and Versed, an anxiolytic.
>
> - Naloxone should always be accessible if urgent reversal of sedation is needed. Flumazenil is another reversal agent, though its application is limited.
> - Several breakthrough trials to be aware of include:
>   - *IN.PACT SFA* and *LEVANT* trials showed significant improvement in patency with drug-coated balloons in comparison with traditional angioplasty.
>   - *SIROCCO* trial showed initial benefit with drug-covered stent, though in-stent restenosis rates equalized between bare stent and drug-covered stent at 18-month follow-up.
>   - *ZILVER PTX* trial showed a greater long-term patency in those treated with the drug-eluting stent in comparison to balloon angioplasty/bare stent.
>   - *EXCITE ISR* trial showed increased efficacy when patients were treated with a combination of atherectomy and angioplasty rather than angioplasty alone.
>   - *DEFINITIVE AR* trial demonstrated higher patency rates in lesions treated with a combination of atherectomy and DCBs rather than DCBs alone.

THROMBECTOMY

- Devices include:
  - Angiojet (Boston Scientific): pharmacomechanical thrombectomy device that uses active aspiration of thrombus and pulsed spray of a tPA solution.
  - Cleaner XT (Argon): mechanical rotational thrombectomy system
  - Arrow-Trerotola PTD (Arrow): mechanical thrombectomy device

REVIEW QUESTIONS

1. A diabetic 69-year-old male has which of the following CHA_2DS_2-VASc scores? What is the appropriate recommendation regarding anticoagulation given his score?
   a. 1; therapy should be considered
   b. 1; therapy is recommended
   c. 2; therapy should be considered
   d. 2; therapy is recommended

2. Which of the following is the most appropriate antibiotic choice prior to percutaneous gastrostomy tube placement?
   a. No antibiotic necessary
   b. Ancef 1 g IV
   c. Vancomycin 1 g PO
   d. Ciprofloxacin 500 mg IV

SUGGESTED READINGS

American College of Radiology Committee on Drugs and Contrast Media. *ACR Manual on Contrast Media*. Version 10.1. http://www.acr.org/Quality-Safety/Resources/Contrast-Manual; Updated 2015. Accessed 9 May 2018.

American College of Radiology Committee on Practice Parameters—Interventional and Cardiovascular Radiology. *ACR-SIR Practice Parameter for Sedation/Analgesia*. https://www.acr.org/-/media/ACR/Files/Practice-Parameters/sed-analgesia.pdf; Revised 2015. Accessed 9 May 2018.

Cho KJ. Carbon dioxide angiography: scientific principles and practice. *Vasc Specialist Int*. 2015;31(3):67–80.

Cho KJ, Hawkins IF. *Carbon dioxide angiography. Medscape (website)*; Updated February 2016. http://emedicine.medscape.com/article/423121-overview#a1. Accessed 9 May 2018.

Cohen J. Adverse events related to procedural sedation for gastrointestinal endoscopy. In: Saltzman JR, Joshi GP, eds. *UpToDate*; Updated March 2016. http://www.uptodate.com/contents/complications-of-procedural-sedation-for-gastrointestinal-endoscopy. Accessed 9 May 2018.

Frank RL. Procedural sedation in adults outside the operating room. In: Wolfson AB, ed. *UpToDate*; Updated June 2017. http://www.uptodate.com/contents/procedural-sedation-in-adults. Accessed 9 May 2018.

Geschwind JFH, Dake MD. *Abrams' Angiography: Interventional Radiology*. 3rd ed. Philadelphia, PA: Wolters Kluwer; 2014.

Greller H, Gupta A. Benzodiazepine poisoning and withdrawal. In: Traub SJ, ed. *UpToDate*; Updated August 2017. http://www.uptodate.com/contents/procedural-sedation-in-adults. Accessed 9 May 2018.

Higgs ZCJ, Macafee DAL, Braithwaite BD, Maxwell-Armstrong CA. The Seldinger technique: 50 years on. *Lancet*. 2005;366 (9494):1407–1409.

Hoffman RJ. Ketamine poisoning. In: Traub SJ, ed. *UpToDate*; Updated August 2017. http://www.uptodate.com/contents/ketamine-poisoning. Accessed 9 May 2018.

Hsu DC, Cravero JP. Procedural sedation in children outside of the operating room. In: Stack AM, Randolph AG, eds. *UpToDate*: Updated August 2017. http://www.uptodate.com/contents/procedural-sedation-in-children-outside-of-the-operating-room. Accessed 9 May 2018.

Hsu DC, Cravero JP. Selection of medications for pediatric procedural sedation outside of the operating room. In: Stack AM, Randolph AG, eds. *UpToDate*; Updated October 2017. http://www.uptodate.com/contents/selection-of-medications-for-pediatric-procedural-sedation-outside-of-the-operating-room. Accessed 9 May 2018.

Inker LA, Perrone RD. Assessment of kidney function. In: Sterns RH, ed. *UpToDate*; Updated March 2017. http://www.uptodate.com/contents/assessment-of-kidney-function. Accessed 9 May 2018.

Kandarpa K, Machan L. *Handbook of Interventional Radiologic Procedures*. 4th ed. Philadelphia, PA: Lippincott Williams & Wilkins; 2011.

Moos JM, Ham SW, Han SM, et al. Safety of carbon dioxide digital subtraction angiography. *Arch Surg*. 2011;146(12):1428–1432.

Rudnick MR. Prevention of contrast nephropathy associated with angiography. In: Palevsky PM, ed. *UpToDate*; Updated March 2018. http://www.uptodate.com/contents/prevention-of-contrast-induced-nephropathy. Accessed 9 May 2018.

Seldinger SI. Catheter replacement of the needle in percutaneous arteriography: a new technique. *Acta Radiol*. 1953;39(5):368–376.

3

Imaging Modalities

Jacob W. Fleming, Jared T. Sokol, Peter R. Bream

This chapter reviews conventional X-rays, fluoroscopy, computed tomography (CT), magnetic resonance imaging (MRI), and positron emission tomography (PET) scans. A proper understanding of these commonly encountered imaging methods is essential to a career in both diagnostic and interventional radiology.

RADIOGRAPHY

- In 1895, Wilhelm Röntgen took the first radiograph of his wife's left hand. He noted that the radiation passed differently through tissue, bone, and metal. This was the birth of radiology and earned Röntgen the first Nobel Prize in Physics.

> ### ⟫ CLINICAL POINT
>
> Just 6 months after Wilhelm Röntgen discovered X-rays, physicians on the battlefields were utilizing the technology to locate bullets in wounded soldiers.

- To perform a **radiograph**, an X-ray beam is directed toward an area of interest. Some radiation is transmitted, and some is absorbed. A digital detector positioned distal to the object captures the transmitted radiation. The information is processed into an image, where dense structures (bone) appear white, softer structures (bowel) appear gray, and the absence of a structure (air) appears black. This method of capturing the radiation "shadow" is called *projection radiography*.
- Radiographs provide moderate resolution in comparison to cross-sectional imaging and are most commonly used to quickly find abnormalities in hard and soft tissue (e.g., bone fractures, lung consolidations, cardiomegaly). It is often the first imaging modality used in many medical scenarios.
- Simple radiographs subject the patient to extremely small amounts of radiation and have minimal cancer risk.

FLUOROSCOPY

- **Fluoroscopy** uses X-rays to create a real-time, live image of the interior of the human body. It is the interventional radiologist's "bread and butter," the imaging modality of choice for many IR procedures.
- Fluoroscopy allows for the visualization of both structure and function—the beating of a heart, the movement of a bone, and the placement of a catheter can all be viewed in real time.
- Use of contrast in fluoroscopy allows for detailed visualization of vascular and digestive structures.
  - Iodinated contrast is used to image the vascular system.
  - Barium is used to image the digestive system.
- Fluoroscopy does expose the patient to significantly more ionizing radiation than a simple single X-ray. Time in the fluoroscopy suite must be monitored judiciously. Excessive radiation exposure in the IR suite may cause cutaneous radiation reactions and skin damage.

COMPUTED TOMOGRAPHY (FIG. 3.1)

- A **CT** scan is essentially a three-dimensional (3D) image that can be viewed as 2D cross-sections. The scanned information can be viewed as high-resolution slices or can be reconstructed into rotatable 3D objects.
- As in fluoroscopy, contrast can be used to highlight certain entities, such as vasculature or the digestive system.
- CT scans carry a significant radiation burden. It is estimated that 1.5% to 2% of all cancers in the United States are due to CT scan radiation. A normal chest CT scan subjects a patient to 70 × the radiation of a simple chest radiograph. It is therefore important for IR physicians to integrate knowledge of radiation exposure into medical decision making.
- CT scans are often used in interventional radiology to understand a patient's anatomy, diagnose pathologies, and to plan for or follow up on a procedure. Recently, CT scans have been brought into the procedure suite in the form of cone beam CTs so physicians can view the most up-to-date anatomy and confirm the location of hardware intraprocedurally.

MAGNETIC RESONANCE IMAGING (FIG. 3.2)

- **MRI** produces high-resolution serial slices of the patient's anatomy, not unlike CT, but there are several key differences. With MRI, no ionizing radiation is used;

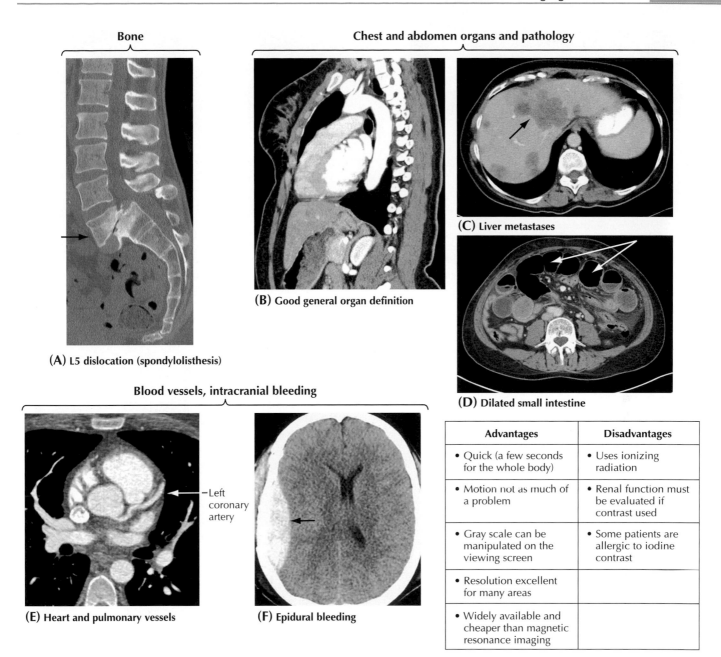

Fig. 3.1 Computed Tomography Uses, Advantages, and Disadvantages. (From Cochard LR, Goodhartz L, Harmath C, et al., eds. *Netter's Introduction to Imaging.* St. Louis: Elsevier; 2012:6).

rather, images are obtained based on proton density and magnetic properties.

- These differences in proton density allow for fantastic soft tissue resolution with MR imaging. Different sequences of pulses are used to focus on different characteristics of anatomy. Some of the more commonly used sequences are T1, T2, inversion recovery sequences such as Short-TI Inversion Recovery (STIR) and Fluid-attenuated inversion recovery (FLAIR), and diffusion-weighted sequences (DWI).

► CLINICAL POINT

T1 and T2 sequences can be easily differentiated by their overt characteristics.
- T1: fat is bright (high proton density)
- T2: water is bright ($H_2O = T_2O$)

- Contrast can be administered intravenously to delineate vascular structures, inflammation, or tumors. In MRI, the contrast agent of choice is gadolinium, a paramagnetic ion that shortens the T1 relaxation time of protons in tissue with which it interacts.
- MRI is preferable to CT in a number of diagnoses including brain tumors, acute ischemic stroke, and early osteomyelitis.
- The downsides to MRI include its long image acquisition time, high cost, loud noise, and less widespread availability than CT. MRIs are contraindicated in patients with many types of implantable devices because of the effect of the magnetic field on ferromagnetic materials.
- Because of issues with timing and magnetism, MRI is not used in many IR procedures. However, it remains an important diagnostic modality for preoperative planning. In particular, MR angiography is a noninvasive method

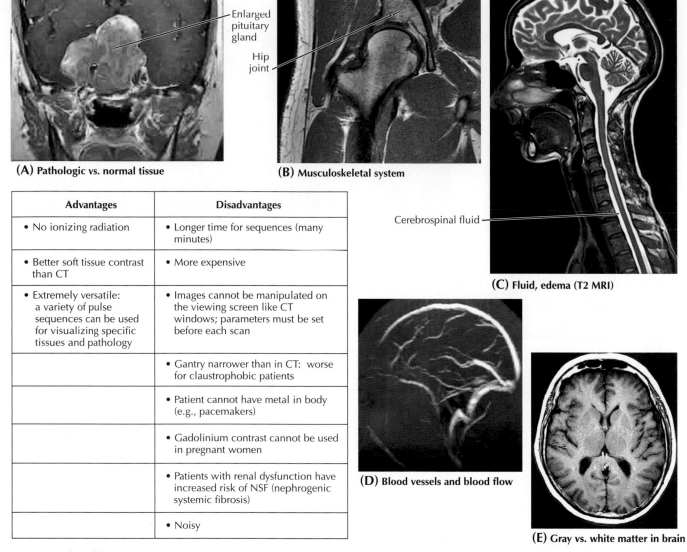

(A) Pathologic vs. normal tissue — Enlarged pituitary gland

(B) Musculoskeletal system — Hip joint

(C) Fluid, edema (T2 MRI) — Cerebrospinal fluid

(D) Blood vessels and blood flow

(E) Gray vs. white matter in brain

Advantages	Disadvantages
• No ionizing radiation	• Longer time for sequences (many minutes)
• Better soft tissue contrast than CT	• More expensive
• Extremely versatile: a variety of pulse sequences can be used for visualizing specific tissues and pathology	• Images cannot be manipulated on the viewing screen like CT windows; parameters must be set before each scan
	• Gantry narrower than in CT: worse for claustrophobic patients
	• Patient cannot have metal in body (e.g., pacemakers)
	• Gadolinium contrast cannot be used in pregnant women
	• Patients with renal dysfunction have increased risk of NSF (nephrogenic systemic fibrosis)
	• Noisy

Fig. 3.2 Magnetic Resonance Imaging Uses, Advantages, and Disadvantages. CT, Computed tomography. (From Cochard LR, Goodhartz L, Harmath C, et al., eds. *Netter's Introduction to Imaging*. St. Louis: Elsevier; 2012:8).

for imaging vasculature that can be employed in patients with allergies to iodinated contrast.
• There has been some use of intraoperative MRI, particularly in high-risk neurovascular cases, but so far very few centers have the necessary equipment to do so. Such suites require nonmagnetic surgical tools.

POSITRON EMISSION TOMOGRAPHY

• PET scan is a modality of **nuclear medicine** meaning that, unlike the modalities already discussed, radiation is produced from inside the body with a PET scan rather than directed at it.
• A pharmaceutical with a radioisotope (e.g., 18-fluorode-oxyglucose) is administered to the patient, and it localizes to areas of high metabolic activity. The radioisotope undergoes

decay, releasing energy in the form of gamma rays, which are detected to produce an image.
• PET scans have poor anatomic detail and are often paired with CT scans for optimal tumor localization.
• Although an important diagnostic study, PET has limited use in IR.

ULTRASOUND (FIG. 3.3)

• **Ultrasound** (US) is unique among imaging modalities in several ways: it does not use radiation or magnetic fields and thus has practically no contraindications; it does not use large stationary equipment and thus can be used in bedside situations; and it is a highly dynamic modality, producing real-time images.

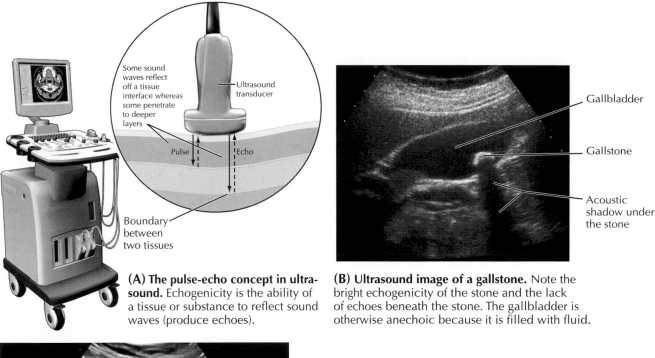

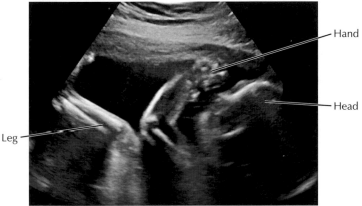

(A) The pulse-echo concept in ultrasound. Echogenicity is the ability of a tissue or substance to reflect sound waves (produce echoes).

(B) Ultrasound image of a gallstone. Note the bright echogenicity of the stone and the lack of echoes beneath the stone. The gallbladder is otherwise anechoic because it is filled with fluid.

(C) Ultrasound image of a second-trimester fetus. Ultrasound is used to monitor prenatal development, detect congenital defects, and determine sex.

Fig. 3.3 **Ultrasound.** (From Cochard LR, Goodhartz L, Harmath C, et al., eds. *Netter's Introduction to Imaging.* St. Louis: Elsevier; 2012:12).

- The principle of US is the conduction of an electrical current through a piezoelectric crystal, which vibrates and produces sound waves. The waves reflect (or "echo") off of the internal anatomy and back to the crystal, creating an electrical signal that a computer converts to an image.
- **Doppler** flow is a mode that calculates velocity of blood flow using calculations based on the Doppler effect and colors the blood flow accordingly. This mode is helpful for assessing blood flow in angioplasty and, vessels to avoid in biopsy cases and is also invaluable in the diagnostic setting (e.g., assess venous flow in the case of suspected deep vein thrombosis (DVT)).
  - The Doppler effect holds that the perceived frequency of a moving wave varies depending on its velocity relative to the velocity of the object detecting the wave.
- The US machine calculates the velocity of blood flow based on the difference between the expected time of arrival of the echo (to the transducer) and the actual time of arrival.
- In IR, US can be used as the primary imaging modality in bedside or office procedures including biopsies, fine-needle aspiration, thoracenteses, and paracenteses.
- It may also be used as an adjunct modality in obtaining initial vascular access or anatomic survey in cases relying on subsequent fluoroscopy or CT use.
- Limitations of US include that it is highly operator dependent, and images can be difficult to interpret without context. Moreover, since US relies on the reflection of sound waves, it works best with solid organs and liquid collections and is limited with gas-filled areas such as the lung.

🏠 TAKE-HOME POINTS

Modality	Primary Uses in Interventional Radiology	Limitations
X-ray	Preoperative planning	Uses ionizing radiation; lower sensitivity than other imaging modalities
Fluoroscopy	Intraoperative real-time visualization of anatomy, supplemented by the use of iodinated contrast	Uses ionizing radiation
CT	Preoperative planning; intraprocedural use (e.g., CT-guided abscess drainage, chest tube placement, mass biopsy)	High dose of ionizing radiation
MRI	Preoperative planning (MRA); soft tissue evaluation	Slow, expensive, loud, and subject to imaging artifacts; cannot be used in patients with certain implanted medical devices
PET	Limited in IR but useful in the evaluation of cancer and treatment progression	High dose of ionizing radiation; poor anatomic detail so it is paired with CT, which exposes the patient to more radiation
Ultrasound	Bedside procedures (e.g., fine needle aspiration (FNA), biopsies, thoracenteses, paracenteses); vascular access in fluoroscopic cases	Highly operator dependent; poor in the evaluation of air/gas-containing structures

CT, Computed tomography; *MRI*, magnetic resonance imaging; *PET*, positron emission tomography.

REVIEW QUESTIONS

1. Which of the following does not appear as the others on a CT scan?
   a. Metal stent
   b. Calcified tumor
   c. Old hemorrhage
   d. Bone
   e. Arterial plaque

2. In MRI, different imaging sequences will highlight different features of anatomy or pathology. Which finding would not appear hyperintense on a T2 sequence in a non-contrast MRI?
   a. Cystic lesion
   b. Cerebrospinal fluid
   c. Acute bleed
   d. Blood vessels
   e. Old bleed

3. Which imaging modality provides the best detail of the vasculature of an anatomic region?
   a. CT angiogram
   b. Angiogram
   c. MR angiogram
   d. PET
   e. Ultrasound

SUGGESTED READING

Cochard LR, Goodhartz L, Harmath C, et al. Introduction to imaging modalities. In *Netter's Introduction to Imaging*. St. Louis: Elsevier; 2012:1–16.

Anatomy

Jacob W. Fleming, Jared T. Sokol, Peter R. Bream

There are few medical specialties where a thorough comprehension of anatomy is as vital as in radiology, and this is especially true in interventional radiology. Interventional radiologists are experts in vascular anatomy, as vascular access and navigation are the bases for many of our procedures. Practitioners must be aware of the typical branching patterns and common variants in a given region. This chapter serves as a cursory overview of vascular anatomy by region.

VASCULAR ANATOMY

The vascular system can be divided into arterial and venous systems, which have important structural and functional differences.

Arterial System

- Gross characteristics
  - The arterial system is the high-pressure side of the vascular circuit. On physical exam, arteries are easily differentiated from veins by palpation because they have pulsatile flow, which is due to the pressure differential between systole and diastole.
  - Because of the high systemic pressure, a punctured artery will bleed much more briskly than a punctured vein.
- Microscopic characteristics
  - Arteries contain three histologic layers: tunica intima (endothelium), tunica media (smooth muscle), and tunica externa (loose fibrous connective tissue). Between the intima and media is a layer of elastin. Outside of the tunica externa is a layer of epithelium called serosa.
  - The elastin layer, which contributes to the elastic recoil that is important to the high-pressure circuit, distinguishes arteries from veins.
  - Weakening of the elastin layer can contribute to gradual dilation of all three layers of the vessel, which is called an **aneurysm**.
  - Aneurysms can dissect and rupture; in the aorta, this is a life-threatening emergency and must be treated surgically.
  - Unruptured aneurysms may be treated prophylactically with either open surgical repair or endovascular stent grafting.

REGIONAL ARTERIAL ANATOMY

Lung

- The **pulmonary artery** is unique among the arterial system because it carries deoxygenated blood (from the right heart to the lungs).
- The pulmonary artery arises from the right ventricle and splits into left and right arteries, easily recognizable on CT angiography.

> ### ▶▶ CLINICAL POINT
>
> A **saddle embolism** is a large clot that straddles the main pulmonary artery trunk at its bifurcation. These occur in approximately 2.6% of patients diagnosed with pulmonary emboli.

- Each pulmonary artery follows the bronchus on its respective side into the hilum of the lung and branches along with it through more than 16 generations, culminating in the microscopic alveolar-capillary interface where blood is oxygenated.
- These capillary beds drain into venules that culminate in two pulmonary veins from each lung, which then course to the left atrium.
- The pulmonary vascular circuit contains anastomotic connections with the bronchial arteries to provide the lung parenchyma with oxygenated blood.
- There are variants of the normal pulmonary artery anatomy. An **aberrant left pulmonary artery** branches from the right pulmonary artery rather than the main and can compress the right main bronchus, causing air trapping in the right lung. This may be associated with tracheal ring stenosis, a condition that can be fatal.

Aorta

- The **aorta** serves as the outflow tract from the left ventricle and provides oxygenated blood throughout the body.
- It consists of *thoracic* and *abdominal* regions; the thoracic aorta can be subdivided into *ascending*, *arch*, and *descending* portions.

Thoracic Aorta

- The **ascending aorta** gives off the coronary arteries that perfuse the heart. Intervention in this area is typically in the realm of vascular surgery and not modern IR.

BOX 4.1   Mnemonic

ABC's: **A**orta, **B**rachiocephalic, **C**ommon carotid, **S**ubclavian

- The **arch** provides arterial supply to the head, neck, and upper extremities.
- The aortic arch begins and ends in the sternal plane, at the level of the second intercostal space. It typically gives off three primary branches: the right-sided **brachiocephalic (innominate) trunk**, **left common carotid**, and **left subclavian** (Box 4.1).
- In this branching pattern, the brachiocephalic trunk usually gives off the **right common carotid** and **right subclavian** arteries. The left common carotid and left subclavian arteries come off directly from the arch.
- This typical branching pattern is seen in about two-thirds of the population.
  - Variants include a **common origin** of the brachiocephalic trunk and left common carotid, seen in approximately 25% of the population, **arch origin of the right vertebral** proximal to the left subclavian, and **arch origin of the right subclavian** distal to the left subclavian.
- Carotid arteries
  - The left common carotid takes off directly from the aortic arch, whereas the right common carotid branches from the brachiocephalic trunk.
  - The carotids provide the majority of the perfusion to the brain with the vertebral arteries (which arise from the subclavians) providing some.
  - Each common carotid gives off external and internal branches; the internal carotid perfuses the brain by way of the circle of Willis, discussed later in this chapter.
- Bronchial arteries
  - The bronchial arteries branch from the descending portion of the thoracic aorta and bring oxygenated blood to the lung parenchyma.
  - Anastomoses exist between the bronchial arteries and the pulmonary arteries such that there is mixing of the oxygenated and deoxygenated blood.
- Arteries of the upper extremity
  - The upper extremities are perfused by the **subclavian artery**, which changes in name as it courses through the axilla and arm. It becomes the **axillary artery** as it passes the lateral margin of the first rib and the **brachial artery** as it passes the inferior edge of the teres major. The brachial then branches into the **radial** and **ulnar arteries**, which anastomose in the arterial arches of the hand.
  - The subclavian artery can be divided into three segments:
    - The first segment (from the origin of the subclavian to the medial margin of the anterior scalene muscle) gives off three branches—**vertebral artery**, **internal thoracic artery**, and **thyrocervical trunk**.

- The thyrocervical trunk in turn divides into the inferior thyroid artery, suprascapular artery, and transverse cervical artery.
    - The second segment (medial to the lateral border of the anterior scalene) gives off the **costocervical trunk**, which in turn divides into the **superior intercostal artery** and **deep cervical artery**.
    - The third segment (from the lateral border of the anterior scalene to the lateral margin of the first rib) gives off the **dorsal scapular artery**.
  - The **axillary artery** is also conceptually divided into three segments (Box 4.2):
    - The first segment gives off the **superior thoracic artery**.
    - The second segment gives off two branches, the **thoracoacromial artery** and **lateral thoracic artery**.
    - The third segment gives off three branches—the subscapular, anterior humeral circumflex, and posterior humeral circumflex arteries (Fig. 4.1).
  - The axillary artery passes the lower border of the teres major to become the **brachial artery** (Fig. 4.2), the major artery of the anterior compartment of the arm. It initially lies medial to the humerus and then moves laterally and posteriorly before branching into the ulnar and radial arteries.
  - Proximal to its bifurcation, it gives off the:
    - **Profunda brachii (deep brachial)**, the major artery of the posterior compartment; it branches off from the posteromedial aspect of the brachial artery around the midpoint of the arm and then courses posteriorly and laterally
    - Nutrient humeral branches
    - Superior and inferior ulnar collateral arteries, which contribute to anastomotic supply around the elbow
    - The brachial bifurcates into the radial and ulnar arteries in the antecubital fossa. These two arteries supply the forearm and hand.

Abdominal Aorta

- The descending thoracic aorta passes through the diaphragm at the level of the T12 vertebra, becoming the abdominal aorta. It is located anterior to the spinal column and behind the parietal peritoneum and is thus retroperitoneal.

BOX 4.2   Mnemonic-Axillary Segments and Branches

- **1st** segment: **1** branch
- **2nd** segment: **2** branches
- **3rd** segment: **3** branches
- "**S**crew **T**he **L**awyers **S**ave **A** **P**atient" (**s**uperior thoracic, **t**horacoacromial, **l**ateral thoracic, **s**ubscapular, **a**nterior humeral circumflex, **p**osterior humeral circumflex)

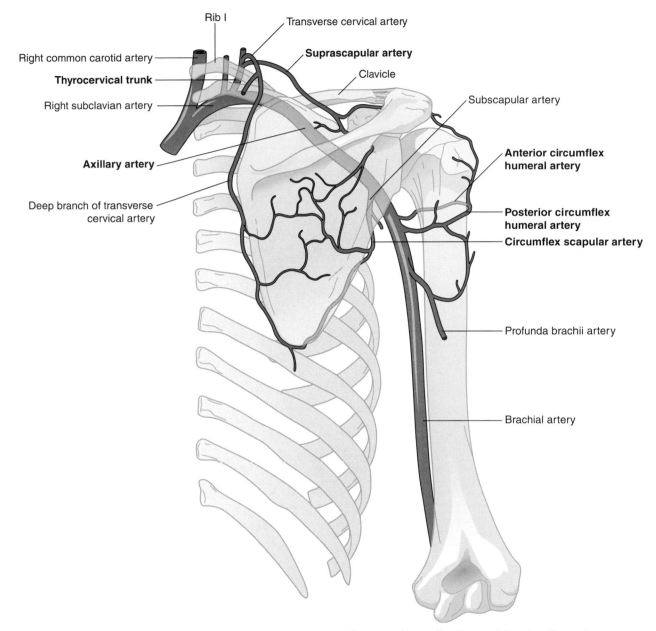

Rib I

Transverse cervical artery

Suprascapular artery

Right common carotid artery

Thyrocervical trunk

Clavicle

Right subclavian artery

Subscapular artery

Axillary artery

Anterior circumflex humeral artery

Deep branch of transverse cervical artery

Posterior circumflex humeral artery

Circumflex scapular artery

Profunda brachii artery

Brachial artery

Fig. 4.1 Subscapular, Anterior Circumflex Humeral, and Posterior Circumflex Humeral Arteries. (Reused with permission from Drake RL, Vogl AW, Mitchell AWM. *Gray's Anatomy for Students.* 3rd ed. Elsevier; Philadelphia, 2015: 683–834, Fig. 7.39.)

- Conceptually, the abdominal aorta gives off three large unpaired arteries, several smaller unpaired arteries, and two pairs of paired arteries.
  - The large unpaired arteries, from superior to inferior, are the **celiac trunk** (or celiac axis), **superior mesenteric artery (SMA)**, and **inferior mesenteric artery (IMA)**.
  - The smaller unpaired arteries include the **inferior phrenic** (T12), **middle suprarenal** (L1), and **median sacral** (L4).
  - The paired arteries are the renal arteries, gonadal arteries, and **common iliac arteries** (the terminal branches of the aorta).
- The **celiac trunk** takes off at the level of the T12 vertebral body. This artery supplies the proximal portion of the

gastrointestinal tract (corresponding to the embryologic foregut) and typically gives off three primary branches—the **left gastric, common hepatic,** and **splenic arteries.**
- The **left gastric artery** gives off an esophageal branch and stomach branch.
- The common hepatic gives off the proper hepatic artery, right gastric artery, and gastroduodenal artery.
  - The **proper hepatic artery** in turn branches into the **left hepatic artery** and **right hepatic artery** (which gives off the **cystic artery** feeding the gallbladder).
- The splenic artery gives off the dorsal pancreatic artery, short gastric arteries, left gastroepiploic artery, and the greater pancreatic artery.
- Common variations of this branching pattern include an **aberrant (or replaced) right hepatic artery** that

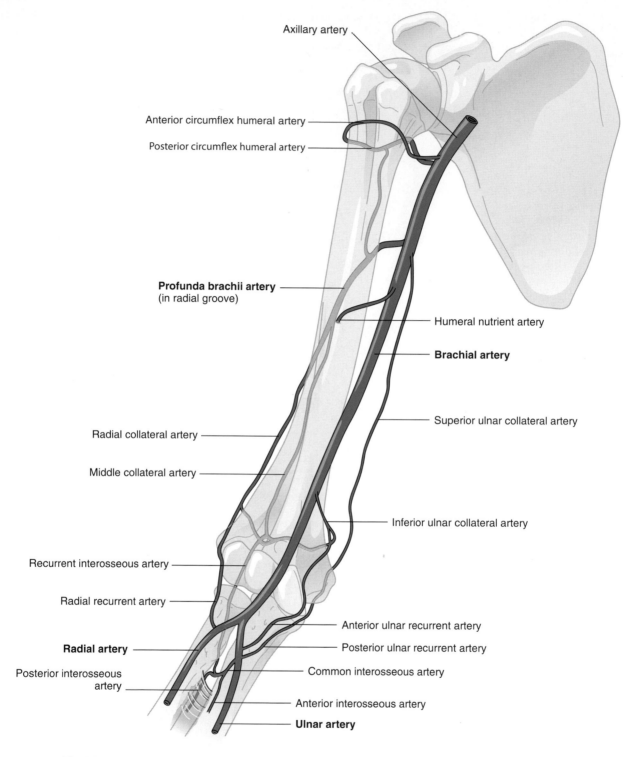

Fig. 4.2 Brachial Artery. (Reused with permission from Drake RL, Vogl AW, Mitchell AWM. *Gray's Anatomy for Students*. 3rd ed. Elsevier; Philadelphia, 2015: 683–834, Fig. 7.66.)

arises from the SMA (rather than the common hepatic) and an **aberrant (or replaced) left hepatic artery** that arises from the left gastric artery (rather than the common hepatic). **Accessory hepatic arteries**, which exist in addition to the normal anatomic pattern, also exist.

- The **SMA** taking off from the abdominal aorta at the L1, just inferior to the take-off of the celiac trunk. It supplies

the portion of the gastrointestinal tract that includes the head of the pancreas and the intestine from the lower duodenum to the distal third of the colon (corresponding to the embryologic midgut). The common branches are the:

- Inferior pancreaticoduodenal artery, intestinal arteries (with jejunal and ileal branches), ileocolic artery, right colic artery, and middle colic artery (with right and left branches).

- An important component of the SMA system is the **marginal artery of Drummond**, which is an anastomotic link with the IMA.
- The **IMA** takes off at L3. It perfuses the distal portion of the gastrointestinal tract that includes the distal transverse colon, descending colon, and rectum (corresponding to the embryologic hindgut). The typical branches are the **left colic artery**, **sigmoid branches**, and **superior rectal artery** (terminal branch of the IMA).
- Before its bifurcation into the common iliac arteries, the abdominal aorta branches off into one final unpaired artery, the **median sacral artery**. This artery, which descends medially past the sacrum and coccyx, is functionally negligible in human anatomy.
- The **renal arteries** branch from the abdominal aorta at approximately right angles between L1 and L2. The right renal artery tends to be longer (as the abdominal aorta is positioned to the left of the IVC) and lower than the left.
  - Each renal artery passes posterior to the corresponding renal vein. Before reaching the kidney hilum, the artery branches in four or five smaller arteries, with the majority passing anterior to the ureter.
  - Each renal artery perfuses the respective kidney, the inferior portions of the adrenal gland (via the **inferior suprarenal arteries**), and the ureter.
  - The renal circulation is voluminous, receiving up to a third of total cardiac output, consistent with the filtering function of the organ.
  - Note that the adrenal glands receive arterial supply by three distinct sources—the **superior suprarenal artery** (branch of **inferior phrenic artery**), **middle suprarenal artery**, and **inferior suprarenal artery**.
  - In 25% to 40% of kidneys, there may be more than one renal artery on a given side, which is termed **supernumerary renal arteries**.
- **Iliac arteries** (Fig. 4.3 and Box 4.3)
  - The abdominal aorta bifurcates into the common iliac arteries at the level of the L4 vertebra. The **common iliac artery** runs inferolaterally and branches into the **external iliac artery**, which continues as the **femoral artery** as it passes under the inguinal ligament, and the **internal iliac**, which provides perfusion to the pelvis.
- Pelvic arteries
  - The internal iliac artery branches from the common iliac anterior to the sacroiliac joint.
  - The branching pattern of the internal iliac is variable, but typically it divides into an anterior and posterior branch.
    - The anterior branch typically gives off the obturator artery, inferior gluteal artery, umbilical artery, uterine artery and vaginal artery (female), inferior vesical artery (male), middle rectal artery, and internal pudendal artery.

- An **aberrant obturator artery** may arise from the inferior epigastric artery.
- The **internal pudendal artery** provides much of the vasculature to the genitalia, and thus the nomenclature of the branches varies by sex. It gives off the **inferior rectal artery, perineal artery, urethral artery, posterior labial/scrotal branches, artery of bulb of the vestibule/penis, dorsal artery of the clitoris/penis**, and **deep artery of the clitoris/penis**.
- The posterior branch gives off the iliolumbar artery, lateral sacral artery, and superior gluteal artery.

> ## ▶▶ CLINICAL POINT

Uterine artery embolization (UAE) can be done for the treatment of uterine leiomyomata (fibroids); the fibroid(s), fed by these branches, become ischemic and shrink by approximately 48%. Emergently, UAE may be done to stabilize a hemorrhaging uterus.

- Lower extremity arteries
  - The lower extremity is perfused by branches of the **external iliac artery**, which passes under the inguinal ligament to become the **superficial femoral artery (SFA)**. This in turn passes through the adductor hiatus to become the **popliteal artery**.
  - The **SFA** gives off several branches:
    - The superficial circumflex iliac artery and inferior epigastric artery, which run superiorly
    - The **superficial external pudendal artery**, which runs medially to supply the labium or scrotum
    - The profunda femoris (deep femoral) artery, which gives off perforating arteries and the medial and lateral femoral circumflex arteries
    - The **descending genicular artery**, which supplies the knee joint
  - The major branches of the popliteal artery are the anterior tibial artery, posterior tibial (PT) artery, and fibular artery.
    - On physical exam, the **popliteal** should be palpable in the popliteal fossa.
    - The **PT** is typically palpable posterior to the medial malleolus.
    - The **anterior tibial** gives off the **dorsalis pedis (DP) artery**, which is typically palpable lateral to the extensor hallucis longus tendon (tendon of the great toe).

Access Points and Landmarks

- **Femoral artery** (Fig. 4.4)
  - The femoral artery is a common access site for arterial interventions because it is easily palpated in most individuals and provides quick navigation to the abdominal aorta.
  - It is found in the femoral sheath, which contains, from lateral to medial, the femoral **nerve**, femoral

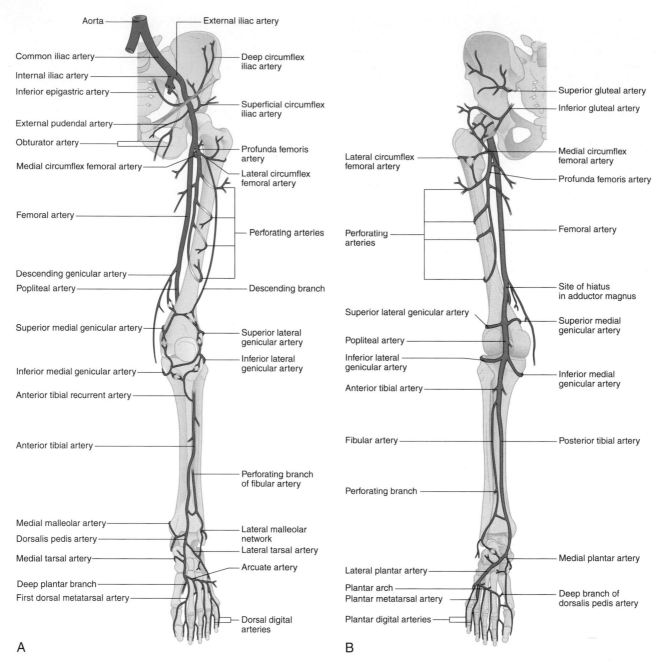

Fig. 4.3 An Overview of the Arteries of the Lower Limb. (A) Anterior aspect. (B) Posterior aspect. (Reused with permission from Susan Standring. *Pelvic Girdle and Lower Limb: Overview and Surface Anatomy in Gray's Anatomy*. 41st ed. Elsevier; Philadelphia, 2015:1314–1333, F78-4.)

BOX 4.3   Mnemonic for Branches of Internal Iliac Artery

"**I** **L**ove **G**oing **P**laces **I**n **M**y **V**ery **O**wn **U**nderwear" (**i**liolumbar, **l**ateral sacral, **g**luteal, internal **p**udendal, **i**nferior vesical, **m**iddle rectal, **v**aginal, **o**bturator, **u**mbilical/**u**terine)

---

artery, femoral **v**ein, and **l**ymphatics (*mnemonic NAVaL*).
- The artery can best be palpated below the inguinal ligament, halfway between the anterior superior iliac spine (ASIS) and the pubic symphysis.

- Radial artery
  - The radial artery has become a popular access point for interventionalists because there is no risk of retroperitoneal hemorrhage, it carries a low risk of thrombosis, and it allows for early ambulation postoperatively.
  - The artery can be palpated at the distal end of the radius between the tendons of the brachioradialis and flexor carpi radialis muscles.

Venous System
- Gross characteristics
  - Unlike the high-pressure elastic arterial system, the venous system is a capacitive system, designed to hold

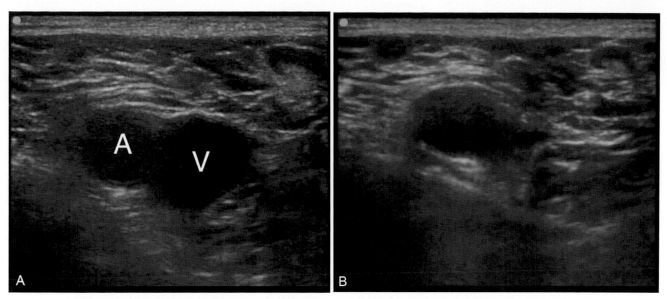

Fig. 4.4 (A) Ultrasound of an uncompressed common femoral artery *(A)* and common femoral vein *(V)*. (B) Ultrasound with compression with only the femoral artery visible. (Courtesy Dr. Peter Bream.)

varying volumes of deoxygenated blood and carry it back to the right heart.

- Because veins are postcapillary in the vascular circuit, they do not display pulsatility and are compressible by palpation or ultrasound compression, which exceeds venous pressure.
- Microscopic characteristics
  - Veins have three histologic layers—the tunica intima (endothelium), tunica media (smooth muscle), and tunica externa (loose fibrous connective tissue). Interspersed between the intima and media is a layer of elastin, much thinner than that found in arteries. As with arteries, a layer of epithelial cells called serosa surrounds the tunica externa.
  - The smooth muscle of the tunica media serves to facilitate vasoconstriction and vasodilation in response to the sympathetic and parasympathetic nervous systems.
  - Major features of the venous system are the interspersed **valves**. Venous blood primarily moves by gravity or against it by the action of contracting muscles. There are several places where valves are absent, such as the portal and azygos systems, allowing for reversible (collateral) flow.

> ## CLINICAL POINT
>
> **Venous insufficiency** is a condition of valvular incompetency, allowing for backflow and pooling of venous blood, typically in the legs. Signs include edema, varicose veins, and venous stasis ulcers. Among the possible interventional treatments are endovenous laser ablation and sclerotherapy of superficial veins.

- Major branches
  - The branches of the venous system mostly correspond to those of the arterial system, but there are several differences.
  - Importantly, there is a superficial venous system that drains into the deep venous system; it is the deep venous system that drains back to the heart.

> ## CLINICAL POINT
>
> **Deep venous thrombosis (DVT)**, clots in the deep system particularly of the lower extremity, may be signified by edema, erythema, and warmth of an occluded limb. DVTs can potentially throw emboli to the pulmonary circulation, which can be fatal. Superficial venous thrombosis, however, is not considered as dangerous because clots in the superficial system will usually be reabsorbed without incident.

- The **superior vena cava** is the major inflow tract from the head, neck, brain, thorax, and upper extremities. It is formed by the confluence of the left and right brachiocephalic veins and drains into the right atrium after being joined by the azygos vein.
- The **inferior vena cava** is the major venous inflow tract for the body inferior to the diaphragm. It is formed by the confluence of the common iliac veins around L5 and parallels the course of the abdominal aorta, lying to its right. As it courses upward, it receives multiple tributaries including the **lumbar veins, renal veins, inferior phrenic vein,** and **hepatic vein**.
- There are several typical cases of asymmetry in the IVC tributaries. The **right gonadal** and **suprarenal veins**

drain directly into the IVC, while their left-sided counterparts first drain into the **left renal vein**.

- The **azygos system** is a collection of collateral vessels involved in draining the thorax. The azygos vein lies to the right of the thoracic spine, formed by the right subcostal vein and ascending lumbar veins at T12. It drains the hemiazygos and accessory hemiazygos veins (its left-sided counterparts). It may receive further tributaries from bronchial veins, pericardial veins, and posterior right intercostal veins.
- The **portal vein** is most typically formed by the confluence of the superior mesenteric vein and splenic vein, with the inferior mesenteric vein usually draining into the splenic.
- The **cephalic, brachial,** and **basilic veins** are the major veins of the upper extremity and are frequently used for the insertion of **peripherally inserted central catheter (PICC) lines**. The cephalic vein lies on the ventral side of the arm, while the basilic vein lies on the medial side. The two veins anastomose via the median cubital vein in the antecubital fossa.

Access Points and Landmarks

- The **internal jugular vein (IJ/IJV)** is one of the major veins draining the head and brain. It is typically found lateral to the common carotid within the carotid sheath, but variations can occur. It is usually best accessed between the sternal and clavicular heads of the sternocleidomastoid muscle; having the patient turn his or her head to the opposite side allows for optimal access.
  - On either side, the internal jugular vein joins the subclavian to form the **brachiocephalic vein**. On

ultrasound, it can be easily distinguished from the carotid due to its compressibility (Fig. 4.5).
- The right IJ is preferred to the left as it provides a relatively straight path into the right atrium for central venous access or through the right atrium into the IVC for access to other venous structures such as the hepatic vein.
- The **femoral vein** is useful for lower body venous interventions or interventions in the pulmonary artery. It is found in the femoral triangle on the medial thigh, located medial to the femoral artery.

COLLATERAL CIRCULATION

- Collateral circulation is reversible blood flow via anastomotic vessels and can be found in both the arterial and venous system.
- This phenomenon allows for alternate flow around high resistance areas such as thromboses, emboli, tumors, or stenotic vasculature. Some systems, such as portosystemic anastomoses, will develop in these settings, while others, like the circle of Willis, are physiologically present.
- **Portal venous circulation** drains the abdominal viscera via the portal vein, which feeds into the hepatic sinusoids of the liver and into the hepatic vein, which feeds into the IVC.
  - In the normal state, this allows for the hepatic processing of nutrients and oral medications.
  - Alternatively, there are **portosystemic anastomoses** that bypass this system by draining the portal vein and its tributaries directly into the IVC. Normally, these pathways receive minimal flow, but in a state of portal

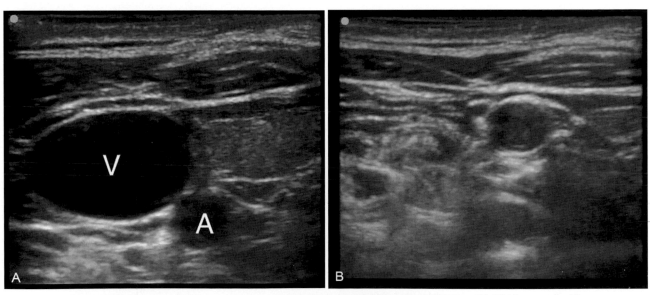

Fig. 4.5 (A) Ultrasound of an uncompressed internal jugular vein *(V)* and carotid artery *(A)*. (B) Ultrasound with compression with only the carotid artery visible. (Courtesy Dr. Peter Bream.)

hypertension, the high resistance to flow in the portal vein causes these anastomoses to swell. These large varicosities, or **varices**, can rupture and result in fatal hemorrhage if not properly managed.

- The most clinically significant varices are **esophageal varices** (engorged esophageal branches of the azygos vein), the rupture of which is the most frequent cause of acute GI bleeding. Rectal varices can result from engorged middle and inferior rectal veins, and engorged paraumbilical veins present as **caput medusae**, a classic physical exam finding of portal hypertension.
- A number of interventional procedures are available to manage portal hypertension and portosystemic varices including **TIPS**, **BRTO**, and **embolization**.
- The **Winslow pathway** is a collateral pathway that develops in the setting of aortoiliac occlusive disease. The clinical syndrome of aortoiliac occlusion is called *Leriche syndrome*, classically presenting as pelvis and thigh claudication, impotence, and absent femoral pulses. In the collateral pathway, arterial blood bypasses the aorta, flowing from the subclavian through the **internal thoracic arteries**, **superficial epigastric arteries**, **inferior epigastric arteries**, and finally into the **external iliacs**.
- The **marginal artery of Drummond** is an arc-shaped anastomotic connection between the branches of the **superior mesenteric** and **inferior mesenteric arteries**. The marginal artery gives off straight branches called *vasa recta* that perfuse the colon, allowing for collateral flow in cases of occlusion or stenosis.
  - One aspect of this system is that it is typically weak or discontinuous around the splenic flexure, the junction of the SMA and IMA. As a result, this region of the colon is a watershed area particularly vulnerable to ischemia in cases of arterial occlusion.
- **The circle of Willis** is a vitally important site of collateral circulation in the brain, consisting of the anastomoses of the anterior cerebral arteries, anterior communicating artery, internal carotid arteries, posterior cerebral arteries, posterior communicating arteries, vertebral arteries, and basilar artery.
  - **Subclavian steal** is a phenomenon where the circle of Willis provides collateral flow to the upper extremity in the case of a proximally occluded subclavian artery. Flow from the contralateral carotid or vertebral artery travels through the circle and down the ipsilateral vertebral artery to the distal subclavian beyond the point of occlusion. In this rare clinical picture, a clinician may detect asynchronous radial pulses, because the radial pulse on the side with subclavian stenosis is delayed as it travels from the contralateral carotid artery.
- The **azygos system** provides an alternate route to the right atrium in the case of vena cava occlusion. Because of the valveless nature of the azygos system, flow is reversible. In the case of IVC obstruction, deoxygenated blood flows upward through the azygos vein and into the SVC, bypassing the blockage. In the case of SVC obstruction, the normal direction of flow is reversed through the azygos and into the IVC.

 CLINICAL POINT

Superior vena cava syndrome occurs when the azygos system fails to compensate for an obstruction of the SVC, commonly lung cancer. Symptoms include facial and upper extremity edema, dyspnea, coughing, and difficulty swallowing. In the acute setting, endovascular stenting of the SVC may mitigate symptoms, although the definitive treatment likely includes surgery.

PARASITIC ARTERIES

- A limiting factor in tumor growth is the acquisition of blood supply. This process is accomplished by angiogenesis and the creation of **parasitic arteries**—arteries that branch from an existing vascular bed but exist solely to nourish the tumor.
- For tumors growing in certain organs, there are often predictable patterns of vessel growth. For example, tumors of the liver tend to be supported by parasitic arteries from the hepatic artery rather than the portal vein; this knowledge allows for tumor embolization via selective catheterization of the hepatic artery.
  - However, these tumors may parasitize extrahepatic arteries (commonly the right inferior phrenic artery), so preoperative angiography is crucial for planning purposes.

VASCULAR MALFORMATIONS

- The description of vasculature presented in this chapter so far has been idealized—in a given patient, there could be many variations of typical branching patterns. In a more select population of patients, there are structural vasculature abnormalities that can be inconvenient and even painful.
- **Venous malformations** are essentially anomalous structures of veins, typically concentrated in a specific area. They can be distressing to patients for cosmetic reasons or may, because of their placement, cause discomfort and pain. Sclerotherapy is the treatment of choice for venous malformations.
- **Arteriovenous malformations** are anomalous connections of the arterial and venous circuit without an intervening capillary bed, causing shunting of oxygenated blood away from the arterial system and into the venous system. AVMs have a predilection for the head and neck and are frequently asymptomatic. However, pulmonary arteriovenous malformations may cause cyanosis and predispose to high-output heart failure and paradoxic pulmonary emboli (venous thromboemboli that bypass the pulmonary capillaries and move through the arterial circulation). Such AVMs can be treated with transcatheter coiling or embolic agents.

TAKE-HOME POINTS

- A **pseudoaneurysm** forms between the two outers layers of an artery, the tunica media and tunica adventitia.
- An **aneurysm** involves dilation of all three layers of the blood vessel.
- The typical aortic arch gives off the right brachiocephalic trunk, left common carotid artery, and left subclavian artery. However, many variants of this configuration exist.
- The **celiac trunk** takes off anteriorly from the abdominal aorta at about the level of the T12 vertebral body. It typically gives off three branches—the left gastric artery, common hepatic artery, and splenic artery—though variants exist.
- The **superior mesenteric artery** takes off anteriorly from the abdominal aorta at about the level of the L1 vertebral body. The **inferior mesenteric artery** takes off at the L3 level. The **marginal artery of Drummond** serves as an important anastomotic link between the two. The splenic flexure is a watershed area particularly vulnerable to ischemia in cases of arterial occlusion.
- The **radial artery** can be palpated at the distal end of the radius between the brachioradialis tendon and flexor carpi radialis muscle. The **femoral artery** can be palpated in the femoral crease, medial to the femoral nerve and lateral to the femoral artery. The **popliteal artery** can be palpated in a flexed popliteal fossa. The **posterior tibial artery** can be palpated posterior to the medial malleolus. The **dorsalis pedia artery** can be palpated lateral to the extensor hallucis longus tendon.

- An *accessory artery* exists in addition to the normal vasculature. An example is an accessory right hepatic artery that comes off the SMA, in addition to the RHA that branches from the common hepatic artery. Should there not be an RHA coming off the CHA, that is termed a *replaced artery*.
  - Variation in hepatic arterial anatomy is seen in 45% of the population.
  - The most common variants are:
    - A replaced right hepatic artery coming off the SMA (13%)
    - A replaced left hepatic artery coming off the left gastric artery (8%)
- Varices develop in cases of portal hypertension, when resistance to flow in the portal vein causes these anastomoses to swell.
  - Rupture of esophageal varices is one of the most common causes of acute GI bleeds.
- The clinical syndrome of aortoiliac occlusion is called **Leriche syndrome**. It presents as pelvis and thigh claudication, impotence, and absent femoral pulses.
- **May-Thurner syndrome** occurs when the right common iliac artery compresses the left common iliac vein as they cross. This can cause lower extremity pain, swelling, discomfort, and deep venous thrombosis in the iliofemoral vein. The DVT has the dangerous potential to embolize to the pulmonary circuit, causing a pulmonary embolism.

REVIEW QUESTIONS

1. An interventionalist is performing a transcatheter arterial chemoembolization (TACE) on a patient with colon cancer that has metastasized to the right lobe of the liver. Which would be a suitable order of access and navigation in the typical anatomy?
   a. Right femoral artery, right common iliac, abdominal aorta, superior mesenteric artery, right hepatic artery
   b. Right femoral artery, right external iliac, right common iliac, abdominal aorta, celiac axis, common hepatic artery, proper hepatic artery, right hepatic artery
   c. Right femoral artery, right external iliac, right internal iliac, abdominal aorta, celiac axis, common hepatic artery, proper hepatic artery, right hepatic artery
   d. Right internal jugular vein, superior vena cava, right atrium, inferior vena cava, common hepatic vein, right hepatic vein

2. In the previously noted patient, which would be the most likely artery providing parasitic blood supply to the right lobe mass?
   a. Right inferior phrenic artery
   b. Cystic artery
   c. Omental artery
   d. Intercostal artery

3. Which method is relatively contraindicated for bronchial artery embolization in cases of hemoptysis?
   a. Coiling
   b. Gelatin sponge
   c. Microspheres
   d. PVA

SUGGESTED READINGS

Ignacio EA, Silva NN, Khati NJ, et al., Vascular anatomy of the pelvis. In: Mauro MA, Murphy KPJ, Thomson KR, et al., eds. *Image-Guided Interventions*. 2nd ed. Philadelphia: Elsevier; 2014:526–541.

Jones A, Pearl MS. Vascular anatomy of the upper extremity. In: Mauro MA, Murphy KPJ, Thomson KR, et al., eds. *Image-Guided Interventions*. 2nd ed. Philadelphia: Elsevier; 2014:143–157.

Ruiz DS, Barnett BP, Gailloud P. Craniocervical vascular anatomy. In: Mauro MA, Murphy KPJ, Thomson KR, et al., eds. *Image-Guided Interventions*. 2nd ed. Philadelphia: Elsevier; 2014:627–647.

Soon KH, Heng RC, Bell KW, et al., Vascular anatomy of the thorax, including the heart. In: Mauro MA, Murphy KPJ, Thomson KR, et al., eds. *Image-Guided Interventions*. 2nd ed. Philadelphia: Elsevier; 2014:575–587.

Neurointerventional Radiology

Zachary Zhang, Kimberly Seifert, Daniel C. Murphy,
Justin Shafa, Jeffrey Carpenter

- Neurointerventional radiologists commonly treat strokes, arteriovenous malformations, brain tumors, and cerebral aneurysms.
- Procedures in this realm are performed by a variety of specialized physicians including radiologists, neurosurgeons, neurologists, and vascular surgeons.
- Trainees specialized must complete additional training in endovascular surgical neuroradiology.

CEREBRAL ANGIOGRAPHY

- **Cerebral angiography** is the **gold standard** in evaluating head and neck vasculature and remains essential in both pretherapeutic planning and treatment follow-up.
- For many indications, noninvasive imaging has replaced traditional catheter angiography.
- **Indications** for **extracranial** craniocervical angiography:
  - Vertebrobasilar insufficiency from subclavian steal
  - Cervical carotid stenosis
  - Neck trauma
  - Cavernous-carotid and dural fistulae
  - Epistaxis
  - Tumor invasion of the carotid artery and tumor embolization
- **Indications** for **intracranial** craniocervical angiography:
  - Spontaneous (nontraumatic) subarachnoid hemorrhage
  - Cerebral aneurysms
  - Arteriovenous malformations and dural fistulae
  - Vasospasm
  - Acute stroke
  - Tumor embolization

PREPROCEDURAL EVALUATION

- **Imaging**
  - Nonenhanced CT, CT angiography, MRI, and MR angiography are complementary modalities used in operative planning.
- **Laboratory data**
  - Standard platelet count, PT, INR, and aPTT to evaluate for a bleeding diathesis. BUN and Cr to evaluate renal function.

- **Physical examination**
  - Focused neurologic examination and documentation of any preprocedural deficits
- **Informed consent** prior to cerebral angiogram should include discussion regarding potential neurologic complications:
  - Cerebral ischemic events secondary to thromboemboli and air emboli (more common) or disruption of atherosclerotic plaque and vessel wall injury (less common)
  - Neurologic deficits occurring within 24 hours of angiography are, by definition, attributable to angiography and are defined by duration and severity:
    - Deficits lasting less than 24 hours are defined as a *transient ischemic attack.*
    - Deficits lasting more than 24 hours are called a *stroke.*
    - Stroke severity should be made by using the National Institutes of Health Stroke Scale.
    - Modified Rankin disability score used to assess the ultimate outcome of procedure-related neurologic complications.
  - Overall rate of neurologic complications is in the range of ~1%.
    - Transient/reversible complications occur at about twice the rate of permanent complications.
- Nonneurologic complications should also be discussed.
  - Complication risk increases with the number of underlying comorbidities; atherosclerotic carotid disease, recent cerebral ischemic event, advanced age, hypertension, diabetes, and renal insufficiency are the most significant.
- See Box 5.1 for risk of complications.

BOX 5.1 Risk of Complications

1. TIA (0.3%–0.4%)
2. Stroke (<0.01%)
3. Cervical dissection (0.3%–0.4%)
4. Groin hematoma (2%–5%)
5. Pseudoaneurysm (0.4%–0.9%)
6. Limb ischemia (0.2%–0.4%)

Basics

- Conventional four-vessel angiogram is considered the **gold standard** for neurovascular lesion detection and characterization.
  - Biplane angiography is typical, as it conserves procedural time and decreases the number of contrast injections by half.
- Access: Femoral approach is typical.
- Catheter selection (Fig. 5.1): Varies, though typically a 4 Fr or 5 Fr is advanced over hydrophilic wires.
- Heparinized saline: Double flush technique at and above the level of the arch

Technique

- A complete vascular evaluation is required in most cases.
  - Bilateral internal and external carotid arteries, with a thorough evaluation of the anterior communicating artery complex
  - Bilateral vertebral arteries including the bilateral posterior inferior cerebellar arteries

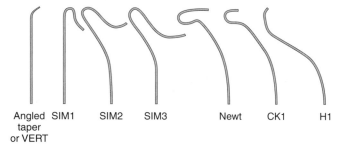

Fig. 5.1 Catheter Selection (Reused from Harrigan MR, Devieikis JP. *Handbook of Cerebrovascular Disease and Neurointerventional Technique.* 2nd ed. New York: Humana Press; 2013.)

- Can be performed via a single dominant vertebral artery in some cases
- Though uncommon, a vertebral artery may not be safely selected.
  - Can perform selective injection of the subclavian artery, aided by inflating a blood pressure cuff to an occlusive pressure on the ipsilateral arm to promote contrast flow into the vertebral artery
- Evaluation of the cervical aortic arch
  - Left anterior oblique position to profile the great vessel origins
  - Injection rate of 20 mL/s for a total of 40 mL at a frame rate of 3 f/s
- Extracranial carotid arteriography
  - Anteroposterior (AP), lateral, and 45-degree bilateral oblique projections are standard.
  - Injection rate of 4 to 5 mL/s for a total of 7 to 9 mL at a frame rate of 3 f/s
  - Radio-opaque calibration markers are useful for cases requiring precise measurements.
- Anterior intracranial angiography (Fig. 5.2)
  - AP (Townes view) and lateral projections are standard.
    - Consider oblique projections to profile overlapping arteries.
      - Submental-vertex view for optimal ACA evaluation
      - Stenvers view for optimal MCA evaluation
  - Injection rate of 4 to 5 mL/s for a total of 20 to 25 mL at 3 f/s
    - Higher frame rate acquisitions are advantageous to evaluate dural AVFs and high flow shunts in AVMs.
- Posterior intracranial (vertebrobasilar artery) angiography (Fig. 5.3)
  - AP (Townes view) and lateral projections, centered caudally and dorsally to cover the PCA distribution
  - Injection rate of 5 to 7 mL/s for 8 to 10 mL at 2 f/s

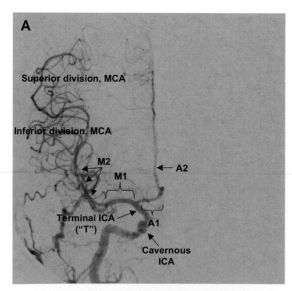

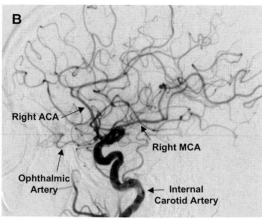

Fig. 5.2 Cerebral angiogram of right internal carotid artery demonstrating segments of the right middle cerebral artery *(MCA)* and right anterior cerebral artery *(ACA).* (A) Anterior projection; (B) lateral projection. *A1 & A2,* Segments of the ACA; *ICA,* internal carotid artery; *M1 & M2,* segments of the MCA. (Reused with permission from Krishnaswamy A, Klein JP, Kapadia SR. Clinical cerebrovascular anatomy. *Catheter Cardiovasc Interv.* 2010;75 (4):530–539, Fig. 5. doi:10.1002/ccd.22299.)

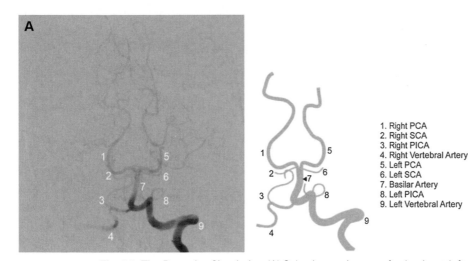
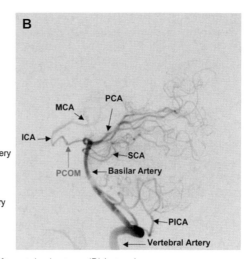

1. Right PCA
2. Right SCA
3. Right PICA
4. Right Vertebral Artery
5. Left PCA
6. Left SCA
7. Basilar Artery
8. Left PICA
9. Left Vertebral Artery

Fig. 5.3 The Posterior Circulation (A) Selective angiogram of a dominant left vertebral artery. (B) Lateral projection of a vertebral artery injection with filling of the anterior circulation via the posterior communicating artery *(PCOM). AICA,* Anterior inferior cerebellar artery; *ICA,* internal carotid artery; *MCA,* middle cerebral artery; *PCA,* posterior cerebral artery; *PICA,* posterior inferior cerebellar artery; *SCA,* superior cerebellar artery. (Reused with permission from Krishnaswamy A, Klein JP, Kapadia SR. Clinical cerebrovascular anatomy. *Catheter Cardiovasc Interv.* 2010;75(4):530–539, Fig. 6. doi:10.1002/ccd.22299.)

- Three-dimensional (3D) rotational angiography reconstruction modeling
  - Higher spatial resolution in comparison to multislice CT scanners
  - Demonstrates collateral circulation and flow dynamics within the corresponding vascular territories
  - Leads to more sensitive/specific aneurysm evaluation, providing invaluable anatomic and geometric information such as aneurysm size, geometry, and neck-to-dome ratio

Pitfalls

- Evaluation and detection of saccular aneurysms are dependent on optimal projections.
- Failure to evaluate the ECA circulation may result in failure to demonstrate a dural AVF as the cause of SAH.
- Digital subtraction angiography is falsely negative in 15% of aneurysmal subarachnoid hemorrhages; one should consider repeating DSA in 5 to 7 days if clinically correlated.
- Nonaneurysmal perimesencephalic subarachnoid hemorrhages are thought to be of venous origin.
  - Up to 95% of these will have a normal cerebral angiogram and fail to identify the source of bleeding.

INTRAARTERIAL THROMBOLYSIS FOR ACUTE ISCHEMIC STROKE

CASE PRESENTATION

A 64-year-old male with a history of hypertension, diabetes mellitus, and smoking presents to the emergency department with aphasia, right facial droop, and right hemiparesis. He was last seen at baseline by his daughter 4 hours prior. NIH stroke

Continued

CASE PRESENTATION—cont'd

scale score was calculated to be 17. Head CT was performed, which demonstrated no acute intracranial hemorrhage with subtle loss of gray-white matter differentiation in the left frontal and parietal lobes. CT angiogram of the head and neck demonstrated occlusion of the M1 segment of the left middle cerebral artery.

- **A Stroke** is classically characterized as a neurologic deficit attributed to an acute focal injury of the central nervous system by a vascular cause, such as cerebral infarction, intracerebral hemorrhage, or subarachnoid hemorrhage. It is a major contributor to disability and death worldwide.
- **Transient ischemic attack (TIA)** is a short (less than 1 hour) episode of neurologic dysfunction resulting from temporary cerebral ischemia not associated with infarction per neuroimaging. Patients who suffer a TIA have a 10% chance of stroke within the subsequent 90 days.

⟫ CLINICAL POINT

The typical patient loses 1.9 million neurons each minute in which a stroke is untreated.

- Intraarterial cerebral fibrinolytic therapy for acute ischemic stroke was first described by Zeumer et al. in 1983.
- In 1999, the Prolyse in Acute Cerebral Thromboembolism (PROACT) II trial was published and prompted many stroke centers to begin performing endovascular stroke therapy.
- In 2013, controversy over the outcomes of endovascular therapy were heightened after the IMS III, MR RESCUE,

and SYNTHESIS clinical trials suggested that endovascular therapy was no more effective than intravenous t-PA alone.

- In 2015, multiple randomized controlled trials demonstrated superior outcomes of endovascular therapy compared with IV-tPA alone for patients with internal carotid or proximal middle cerebral artery occlusions up to 6 hours after onset.
- Various imaging modalities are being investigated for their potential to select patients who would benefit from endovascular therapy by evaluating the size of the infarction zone and penumbra. This includes noncontrast CT (ASPECTS score), multiphase CT angiogram (collateral vessel scoring), CT perfusion, and MR perfusion imaging.
  - MRI with diffusion-weighted imaging remains the gold standard for determining infarction size.

◎ KEY DEFINITION

Penumbra is brain tissue that is ischemic but not yet infarcted and is therefore at risk for further damage unless flow is rapidly restored.

Indications

- Updated 2015 guidelines from the American Heart Association/American Stroke Association state that endovascular therapy is recommended in patients who meet all of the following criteria (Class I; Level of Evidence A):
  - Prestroke mRS score of 0 to 1
  - Acute ischemic stroke who receive intravenous recombinant-tPA within 4.5 hours of onset
  - Causative occlusion of the internal carotid artery or proximal MCA (M1)
  - Age ≥ 18 years
  - NIHSS score of ≥6
  - ASPECTS of ≥6

- Treatment that can be initiated (groin puncture) within 6 hours of symptom onset
- Additional indications that may be considered:
  - Patients with contraindications to IV-tPA presenting within 6 hours of symptom onset
  - Patients with occlusion of the anterior cerebral artery, M2 or M3 segments of the middle cerebral artery, vertebral, basilar, or posterior cerebral arteries

Contraindications

- There are currently no standard contraindications for endovascular treatment, as risks and benefits of therapy must be evaluated on a case-by-case basis. However, some risk factors to consider include
  - Rapidly improving NIH stroke scale ≤4
  - INR > 3.0
  - Thrombocytopenia <50,000 platelets
  - Blood glucose <50 mg/dL or >400 mg/dL despite treatment
  - Systolic blood pressure >185 mm Hg or diastolic blood pressure >110 mm Hg despite treatment
  - Intracranial hemorrhage or mass

Equipment

- *Mechanical Embolus Removal in Cerebral Ischemia (MERCI) retriever* (Fig. 5.4A)—the first FDA-approved device to remove acute clots in patients presenting with ischemic stroke
- *5MAX DDC*—applies direct aspiration at the site of occlusion to optimize thrombus removal
- *Solitaire FR Revascularization Device* (Fig. 5.4B)—mechanical thrombectomy device
- *Trevo XP ProVue Retriever* (Fig. 5.4C)—mechanical thrombectomy device with improved accuracy and speed in removing thrombus

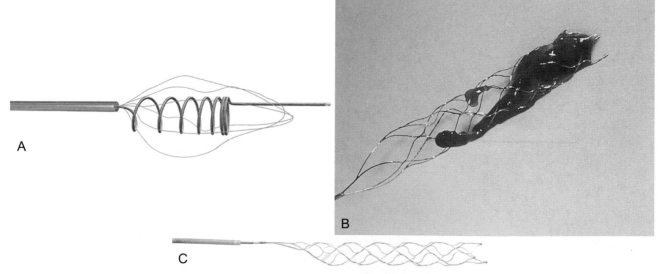

Fig. 5.4 (A) MERCI retriever—mechanical embolus removal in cerebral ischemia. (B) Solitaire FR with clot. (C) Trevo XP ProVue Retriever. (A, Courtesy of Stryker Corporation. B, From Dávalos A, Pereira VM, Chapot R, et al. Retrospective multicenter study of Solitaire FR for revascularization in the treatment of acute ischemic stroke. *Stroke.* 2012;43:2699–2705. C, Courtesy Stryker Neurovascular, Fremont, CA.)

BOX 5.2 mTICI Grades

- **Grade 0:** No perfusion
- **Grade 1:** Antegrade reperfusion past the initial occlusion but limited distal branch filling with little or slow distal reperfusion
- **Grade 2A:** Antegrade reperfusion of less than half of the occluded target artery previously ischemic territory (e.g., in one major division of the MCA* and its territory)
- **Grade 2B:** Antegrade reperfusion of more than half of the previously occluded target artery ischemic territory (e.g., in two major divisions of the MCA* and its territories)
- **Grade 3:** Complete antegrade reperfusion of the previously occluded target artery ischemic territory, with absence of visualized occlusion in all distal branches

* indicates middle cerebral artery, and mTICI is modified treatment in cerebral ischemia scale.

Anatomy

- Review of patient anatomy with either a CT angiogram of the head and neck or cerebral angiogram is essential prior to revascularization treatment.
- 90% of the population has a dominant left hemisphere.
- Posterior circulation supplies the brainstem, cerebellum, and occipital cortex. Symptoms of posterior occlusion frequently involve the 5 Ds (dizziness, diplopia, dysarthria, dysphagia, and dystaxia).
- The hallmark of a posterior circulation stroke is crossed findings, with cranial findings on the ipsilateral side of the occlusion and motor/sensory findings on the contralateral side. The exact symptoms depend on the precise level of the infarct.

Procedural Steps

Stent Retriever System

1. Right common femoral artery access is favored.
2. A large 8- to 9-Fr sheath with a 6- to 7-Fr balloon guiding catheter is used.
3. Infusion of a mixture of heparin and normal saline through the guiding catheter is useful in preventing occurrence of a new thromboembolic event during the procedure.
4. The balloon guiding catheter is ideally placed in the ICA and is used to reverse flow at the time of clot retrieval. Using angiography, the thrombolysis in cerebral infarction (TICI) score of the occluded vessel is determined (<3 is abnormal) (Box 5.2).
5. After placement of the guiding catheter is confirmed, a microwire and microcatheter are used to traverse the clot using roadmapping. The balloon guiding catheter is inflated to stop blood flow within the artery.
6. Microwire is removed and replaced with the stent retriever (e.g., Solitaire or Trevo). The stent retriever is deployed within the clot by withdrawing the microcatheter over the stent retriever.
7. The stent is left in place for at least 3 minutes, which allows the stent to better grasp the clot upon retrieval. Stent deployment allows for partial antegrade blood flow to the ischemic tissue.

8. Once the stent is adequately positioned, the entire system (stent and microcatheter) is withdrawn under negative suction using a 50-mL syringe, applied at the level of the guiding catheter to prevent emboli.
9. This procedure should be repeated 2 to 3 times until a TICI score of ≥ 2b is achieved in the previously occluded vessel.
10. Manual compression or closure device is used for the groin puncture.

Penumbra Aspiration System

1. A large guide sheath is delivered as far distally as possible, usually in the cervical internal carotid artery. A balloon guide catheter may be used if stent retriever use is anticipated.
2. A diagnostic angiogram is performed.
3. The aspiration catheter is selected for vessel size and delivered over a medium catheter and microwire to the clot face.
4. The inner catheter and guidewire are removed, and suction is activated. The canister and tubing should be monitored carefully for cessation of flow or clot removal. If flow ceases for greater than 2 minutes, the aspiration catheter is carefully withdrawn, as the clot may be engaged at the tip of the catheter.
5. Several passes can be made with the aspiration catheter, or other devices such as a stent retriever may be used.
   Post procedure Care.

- Close monitoring in a neuro-ICU is warranted.
- Appropriate blood pressure control for patients that have been successfully recanalized. Permissive hypertension can be considered if residual occlusion persists.
- Close interval imaging follow-up to evaluate for hemorrhagic conversion of the infarct is needed.

▶▶ CLINICAL POINT

Permissive hypertension: Patients with acute stroke may be allowed to maintain blood pressure up to 200 mm Hg to allow collateral flow to ischemic tissue.

Complications

- Distal thrombus embolization or embolization to new vascular territories
- Intracranial hemorrhage
- Air embolism
- Arterial dissection
- Vasospasm

Alternate Treatments

- Intravenous tPA is an FDA-approved treatment for ischemic stroke if administered within 3 hours (up to 4.5 hours in certain patients) of symptom onset. However, many patients present outside of this time frame or have contraindications to systemic thrombolysis.
- Intraarterial tPA is rarely used but may be considered in cases where mechanical thrombolysis device delivery is limited by patient anatomy.

PERCUTANEOUS VERTEBROPLASTY AND KYPHOPLASTY

CASE PRESENTATION

A 75-year-old female with a history of osteoporosis presented to her primary care physician with intense back pain after a ground-level fall. The patient was examined and found to have no focal neurologic deficits or cord compression symptoms. Her primary care physician tried to manage her pain with NSAIDs and physical therapy; however, the patient did not have any improvement. X-rays were obtained that showed an acute L2 compression fracture. The patient was referred to interventional radiology for possible percutaneous vertebroplasty or kyphoplasty.

- **Percutaneous vertebroplasty** (PVP) and **kyphoplasty** (KP) are similar procedures used to treat symptomatic vertebral compression fractures (VCF) and vertebral angiomas.
  - PVP is a minimally invasive procedure that involves the injection of cement into a fractured vertebra to help stabilize the vertebra and potentially relieve pain.
  - KP also involves injecting cement into the vertebra. First, however, a balloon is inserted into the vertebra and inflated to restore the height of the vertebra and create a cavity for the cement to fill. KP is also called "balloon-assisted vertebroplasty."
- PVP was first done in 1984 in France by Dr. Herve Deramond and was described by Drs. Galibert, Deramond, and Rosat in 1987. This initial procedure was performed for a vertebral angioma.
- The PVP technique was brought to the United States in 1993 and first reported in 1997.
- KP was conceived by orthopedic surgeon Dr. Mark Reiley in the early 1990s; the initial concept was to restore vertebral body height to reduce the kyphotic deformities associated with VCF.

Indications

- Spontaneous VCF due to osteoporosis is the most common indication. VCF secondary to trauma is also seen.
- Palliative pain relief in patient with VCF caused by spinal metastases.
- Pain from VCF refractory to medical therapy
  - Failure of medical therapy includes patients becoming nonambulatory due to pain, intolerance to physical therapy due to pain, and/or side effects (sedation, confusion, GI bleeding, and constipation) from high doses of analgesics
- In some instances, focal symptomatic vertebral hemangiomas can be treated.
- Patients with symptomatic microfractures as seen on imaging, despite the absence of vertebral body compression.

CLINICAL POINT

Clinical studies are ongoing regarding the prophylactic use of PVP and KP in osteoporotic patients. These studies are evaluating whether there is a decrease in the occurrence of future compression fractures when cement is injected in vertebra adjacent to the compression fraction being treated.

Contraindications

- Absolute contraindications:
  - Septicemia
  - Active osteomyelitis at site of planned procedure
  - Allergy to cement agent
  - Uncorrectable coagulopathy
- Relative contraindications:
  - Radiculopathy not caused by the compression fracture
  - Retropulsion of a fracture fragment causing compromise of the spinal cord
  - Epidural tumor with compromise of the spinal cord
  - Active systemic infection
  - Symptomatic improvement with conservative therapies
  - Myelopathy at the fracture level

Equipment

- Most commonly done under fluoroscopy, though CT-guided PVP/KP is possible
  - Rapid access to CT and MRI is required to evaluate complications if they arise.
- Key equipment
  - Trocar needle (Fig. 5.5A)
  - A delivery device (see Fig. 5.5B) that injects orthopedic cement through the trocar

Anatomy

- Proper positioning of the trocar needle in the vertebral body is shown in Fig. 5.6. The trocar is placed at an angle to avoid injury to the spinal cord.

Procedural Steps

1. The skin overlying the fracture vertebra is cleaned and sterilely prepped. Local anesthetic is injected at the site.
2. A small incision is made in the skin that overlies the fractured vertebra.
3. The trocar is guided under either fluoroscopy or CT into the correct portion of the vertebra. It is vital to angle the trocar so that the spinal cord is not damaged.
   a. The trocar may need extra work to enter the vertebra. A twisting motion can be helpful, but sometimes this requires using a mallet to advance the trocar.
4. If kyphoplasty is being performed:
   a. A drill is placed through the trocar and used to create a channel for the balloon.
   b. The balloon is inserted through the trocar and inflated in the vertebra (Fig. 5.7).
   c. The balloon is removed.

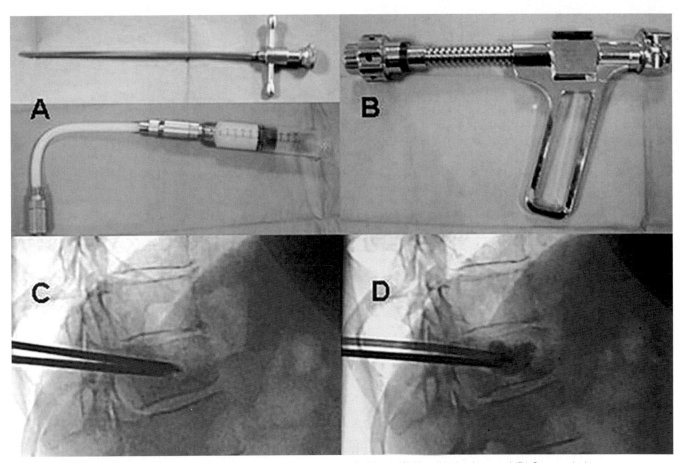

Fig. 5.5 (A) Needle, detachable syringe, and connection. (B) Pistol. (C) Needles in place and (D) Cement being injected during vertebroplasty. (Reused with permission from Santiago FR, Abela AP, Alvarez LG, et al. Pain and functional outcome after vertebroplasty and kyphoplasty. A comparative study. *Eur J Radiol.* 2010;75(2):e108–e113.)

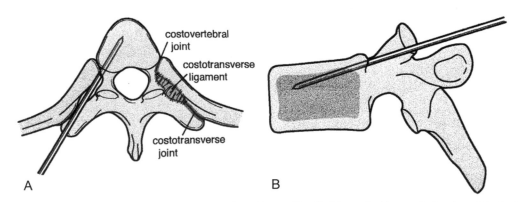

Fig. 5.6 Vertebra Anatomy With Placement of the Trocar Needle (Reused with permission from Mathis J, Wong W. Percutaneous vertebroplasty: technical considerations. *J Vasc Interv Radiol.* 2003;14(8):953–960.)

5. Cement is injected into the vertebra through the trocar. Imaging is used to ensure that the cement is entering the correct position.
6. After cement has been injected, final images are obtained and the trocar is removed.
7. Pressure is applied if there is any bleeding. A sterile dressing is applied.

Alternate Treatments

• Conservative pain management, including bed rest, pain medication, physical therapy, and back support

• Invasive surgical procedures by orthopedic surgeons or neurosurgeons can be performed to stabilize the fractured vertebra.

Complications

• In patients whose condition is secondary to osteoporosis, major complications occur in less than 1%.
• In patients with neoplastic disease, the complication rate increases to 5%.
• Table 5.1 details specific complications in vertebral augmentation.

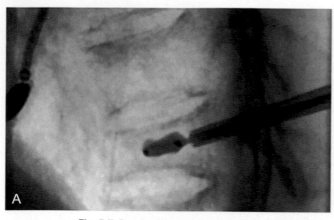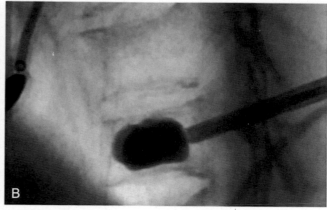

Fig. 5.7 Precise Placement of the Balloon Bone Tamp Facilitates Fracture Reduction (From Tong SC, Eskey CJ, Pomerantz SR, Hirsch JA. "SKyphoplasty": a single institution's initial experience. *J Vasc Interv Radiol.* 2006;17(6):1025–1030.)

TABLE 5.1   Specific Complications for Vertebral Augmentation

Specific Complication	Published Rates
Transient neurologic deficit (within 30 days of procedure)	
Osteoporosis	1%
Neoplasm	10%
Permanent neurologic deficit (within 30 days of the procedure or deficits requiring surgery)	
Osteoporosis	<1%
Neoplasm	2%
Fracture of rib, sternum, or vertebra	1%
Allergic or idiosyncratic reaction	<1%
Infection	<1%
Symptomatic pulmonary material embolus	<1%
Significant hemorrhage or vascular injury	<1%
Symptomatic hemothorax or pneumothorax	<1%
Death	<1%

CAROTID ARTERY STENTING

CASE PRESENTATION

A 69-year-old man presents to the Emergency Department having suffered his second TIA in 2 weeks. After the first, which caused transient left leg weakness, his primary care physician prescribed aspirin and Plavix. The second TIA caused right hemiparesis and prompted urgent presentation to the local ED. Duplex ultrasound of his bilateral carotid arteries shows 85% narrowing of the right internal carotid artery and near total occlusion of the left internal carotid artery. A discussion is held as to whether the patient should undergo endovascular carotid artery stenting or open carotid endarterectomy.

- Just as any other blood vessel, the carotid arteries can develop atherosclerosis over time, decreasing blood flow to the brain and potentially leading to a stroke.
- In 1995, carotid artery stenting (CAS) was first introduced as an investigational treatment for carotid artery disease.

- In 2004, the FDA approved CAS as a treatment option for patients who have carotid artery stenosis and meet the following criteria:
  - Experiencing symptoms from the stenosis
  - Have greater than 70% blockage
  - Where open surgical intervention poses a major risk
- Many major studies have compared CAS and carotid endarterectomy (CEA), including the Stent-Protected Angioplasty Versus Carotid Endarterectomy (SPACE) trial and the Carotid Revascularization Endarterectomy Versus Stent (CREST) trial.
- Multiple imaging studies are used to assess the patency of the carotid arteries:
  - Carotid artery duplex is typically the cheapest, quickest, and least invasive method
  - CT angiogram (Fig. 5.8)
  - MR angiogram (Fig. 5.9)
  - Carotid angiogram (Fig. 5.10) is the **gold standard** but the most invasive

Indications

- Asymptomatic high-grade (>60%) internal carotid artery stenosis
- Symptomatic internal carotid artery stenosis
  - Defined as the acute onset of neurologic symptoms, TIAs, and/or stroke on the side of atherosclerosis

Contraindications

- Absolute
  - Active infection
  - Thrombus within the internal carotid artery visible on ultrasound
- Relative
  - Circumferential plaque buildup
  - Near complete occlusion of the carotid artery, shown by the so-called string sign (Fig. 5.11)
  - Severe calcification of existing plaque
  - Severe carotid artery tortuosity
  - Calcified aortic arch

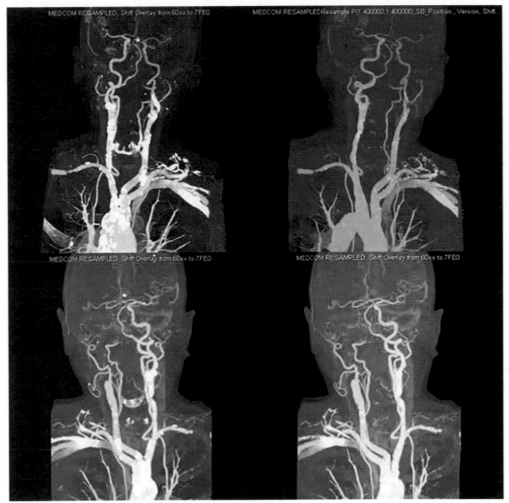

Fig. 5.8 Three-Dimensional Reconstructed CT Angiogram Note lack of flow through the right carotid artery compared to the left. (Reused with permission from Barone DG, Jones R, Trivedi R. Surgical and non-surgical management of carotid atherosclerosis. *Neurosurgery.* 2013;13[1]. Available at http://www.acnr.co.uk/2013/03/surgical-and-non-surgical-management-of-carotid-atherosclerosis/.)

- Inability to deploy an embolic protection device
- Patients 80 years of age and older

Equipment

- There are two types of carotid stents:
    - Open-cell stents: greater flexibility and used for highly angulated lesions
    - Closed-cell stents: characterized by smaller free cell areas between the struts
- Drug-eluting stents are not commonly used in CAS given low restenosis rates.
- The embolic protection device (EPD) (Fig. 5.12) is a device that is temporarily installed in the carotid artery beyond the area of blockage. It is designed to catch any dislodged particles, preventing them from traveling into the brain and thereby reducing the risk of embolic strokes during carotid artery stenting.
    - There are two types of EPDs:
        - Filter devices (more common) allow continued antegrade flow during CAS.
        - Retrograde flow devices reverse flow of blood and particulates away from the ICA.

- Issues with EPD deployment include that they:
    - Must pass across the stenosis, possibly dislodging emboli in the process
    - May cause vasospasm, leading to stroke if for a prolonged duration
    - May cause vessel wall injury or be difficult to remove

Anatomy

See Fig. 5.13.
- The right common carotid branches off the right brachiocephalic trunk (along with the right subclavian artery). The left common carotid typically originates off the aortic arch.
    - Variations do exist, such as a bovine aortic arch (Fig. 5.14), where the left common carotid artery branches off the brachiocephalic.
- The common carotid arteries divide into the internal and external carotid arteries (Box 5.3) at the level of the C3/C4 vertebrae, corresponding to the superior border of the thyroid cartilage.
- The carotid bifurcation, often with extension into the proximal internal carotid artery, is most commonly affected by atherosclerosis.

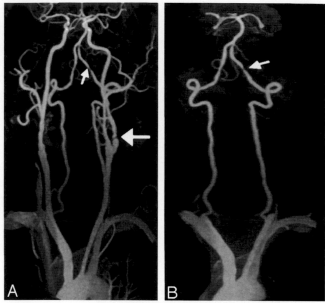

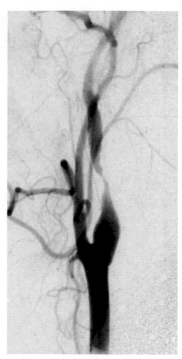

Fig. 5.9 (A and B) MRA showing stenosis of the left ICA *(large arrow)* as well as the left vertebral artery *(small arrow)*. (Reused with permission from Yang CW, Carr JC, Futterer SF, et al. Contrast-enhanced MR angiography of the carotid and vertebrobasilar circulations. *AJNR Am J Neuroradiol.* 2005;26[8]:2095–2101, Fig. 1.)

Fig. 5.10 Lateral right common carotid artery angiogram shows a severe stenosis approximately 2 cm above the carotid bifurcation. (Reused with permission from Stetler W, Gemmete JJ, Pandey AS, et al. Endovascular treatment of carotid occlusive disease. *Neuroimaging Clin N Am.* 2013;23/4:637–652, Fig. 2.)

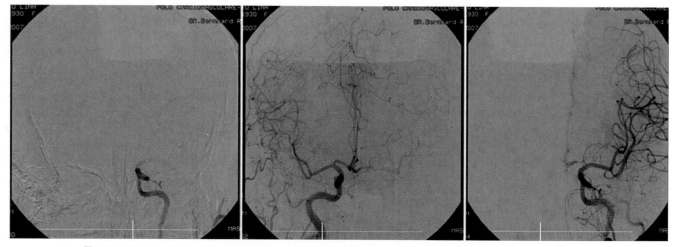

Fig. 5.11 Intracerebral angiography before and after carotid stenting in a patient with string sign. (Reused with permission from Nikas DN, Ghany MA, Stabile E, et al. Carotid artery stenting with proximal cerebral protection for patients with angiographic appearance of string sign. *JACC: Cardiovasc Interv.* 2010;3[3]:298–304, Fig. 3.)

Procedure Steps
Preoperative Management
- Antibiotic prophylaxis: cefazolin 2 to 3 g IV
- Anticoagulation: dual antiplatelet therapy with aspirin and Plavix pre- and postoperatively is recommended
1. A femoral, upper extremity, or transcervical approach can be taken. The area is prepped, lidocaine is injected, and the chosen artery is accessed.
   a. If the right femoral artery is accessed, arch aortogram will be required to identify the arch's anatomy, possible variants, and degree of calcification.

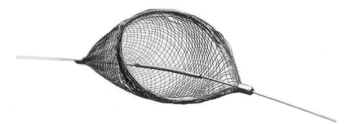

Fig. 5.12 SpiderFX EPD Filter (© 2018 Medtronic. All rights reserved. Used with the permission of Medtronic.)

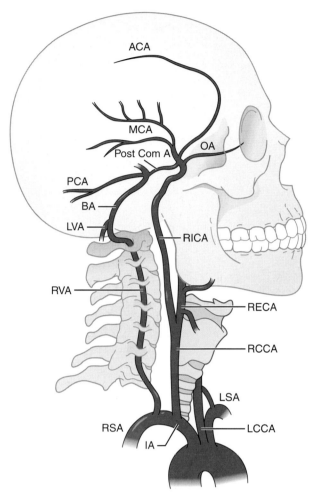

Fig. 5.13 Anatomy of the extracranial cerebral-bound arteries and their main intracranial supplies, lateral view from the right. *ACA*, Anterior cerebral artery; *BA*, basilar artery; *IA*, innominate artery; *LCCA*, left common carotid artery; *LSA*, left subclavian artery; *LVA*, left vertebral artery; *MCA*, middle cerebral artery; *OA*, ophthalmic artery; *PCA*, posterior cerebral artery; *Post Com A*, posterior communicating artery; *RCCA*, right common carotid artery; *RECA*, right external carotid artery; *RICA*, right internal carotid artery; *RSA*, right subclavian artery; *RVA*, right vertebral artery. The anterior choroidal artery is not depicted. (Reused with permission from Gautier JC, Mohr JP. Ischemic stroke. In: Mohr JP, Gautier JC, eds. *Guide to Clinical Neurology*. New York: Churchill Livingstone; 1995:543.)

> ### ⟫ CLINICAL POINT
>
> Some patients may have a temporary pacemaker wire inserted through a venous sheath to regulate heart rhythm during the procedure if the femoral approach is selected.

2. A short sheath is then inserted over the wire.
3. A catheter is inserted through the sheath and is guided through the aorta under fluoroscopy up to the carotid artery.
4. Cerebral angiography is performed.

> ### ⟫ CLINICAL POINT
>
> Before any wire is inserted into the carotid artery, the patient should be anticoagulated with heparin to maintain an activated clotting time (ACT) between 4 and 5 minutes.

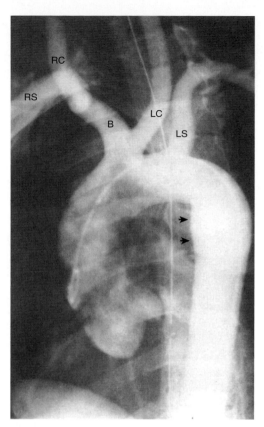

Fig. 5.14 Common origin of left common carotid and brachiocephalic arteries (i.e., bovine arch). Left anterior oblique arch aortogram of a bovine arch. *B*, Brachiocephalic artery; *LC*, left carotid; *LS*, left subclavian artery; *RC*, right carotid; *RS*, right subclavian artery. (Reused with permission from Kadir S. *Atlas of Normal and Variant Angiographic Anatomy*. Philadelphia: WB Saunders; 1991.)

> ### BOX 5.3   Mnemonic: Branches of the External Carotid Artery
>
> "**S**ome **A**natomists **L**ike **F**reaking **O**ut **P**oor **M**edical **S**tudents" (**s**uperior thyroid, **a**scending pharyngeal, **l**ingual, **f**acial, **o**ccipital, **p**osterior auricular, **m**axillary, and **s**uperficial temporal arteries)

5. A guidewire with the embolic protection device is inserted beyond the site of narrowing to reduce the risk of embolic events. EPD is deployed when in proper position.
6. An angioplasty balloon is guided to the site of blockage and the stenotic region is predilated.

> ### ⟫ CLINICAL POINT
>
> Balloon inflation at this stage can potentially lead to excessive stimulation of the adjacent carotid baroreceptor, resulting in bradycardia and hypotension.

7. The carotid stent (Fig. 5.15) is then positioned and deployed.
8. Poststenting angioplasty is performed to ensure deployment and apposition of the stent against the arterial wall. If needed, repeat angioplasty can be done to further expand the stent.

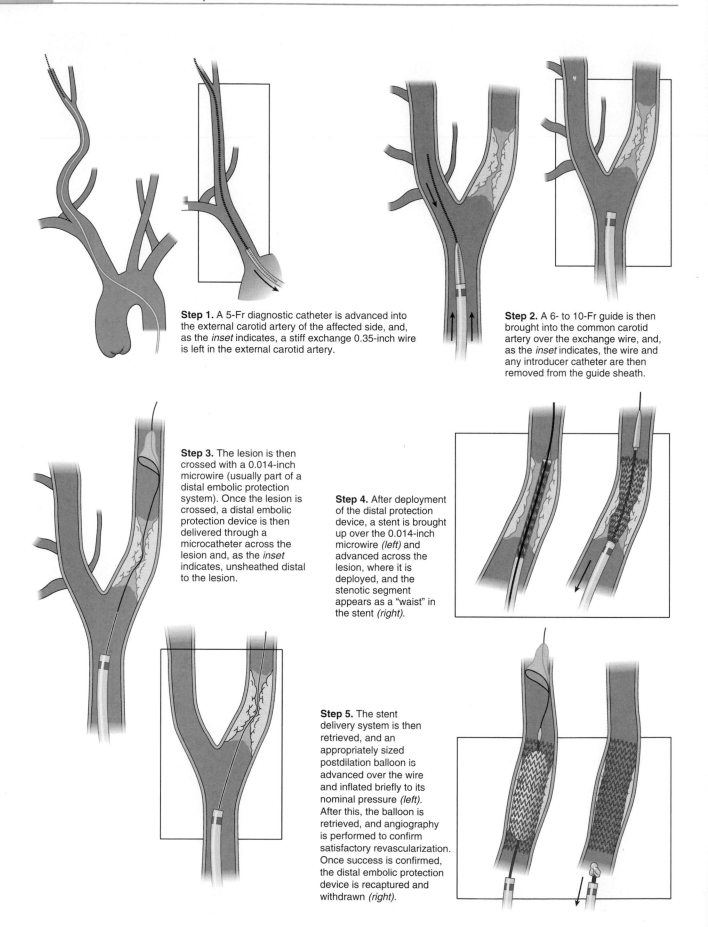

Step 1. A 5-Fr diagnostic catheter is advanced into the external carotid artery of the affected side, and, as the *inset* indicates, a stiff exchange 0.35-inch wire is left in the external carotid artery.

Step 2. A 6- to 10-Fr guide is then brought into the common carotid artery over the exchange wire, and, as the *inset* indicates, the wire and any introducer catheter are then removed from the guide sheath.

Step 3. The lesion is then crossed with a 0.014-inch microwire (usually part of a distal embolic protection system). Once the lesion is crossed, a distal embolic protection device is then delivered through a microcatheter across the lesion and, as the *inset* indicates, unsheathed distal to the lesion.

Step 4. After deployment of the distal protection device, a stent is brought up over the 0.014-inch microwire *(left)* and advanced across the lesion, where it is deployed, and the stenotic segment appears as a "waist" in the stent *(right)*.

Step 5. The stent delivery system is then retrieved, and an appropriately sized postdilation balloon is advanced over the wire and inflated briefly to its nominal pressure *(left)*. After this, the balloon is retrieved, and angiography is performed to confirm satisfactory revascularization. Once success is confirmed, the distal embolic protection device is recaptured and withdrawn *(right)*.

Fig. 5.15 Carotid Artery Stenting Procedure (Reused with permission from Munich SA, Mokin M, Krishna C, et al. Carotid artery angioplasty and stenting. In: Winn HR, ed. *Youmans and Winn Neurological Surgery.* 7th ed. Philadelphia, PA: Elsevier; 2017: 3107–3123.e4, F367-1–367-5.)

9. The embolic protection device is removed.
10. Repeat carotid angiography should demonstrate improved flow through the stenosis (Fig. 5.16). Repeat cerebral angiography can be compared with presenting angiogram for evidence of embolic debris.
11. Pressure is held over the access site, or an arterial closure device can be used.

Postprocedure Care

- Patient should be closely monitored with frequent vitals to assess hemodynamic instability and frequent neurologic assessments of overall functioning.
- Patients can typically be discharged within 1 to 2 days.
- Repeat carotid artery duplex ultrasound should be done at 3 to 6 weeks to establish the patient's new baseline.

Treatment Alternatives

- Carotid endarterectomy (CEA)
  - Preferred treatment in patients with symptomatic carotid disease
  - Commonly performed by vascular surgeons
  - In a select group of symptomatic patients, CAS is preferred to CEA. This includes patients in whom:
    - Artery is not suitable for open surgical access
    - Stenosis is radiation-induced
    - Artery has restenosed after previous CEA
    - Surgery and/or anesthesia poses a high risk
  - The CREST trial compared CAS to CEA and found no significant difference in major risks of the two treatments. Both procedures achieve similar long-term outcomes for patients with symptomatic disease. CAS has a greater 30-day postprocedure stroke and death rate than CEA.
- Medical management
  - Dual antiplatelet therapy—aspirin and Plavix
  - Antihypertensive agents
  - Statins

Complications

- Neurologic sequelae—namely, stroke. This can be due to a number of factors, including distal embolization during and after the procedure, hypoperfusion secondary to baroreceptor stimulation, hemorrhage, and/or cerebral hyperperfusion.
- Older patients and those with heavily calcified aortic arches are at greatest risk
- Stroke risk is greater in patients undergoing CAS than in patients undergoing CEA.

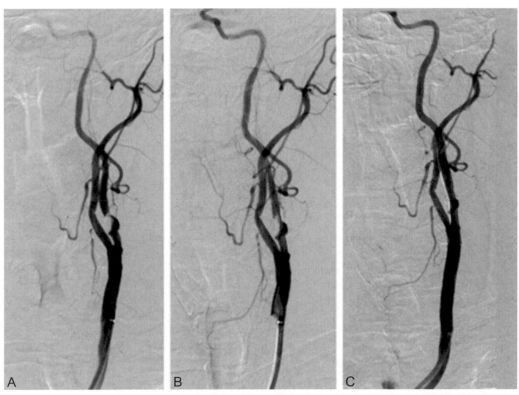

Fig. 5.16 A, selective angiogram that shows a high-grade stenosis of >90% in the left internal carotid artery due to a great atheromatous plaque with calcification. B, After sent deployment (7 × 40 mm Carotid Wallstent), a significant residual stenosis is revealed despite performing a postdilation with a 4 × 20 mm balloon. C, Final result after a second overlapped stent placement with no residual stenosis. (Reused with permission from Oteros R, Jimenez-Gomez E, Ochoa JJ, et al. Unprotected Carotid Artery Stenting in Symptomatic Patients with High-Grade Stenosis: Results and Long-Term Follow-Up in a Single-Center Experience. *Am J Neuroradiol.* 2012;33(7):1285–1291. Figure 2).

⌖ LITERATURE REVIEW

A 2012 study by Bijuklic et al. of CAS in 728 patients with embolic protection devices found new ipsilateral ischemic brain lesions in 32.8%, contralateral lesions in 25%, and a stroke rate of 1.9%.

- Hemodynamic instability
  - Due to baroreceptor stimulation during balloon inflation
  - Some degree of bradycardia and/or hypotension occurs in up to 68% of patients
- Hyperperfusion syndrome
  - Sequelae of ipsilateral headache, motor seizures, and intracerebral hemorrhage
  - Typically follows one-sided correction of severe carotid artery stenosis in patients with severe bilateral stenosis
  - Often preceded by marked hypertension
- Restenosis of the target artery
  - Reported in up to 5% of patients undergoing CAS
  - Acute (<30 days) thrombosis typically due to inadequate antiplatelet therapy
  - Subacute (>30 days) restenosis due to neointimal hyperplasia
- Stent fracture—common complication with unknown clinical significance
- Myocardial infarction—1%–4% of patients
- Renal failure—due to contrast-induced nephropathy, renal atheroemboli, or renal hypoperfusion
- Access-related problems, the most common complication

🏠 TAKE-HOME POINTS

Intraarterial Thrombolysis for Acute Ischemic Stroke
- With improvements in device development and our understanding of stroke pathophysiology, endovascular treatment options have become a valuable treatment alternative in patients with large proximal arterial thrombosis.
- Recent multicenter randomized control trials have demonstrated significant functional benefit for select patients with

🏠 TAKE-HOME POINTS—cont'd

large acute territorial infarcts who present in a timely manner.
- Many areas of further investigation remain regarding the impact of imaging predictors, alternative procedural techniques, and demographic factors on outcomes following endovascular thrombolysis.
- IV-tPA remains an FDA-approved option in patients without contraindications to systemic thrombolysis who present within 3 to 4.5 hours after cerebrovascular accident.

Percutaneous Vertebroplasty and Kyphoplasty
- Percutaneous vertebroplasty and kyphoplasty are performed to help relieve pain associated with compression fractures from osteoporosis or malignancy or pain associated with vertebral angiomas.
- Imaging with fluoroscopy or CT is used to help guide the trocar needle and avoid injuring the spinal cord. Fluoroscopy is more commonly employed.
- These are considered safe procedures with low complication rates—less than 1% in osteoporotic patients and less than 5% in fractures associated with malignancy. The most common complications involve neurologic deficits that commonly resolve within 30 days post procedure.

Carotid Artery Stenting
- In patients with bilateral carotid stenosis, a staged approach (separate operations for each side) is preferred to a simultaneous approach (operating on both sides together).
  - This reduces the risk of hyperperfusion syndrome and hemodynamic instability.
- Hemodynamic instability is due to carotid baroreceptor stimulation during balloon inflation. Clinical signs include hypotension and bradycardia, and serious cases may require atropine administration.
- The most serious complication of CAS is stroke.
  - This risk can be lessened with dual antiplatelet therapy before and after surgery.
  - Embolic protection devices theoretically reduce the risk of embolic material reaching the brain. However, their benefit has not been established.
- Alternatives to CAS include medical management and CEA, an operation commonly performed by vascular surgeons.

REVIEW QUESTIONS

1. Mrs. Jones has a scheduled vertebroplasty for L3. What could prevent her from having this procedure?
   a. Mrs. Jones no longer has pain.
   b. Mrs. Jones developed an infection of L3.
   c. A piece of her fracture has moved and is compressing the spinal cord.
   d. Vertebroplasty is not indicated in the treatment of acute compression fractures.
   e. None of the above
2. What is the most common complication of vertebroplasty?
   a. Pulmonary embolism
   b. Pneumothorax
   c. Transient neurologic deficit
   d. Permanent neurologic deficit
   e. Infection

3. What is the most common imaging modality used for vertebroplasties?
   a. MRI
   b. Ultrasound
   c. Fluoroscopy
   d. CT
4. What is the difference between vertebroplasty and kyphoplasty?
   a. Vertebroplasty uses a balloon to restore the height of the vertebra.
   b. Kyphoplasty is used for asymptomatic fractures.
   c. Vertebroplasty is used for asymptomatic fractures.
   d. Kyphoplasty uses a balloon or similar device to restore the height of the vertebra.

5. What imaging modality is typically the first choice in the diagnosis of carotid artery disease? What modality is considered the gold standard?
   a. Carotid artery duplex ultrasound; carotid artery duplex ultrasound
   b. CT angiogram; carotid artery duplex ultrasound
   c. MR angiogram; carotid angiogram
   d. Carotid artery duplex ultrasound; carotid angiogram

6. Which of the following is the only absolute contraindication to carotid artery stenting?
   a. Severe tortuosity of the carotid artery
   b. Anatomy unfavorable to the deployment of an embolic protection device
   c. Circumferential plaque buildup
   d. Thrombus visible within the carotid artery
   e. Bilateral carotid artery disease >85%

SUGGESTED READINGS

Ahn SH, Prince EA, Dubel GJ. Basic neuroangiography: review of technique and perioperative patient care. *Semin Intervent Radiol.* 2013;30:225–233.

Ahn SH, Prince E, Dubel G. Carotid artery stenting: review of technique and update of recent literature. *Semin Intervent Radiol.* 2013;30(3):288–296.

American College of Radiology. *ACR–ASNR–ASSR–SIR–SNIS Practice Parameter for the Performance of Vertebral Augmentation.* Revised 2017. Available at https://www.acr.org/-/media/ACR/Files/Practice-Parameters/verebralaug.pdf. Accessed May 11, 2018.

Arnaout OM, Rahme RJ, Ahmadieh TY, et al. Past, present, and future perspectives on the endovascular treatment of acute ischemic stroke. *Tech Vasc Interv Radiol.* 2012; 15(1):87–92.

Aziz F. Carotid artery stenting technique. In: Peter K, ed. *Medscape.* Available at emedicine.medscape.com/article/1839544-tech nique#showall. Updated April 2016. Accessed May 11, 2018.

Berkhemer OA, Fransen PS, Beumer D, et al. A randomized trial of intraarterial treatment for acute ischemic stroke. *N Engl J Med.* 2015;372(1):11–20.

Bijuklic K, Wandler A, Hazizi F, Schofer J. The PROFI study (Prevention of Cerebral Embolization by Proximal Balloon Occlusion Compared to Filter Protection during Carotid Artery Stenting): a prospective randomized trial. *J Am Coll Cardiol.* 2012;59(15):1383–1389.

Brott TG, Hobson RW 2nd, Howard G, et al. Stenting versus endarterectomy for treatment of carotid-artery stenosis. *N Engl J Med* 2010;363(1):11–23.

Campbell BC, Mitchell PJ, Kleinig TJ, et al. Endovascular therapy for ischemic stroke with perfusion-imaging selection. *N Engl J Med.* 2015;372(11):1009–1018.

Citron SJ, Wallace RC, Lewis CA, et al. Society of Interventional Radiology; American Society of Interventional and Therapeutic Neuroradiology; American Society of Neuroradiology: Quality improvement guidelines for adult diagnostic neuroangiography. Cooperative study between ASITN, ASNR, and SIR. *J Vasc Interv Radiol.* 2003;14(9, Pt 2):S257–S262.

Fairman RM. Carotid artery stenting and its complications. In: Kasner SE, Eidt JF, Mills JL Sr, eds. UpToDate. Available at uptodate.com/contents/carotid-artery-stenting-and-its-complications?source=search_result&search=carotid+artery+stenting&selectedTitle=1~37.

Goyal M, Demchuk AM, Menon BK, et al. Randomized assessment of rapid endovascular treatment of ischemic stroke. *N Engl J Med.* 2015;372(11):1019–1030.

Hassan AE, Rostambeigi N, Chaudhry SA, et al. Combination of noninvasive neurovascular imaging modalities in stroke patients: patterns of use and impact on need for digital subtraction angiography. *J Stroke Cerebrovasc Dis.* 2013;22:e53–e58.

Hui FK, Yim J, Spiotta AM, et al. Intermediate catheter injections in closed segments during acute stroke intervention: a cautionary note. *J Neurointerv Surg.* 2012;4(6):e39.

Rosen H, Walega DR. Osteoporotic thoracolumbar vertebral compression fractures: clinical manifestations and treatment. In: Rosen CJ, ed. Available at https://www.uptodate.com/contents/osteoporotic-thoracolumbar-vertebral-compression-fractures-clinical-manifestations-and-treatment.

Santiago FR, Abela AP, Alvarez LG, et al. Pain and functional outcome after vertebroplasty and kyphoplasty. A comparative study. *Eur J Radiol.* 2010; 75(2):e108–e113.

Saver JL. Time is brain—quantified. *Stroke.* 2015;37(1):263–266.

Saver JL, Goyal M, Bonafe A, et al. Stent-retriever thrombectomy after intravenous t-PA vs. t-PA alone in stroke. *N Engl J Med.* 2015;372(24):2285–2295.

Wojak JC, Abruzzo TA, Bello JA, et al. Quality improvement guidelines for adult diagnostic cervicocerebral angiography: update. *J Vasc Interv Radiol.* 2015;26:1596–1608.

Zeumer H, Hacke W, Ringelstein EB. Local intraarterial thrombolysis in vertebrobasilar thromboembolic disease. *AJNR Am J Neuroradiol.* 1983;4:401–404.

6

Interventional Oncology

Philip Yue-Cheng Cheung, Lourdes Alanis, Jason Chiang, Junjian Huang, Eric vanSonnenberg

Interventional oncology encompasses a wide spectrum of care for the cancer patient, from port placement for chemotherapy administration, to percutaneous drainage for management of renal or biliary obstruction, to tumor ablation and arterial embolization to treat a host of solid tumors. Interventional radiologists function as part of a multidisciplinary team, working closely with oncologists, surgeons, internists, radiation oncologists, and other specialists to provide optimal patient care.

Herein we provide an introduction to the principles, technology, and approach that interventional radiologists use in the treatment of solid tumors. Selected cases of malignancy in different organs will be presented, along with a discussion of the most commonly used ablative and embolic therapeutic techniques.

OVERVIEW OF TUMOR ABLATION

- Ablation refers to directed focal destruction of solid tumors and can be broadly divided into chemical-based and energy-based techniques.
- Chemical-based methods involve direct exposure of tumors to damaging chemicals
- Energy-based methods (typically termed "thermal ablation") are divided into hyperthermic and hypothermic techniques. Newer approaches induce coagulation necrosis primarily through nonthermal means as well.
  - Hypothermic methods are termed cryoablation.
  - Hyperthermic methods include radiofrequency (RF), microwave (MW), ultrasound (US), and laser ablation.
  - Irreversible electroporation (IRE) is a nonthermal ablative technique that induces tissue necrosis by disrupting cellular homeostatic mechanisms.

Chemical Ablation

Chemical ablation is used primarily in patients with hepatocellular carcinoma (HCC). It involves the direct instillation of damaging chemical agents into neoplastic tissue. HCC typically arises in the context of cirrhotic liver morphology, and the fibrotic liver capsule that surrounds the mass tends to contain the chemicals within the tumor (Fig. 6.1).

- **Ethanol** (ETOH) is the major agent used for chemical ablation. It produces an ablative effect through two mechanisms:
  - Diffusion across the cytoplasmic membrane to cause immediate cellular dehydration, resulting in coagulation necrosis of tumor cells
  - Damaging of endothelial cells in the local vasculature, leading to local thrombosis and ischemic injury to the tumor
- **Acetic acid** (Fig. 6.2) has been explored as an alternative to ETOH but rarely is.
  - Mechanism of action is identical to that of ETOH, and some studies have shown greater coagulation necrosis when using acetic acid compared with EtOH.

Energy-Based Ablation

- Used most commonly in cases of percutaneous tumor ablation.
- **Thermal** ablation induces extreme temperature variations to produce irreversible cellular injury.
- **Nonthermal** approach of IRE applies energy to induce cell death through mechanisms other than thermal injury.

Mechanisms of Thermal Ablation
Hypothermic Cellular Injury (Cryoablation)
- Modern argon gas systems use the **Joule-Thomson effect**.
  - Forced expansion of a *real* gas under adiabatic conditions (i.e., heat does not enter or leave the system) creates rapid changes in the temperature of the gas.
- Direct tissue cooling produces initial injury.
  - At low cooling rates, freezing propagates *extracellularly*, drawing water out from cells through osmotic dehydration and injuring the cellular membrane.
  - At very low temperatures, freezing propagates *intracellularly*. Formation of ice crystals within cells directly damages organelles, a process that is highly lethal.
    - Intracellular ice formation begins at temperatures as high as $-15°C$ and is virtually guaranteed at $-40°C$
    - Commercial cryoprobes reach temperatures as low as $-190°C$
- Vascular injury produces further damage to neoplastic tissue.
  - *Endothelial injury* resulting from direct tissue cooling causes thrombus formation, *mechanical damage* from

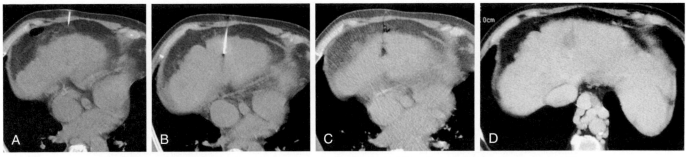

Fig. 6.1 Ethanol Ablation of Hepatocellular Carcinoma. (A and B) Needle is positioned in a very small hepatocellular carcinoma in a patient with alpha-fetoprotein (AFP) of 600. (C) Immediately after ablation, an area of low density has replaced the tumor. (D) Three-month follow-up imaging demonstrates no evidence of recurrence. AFP had decreased to 5 ng/mL. (From Weintraub JL, Ward TJ, Rundback JH. Chemical ablation of liver lesions. In: Mauro MA, Murphy KPJ, Thomson KR, et al., eds. *Image-Guided Interventions*. 2nd ed. Philadelphia: Elsevier; 2014:1061–1067.)

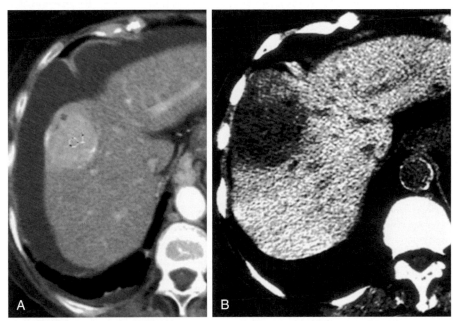

Fig. 6.2 Results of Acetic Acid Ablation for Hepatocellular Carcinoma in a 76-Year-Old Woman. (A) Initial computed tomography (CT) demonstrates a capsular lesion with marked enhancement. (B) CT performed at 1 month post treatment shows no area of enhancement, consistent with complete necrosis. (From Weintraub JL, Ward TJ, Rundback JH. Chemical ablation of liver lesions. In: Mauro MA, Murphy KPJ, Thomson KR, et al., eds. *Image-Guided Interventions*. 2nd ed. Philadelphia: Elsevier; 2014:1061–1067.)

ice formation increases vascular permeability, and *reperfusion injury* leads to increased generation of reactive oxygen species, all resulting in ischemic injury to the tumor.

Hyperthermic Cellular Injury

- Sustained high-temperature exposure greater than 46°C produces irreversible cellular injury that leads to cellular death. This process occurs more rapidly with increasing temperature, and cell death is essentially instantaneous at temperatures above 53 degrees.
- Extremely high temperatures (approximately 100°C and greater) vaporize and carbonize tissue to produce char that limits RF-based systems.
- Optimal temperatures for most hyperthermic approaches range from 50°C to 100°C, with 90°C a common target temperature.

- *Coagulative necrosis* has a characteristic histologic appearance that is defined, in part, by dead cells with absent nuclei.
- *Thermal fixation* results in the preservation of normal-appearing cellular architecture despite definitive cellular death and is typically associated with MW-based methods.
- Given the frequent lack of the histologic hallmarks of coagulative necrosis in adequately ablated tissues, the preferred term for the effect of thermal ablation is "coagulation" or "coagulation necrosis."
- The bioheat equation, as described by Pennes, defines the gradient of temperatures through tissue as a function of heat delivery and local physiologic characteristics. Simplified, the bioheat equation is approximated as:
  Coagulation necrosis = energy deposited × local tissue interactions − heat loss

RADIOFREQUENCY ABLATION

- Radiofrequency ablation (RFA) involves the conduction of alternating current through tissue to produce thermal injury and cell death.
- An array of applicators, spaced to allow optimal overlap of energy delivery, allows for ablation of different shapes and volumes.
- RFA is limited by the potential for char formation/local tissue desiccation that substantially increases tissue impedance and interferes with the propagation of heat energy (Fig. 6.3).
  - Optimal tissue temperatures range between 50°C and 100°C, with 90°C being most common.
- **Internally cooled electrodes** reduce adjacent heat damage, improve energy deposition in tissue, and increase the zone of coagulation.
- **Arrays** of clustered internally cooled electrodes generate larger area of necrosis than using either arrays or internally cooled electrodes alone.
- **Pulsed** delivery involves alternating periods of high-energy deposition with low-energy deposition as a means of maximizing energy delivery.
  - High-energy periods rapidly induce tissue coagulation.
  - Low-energy periods allow adjacent tissue to cool, thereby decreasing charring and vaporization.
  - Pulsed delivery can be combined with internally cooled electrodes.
- **Perfusion** electrodes deliver saline solution into tissue to decrease resistance along the electrical path, thereby increasing thermal delivery and augmenting the zone of necrosis.
- It is hypothesized that the ionicity of saline provides a medium for improved current flow by reducing impedance.

> ## ▶ CLINICAL POINT
>
> Delivered energy can be absorbed by blood and siphoned away, inhibiting the hyperthermic ablative effect that the operator is trying to achieve. Alternatively, fluid flow may deliver heat to an area undergoing cryoablation, inhibiting the effectiveness of tissue cooling in an analogous manner. This phenomenon, called the *heat sink effect* and *cold sink effect*, respectively, has been described extensively in the literature, particularly relating to RFA of vascularized tumors.

- Many approaches have been described to reduce the vascular perfusion of the target region to diminish the heat sink effect.
  - Intraoperatively, the Pringle maneuver (compression of the portal vasculature) can reduce flow to the liver in the treatment of hepatic malignancies.
  - Temporary balloon tamponade of portal vessels permits a similar degree of rapidly adjustable vascular flow control.
  - Preemptive coil embolization of vessels perfusing the tumor provides permanent reduction in flow.
- Pharmacologic modulation using agents such as epinephrine, halothane, or vasopressin is less invasive than those approaches described earlier.

MICROWAVE ABLATION

- MW ablation (MWA) heats tissue with an alternating electric field. It is capable of propagating through a variety of tissues through a process called *dielectric hysteresis*. MW energy can heat tissue to greater temperatures than can RFA, leading to larger and more homogeneous ablation zones, even in the presence of larger vasculature.
- MW energy is capable of heating through desiccated and charred tissue, allowing ablation zones to reach larger sizes and hotter temperatures compared with that of RFA. As a result, MWA has been shown to be effective in creating ablation zones even in the presence of large hepatic vasculature that otherwise might produce heat sink effects.
- The rapid and high heating rate associated with MWA causes multiple physical changes to occur, including water vaporization, desiccation, and dehydration. These changes can be observed under imaging.
- *Water vaporization*: an early indication of rapid heating in liver tissue is the formation of water vapor, identifiable under real-time US imaging as a hyperechoic interface that can be used as a marker to evaluate the ablation progress. On computed tomography (CT), the vapor appears as a hypoattenuating lesion against background liver parenchyma.
- A metric of technical success when creating ablation zones is to calculate the volume of ablated tissue around the tumor boundary.
- Studies have detailed the amount of tissue contraction that occurs during thermal ablation. It is hypothesized that the zone of contraction is a consequence of collagen shrinkage during heating. These contractions can lead to ablation dimensions over 50% smaller than expected based on postprocedural CT.
- Understanding the potential for error when evaluating technical success of an MWA zone can prevent overtreatment of tumors located near critical liver anatomy.
- MWA systems have the high potential for undesired off-target injury to neighboring structures given the energy and heat involved. Damage to intrahepatic and extrahepatic structures, including bowel perforation, duct injury, peritoneal burns, and diaphragmatic burns, has been reported.
- The use of "physical displacement strategies" minimizes the risk of off-target injury. One such technique, hydrodissection, displaces nearby structures away from the ablation zone by injecting fluid (5% dextrose or 0.9% saline) into the adjacent potential space.
- Multiple MW antenna arrays are used to create larger ablation zones. Doing so is essential in making ablation zones large enough to maintain adequate tumor margins and to reduce rates of local tumor progression.

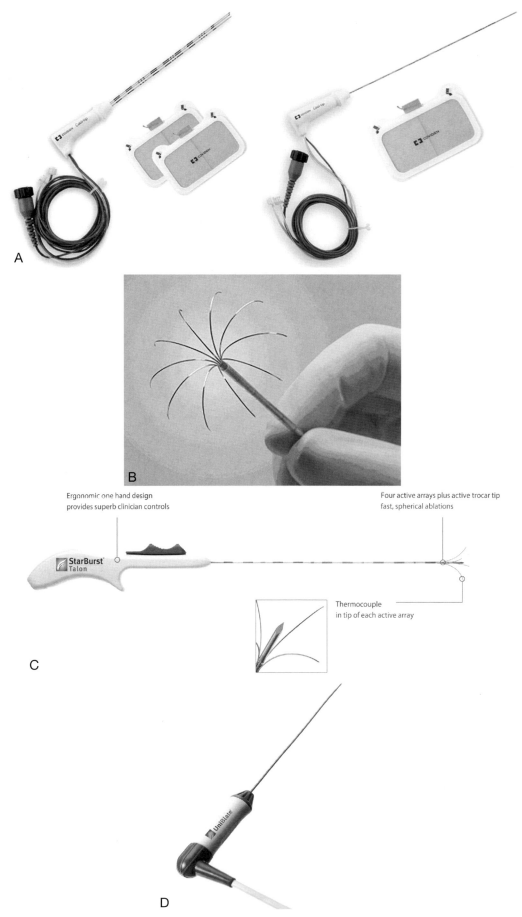

Fig. 6.3 Examples of Commercial Radiofrequency Ablation Probes. (A) Medtronic CoolTip internally cooled single and cluster electrodes. (B) Boston Scientific LeVeen needle electrodes. (C) AngioDynamics StarBurst array electrodes. (D) AngioDynamics UniBlate perfusion electrode. ([A] Courtesy Medtronic, Minneapolis, MN; [B] Courtesy Boston Scientific, Marlborough, MA; [C and D] Courtesy AngioDynamics, Latham, NY.)

Ergonomic one hand design
provides superb clinician controls

Four active arrays plus active trocar tip
fast, spherical ablations

Thermocouple
in tip of each active array

OTHER ABLATION TECHNIQUES

High-Intensity Focused Ultrasound

- US ablation, often referred to as high-intensity focused ultrasound (HIFU), involves the focal application of acoustic energy to generate local tissue heating and coagulation.
- HIFU differs from diagnostic US in that HIFU concentrates US waves into a focal region, delivering an acoustic intensity to the region that can be several hundred times stronger than that experienced by overlying tissue.
- Like other ablation techniques, HIFU can generate coagulation necrosis through hyperthermic injury at temperatures ranging between 50°C and 100°C. However, its acoustic mechanism introduces the following additional consideration:
  - At temperatures greater than 100°C, the boiling of water contained within tissues creates gas bubbles that can significantly disrupt further delivery of acoustic energy. The disruption of the US field by these microbubbles is a process referred to as *acoustic cavitation*. These microbubbles may collapse, generating shear forces that create direct mechanical tissue trauma.
- US devices may be divided as follows:
  - **Transcutaneous** devices ablate a wide variety of lesions using an applicator or probe placed on the skin surface.
  - **Interstitial** devices are inserted percutaneously or laparoscopically to transduce acoustic energy from within tissues (e.g., esophageal tumors and tumors of the biliary system)
  - **Transrectal** devices are designed specifically for the ablation of prostate masses.

Laser Ablation

- Laser ablation systems deliver high-intensity photons into tissue through fiberoptic cables. These photons strike tissue molecules, causing molecular excitation and generation of heat.
- Wavelengths in the near-infrared spectrum (1000–1100 nm) permit maximal penetration.
- Laser ablation is under active investigation in virtually all solid tumors.
  - MR-guided laser ablation seems to have found a unique niche in treating brain pathology, including selected neoplasms and epilepsy.

◎ LITERATURE REVIEW

A 2015 study by Medvid et al. suggests that the safety profile of this technique is sufficiently low to justify its use as a palliative option in malignant brain neoplasms. The most commonly reported complications in this review were transient neurologic deficits (13%), followed less commonly by progressive or persistent neurologic deficits (3%), intracranial hemorrhage (2.5%), infection (2.5%), and deep venous thrombosis (2.5%).

Irreversible Electroporation

- The application of short (microsecond to millisecond) pulses of high-voltage direct current is thought to destabilize the phospholipid bilayer of the cell membrane, resulting in the formation of nanopores that fenestrate the membrane.
- Although some degree of heat generation occurs, the primary mechanism of cellular injury is believed to be a direct result of the loss of homeostatic mechanisms secondary to pore formation.
- Due to its nonthermal mechanism, IRE may not be susceptible to the heat sink effect that limits RF, MW, and cryoablation methods.
- A relative disadvantage of IRE is the need for neuromuscular blockade in addition to general anesthesia to prevent severe muscular contraction in response to delivery of the electrical current.

ANGIOGRAPHIC TECHNIQUES FOR TUMOR THERAPY

Embolization

Embolization refers to occlusion of a blood vessel via an intravascular means (i.e., intentional production of physical blockage or an embolus). Simple transarterial embolization (TAE) is sometimes termed *bland embolization*, in contrast to methods for embolization with concomitant delivery of chemotherapeutic agents (*chemoembolization*). Embolization is used in a variety of clinical settings, both oncologic and nononcologic, including:

- **Hepatic arterial embolization** in the context of HCC. Partial or total occlusion reduces blood flow to the target area, producing ischemia in tumor cells and leading to growth arrest and/or necrosis.
- **Portal venous occlusion** causes atrophy of hepatic regions downstream from the occlusion and compensatory hypertrophy in other regions. This effect is exploited as a prophylactic procedure to improve outcomes in patients requiring hepatectomy.
- **Renal arterial embolization** is used to reduce operative blood loss in patients with locally advanced renal cell carcinoma (RCC) and as a palliative or cytoreductive procedure in those who have inoperable disease.
- **Uterine artery embolization** is used to treat benign uterine leiomyomas and adenomyosis.

Embolic Agents

- Many agents are used commonly; they may best be grouped by their duration of action and their physical characteristics.
- **Temporary embolic agents** degrade over time, allowing recanalization of occluded vessels and restitution of blood flow. The most widely used agent, *gelatin sponge* (Gelfoam), produces an occlusion that typically lasts 3 to 6 weeks. It is available as a powder, in sheets, or as sponge blocks. Powder is rarely used due to risk of off-target tissue infarction. Sponges are widely available, relatively inexpensive, and easy to manipulate.

- **Permanent embolic agents** may be divided into nonabsorbable microparticles, mechanical agents, and physical agents.
  - **Nonabsorbable microparticles** encompass a variety of microspheres that generate permanent occlusion of vessels by inducing an inflammatory reaction that leads to vessel fibrosis. A variety of microspheres with differing compositions, mechanical properties, and sizes have been developed. Some microparticles have additionally been modified to transport chemotherapeutic or radioactive agents.
  - **Mechanical embolization devices** are intravascularly deployed coils or plugs designed to occlude cross-sectional flow through a vessel, producing permanent occlusion through thrombosis.
    - Several deployment systems are in use. Coils may be loaded into a catheter and delivered via a pushing wire (*pushable coils*) or saline flush (*injectable coils*). Detachable coils are designed to allow recapture and repositioning before final release, allowing optimal positioning.
    - The simplest devices are *bare metal coils* made of steel or platinum; steel coils exhibit greater strength and are less likely to migrate than platinum under high-flow conditions, whereas platinum coils are more malleable and radiopaque.
    - *Coated coils* have greater thrombogenicity than bare metal coils due to the addition of coating fibers made from polyester, nylon, or silk.
    - *Hydrogel coils* are platinum coils coated with highly hydrophilic polymers that expand to nine times the original coil diameter on exposure to blood. This property allows for a greater degree of immediate flow occlusion.
    - The Amplatzer *vascular plug* is a nitinol mesh that self-expands to provide cross-sectional occlusion of a vessel.
  - **Liquid embolic agents** are difficult to control but carry the advantage of not having to rely on an intact coagulation system. Agents include:
    - *Sclerosants* induce vascular endothelial injury (hardening). Examples include absolute ETOH and sodium tetradecyl sulfate.
    - *Polymers* such as *N*-butyl-2-cyanoacrylate (NBCA) and ethylene vinyl alcohol copolymer (Onyx). NBCA is an adhesive, often referred to as "glue," that rapidly polymerizes upon exposure to ionic solutions (such as blood) to occlude the vessel. Onyx is a nonadhesive embolic agent with slower polymerization time.

Chemoembolization

- **Chemoembolization** (often referred to as transarterial chemoembolization [**TACE**]) refers to the combination of embolization with direct intraarterial delivery of chemotherapeutic agents into the tumor.
- TACE is considered to be the standard of care for intermediate-stage HCC.

- *Lipiodol* or ethiodized oil, an iodinated poppy seed oil, is considered to be the first "chemoembolic" agent and remains one of the most widely used agents.
  - Lipiodol readily adheres to tumor cell walls, where it is actively transported into the cell, eventually producing cell lysis.
- In the 1970s and 1980s, interventional radiologists explored the local delivery of lipiodol mixed with chemotherapeutic agents (often doxorubicin, cisplatin, and/or mitomycin C) followed by vessel embolization to maximize local delivery of chemotherapy while minimizing systemic exposure.
- In the mid-2000s, new vehicles were developed to realize the goal of sustained local chemotherapeutic delivery. **Drug-eluting beads (DEBs)** contain chemotherapeutic agents (commonly doxorubicin) and were designed to slowly release agents and maximize contact time with tumor cells.
- In DEB-TACE, beads are delivered intraarterially to the tumor followed by embolization to maximize entrapment of beads within the tumor vasculature.
  - In vivo studies have validated that beads are capable of eluting chemotherapeutic agents over approximately 7 days, with peak systemic levels approximately 5% of equivalent systemic chemotherapy dosing.
- Although TACE is presently regarded as the standard of care for unresectable intermediate stage HCC, there is a lack of evidence supporting TACE as superior to bland embolization.
  - All existing randomized clinical trials comparing Transarterial embolization (TAE) and TACE in HCC have found no statistically significant differences in overall survival.
  - Some argue that a lack of standardization in techniques has obscured benefit, citing secondary measures including tumor response and time to progression as evidence of superiority.
  - Others note that the lack of benefit from adding chemotherapeutic drugs to TAE adds unnecessary expense and exposes patients to risks that are not balanced by benefits.

PERCUTANEOUS TUMOR ABLATION

Equipment

- Standard set (10-mL syringes, local anesthetic, 25-G needle, 22-G needle, #11 blade, hemostat)
- 15-cm 22-G needle, used as a guide needle
- Ablation system and probe(s)
- Sterile probe cover if using US guidance

General Image-Guided Percutaneous Ablation Procedure Steps

1. Provide appropriate anesthesia; conscious sedation is often preferred over general anesthesia but is at the discretion of the interventional radiologist.
2. Perform immediate preprocedural imaging to localize the tumor and finalize access route planning.

a. If using CT, place a CT grid on the patient's skin overlying the region of the lesion to assist in localization.
3. Mark the skin to indicate the intended trajectory.
4. After prepping the patient and administering lidocaine, insert a guide needle into the patient's skin along the planned trajectory, ascertaining, as necessary, the position of the guide needle under imaging.
5. Administer local anesthetic in deeper tissues along the final probe trajectory, particularly into sensitive layers such as the parietal pleura, liver capsule, periosteum, or parietal peritoneum.
6. Perform a dermatotomy (skin nick) using a #11 blade to facilitate insertion of the ablation probe.
7. Introduce the ablation probe alongside the guide needle (referred to as the "tandem approach"), confirming appropriate positioning of the ablation probe with imaging guidance.
8. If needed for safety reasons, perform hydrodissection by injecting 5% dextrose in water (D5W; for RFA) or normal saline (acceptable with most other modalities) to displace normal structures such as bowel away from the ablation zone.

> ### ▶▶ CLINICAL POINT
>
> Deflection of normal structures away from the ablation path using a gas, such as CO_2, is referred to as *pneumodissection*. It is less commonly performed than *hydrodissection*.

9. The manufacturer-specified ablation protocol should be used when probe position is confirmed. Ablation beyond the visualized tumor margin should be achieved to ablate microinvasive disease and provide a 1-cm circumferential margin.
10. Obtain postprocedure imaging to document ablation efficacy and assess for complications.
11. Follow-up with serial imaging. A reasonable general approach includes short-term imaging at 6 weeks, 3 months, and 6 months post procedure. Surveillance intervals may lengthen to every 6 months until 2 to 3 years post procedure with annual imaging thereafter if no evidence of recurrence or spread has been found.

RENAL CELL CARCINOMA

> ### CASE PRESENTATION
>
> A 45-year-old man presents to the emergency department with hematuria. He denies fever, chills, and flank pain. His past surgical history is relevant for a right partial nephrectomy for papillary renal cell carcinoma (RCC). Renal protocol CT demonstrates a 3-cm Bosniak III lesion adjacent to the surgical bed of the right partial nephrectomy. Further evaluation reveals that the patient has HPRC gene mutations in the tyrosine kinase region of the met proto-oncogene consistent with type 1 hereditary papillary RCC. The urologist refers the patient to interventional radiology for percutaneous tumor ablation for maximal renal sparing due to high risk of recurrent tumor growth.

- RCC develops in the proximal renal tubular epithelium. Both sporadic and hereditary variants are associated with mutations in chromosome 3p.
  - Hereditary syndromes include:
    - Von Hippel-Lindau
    - Hereditary papillary RCC
    - Familial renal oncocytoma
    - Hereditary RCC
  - Risk factors for sporadic development include:
    - Tobacco
    - Obesity
    - Polyaromatic hydrocarbons
    - Dialysis (acquired polycystic kidney disease)
- 25% to 30% of cases are diagnosed incidentally, usually on CT. The classic triad of symptoms, indicative of late stage disease, is seen only in 10% of patients:
  - Hematuria—40%
  - Flank pain—40%
  - Palpable flank mass—25%
- Approximately 63,000 new cases and 14,000 deaths per year from RCC in the United States
- The first percutaneous renal RFA was reported by Zlotta et al. in 1997 in which three tumors were ablated and subsequently resected.
- In 1999, McGovern et al. reported the first in situ renal RFA.

Indications

- Small renal masses, T1a (<4 cm) and T1b (<7 cm), are amenable to ablation with outcomes similar to surgery.
- Poor surgical candidates—those with significant comorbidities, multiple prior abdominal operations, or pelvic or horseshoe kidney variants
- Patients in whom maximal renal sparing is needed such as those with prior nephrectomy, a solitary kidney, or multiple tumors

> ### ◎ LITERATURE REVIEW
>
> Studies by Georgiades et al. in 2014 and Thompson et al. in 2015 demonstrated comparable 5-year oncologic control between partial nephrectomy, percutaneous cryoablation, and RFA in nearly 2000 patients with primary cT1N0M0 renal masses.

Contraindications

- Absolute contraindications
  - Uncorrectable coagulopathy
  - Recent myocardial infarction
  - Acute systemic infection
- Relative contraindications
  - Proximity to the central collecting system
  - Proximity to solid visceral organs (bowel, pancreas, adrenal, liver, or gallbladder)

Equipment

See General Equipment listed under "**Percutaneous Tumor Ablation.**"

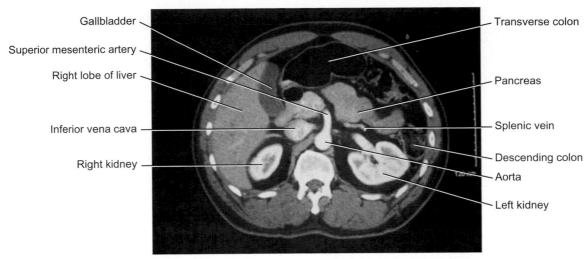

Gallbladder — Transverse colon
Superior mesenteric artery
Right lobe of liver
— Pancreas
Inferior vena cava — Splenic vein
— Descending colon
Right kidney — Aorta
— Left kidney

Fig. 6.4 Axial CT image of mid-abdomen. (Reused with permission from Netter FH, Atlas of Human Anatomy, 7th edition, Elsevier, 2018, Plate 326).

Anatomy

- The right kidney typically is located more inferior than the left (Fig. 6.4).
- Normal vascular supply is a single renal artery and vein to and from each kidney, but variants are common.
- Posteriorly located tumors have increased risk of ilioinguinal nerve injury from ablation due to proximity to the psoas muscle, but this complication is uncommon (4%).
- Tumors located near the renal sinus are subject to the *heat sink phenomenon* due to the nearby flow of urine and adjacent large vessels.

Procedure

- See steps described previously under "Percutaneous Tumor Ablation."

Renal Cell Carcinoma–Specific Procedural Considerations

- Cryoablation and RFA are the most commonly used ablation methods.
- Principle is to keep bowel and skin at least 2 cm away from the peripheral edge of the ablation zone to prevent bowel and skin necrosis.
  - Hydrodissection can protect adjacent viscera
  - Saline compresses or warming pads placed on skin can prevent injury during treatment of superficial renal masses
  - Preoperative stent placement can protect the ureter from injury
- Imaging modalities include US, CT, and MRI.
- For CT-guided procedures:
  - Noncontrast CT typically is used for preprocedure and intraprocedure imaging.
  - Contrast-enhanced CT is used postprocedurally to demonstrate the ablation zone, rule out residual tumor, and assess for complications (Fig. 6.5).

Alternative Treatments

- Radical nephrectomy
- Partial nephrectomy
- Laparoscopic ablation

Complications
Cryoablation

- Relative risk factors include advanced patient age, large tumor size, and tumor location (peripheral versus central [Fig. 6.6])
- General complication rate is approximately 12%. Common complications include:
  - Retroperitoneal hematoma (5%) typically is seen with peripheral tumors.
  - Hematuria (3%) typically is seen with central tumors. Minor hematuria is relatively common.

Radiofrequency Ablation

- Complication rate is approximately 10%. Common complications include:
  - Nerve injury (4%) is typically seen with peripheral tumors abutting the psoas muscle
  - Urinary tract injury (2%) is seen with central tumors

HEPATOCELLULAR CARCINOMA

CASE PRESENTATION

A 64-year-old man presents to his primary care physician with complaints of fatigue and weight loss. Examination reveals mild scleral icterus but is otherwise unremarkable. Work-up reveals Child-Pugh class A cirrhosis in the context of chronic hepatitis C infection. Triple-phase CT imaging reveals a focal 1.4-cm mass in segment IVb of the liver with early arterial enhancement and washout, consistent with a diagnosis of hepatocellular carcinoma. The case is discussed at a multidisciplinary tumor board meeting, and interventional radiology is consulted for ablation.

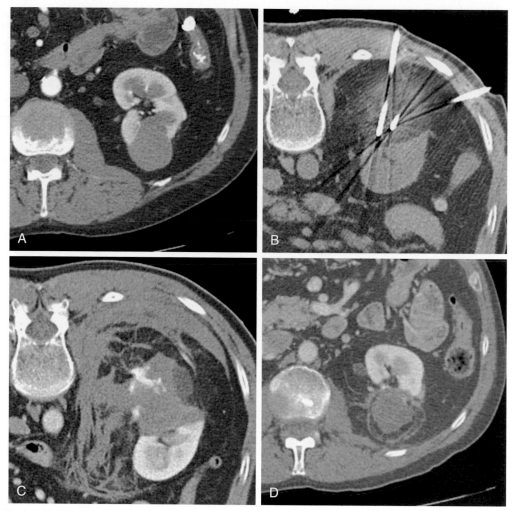

Fig. 6.5 (A) This 53-year-old man with history of esophageal cancer was found to have a 3.6-cm left renal tumor, diagnosed as renal cell carcinoma, papillary type 1. (B) Axial computed tomography (CT) image of the kidney during cryoablation shows three of the four cryoprobes engulfed in a low-density ice ball. (C) Immediately after two freeze/thaw cycles, contrast-enhanced CT showed active extravasation and associated retroperitoneal hematoma. Selective embolization (not shown) was promptly performed because of dropping blood pressure. (D) Contrast-enhanced follow-up CT image at 12 months shows zone of ablation with no evidence of residual disease. (From Ahrar K, Matin SF, Wallace MJ. Thermal ablation of renal cell carcinoma. In: Mauro MA, Murphy KPJ, Thomson KR, et al., eds. *Image-Guided Interventions.* 2nd ed. Philadelphia: Elsevier; 2014:1098–1110. Copyright Kamran Ahrar.)

- HCC accounts for 85% to 90% of primary liver cancers.
- Worldwide, HCC is the fifth most common primary malignancy and the third leading cause of cancer mortality, responsible for approximately 1 million deaths per year.
- Worldwide, the most common etiology is hepatitis B virus (HBV), which accounts for greater than 50% of all HCC cases.
- In the United States the most common cause of HCC is hepatitis C virus (HCV).
- The remainder of HCC patients who do not have HBV or HCV infection are likely to suffer from nonalcoholic steatohepatitis (NASH, or colloquially "fatty liver disease") as a result of obesity, diabetes mellitus type 2, or metabolic syndrome.
- Despite the frequency with which HCC is seen, the majority of hepatic malignancies in the United States are metastases from extrahepatic primary tumors.

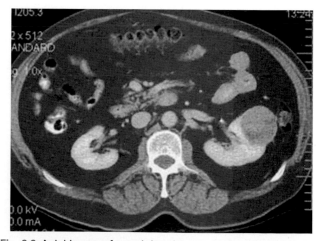

Fig. 6.6 Axial image of a peripheral tumor in the left kidney.

- The most common primaries are the breast, lung, colon, and rectum.
- Prognosis and management of secondary hepatic malignancies depend on the type of primary lesion and the extent of secondary involvement.
- The pathogenesis of HCC is under active investigation. The most accepted hypothesis describes a step-by-step process in which persistent regenerative stimuli induce genetic alterations:
  - Chronic inflammation leads to fibrosis, cirrhosis, and eventual cell death.
  - New cell proliferation results in small cell dysplasia or, if surrounded by fibrotic ring, low-grade dysplastic nodule (LGDN) to high-grade dysplastic nodule (HGDN). HGDN is the preneoplastic lesion that can lead to HCC in 30% of patients within 5 years.

Staging and Prognosis of Hepatocellular Carcinoma

- Multiple staging systems have been developed for HCC. The Barcelona Clinic Liver Cancer (BCLC) guideline provides prognosis and a suggested treatment algorithm that remains the standard of care in most settings (Fig. 6.7).
  - Very early-stage HCC (stage 0) offers the best prognosis but is difficult to diagnose due to lack of symptoms. Surgical resection is the preferred treatment option. This stage applies to:
  - Single lesions smaller than 2 cm in diameter
- Early-stage HCC (stage A) has a 5-year survival rate of 50% to 75%. Recommended therapy, if transplant is not readily available, is surgical resection or ablation. This stage applies to:
  - Solitary lesion less than 5 cm in diameter or up to three lesions, each less than 3 cm in diameter, in a patient with preserved liver function (Child-Pugh class A or B) and satisfactory performance status (ECOG 0–2)
- Intermediate-stage (B) and advanced-stage (C) HCC have a 3-year survival rate of 20% to 40%. Recommended therapy is TACE for stage B HCC and targeted molecular therapy for stage C HCC.
  - Stage B applies to:
    - Multinodular HCC with no vascular invasion in patients with preserved liver function (Child-Pugh class A or B) with satisfactory performance status (ECOG 0–2)
  - Stage C applies to:
    - Multinodular HCC with vascular invasion or extrahepatic spread in patients with satisfactory performance status (ECOG 0–2)

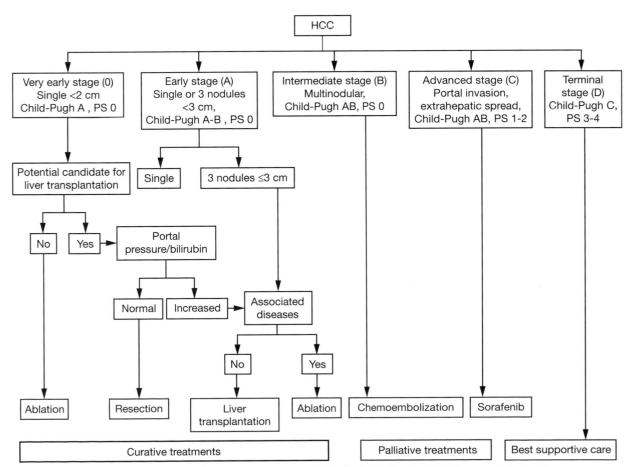

Fig. 6.7 Barcelona Clinic Liver Cancer Staging and Treatment Strategy. *HCC*, Hepatocellular carcinoma. (Modified from Forner A, Reig ME, de Lope CR, et al. Current strategy for staging and treatment: the BCLC update and future prospects. *Semin Liver Dis.* 2010;30(1):61–74.)

ECOG PERFORMANCE STATUS

Grade	ECOG
0	Fully active, able to carry on all pre-disease performance without restriction
1	Restricted in physically strenuous activity but ambulatory and able to carry out work of a light or sedentary nature, e.g., light house work, office work
2	Ambulatory and capable of all selfcare but unable to carry out any work activities. Up and about more than 50% of waking hours
3	Capable of only limited selfcare, confined to bed or chair more than 50% of waking hours
4	Completely disabled. Cannot carry on any selfcare. Totally confined to bed or chair
5	Dead

(Reused with permission from Oken M, Creech R, Tormey D, et al. Toxicity and response criteria of the Eastern Cooperative Oncology Group. *Am J Clin Oncol.* 1982;5:649–655.)

- Terminal stage (D) HCC has a 1-year survival rate of 10% to 20%. It applies to:
  - Multinodular HCC with vascular invasion or extrahepatic spread in patients with Child-Pugh class C and compromised performance status (ECOG > 2)

Indications

- Patient selection factors:
  - Poor surgical candidates due to poor liver reserve or significant comorbidities
  - Inoperable tumor due to anatomic involvement such as invasion of hepatic vasculature
  - Surgical candidates who wish to defer surgery to minimize the number of hepatectomies performed
  - Surgical candidates who decline surgical intervention
- Indications for primary HCC:
  - **As neoadjuvant therapy** to reduce the size of initially inoperable tumors, making them amenable to surgical resection
  - **As a bridge to transplantation**, by delaying tumor progression and maintaining eligibility for potentially curative liver transplantation
  - **For reduction of tumor burden**
    - May confer a survival benefit to patients and can provide palliation of pain or obstructive symptoms resulting from tumor mass effect
  - **As curative treatment** in patients with:
    - Very early- or early-stage HCC
    - Inoperable tumors at these stages are well-accepted indications for ablation under the BCLC guidelines.
      - Data from multiple studies show near equivalence between surgical resection and RFA for patients with HCC at these stages. Ablation preserves hepatic reserve more so than surgical resection, which is why some investigators advocate for ablation in early-stage HCC even if surgery is an option.

▶▶ **CLINICAL POINT**

The presence of a cirrhotic capsule is beneficial for ablation because it creates an "oven effect" due to the lack of significant vascular perfusion and retains heat within the tumor. See the bioheat equation discussed previously.

- Indications for liver metastases:
  - Colorectal primary: palliative treatment—treating these patients with RFA and systemic chemotherapy has demonstrated a survival benefit in randomized control trials
  - Neuroendocrine primary: treatment of hormonal symptoms and pain
  - Sarcoma primary: symptomatic control—TACE is the preferred intervention

Contraindications

- Absolute
  - Uncorrectable coagulopathy
  - Single lesion >5 cm or multiple lesions each >3 cm in size
  - Cirrhosis, if insufficient hepatic reserve
  - BCLC stage C or D
  - Biliary obstruction
- Relative
  - Patients with pacemakers
  - Tumor position
    - HCCs near the body wall or diaphragm may not be amenable to a percutaneous approach (or may require hydrodissection or pneumodissection as an adjunctive measure)
    - Perivascular tumors are more susceptible to the heat sink effect and are at increased risk of vascular occlusion or hepatic infarct if ablated

Equipment

See General Equipment listed under **"Percutaneous Tumor Ablation."**

Anatomy
Liver Anatomy

- Couinaud, a French surgeon and anatomist, described the division of the liver into eight anatomic segments, each with independent vascular supply, outflow, and biliary drainage (Figs. 6.8 and 6.9).
  - The middle hepatic vein divides the left and right hepatic lobes.
  - The falciform ligament divides the left lobe into a medial segment (IV) and lateral segments (II and III).
  - The right hepatic vein divides the right hepatic lobe into anterior and posterior segments.
  - The portal vein divides the liver into superior and anterior segments.
- Having thus been divided, the eight segments are numbered as follows:

- Segment I is the caudate lobe.
- The remaining seven segments are numbered II through VIII in clockwise fashion.
- Segment IV is commonly divided into a superior portion (IVa) and inferior portion (IVb).

Neighboring Structures

- The liver is adjacent to many structures that are at risk of injury during ablation (Fig. 6.10).
  - The diaphragm borders the liver superiorly.
  - The right kidney and adrenal gland are immediately posterior and inferior to hepatic segment VII.

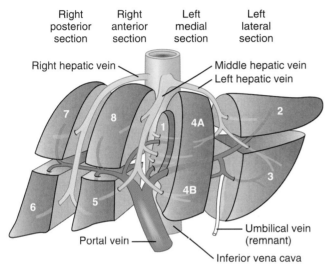

Fig. 6.8 Segmental anatomy of the liver depicting the segments of the liver and vascular and biliary anatomy. (Reused with permission from Hertzberg BS, Middleton WD. *Ultrasound: The Requisites (Requisites in Radiology)*. 3rd ed. Philadelphia: Elsevier; 2015, F3-1).

- The inferior vena cava (IVC), stomach, pylorus, and intraperitoneal portion of the duodenum are posterior and medial to the left lobe of the liver.

Procedure

See general steps under "Percutaneous Tumor Ablation."

Procedural Choices

- In focal hepatic tumors, RFA has been the most widely studied thermal ablative technique.
  - Its effectiveness is limited by the heat sink effect given a large volume of hepatic blood flow.
  - Adjunctive techniques to reduce vascular perfusion to the tumor—preablation embolization, temporary balloon tamponade, the Pringle maneuver, and pharmacologic flow modulation—all have enhanced the efficacy of thermal ablation.
- With the advent of second-generation MWA devices that are less susceptible to the heat sink effect, MWA is supplanting RFA at many centers.
- Cryoablation also is commonly used for hepatic tumor ablation.
- Chemical ablation with EtOH or acetic acid is particularly effective in treating HCC surrounded by a fibrotic capsule. It is uncommonly performed in the United States; however, because it is inexpensive, it is used to good effect around the world.

Technical Considerations

- See Figs. 6.11 and 6.12.
- Approach the ablation in a way that minimizes damage to the biliary system.
- Superficial lesions should be targeted by traversing an area of normal hepatic parenchyma, if possible.

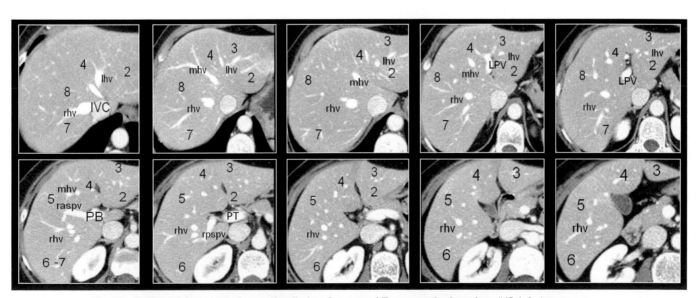

Fig. 6.9 Couinaud Segmentation as Applied to Computed Tomography Imaging. *IVC*, Inferior vena cava; *lhv*, left hepatic vein; *LPV*, left portal vein; *mhv*, middle hepatic vein; *PB*, portal bifurcation; *PT*, portal trunk; *raspv*, right anterior sectorial portal vein; *rhv*, right hepatic vein; *rpspv*, right posterior sectorial portal vein; 1–8, segments' numbering system according to Couinaud. (Reused with permission from Majno P, Mentha G, Toso C, et al. Anatomy of the liver: an outline with three levels of complexity—a further step towards tailored territorial liver resections. *J Hepatol.* 2014;60[3]:654–662.)

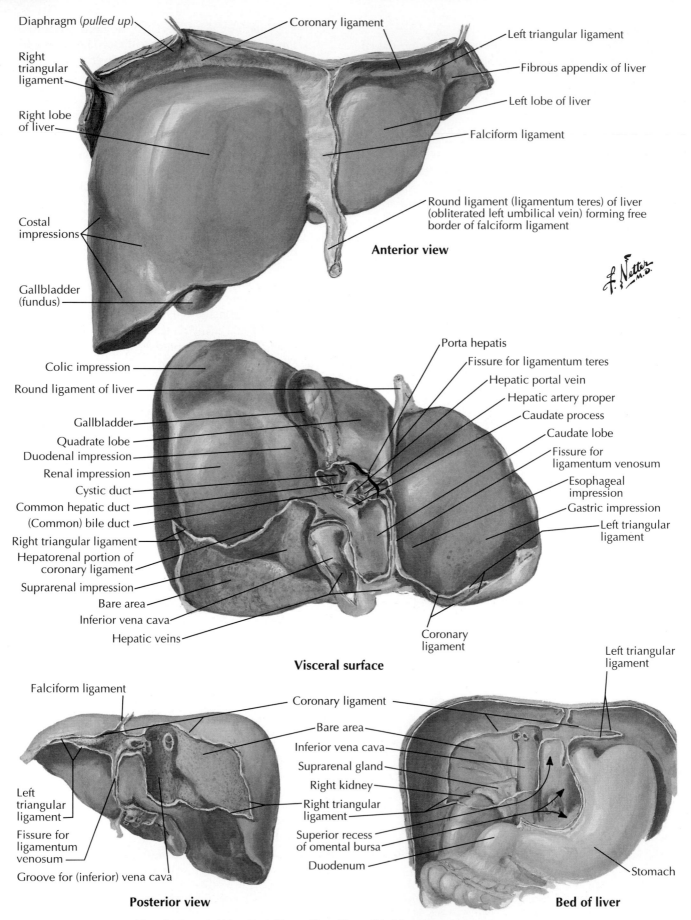

Diaphragm (*pulled up*)

Coronary ligament

Left triangular ligament

Right triangular ligament

Fibrous appendix of liver

Left lobe of liver

Right lobe of liver

Falciform ligament

Costal impressions

Round ligament (ligamentum teres) of liver (obliterated left umbilical vein) forming free border of falciform ligament

Gallbladder (fundus)

Anterior view

Colic impression

Porta hepatis

Fissure for ligamentum teres

Round ligament of liver

Hepatic portal vein

Hepatic artery proper

Gallbladder

Caudate process

Quadrate lobe

Caudate lobe

Duodenal impression

Fissure for ligamentum venosum

Renal impression

Cystic duct

Esophageal impression

Common hepatic duct

Gastric impression

(Common) bile duct

Left triangular ligament

Right triangular ligament

Hepatorenal portion of coronary ligament

Suprarenal impression

Bare area

Inferior vena cava

Hepatic veins

Coronary ligament

Visceral surface

Falciform ligament

Left triangular ligament

Coronary ligament

Bare area

Inferior vena cava

Suprarenal gland

Left triangular ligament

Right kidney

Fissure for ligamentum venosum

Right triangular ligament

Superior recess of omental bursa

Groove for (inferior) vena cava

Duodenum

Stomach

Posterior view

Bed of liver

Fig. 6.10 Liver Surface and Liver Bed. (Reused from Netter FH. *Atlas of Human Anatomy*. 7th ed. Philadelphia: Elsevier; 2019.)

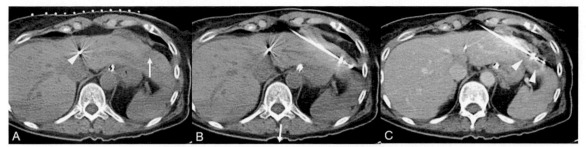

Fig. 6.11 Computed Tomography (CT)-Guided Microwave Ablation of Recurrent Cholangiocarcinoma in a 65-Year-Old Woman. The patient previously underwent stereotactic body radiotherapy for the primary tumor at the hepatic venous confluence. (A) Planning CT image demonstrates the hypodense metastasis *(arrow)* in segment II and metallic fiducial marker *(arrowhead)* used for prior radiation therapy. (B) The microwave applicator has been placed into the tumor from an epigastric approach. (C) Contrast-enhanced CT obtained immediately after microwave ablation demonstrates satisfactory ablation zone *(arrowheads)* coverage of the tumor. (Courtesy Paul B. Shyn, MD.)

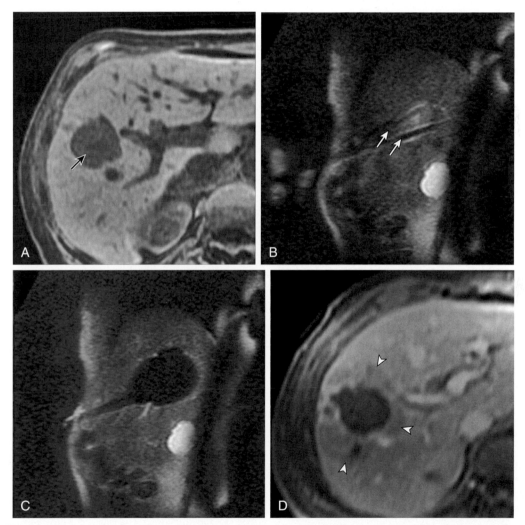

Fig. 6.12 (A) Axial contrast-enhanced magnetic resonance imaging (MRI) shows a large minimally enhancing liver metastasis *(arrow)* from a primary breast cancer. (B) T2 oblique sagittal image shows intraprocedural MRI-guided placement of multiple cryoprobes *(arrows)* into hyperintense tumor. (C) T2 oblique sagittal image shows a hypointense iceball after 15 minutes of freezing. (D) Axial contrast-enhanced MRI shows treated tumor surrounded by a nonenhancing margin of ablated normal tissue *(arrowheads)* 24 hours after procedure. (Reused with permission from Mamlouk MD, vanSonnenberg E, Silverman SG, et al. Cryoablation of liver tumors. In: Mauro MA, Murphy KPJ, Thomson KR, et al., eds. *Image-Guided Interventions*. 2nd ed. Philadelphia: Elsevier; 2014:1055–1061.)

- Normal parenchyma holds the ablation probe in place and may tamponade any bleeding.
- Normal parenchyma can be cauterized as the probe is removed, termed *tract ablation*, to minimize hemorrhage and reduce the risk of tumor seeding the probe tract.

Alternative Treatments

- Liver transplant is considered the gold standard treatment for HCC, providing 5-year survival of up to 75%.
- Given the lack of donor livers relative to the number of pending recipients, surgical resection has been the de facto option for most patients with HCC.
- The presence of cirrhosis is a critical determinant of treatment approach for patients with HCC
  - Those without cirrhosis are more likely to do well and are treated preferentially with resection.
  - The presence of cirrhosis makes definitive transplantation the better option.
- For those patients with early-stage HCC who are ineligible for transplantation and whose HCC is not amenable to surgical resection, a growing body of evidence supports the use of ablation as a first-line therapy.

Complications

- Complications are seen in approximately 7% of hepatic RFA cases
- Minor hemorrhage around the ablation zone is common; however, major bleeding requiring transfusion or procedural hemostasis occurs in <1% of cases
- Other complications include:
  - Abscess formation, which is more likely after bowel manipulation or in the context of biliary obstruction
  - Bowel perforation
  - Abdominal wall injury
  - Diaphragmatic injury
  - Seeding of the applicator tract. This is rare but is more commonly seen with superficial tumors when healthy liver is not transversed by the probe.

MUSCULOSKELETAL ONCOLOGY

CASE PRESENTATION

A 15-year-old male presented to his pediatrician with left lower leg pain for the past 3 months. He reported the pain was more severe at night and found relief only with aspirin. His pediatrician requested radiographs of his left tibia-fibula, which revealed a well-defined radiolucency within a sclerotic area in the anterior aspect of the distal tibia. The pediatrician then referred the patient to an orthopedic surgeon who determined the bone lesion to be an osteoid osteoma, based on the patient's age, symptoms, and imaging features. The orthopedic surgeon requested an interventional radiology consult to discuss treatment of the osteoid osteoma with RFA.

- Work-up of benign and malignant bone lesions includes the patient's age, clinical presenting symptoms, imaging features, and histology.
- Benign, malignant, and metastatic skeletal lesions can all result in pain, pathologic fracture, and neurovascular compromise.
- Patients with primary breast, prostate, or lung cancer with metastatic skeletal lesions have a poor prognosis, with median survival of 3 years or less.
- The original application of RFA in skeletal oncology was to treat osteoid osteomas; it is currently the standard of care for these benign osseous tumors. It is also used in the treatment of various painful, small (3–5 cm) bone lesions and as palliation for larger lesions by minimizing further spread into bone.
  - RFA can be used alone or as an adjunct to surgical resection, with or without cementoplasty.

Bone Tumors and Tumor-like Conditions That May Be Treated With Image-Guided Interventions
Bone-Forming Lesions

- **Osteoid osteomas** (Fig. 6.13)
  - Comprise 10% of benign bone tumors, usually occurring in the femur or tibia
  - Seen more in men
  - Most commonly seen in 10- to 35-year-olds
  - Classically presents with pain at rest that worsens at night and responds well to NSAIDs (nonsteroidal anti-inflammatory drugs)
  - Well characterized on CT and X-ray, appearing as a small (less than 1 cm), well-defined lesion with a nidus of osteoid tissue that may be radiolucent or have a sclerotic center
- **Osteoblastomas** (Fig. 6.14)
  - Comprise 3% of benign bone tumors
  - 75% of cases present in the first through third decades of life
  - Histologically similar to osteoid osteomas but are typically larger than 2 cm, progress in size, and behave aggressively
  - Patients may be asymptomatic or present with pain not relieved by NSAIDs.
  - Radiographic appearance may be similar to a large osteoid osteoma, mimic an expansile lesion similar to an aneurysmal bone cyst, or appear as an aggressive lesion.
  - May be treated with RFA, surgical excision, or curettage

Lesions of Cartilaginous Origin

- **Enchondroma** (Fig. 6.15)
  - Second most common benign bone tumor, typically occurring in the short (phalanges and metacarpals) and long (humerus and femur) tubular bones
  - Seen during the second through fourth decades of life
  - Patients may be asymptomatic or present with pain secondary to a pathologic fracture.
  - In the short bones, enchondromas may be entirely radiolucent, whereas long bone enchondromas may have visible calcifications.

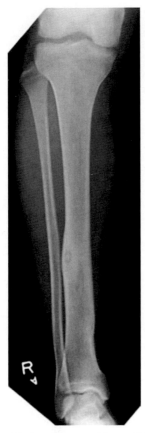

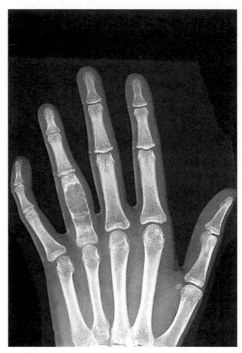

Fig. 6.15 Enchondroma of the Proximal Phalanx of the Ring Finger. (Reused with permission from Bullough PG, Adams JE, Jackson SJ. Cartilage-forming tumors and tumor-like conditions. In: *Orthopaedic Pathology*. 5th ed. St. Louis: Mosby; 2010:399–428.)

Fig. 6.13 Radiographic Appearance of Osteoid Osteoma Involving the Distal Tibia. (Courtesy Cincinnati Children's Hospital Medical Center, Department of Pediatric Orthopaedics.)

- **Chondroblastomas** (also known as Codman tumors) (Fig. 6.16)
  - Represent less than 1% of all primary bone lesions
  - Occur in the epiphysis of immature long bones such as the humerus, tibia, and femur
  - Patients present with pain
  - On imaging, they are located eccentrically, have a sclerotic border, and may demonstrate matrix calcifications
  - May require RFA with bone grafting to avoid articular collapse
- **Chondromyxoid fibromas** (Fig. 6.17)
  - Represent less than 1% of all primary bone lesions
  - Presents in adolescents and young adults, males more so than females
  - Range in size from 1 to 10 cm (average 3–4 cm) and are frequently located in the proximal tibia or distal femur
  - Patients may present with local pain and swelling as a result of mass effect on adjacent neurovascular structures.
  - Appear radiographically as eccentric, radiolucent lesions with a sclerotic, scalloped margin that may erode or balloon out of the cortex

Fibrous, Fibro-osseous, and Fibrohistiocytic Lesions

- **Fibrous cortical defects and nonossifying fibromas** (Fig. 6.18)
  - Relatively common in children and adolescents; considered to be a developmental defect rather than a true bone tumor with a tendency to spontaneously involute

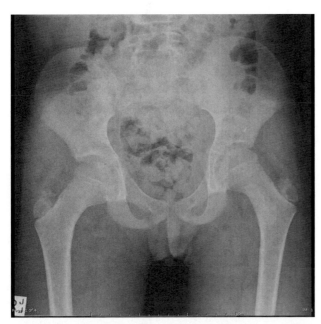

Fig. 6.14 Osteoblastoma of the Left Proximal Femur. (Reused with permission from Riley ND, Camilleri D, McNally MA. Osteoid osteoma following fracture of the distal tibia: a case report and literature review. *Injury Extra*. 2014;45(9):69–72.)

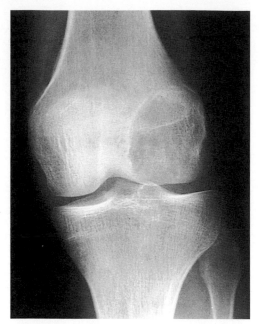

Fig. 6.16 Chondroblastoma of the Left Distal Femur. (Courtesy Mark R. Wick. Pernick N. Bone. Cartilaginous tumors other than chondrosarcoma. Chondroblastoma. *PathologyOutlines.com* [website] 2016. http://www.pathologyoutlines.com/topic/bonechondroblastoma.html.)

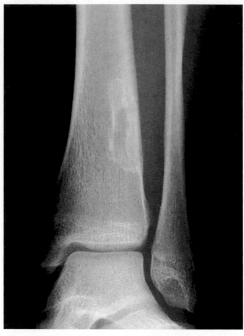

Fig. 6.18 Nonossifying Fibroma of the Distal Tibia. (Printed with permission from Toy PC, Heck RK. General principles of tumors. In: Azar FM, Beaty JH, Canale ST, eds. *Campbell's Operative Orthopaedics.* 13th ed. 2017: Philadelphia, PA: Elsevier/Mosby, 829–5.)

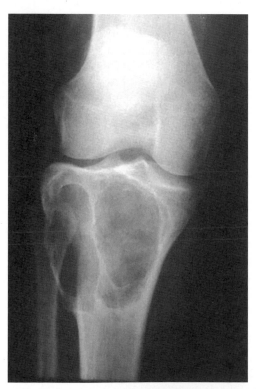

Fig. 6.17 Chondromyxoid Fibroma of the Proximal Tibia. (Reused with permission from Weidner N, Lin GY, Kyriakos M. Joint and bone pathology. In: Weidner N, Cote RJ, Suster S, et al., eds. *Modern Surgical Pathology.* 2nd ed. Philadelphia: Saunders; 2009:1784–1840.)

- Commonly located in long bones (femur and tibia), occurring more commonly in males
- Appear as elliptical, radiolucent lesions with a scalloped sclerotic border
- **Fibrous dysplasia**
  - May affect one bone (monostotic form) or several bones (polyostotic form)
  - Characterized by the replacement of lamellar cancellous bone with abnormal fibrous tissue with a typical "ground-glass" appearance on imaging
  - Patients are usually asymptomatic but may experience pain secondary to pathologic fractures
  - Usually requires surgical fixation if symptomatic

Miscellaneous Lesions

- **Giant cell tumors**
  - Aggressive lesions composed of highly vascularized tissue
  - Represent 5% to 9% of primary bone tumors and 23% of benign bone tumors
  - Present after skeletal maturity and affect women more than men
  - Occur at the articular ends of long bones (proximal humerus, distal radius, proximal tibia, and distal femur)
  - Appear radiographically as radiolucent lesions without sclerotic or periosteal reaction
- **Hemangiomas**
  - Represent 2% to 3% of all spinal tumors

- Occur more often in females and incidence increases with increasing age
- Commonly found in the vertebral body but may extend into the pedicle and lamina
- Composed of abnormal vascular channels with high osteoclast concentration at the bone-tumor interface
- Coarse vertical striations on radiograph and coarse punctate densities on CT within the vertebral body are characteristic

Indications
- Nonsurgical candidates including patients with advanced bone lesions, comorbidities, and high likelihood of postoperative morbidity
- Patients with previous surgery in the area of question
- Patients with risk of future pathologic fracture or direct invasion into surrounding critical tissue
- Patients with painful, localized metastases refractory to conventional therapy

Contraindications
- Absolute
  - Uncorrectable coagulopathy
  - Active infection
  - Severe immunosuppression
  - Inability to access the target lesion safely
- Relative contraindications include:
  - Diffuse skeletal or soft tissue metastases where a systemic approach would be more appropriate
  - Location of the bone lesion (proximity to skin, surrounding critical structure, etc.)
  - Bone that cannot be cemented post RFA for stability

Equipment
- See General Equipment listed under "**Percutaneous Tumor Ablation.**"
- To access the target lesion, options include hand drills, Steinmann pins, Stryker 4200 cordless drill, and mallets/trocars. Alternatively, a bone biopsy kit may be used. Available biopsy needles include:
  - 14-G Bonopty needle
  - Laurane biopsy needle
  - 11- or 13-G Osteosite M2 bone biopsy needle

Anatomy
- Local anatomy surrounding the target lesion should be evaluated for its proximity to critical structures (i.e., major neurovascular bundles, nerve roots, spinal cord, artery of Adamkiewicz, bowel, bladder, and skin).
- Central neural structures may be better visualized with preprocedural intrathecal contrast imaging, oblique planar imaging, CT gantry angulation, or MRI.
- At least 2 cm of surrounding subcutaneous fat is advised to avoid skin burns.

Procedure
See general steps under "Percutaneous Tumor Ablation."

Procedural Considerations
- All ablation techniques may be used; however, RFA is used most commonly.
- General, epidural, or spinal anesthesia may be preferred to decrease patient movement, anxiety, and pain during the procedure.
- Bone lesions within 1 cm of a critical structure require additional precautions, such as:
  - Use of a thermocouple, which is placed adjacent to the treatment zone to monitor temperature during ablation
    - Temperature should be >45°C in RFA and laser ablation or <8°C in cryoablation.
  - Carbon dioxide pneumodissection (Fig. 6.19)
    - Instilled via a 21- or 22-G spinal needle placed between the bone lesion and adjacent vital structures
    - Depending on the lesion location, the total volume of gas injected can range from a few milliliters (in the epidural space) to almost 2 L (in the peritoneal cavity).
  - Hydrodissection (Fig. 6.20)
    - Either sterile saline or D5W with a small amount of dilute contrast added for increased visualization.
    - Not recommended with cryoablation because the fluid may freeze and increase the risk for thermal damage.
    - To prevent skin burns or frostbite during ablation of superficial lesions, a subdermal injection with sterile water or lidocaine 1% can be used for insulation.
  - Continuous neural monitoring with somatosensory evoked potentials (SSEPs)
    - Potential neural injury can be prevented if any changes in the wave parameters are detected during ablation.
- The shortest possible trajectory should be chosen when crossing normal bone.
- Vertebral bodies are accessed via an anterior approach at the cervical level, intercostopedicular approach at the thoracic level, and via a transpedicular approach at the lumbar level (Fig. 6.21).
- The sacrum is approached posteriorly (Fig. 6.22), whereas the periacetabular region is approached anterolaterally or posterolaterally to avoid the sciatic and femoral nerves.

Alternative Treatments
- Treatments for bone lesions include palliative analgesics, radiation therapy, surgery, chemotherapy, ablation (RF, MW, cryo, laser, ETOH), HIFU, arterial embolization, cementoplasty, and combination therapy.
  - Bone tumors are more sensitive to RFA, in comparison to chemotherapy and radiation therapy, because of their hypoxic state and limited blood supply.

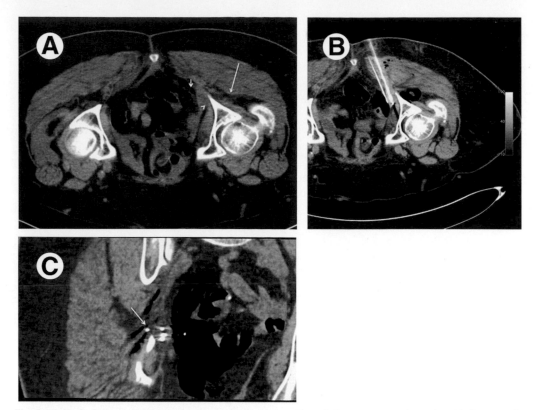

Fig. 6.19 (A–C) Carbon dioxide dissection used to displace the sciatic nerve away from the ablation zone for treatment of an ischial spine metastasis. (From Tsoumakidou G, Buy X, Garnon J, et al. Percutaneous thermal ablation: how to protect the surrounding organs. *Tech Vasc Interv Radiol.* 2011;14[3]:170–176.)

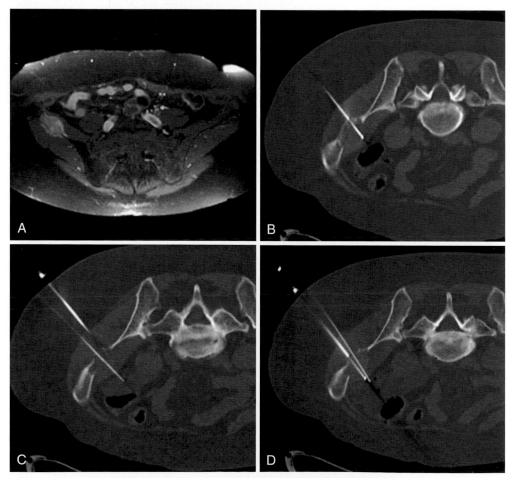

Fig. 6.20 (A–D) Hydrodissection with dextrose 5% in water to insulate and displace the colon away from the ablation zone. (Reused with permission from Tutton SM, Zvavanjanja RC, Tam AL. Musculoskeletal interventions for benign bone lesions. In: Kee ST, Murthy R, Madoff DC, eds. *Clinical Interventional Oncology.* Philadelphia: Elsevier; 2014:302–319.)

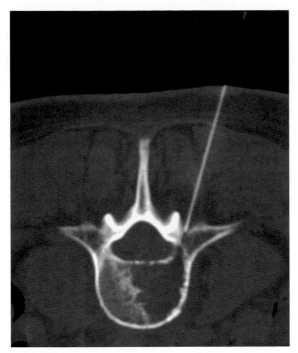

Fig. 6.21 Transpedicular Approach for Lumbar Vertebral Bodies. (Reused with permission from Shaw C, Zoga A. Percutaneous musculoskeletal biopsy. In: Kee ST, Murthy R, Madoff DC, eds. *Clinical Interventional Oncology*. Philadelphia: Elsevier; 2014: 281–301.)

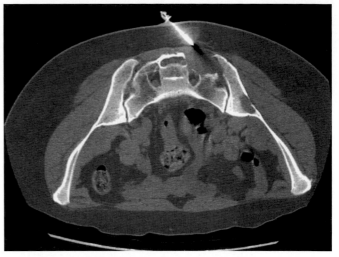

Fig. 6.22 Sacral Posterior Approach. (Reused with permission from Shaw C, Zoga A. Percutaneous musculoskeletal biopsy. In: Kee ST, Murthy R, Madoff DC, eds. *Clinical Interventional Oncology*. Philadelphia: Elsevier; 2014:281–301.)

- In addition to more commonly used ablation approaches, coblation is a new plasma-based option.
  - Uses RF energy to excite electrolytes in an electric conductive fluid (e.g., saline solution). This can cause the tumor to dissolve at low temperatures between 40°C and 70°C, resulting in minimal thermal damage to surrounding nontarget soft tissues.

- Surgery for certain lesions such as osteoblastoma
- Systemic chemotherapy for diffuse metastatic disease
- Cementoplasty, osteoplasty, or vertebroplasty
  - More often used as an adjunct after ablative techniques to provide structural support to weakened bone (Fig. 6.23)

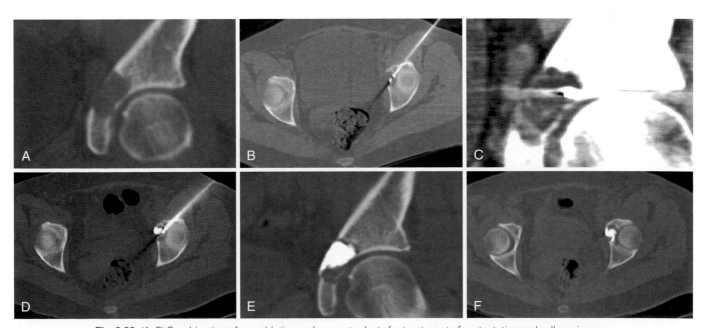

Fig. 6.23 (A–F) Combination of cryoablation and cementoplasty for treatment of metastatic renal cell carcinoma. Following cryoablation of the left acetabulum, cementoplasty was done to provide structural support of this weight-bearing region. (Reused with permission from Kurup AN, Callstrom MR. Ablation of musculoskeletal metastatic lesions including cementoplasty. In: Kee ST, Murthy R, Madoff DC, eds. *Clinical Interventional Oncology*. Philadelphia: Elsevier; 2014:320–334.)

Complications

- The following complications are paired with appropriate management:
  - Bleeding: monitoring vital signs, IV fluids, transfuse as needed
  - Radiculopathy (e.g., from leaked cement): expectant management
  - Skin burn and frostbite: treat with topical agents (e.g., silver sulfadiazine)
  - Nerve damage (e.g., weakness, paralysis, dysesthesia, or paresthesias): may require neuropathic pain medications
  - Infection of skin or bone: long-term antibiotics
  - Bowel or bladder injury (e.g., perforation, infection, or fistula): may require catheter drainage and/or surgical repair
  - Postablation edema and soft tissue inflammation: postprocedural steroids and/or supportive care
  - Pathologic fracture: surgical fixation and/or cementoplasty

PULMONARY MALIGNANCIES

CASE PRESENTATION

A 72-year-old smoker with a history of CHF and recent MI status post four-vessel CABG presents to his primary care physician with complaints of malaise, weight loss, fatigue, and pallor. He admits recent hemoptysis. CT of the chest, abdomen, and pelvis reveals a 5-cm mass involving the ascending colon and a 2-cm peripheral nodule in the right lower lobe of the lung. Biopsy of the nodule is consistent with a metastatic colorectal carcinoma. Given limited metastatic spread to a single distant organ, this patient meets criteria for stage IVa colon carcinoma. The colorectal surgeon plans for total abdominal resection of the primary colonic tumor. She has requested input from interventional radiology regarding potential treatment of the pulmonary metastasis.

Primary Malignancy

- Lung cancer is the second most common primary malignancy in both men and women and is the leading cause of cancer death in the United States.
- In 2015, lung cancer mortality was estimated to exceed 158,000 patients in the United States.
- Primary pulmonary malignances may be divided into small cell lung cancer (SCLC) and non–small cell lung cancer (NSCLC).
  - SCLC is highly malignant, often has neuroendocrine cell characteristics, and accounts for approximately 15% of all primary lung cancers.
  - NSCLC makes up the remaining 85% and is divided into three pathologic subtypes: squamous cell carcinoma, adenocarcinoma, and large cell carcinoma. Up to a third of NSCLCs are unresectable at presentation.
    - Squamous cell carcinoma was historically the most common subtype of lung cancer; it currently accounts for 20% of lung cancer cases.
    - Adenocarcinoma incidence increased greatly over the past four decades and accounts for approximately 39% of lung cancer cases.
    - Changes in long-term smoking trends are thought to account for these shifts in incidence.

> ### ►► CLINICAL POINT
>
> Bronchoalveolar carcinoma (BAC) was previously regarded as a fourth subtype of NSCLC. Adenocarcinoma in situ, minimally invasive adenocarcinoma, and invasive adenocarcinoma of the lung are revised classifications that superseded the term BAC in 2011. However, the term BAC remains in common use.

- Smoking and lung cancer
  - Smoking is well known to be the strongest modifiable risk factor for the development of lung cancer.
  - Although smoking increases the risk of all subtypes of lung cancer, the association is strongest with SCLC and squamous cell carcinoma.
  - In nonsmokers, adenocarcinoma is the most common subtype.

Lung Metastases

- The lungs are among the most common sites for solid tumor metastasis.
- Prognosis and management strategies for pulmonary metastases depend on the primary lesion type.
- Almost all types of cancers can metastasize to the lung.
- For patients with colorectal cancer metastases to the lung, RFA is a well-accepted treatment for the metastatic burden. Patient selection factors include fewer than three metastases, each no larger than 3 cm in diameter.

Indications (Fig. 6.24)

- Unresectable primary bronchopulmonary carcinoma
- Oligometastatic (<5 total metastases) pulmonary lesions
- Nonsurgical patients with primary colorectal cancer and secondary metastases
- Palliation of painful tumors locally invading into the thoracic wall or ribs
- Previous surgical resection with disease recurrence

Contraindications

- Uncorrectable coagulopathy
- Tumor invasion into the mediastinum or hilum
- Tumors located <1 cm from the trachea, main bronchi, esophagus, heart, aorta, aortic arch branches, or pulmonary arteries

Equipment

See General Equipment listed under "Percutaneous Tumor Ablation."

Anatomy

- The right lung has three lobes, divided by two fissures:
  - The horizontal (or minor) fissure divides the upper lobe from the middle lobe.

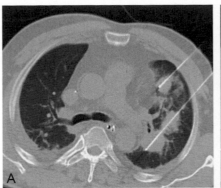 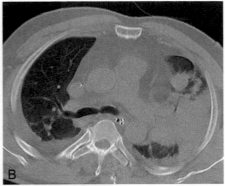

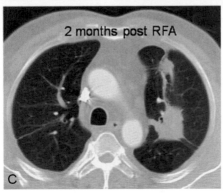

Fig. 6.24 Radiofrequency ablation of lung tumors. A) Radiofrequency ablation of two pulmonary metastases in the left upper lobe. Parenchymal hemorrhage is seen anterior to the more posterior lesion but did not preclude radiofrequency probe insertion. (B) Pulmonary hemorrhage in the left upper lobe seen immediately following ablation. (C) Follow-up CT scan 2 months after ablation demonstrates interval resolution of the parenchymal hemorrhage. (Reused with permission from Casal RF, Tam AL, Eapen GA. Clinics in Chest Medicine, Volume 31, Issue 1, 2010, Pages 151–163, Fig. 4)

- The right oblique (or major) fissure separates the upper lobe from the lower lobe superiorly and the middle lobe from the lower lobe inferiorly.
- The left lung has only two lobes:
  - The left oblique fissure separates the lung into an upper and lower lobe.
  - The lingula is a structure that is homologous to the right middle lobe.
  - The lungs have a dual vascular system:
  - Pulmonary system
    - Pulmonary arteries receive deoxygenated blood from the right ventricle.
    - Pulmonary veins return oxygenated blood to the left atrium from the lungs.
  - Bronchial system
    - Bronchial arteries are branches of the thoracic aorta that provide oxygenated blood to the lung parenchyma.
    - Bronchial veins drain to the pulmonary veins, the superior vena cava (SVC), and the azygos system.
- The pleura consists of two layers, parietal and visceral.
  - The visceral pleura is attached directly to the lung surface.

- The parietal pleura is attached to the thoracic wall, receives somatic sensory innervation, and is exquisitely sensitive.
- The intercostal spaces are commonly used for percutaneous access to lung or pleural lesions. There are three layers of intercostal muscles—external, internal, and innermost.
  - The primary neurovascular bundle is located between the internal and innermost intercostal muscles, shielded by the costal groove of the superior rib (i.e., the bundle rests along the lower border of each rib). It is comprised of, from superior to inferior, an intercostal vein, artery, and nerve at each interspace.

Procedure

- See general steps under "**Percutaneous Tumor Ablation.**"
- Procedural considerations:
  - If lesions are not easily accessible in a prone or supine position, it is preferable to oblique the patient with the unaffected (or healthier) lung in a superior position to avoid inhibiting ventilation in case of complications.

- If using an intercostal route, avoid injury to the primary intercostal neurovascular bundle, which is located along the inferior border of each rib, by puncturing above the rib.
- For tumors shielded by a rib (and therefore not amenable to intercostal access), transcostal access using a Bonopty needle can be considered.

Complications

- Pneumothoraces are common, with a reported incidence between 11% and 52%.
  - Chest tube placement is necessary in 6% to 29% of cases.
  - Delayed development of pneumothoraces is possible and occurs in approximately 10% of cases.
- Aseptic pleuritis or pleural effusion (6%–19%)
- Pulmonary hemorrhage (6%–18%)—rarely clinically significant
- Air embolism (<1%)
- Pseudoaneurysm (<1%)
- Acute interstitial pneumonitis (<1%)
- Bronchopleural fistula (<1%)
- Injury to surrounding structures—variable, dependent on tumor location

Alternative Treatments

- For primary pulmonary malignancies:
  - Stereotactic body radiotherapy (SBRT)
  - Surgical sublobar resection
  - High-dose targeted radiotherapy
- For pulmonary metastases:
  - Surgical sublobar resection

ADRENAL TUMORS

CASE PRESENTATION

A 57-year-old woman was diagnosed with locally invasive lung adenocarcinoma 4 years ago. She underwent multimodality treatment with chemoradiotherapy and subsequent lobectomy with good response. She now presents with intractable back pain and confusion. Imaging reveals multifocal disease in the brain, along with a presumed adrenal metastasis. IR has been consulted for tissue diagnosis of the adrenal lesion and ablation, if indicated.

- Adrenal masses are common and may be found incidentally in up to 8.7% of patients undergoing abdominal imaging.
- The vast majority are benign, asymptomatic lesions, colloquially described as *adrenal incidentalomas*.
- Imaging (CT with adrenal protocol or chemical shift MRI) characteristics often permit the radiologist to distinguish benign adrenal adenomas from malignancies.

Primary Neoplasms

- Adrenal tumors are best divided into functional (i.e., hormone producing) and nonfunctional lesions. Due to the unique endocrine functions of the gland, a broad spectrum of neoplasms with widely varying manifestations, prognoses, and therapeutic options may occur.

Nonfunctional Tumors

- Adrenal adenomas are the most common adrenal mass. They are benign, and no treatment is indicated.
- Primary adrenocortical carcinoma is a rare but aggressive malignancy. Up to two-thirds of cases have metastasized from the adrenal gland at the time of diagnosis. No chemotherapeutic or radiation regimen has been shown to improve survival.

Functional Tumors

- Aldosteronomas are associated with hypertension, metabolic alkalosis, and hypokalemia.
- Cortisol-secreting adenomas are the most common endogenous cause of Cushing syndrome. Manifestations include obesity, formation of abdominal striae, insulin resistance, hypertension, and depression.
- Pheochromocytomas are rare malignancies that secrete high levels of catecholamines, classically presenting with headache, anxiety, hypertension, tachycardia, and diaphoresis.

Adrenal Metastases

- The adrenal gland is the fourth most common site for tumor metastasis.
- Approximately 27% of adrenal masses found in the context of known malignancy elsewhere represent metastatic spread.
- The most common primary malignancies that metastasize to the adrenal gland are bronchogenic carcinoma, colorectal carcinoma, RCC, HCC, and malignant melanoma.

Indications

- Symptoms refractory to medical therapy
- Patients with primary or metastatic disease who refuse surgery or are poor surgical candidates due to comorbidities
- Patients with painful metastases
- Specifically for pheochromocytoma, additional indications include:
  - Palliative management of painful or life-threatening metastases
  - Palliative tumor debulking to reduce hormonal load

Contraindications

- Uncorrectable coagulopathy

Equipment

See General Equipment listed under "Percutaneous Tumor Ablation."

Anatomy

- The adrenal glands are located superoanteriorly to the kidneys.
- The right adrenal gland is posterior to and to the right of the IVC.
- The left adrenal gland is lateral to the abdominal aorta.
- Each adrenal gland has three primary feeding arteries:
  - Superior suprarenal arteries—terminal branches of the inferior phrenic arteries that arise from the abdominal aorta at the aortic hiatus
  - Middle suprarenal arteries—arise from the abdominal aorta lateral to the origin of the celiac trunk
  - Inferior suprarenal arteries—terminal branches of the renal arteries
- Venous drainage from each adrenal gland is primarily through a single suprarenal vein, which drains into the respective renal vein.

Procedure

See general steps under "Percutaneous Tumor Ablation."

Procedural Considerations

- Preprocedural planning is critical due to the proximity of the adrenal glands to vulnerable structures such as the liver, kidney, inferior vena cava, and aorta. A variety of approaches are possible (Fig. 6.25).

- Control of the extent of ablation is similarly critical due to narrow margins of safety with respect to surrounding structures.
- The possibility of hypertensive crisis in patients with pheochromocytoma should be planned for and prophylaxis—preprocedural α- and β-blockade—should be administered.
- Prophylaxis against hypertensive crisis in patients with nonpheochromocytoma adrenal tumors is controversial. Adequate intraprocedure blood pressure is usually achieved with calcium channel blockers.

Complications

- Hypertensive crisis is a complication unique to the treatment of adrenal malignancies, particularly with pheochromocytoma.
- Adrenal insufficiency
- Bleeding
- Infection
- Tumor seeding of the applicator tract

Alternative Treatments

- Surgery is preferred for all resectable adrenal malignancies.
- Medical management may provide symptomatic relief for unresectable functional tumors.
  - Mineralocorticoid receptor antagonists such as spironolactone and eplerenone may be used for aldosteronomas.
  - β-Blockers may be used for control of pheochromocytoma symptoms. α-Blockade is also an option for α-producing tumors.

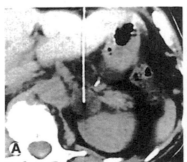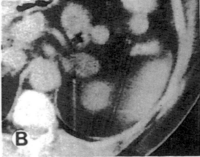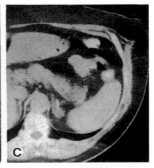

Fig. 6.25 Various Approaches to the Left Adrenal Gland Demonstrated by Computed Tomography Guidance. (A) Anterior approach. (B) Straight posterior approach obtained during exhalation in this patient with normal lungs. (C) Posterior angled approach performed in a patient with hyperexpanded emphysematous lungs. (Reused with permission from Koenker RM, Mueller PR, vanSonnenberg E. Interventional radiology of the adrenal glands. *Semin Roentgenol.* 1988;23[4]:314–322, Fig. 2.)

TAKE-HOME POINTS

Renal Cell Carcinoma
- Cryoablation and RFA have comparable outcomes to partial nephrectomy in cases of cT1 RCC.
- Renal ablation is a viable option in patients who are poor surgical candidates due to comorbidities, prior abdominal surgeries, anatomic considerations, or high likelihood of recurrence.
- Adjunctive maneuvers such as hydrodissection facilitate probe placement and decrease risk of damage to adjacent critical structures.

Hepatocellular Carcinoma
- Ablation is an accepted first-line treatment for BCLC stage 0 or stage A HCC. Ablation may be considered for tumor debulking.
- Adjunctive embolization techniques to reduce hepatic tumor perfusion (and the *heat sink effect*) may be beneficial, particularly prior to thermal ablation.

Musculoskeletal Oncology
- A variety of interventional approaches can be considered when treating bone lesions, including RFA, MWA, cryoablation, laser ablation, ETOH ablation, HIFU, embolization, and cementoplasty.
- Indications include curative treatment, palliation of pain, prevention of local tumor spread into adjacent critical structures, and as an adjuvant for surgical intervention.

- Preoperative imaging is imperative to evaluate surrounding critical structures (large vessels, bowel, or nerves), assess lesion configuration, and plan the approach.
- Carbon dioxide insulation, use of a thermocouple, hydrodissection, and SSEP monitoring offer protective measures when ablating near vital structures or neurovascular bundles.

Pulmonary Malignancies
- For primary lung cancer, ablation is reserved for early-stage NSCLC patients who are not surgical candidates.
- For patients with primary colorectal cancer metastatic to the lung, RFA is an accepted treatment modality when there are fewer than three lesions to each lung, none larger than 3.5 cm in diameter.

Adrenal Tumors
- Although resection is the standard, ablation of adrenal tumors is a viable approach in patients who are not surgical candidates.
- Hypertensive crisis is a unique complication associated with the treatment of pheochromocytomas; however, it has been reported in hyperthermic ablation of other adrenal malignancies, albeit rarely.

REVIEW QUESTIONS

1. Which of the following gases can be used during the active thawing process of cryoablation?
   a. Oxygen, nitrogen, and fluorine
   b. Xenon, radon, and boron
   c. Hydrogen, helium, and neon
   d. Argon, krypton, and chlorine
2. A 56-year-old woman presents to the emergency department with severe (right upper quadrant abdominal) pain, jaundice, and fever. On ultrasound, two hypoechoic 2-cm nodules are incidentally found in the liver parenchyma. Contrast-enhanced CT shows that these lesions exhibit early arterial enhancement with early washout with one lesion appearing to invade the portal vein. Which of the following therapies is most appropriate?
   a. Tumor ablation
   b. Surgical resection
   c. Transplant
   d. Medical therapy
   e. TACE
3. If the patient from question 2 were to receive ablation, which of the following potential complications is she at increased risk for?
   a. Ablation tract seeding
   b. Abdominal wall injury
   c. Biloma
   d. Hepatic abscess

SUGGESTED READINGS

Ahmed M, Brace CL, Lee Jr. FT, et al. Principles of and advances in percutaneous ablation. *Radiology.* 2011;258(2):351–369.

Ahmed M, Goldberg SN. Image-guided tumor ablation: basic science. In: vanSonnenberg E, McMullen W, Solbiati L, eds. *Tumor Ablation: Principles and Practice.* New York: Springer; 2005.

Brown DB, Geschwind JH, Soulen MC, et al. Society of Interventional Radiology position statement on chemoembolization of hepatic malignancies. *J Vasc Interv Radiol.* 2006;17(2 Pt 1):217–223.

Erinjeri JP, Clark TW. Cryoablation: mechanism of action and devices. *J Vasc Interv Radiol.* 2010;21(8 suppl):S187–S191.

Ethier MD, Beland MD, Mayo-Smith W. Image-guided ablation of adrenal tumors. *Tech Vasc Interv Radiol.* 2013;16(4):262–268.

Foltz G. Image-guided percutaneous ablation of hepatic malignancies. *Semin Intervent Radiol.* 2014;31(2):180–186.

Georgiades CS, Rodriguez R. Efficacy and safety of percutaneous cryoablation for stage 1A/B renal cell carcinoma: results of a prospective, single-arm, 5 year study. *Cardiovasc Intervent Radiol.* 2014;37:1494–1499.

Gervais DA, Goldberg SN, Brown DB, et al. Society of Interventional Radiology position statement on percutaneous radiofrequency ablation for the treatment of liver tumors. *J Vasc Interv Radiol.* 2009;20(7 suppl):S342–S347.

Gervais DA, McGovern FJ, Arellano RS, et al. Radiofrequency ablation of renal cell carcinoma. *AJR Am J Roentgenol.* 2005;185(1):64–80.

Medsinge A, Zajko A, Orons P, et al. A case-based approach to common embolization agents used in vascular interventional radiology. *AJR Am J Roentgenol.* 2014;203(4):699–708.

Medvid R, Ruiz A, Komotar RJ, Jagid JR, Ivan ME, Quencer RM, et al. Current applications of MRI-guided laser interstitial thermal therapy in the treatment of brain neoplasms and epilepsy: a radiologic and neurosurgical overview. *AJNR Am J Neuroradiol.* 2015;36(11):1998–2006.

Orsi F, Arnone P, Chen W, et al. High intensity focused ultrasound ablation: a new therapeutic option for solid tumors. *J Cancer Res Ther.* 2010;6(4):414–420.

Silk M, Tahour D, Srimathveeravalli G, et al. The state of irreversible electroporation in interventional oncology. *Semin Intervent Radiol.* 2014;31(2):111–117.

Smith SL, Jennings PE. Lung radiofrequency and microwave ablation: a review of indications, techniques and post-procedural imaging appearances. *Br J Radiol.* 2015;88(1046):20140598.

Tutton SM, Zvavanjanja RC, Tam AL. Musculoskeletal interventions for benign bone lesions. In: Kee S, Murthy R, Madoff DC, eds. *Clinical Interventional Oncology.* Philadelphia: Elsevier; 2014:302–319.

Thompson RH, Atwell T, Schmit G, et al. Comparison of partial nephrectomy and percutaneous ablation for cT1 renal masses. *Eur Urol.* 2015;67:252–259. https://doi.org/10.1016/j.eururo.2014.07.021.

7

Surgery

Kimberly McFarland, Vincent Gallo, Akhil Khetarpal, Nathan Cornish, James Walsh

This chapter details the intimate relationship between interventional radiology and surgery. In the context of trauma and acute care surgery, cases of gastrointestinal bleeds (GIBs), splenic artery embolization, and pelvic embolization are discussed. The transplant section details procedures typically done by the interventionalist on liver and renal transplant candidates and recipients. The vascular surgery section describes the close, often overlapping relationship between the two fields.

INTERVENTIONAL RADIOLOGY AND VASCULAR SURGERY

- Endovascular treatment of vascular disease is based on the principle of angiography with or without intervention. This includes:
  - Angiography solely for diagnostic purposes
  - Angiography followed by endovascular treatment
  - Angiography followed by open surgical treatment
- Multiple major disease processes have overlap between interventional radiology (IR) and vascular surgery
  - Peripheral arterial disease (PAD): acute and chronic limb ischemia
  - Aortic disease: aortic dissections and abdominal/thoracic aortic aneurysms
  - Venous disease: venous insufficiency and deep venous thrombosis
  - Renal disease: arteriovenous fistula/graft evaluation and intervention
- Patients with significant vascular disease often have multiple associated medical comorbidities that the interventionalist must be comfortable recognizing and managing. This includes:
  - Coronary artery disease (CAD)
  - Hyperlipidemia
  - Diabetes
  - Hypertension
  - Renal failure
  - Hyper- and hypocoagulopathic states
  - Genetic collagen abnormalities (e.g., Marfan disease and Ehlers-Danlos syndrome)
  - Smoking
- Practitioners in both fields are adept at percutaneous access and closure. Vascular surgeons can perform a femoral artery cutdown when necessary.

- *Cutdown* describes open surgical exposure of the femoral artery with direct puncture and/or closure.
- Certain risk factors may make a femoral artery cutdown necessary, including
  - Densely calcified or femoral arteries of very small caliber
  - Severe aortic or iliac kinking
  - Excessive groin scarring
  - Obesity

Outpatient Workup of Vascular Disease
Physical Exam Principles
- Examination of the extremities for discoloration, ulcerations, and gangrene
- Palpation of peripheral pulses
  - Systematic evaluation of radial, femoral, popliteal, dorsalis pedis, and posterior tibial pulses
- Palpation and auscultation of the abdominal aorta to examine for bruits and aneurysm
- Auscultation of the carotid arteries to examine for bruits

Noninvasive Vascular Testing
- Noninvasive imaging includes duplex ultrasound, computed tomography angiography (CTA), and magnetic resonance angiography (MRA).

Doppler Examination
- Doppler probe placed over the vessel of interest
- Triphasic flow
  - Seen in normal peripheral arteries
  - Composed of three signal components—forward flow in systole, early reversal of flow in diastole, and late forward flow in diastole
- Biphasic flow
  - Seen in normal carotid arteries and early PAD
  - Composed of two signal components—forward systolic flow and forward diastolic flow
- Monophasic flow
  - Usually seen in vessels with significant stenosis
  - Composed of one signal component—forward systolic flow

Ankle-Brachial Index

- Steps:
  1. Doppler signal is identified in the ankle of the lower extremity being evaluated.
  2. Blood pressure cuff placed around the calf is inflated until the Doppler signal disappears and then deflated until the signal returns. The pressure at which the signal returns is recorded.
  3. Brachial artery pulse is auscultated.
  4. Blood pressure cuff placed around the upper arm is inflated until the pulse disappears and then deflated until the pulse returns. The pressure at which signal returns is recorded. Both arms are tested, and the highest value is used.
  5. Ankle-brachial index (ABI) = result of step 2/result of step 4.
- ABI greater than 1.4 suggests noncompressible arteries as seen with severe atherosclerotic disease.
- ABI between 0.9 and 1.4 is normal.
- ABI between 0.4 and 0.9 suggests chronic claudication.
- ABI less than 0.4 is concerning for critical limb ischemia.

Commonly Encountered Medications

- It is vitally important to understand the mechanism, metabolism, and clearance of common anticoagulants and antiplatelet agents.
- Anticoagulants include
  - Warfarin (Coumadin)
    - Mechanism: inhibits vitamin K epoxide reductase
    - Metabolism: hepatic
    - Clearance: predominantly renal
  - Enoxaparin (Lovenox)
    - Mechanism: inhibits factor Xa
    - Metabolism: hepatic
    - Clearance: predominantly renal
  - Dabigatran (Pradaxa)
    - Mechanism: inhibits factor IIa
    - Metabolism: hepatic
    - Clearance: 80% renal, 20% gastrointestinal
  - Rivaroxaban (Xarelto)
    - Mechanism: inhibits factor Xa
    - Metabolism: hepatic
    - Clearance: 66% renal, 33% gastrointestinal
  - Apixaban (Eliquis)
    - Mechanism: inhibits factor Xa
    - Metabolism: hepatic
    - Clearance: 27% renal, 63% gastrointestinal
- Antiplatelet agents include
  - Clopidrogel (Plavix)
    - Mechanism: prevents binding of adenosine diphosphate to the platelet P2Y12 receptor, which interferes with the glycoprotein GPIIb/IIIa complex and thus inhibits platelet aggregation
    - Metabolism: hepatic
    - Clearance: 50% renal, 46% gastrointestinal
  - Aspirin
    - Mechanism: blocks formation of thromboxane A2 and thus inhibits platelet aggregation
    - Metabolism: hepatic
    - Clearance: predominantly renal

INTERVENTIONAL RADIOLOGY AND TRANSPLANT SURGERY

- The care of complex transplant patients involves a multidisciplinary team, including the medical subspecialty (nephrology, hepatology, pulmonology, etc.), surgical subspecialty (urology, liver transplant surgery, cardiothoracic surgery, etc.), immunology, infectious disease, and, of course, IR.
- Kidneys are the most common transplanted organs worldwide, followed by the liver, heart, lungs, pancreas, and intestine.
- Advancements in endovascular and minimally invasive therapy have played a significant role in the management of transplant patients and their outcomes. The varied role of the interventionalist in the care of transplant patients includes
  - Preprocedural management and risk stratification
  - Therapeutic techniques prior to transplant surgery
  - Providing pre- and postoperative diagnostic imaging
  - Diagnosing organ failure and transplant rejection by biopsy
  - Managing postoperative complications

LIVER TRANSPLANTATION

- The etiology of liver failure includes
  - **Hepatocellular** causes, such as chronic hepatitis C (the most common cause) or hepatitis B virus (HBV); hepatocellular carcinoma; and cryptogenic, autoimmune, alcoholic, metabolic, or fulminant cirrhosis
  - **Biliary** causes such as primary sclerosing cholangitis and primary biliary cirrhosis
- The general indication for transplantation is a qualified patient with acute or chronic liver disease that cannot sustain a normal quality of life and/or has life-threatening complications.
  - Qualifications include having a strong social support network, pledging to abstain from alcohol and drugs, and having suitable surgical anatomy.

> ◎ **KEY DEFINITIONS**
>
> - **Acute liver failure (ALF)** is the development of severe acute liver injury with encephalopathy and impaired synthetic function (international normalized ratio [INR] of ≥1.5) in a patient without preexisting liver disease.
> - **Fulminant hepatic failure** is ALF and encephalopathy within 8 weeks of the initial development of symptoms.

- Absolute contraindications to surgery include spontaneous bacterial peritonitis or another active infection, advanced cardiopulmonary disease, incurable extrahepatic malignancy, intrahepatic cholangiocarcinoma, and AIDS.

- Relative contraindications include chronic kidney disease (CKD; may be a candidate for combined transplant), portal vein thrombosis, multisystem organ failure, and medication-resistant HBV cirrhosis.
- The Milan Criteria determine the need for transplantation in patients with hepatocellular carcinoma.
  - Either a single lesion up to 5 cm or two to three lesions up to 3 cm
  - No vascular invasion and extrahepatic spread
- Diagnostic imaging allows for improved candidate selection and a reduction in operative complications rates.
  - Imaging should assess the parenchyma, biliary tree, and vasculature to ensure that there are no anatomic barriers to transplantation.
  - Potential modalities include:
    - Doppler ultrasound
    - Hepatic-protocol computed tomography (CT) with intravenous contrast
    - Magnetic resonance imaging (MRI)
    - CTA/MRA to assess the vasculature
    - Magnetic resonance cholangiopancreatography (MRCP) to assess biliary anatomy

Model for Scoring End-Stage Liver Disease (MELD)

- The main scoring system used for determining liver transplantation candidates
  - Prioritizes patients on the transplant list based on disease severity and mortality risk.
  - Predicts mortality following transjugular intrahepatic portosystemic shunt (TIPS) placement.
  - Has predictive value for outcomes in patients with cirrhosis undergoing procedures other than transplantation.
- Uses three laboratory values to prognosticate outcomes in patients with cirrhosis—INR, serum creatinine, and total serum bilirubin.
  - Some conditions impair survival but are not accounted for in the model for end-stage liver disease (MELD) calculation. The following conditions are eligible for additional points, termed *MELD exception points*:
    - Hepatocellular carcinoma (HCC)
    - Hepatopulmonary syndrome
    - Familial amyloidosis
    - Primary hyperoxaluria
    - Cystic fibrosis
    - Hilar cholangiocarcinoma
    - Hepatic artery thrombosis
- Transplant evaluation is initiated when the MELD score is greater than 10. This allows sufficient time for a complete evaluation and for interventions to address relative contraindications prior to the development of end-stage disease. Patients are candidates for transplants with MELD scores of 15 or greater.

SURGICAL TECHNIQUES IN SOLID ORGAN TRANSPLANTATION

Liver Transplantation Types

- Living donor liver transplant (LDLT):
  - A living donor donates a portion of his or her liver to the transplant recipient.
  - This accounts for only 10% of liver transplants in adults; recipients usually have an urgent need.
  - The most common technique is a left lateral hepatectomy where segments II and III of the liver are resected.
- Split liver transplant (SLT):
  - A donor liver from a deceased adult is divided between a pediatric recipient and an adult recipient. This originated as a solution to a limited donor pool.
  - The most common technique is the left lateral split performed at the falciform ligament.
    - Segments I and IV through VIII are used in the adult.
    - Segments II and III are used in the child.
- Orthotopic liver transplant (OLT):
  - The most common type of transplantation
  - A liver from a deceased donor is transplanted into its normal position in the body of the recipient.

Anastomoses

Inferior Vena Cava Anastomosis: Two Techniques

- Classic technique
  - The donor's inferior vena cava (IVC) is anastomosed to the recipient's suprahepatic and infrahepatic IVC, maintaining the normal anatomic relationship and angulation.
- Piggyback technique (Fig. 7.1)
  - The donor's IVC is anastomosed to the side of the recipient's IVC.
  - This may produce an acute takeoff of the hepatic vein from the IVC, making catheterization more difficult for future interventional procedures.
  - Reasons for the piggyback technique:

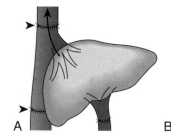
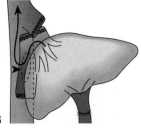

Fig. 7.1 (A) Classic technique. The recipient's inferior vena cava (IVC) is resected and replaced with the donor IVC, retaining the anatomic relationships. (B) Piggyback technique. The recipient's IVC is retained and the donor's IVC is sutured to the side of the recipient's IVC in the location of the native hepatic veins. Curved arrows indicate hepatic venous flow. (Modified from Kaufman JA, Bromley PJ. Portal and hepatic veins. In: Kaufman JA, Lee MJ, eds. *Vascular and Interventional Radiology: The Requisites.* 2nd ed. Philadelphia: Elsevier; 2014.)

- It minimizes hemodynamic disturbances during the procedure.
- It decreases warm ischemia time, as only one caval anastomosis is needed.
- There is less blood loss and a decreased need for retroperitoneal dissection.
- It allows for adjustment of vessel size between the donor and recipient.

> **◎ KEY DEFINITION**
>
> **Warm ischemia time** is the time the organ remains at body temperature after its blood supply is cut off until it is cooled or reconnected to a blood supply.

Portal Anastomosis

- Usually an end-to-end recipient-to-donor portal vein anastomosis

Hepatic Artery Anastomosis: Two Techniques

- End-to-end anastomosis
  - Donor to recipient hepatic artery anastomosis
- Aortic conduit
  - The donor iliac artery is used as an interposition graft.
  - Done when there is a history of arterial disease in the recipient's hepatic artery or celiac trunk.

Biliary Anastomosis—Two Techniques

- Duct-to-duct anastomosis (choledochocholedochostomy)
  - Preferred and most widely used technique
- Roux-en-Y hepaticojejunostomy (hepatic duct anastomosed to the jejunum) or choledochojejunostomy (common bile duct anastomosed to the jejunum); performed if
  - The bile duct in the donor and/or recipient is too short.
  - There is a severe mismatch in size between the common bile ducts of the donor and recipient.
  - There is disease of the extrahepatic bile ducts, biliary atresia, or bile duct injury.

Recognizing the Signs and Symptoms of Transplant Rejection

- Routine laboratory surveillance should be performed.
- Signs of liver/graft failure must be watched for, including:
  - Increasing scores on liver function tests (LFTs)

- Hepatocyte damage (ALT, AST)
- Cholestasis (ALP, GGT, bilirubin)
- Synthetic function (albumin, protein, INR)
- Symptoms of liver/graft failure
  - Jaundice, abdominal pain, and ascites
- If there are signs of rejection/failure
  - Obtain imaging beginning with (1) an ultrasound, (2) CT and MRI scans, and (3) angiography.
  - Obtain an organ biopsy, which is the gold standard for diagnosis.

Vascular Complications After Liver Transplantation

- Up to 15% of liver transplant recipients develop vascular complications, including bleeding, stenosis, and thrombosis.
- Hepatic artery thrombosis (HAT) and portal vein thrombosis are the most common vascular complications overall.
- HAT has a high mortality rate (33%) and can lead to graft loss and the need for retransplantation.
  - HAT is often preceded by hepatic artery stenosis (Fig. 7.2).
- Stenoses typically occur at the sites of anastomoses, as described earlier.
- Causes of vascular complications include:
  - Surgical error or injury to the artery during anastomosis
  - Kinking of the anastomosis
  - Extrinsic compression on the artery
  - Dissection of the vessel
  - Transplant rejection
  - Differences in diameter between the donor and recipient vessels
  - Intimal hyperplasia and fibrosis (late complication)
- Clinical presentation of vascular compromise:
  - Can be asymptomatic or suspected by abnormal LFTs.
  - Portal vein stenosis may present with symptoms of portal hypertension, such as ascites, variceal bleeding, and splenomegaly.
  - Occlusion of the IVC and hepatic vein can present with renal dysfunction and lower extremity swelling.
  - The biliary tree is almost completely dependent on flow through the hepatic artery. Compromise of this flow can lead to severe consequences, including:
    - Biliary ischemia, biliary stricture, biliary necrosis, biloma formation, fulminant hepatic failure, and bacteremia

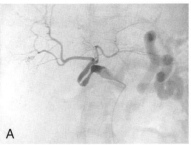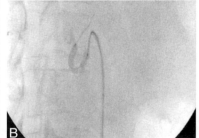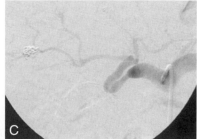

Fig. 7.2 Digital Subtraction Angiogram Demonstrating Hepatic Artery Stenosis (A) Surgical anastomosis treated (B) with balloon angioplasty. (C) Digital subtraction angiogram after angioplasty showing a widely patent hepatic artery. (Courtesy Dr. James Walsh, Kings County Hospital, Brooklyn, NY.)

Diagnostic Imaging of Vascular Complications

- Doppler ultrasound is typically the first-line choice.
- CTA or MRA may also be used.
- If the noninvasive studies mentioned earlier are equivocal, catheter angiography can be performed. This is the gold standard and has an added benefit of making it possible to perform therapeutic interventions at the same time as determining the diagnosis.
- Tissue biopsy is the gold standard for the evaluation of transplant rejection and should be obtained after imaging.

Treatment of Vascular Complications

- Surgical exploration with anastomotic revision and open thrombectomy to remove clots
- Endovascular intervention
  - Thrombolysis to dissolve clots
  - Angioplasty to treat stenosis
  - Stent placement for cases refractory to angioplasty
- Systemic anticoagulation for thrombosis
- Retransplantation

Biliary Complications After Liver Transplantation

- These occur in 5% to 30% of patients after liver transplantation. Graft loss can occur in 3% to 12% of these patients.
- Complications include:
  - Biliary strictures (most common)
  - Bile leaks
  - Biloma formation
  - Sphincter of Oddi dysfunction
  - Stone and sludge formation in the biliary tree
- Causes of complications:
  - Surgical error or technique, such as kinking or narrowing at the anastomosis
  - Compromise to the arterial blood supply
- Clinical presentation and imaging evaluation:
  - Asymptomatic or with jaundice, raised scores on LFTs, abdominal pain, fever, and/or cholangitis
  - An ultrasound or CTA of the abdomen should be obtained to rule out arterial complications
  - MRCP, which may show dilation of the biliary duct, is the imaging modality of choice for biliary complications.
  - Liver biopsy may show histology consistent with cholestasis due to biliary obstruction.
- Treatment of biliary complications:
  - Endoscopic retrograde cholangiopancreatography (ERCP)-guided drainage, which is both diagnostic and therapeutic (Figs. 7.3 and 7.4)
  - Percutaneous transhepatic biliary drainage (PTBD)
  - Transhepatic catheter placement and balloon angioplasty to widen strictures
  - Surgical drainage/revision

Related Therapies Offered by Interventional Radiography

These procedures are discussed in detail in other chapters.

- **Transcatheter arterial chemoembolization (TACE)** may be performed in cases of large unresectable HCCs or in patients awaiting transplant to reduce tumor progression.

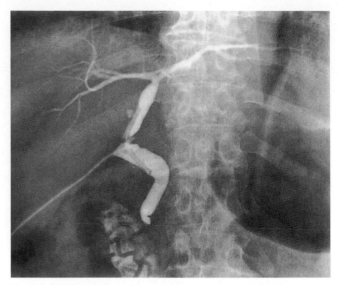

Fig. 7.3 Cholangiogram Showing an Anastomotic Stricture in the Common Bile Duct (From Gomes AS. Radiological evaluation in transplantation. In: Busuttil RW, Klintmalm GBG, eds. *Transplantation of the Liver*. 3rd ed. Philadelphia: Elsevier; 2015:455–477.)

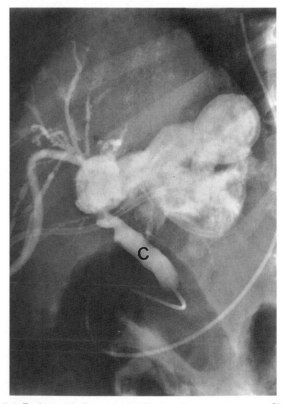

Fig. 7.4 Endoscopic Retrograde Cholangiopancreatogram Shows Filling of the Common Bile Duct and Right Biliary Ducts The left biliary ducts are in communication with a large biloma. (From Gomes AS. Radiological evaluation in transplantation. In: Busuttil RW, Klintmalm GBG, eds. *Transplantation of the Liver*. 3rd ed. Philadelphia: Elsevier; 2015:455–477.)

- **Radiofrequency ablation (RFA)** may be used to ablate small liver tumors in patients who do not meet resectability criteria or who are on the waiting list for transplant to prevent tumor progression.

- **Yttrium-90 radioembolization** can induce tumor necrosis in patients with unresectable tumors, most commonly HCCs.
- **Paracentesis** is performed to relieve abdominal pressure from ascites and for the removal of fluid that precludes percutaneous procedures.
- **TIPS** is performed to relieve portal pressure in cirrhosis (both in liver failure and posttransplant patients) that would otherwise cause life-threatening variceal bleeding.

KIDNEY TRANSPLANTATION

- The most common causes of end-stage renal disease in adult patients awaiting transplant are:
  - Diabetes > hypertension > glomerulonephritis > other or unknown causes > polycystic kidney disease
- Indications for transplantation are:
  - CKD
  - Renal tumors

> ◎ **KEY DEFINITION**
>
> Chronic kidney disease requires the presence of kidney damage or decreased kidney function for 3 or more months irrespective of the cause.

- Contraindications to transplantation:
  - Absolute
    - Metastatic cancer
    - Reversible renal failure
    - Low life expectancy despite transplant
    - Serious cardiac or peripheral vascular disease
    - Hepatic insufficiency, although such patients may be candidates for combined liver-kidney transplantation
  - Relative
    - Malnutrition
    - Primary hyperoxaluria
    - Active systemic diseases that may have caused kidney failure
    - Systemic amyloidosis
  - HIV is not a contraindication as long as certain criteria are met.
- Potential transplant patients are risk-stratified according to CKD stage, which is based on the glomerular filtration rate (GFR) (Table 7.1).

TABLE 7.1 Stages of Chronic Kidney Disease With Glomerular Filtration Rate

CKD Stage	GFR (mL/min/1.73 m^2)
1	$\geq$90
2	60–89
3a	45–59
3b	30–44
4	15–29
5	<15 or on dialysis

CKD, Chronic kidney disease; *GFR*, glomerular filtration rate.

- Mortality increases as GFR declines.
- Estimated GFR below 30 mL/min/1.73 m^2 is the accepted cutoff for referral for transplantation.
- Preoperative imaging allows for the evaluation of the renal vasculature, parenchyma, potential masses, stones, and ureteral anatomy. Imaging should ensure that there are no anatomic barriers to transplantation.
- Imaging modalities include:
  - Doppler ultrasound
  - CT without contrast
  - CTA
- Renal anatomy overview (Fig. 7.5)

Surgical Technique for Renal Transplantation

- Combines elements of both vascular surgery and urology.
- The transplanted kidney is placed in the right or left iliac fossa; native kidneys are typically left in situ unless they are causing mass effect or physical discomfort.
- Typically this procedure involves an end-to-side anastomosis between the transplanted renal artery and native right external iliac artery and transplanted renal vein and native right external iliac vein (Fig. 7.6).
- Urinary tract reconstruction, termed *ureteroneocystostomy*, is the surgical transplantation of the transplanted ureter into a new site in the bladder.
- Signs of transplant rejection:
  - Increasing creatinine and proteinuria
  - Decreased urine output
  - Hematuria
  - Increased blood pressure
  - Increase in weight or ankle swelling
- If there are signs of rejection/failure: not

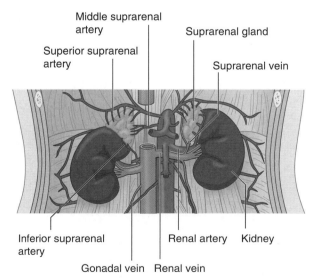

Fig. 7.5 Vascular Anatomy of the Human Kidney Note that the renal artery arises from the aorta and the renal vein from the inferior vena cava. (From Moses KP, Banks JC, Nava PB, et al. Abdominal organs. In: Moses, Nava, Banks, and Petersen, *Atlas of Clinical Gross Anatomy.* 2nd ed. Philadelphia: Elsevier; 2013: 418–431.)

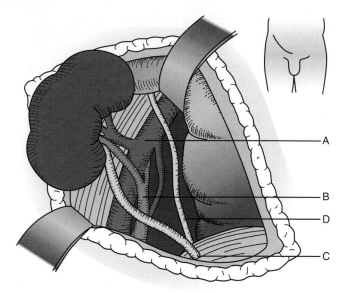

Fig. 7.6 Basic Surgical Vascular Anatomy of a Right-Lower-Quadrant Kidney Transplant (A) External iliac artery anastomosed end to side with the renal artery. (B) External iliac vein anastomosed end to side with the renal vein. (C) Implanted donor ureter. (D) Native ureter. (From Lenihan CR, Busque S, Tan JC. Clinical management of the adult kidney transplant recipient. In: Skorecki K, Chertow GM, Marsden PA, et al., eds. *Brenner and Rector's The Kidney.* 10th ed. Philadelphia: Elsevier; 2016:2251–2292.)

- Imaging should be obtained, beginning with an ultrasound. Then CT, MRI, or angiography can be obtained as indicated.
- Consider renal biopsy, which is the gold standard for diagnosis.

Related Therapies Offered by Interventional Radiology

- **Radiofrequency ablation** can ablate small renal tumors in patients who do not meet resectability criteria or to prevent tumor progression in patients who are on the transplant waiting list.

INTERVENTIONAL RADIOLOGY, TRAUMA, AND LOWER GASTROINTESTINAL BLEEDS

CASE PRESENTATION

An 81-year-old female with dementia was admitted for bright red blood per rectum (BRBPR) with clinical suspicion for a lower gastrointestinal bleed (GIB). She was found to have a hemoglobin of 7.0 mg/dL. Upper endoscopy and colonoscopy were negative. The patient was initially treated conservatively and responded appropriately to blood transfusions as her hemoglobin increased to 10.0 after three units of packed red blood cells. On hospital day 2, the patient had a large amount of BRBPR; repeat hemoglobin was 7.2, and she was tachycardic. Interventional radiology was consulted for an emergent pelvic angiogram for presumed acute lower GIB.

- Embolotherapy for a GIB was first performed in 1974 by Joseph Bookstein, who used an autogenous clot to stop a bleed.
  - In 1975, Cesare Gianturco described the first coil embolization for a GIB.
- Arterial GIBs can be divided into two location-based categories—upper and lower.
  - Upper GIBs (UGIB) occur proximal to the duodenojejunal junction (ligament of Treitz).
  - Lower GIBs (LGIB) include any bleed distal to the ligament of Treitz.
- Causes of LGIBs include but are not limited to diverticular disease, inflammatory bowel disease, coagulopathy, malignant neoplasms, hemorrhoids, and arteriovenous malformations.
- The incidence of LGIB increases markedly with age. Mortality is greatest in patients 70 years of age and older, those with intestinal ischemia, and those with multiple comorbidities.
- The role of IR in an LGIB is to isolate the site of bleeding using arteriography and to get as close to the bleed as possible using a superselective catheter to avoid nonselective embolization (which leads to bowel ischemia).
- The choice of embolic agents is multifactorial. Considerations include the size of the artery and whether embolization is permanent or temporary.
- Commonly used embolic agents include microcoils, Gelfoam, polyvinyl alcohol, and Embospheres.
- For a hemodynamically stable patient with a GIB, noninvasive imaging should be used to try to identify the location of the bleed.
  - The type of imaging study to be used often depends on what is available at a given hospital and on the suspected rate of bleeding.
    - A radionuclide 99mTc-tagged reb blood cell (RBC) scan (most sensitive) can identify active bleeds with a rate as low as 0.1 mL/min.
    - CTA can identify active bleeds with rates of 0.5 to 1.0 mL/min.
    - Catheter angiography can detect bleeding rates as low as 0.5 mL/min.
  - Given the often intermittent course of bleeds, it is best, if possible, to image the patient when he or she is actively bleeding in order to avoid a false-negative study.

Indications

- Acute GIBs that fail medical treatment (defined as the requirement of more than 2 units packed red blood cells [PRBCs] within 24 hours or a drop in hemoglobin by at least 2 g/dL) and are not amenable to endoscopic/colonoscopic intervention (most often because the bleed is not visualized) are candidates for IR intervention.
- Since most GIBs are intermittent, they are often difficult to visualize.
  - In some cases, repeat endoscopy/colonoscopy is warranted.

- However, after one failed attempt by the GI service, it is appropriate to consider angiography as clinically indicated.

Contraindications

- The only absolute contraindication is the acutely unstable patient.
  - Aggressive resuscitation and/or surgery are appropriate options in these patients.
- Relative contraindications include contrast allergy, renal impairment, uncorrectable coagulopathy, an uncooperative patient, and a pregnant patient.

Equipment

- Micropuncture set
- 5-Fr sheath and J-wire
- Multiple catheter options (e.g., Contra 2 catheter) and a variety of microcatheters
- A 0.035-inch guidewire

- Choice of embolic agent between microcoils, Gelfoam, polyvinyl alcohol, and Embospheres

Anatomy

- For LGIB arteriograms, the common femoral artery (CFA) is typically accessed at the level of the femoral head.
- For LGIBs, the two most important branches of the abdominal aorta to investigate are the **superior mesenteric artery** (SMA) and the **inferior mesenteric artery** (IMA) (Fig. 7.7). The SMA perfuses the small bowel, ascending colon, and part of the transverse colon, whereas the IMA perfuses the colon from the splenic flexure to the anus.
  - Most LGIBs occur in third-order branches off of the SMA or IMA (see Fig. 7.7).
    - Multiple arteriograms are often required to isolate the actively bleeding artery. In these cases, a previously performed CTA can be helpful in guiding the interventionalist to the likely area of bleeding.

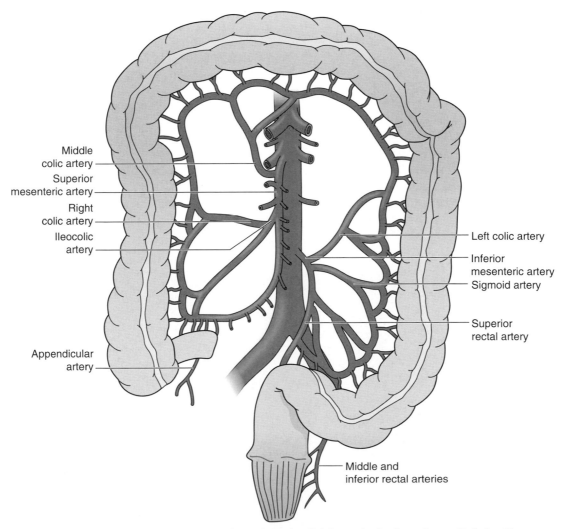

Fig. 7.7 The Arterial Blood Supply to the Large Intestine Originates in the Superior and Inferior Mesenteric Arteries The superior mesenteric artery feeds branches supplying the right and transverse segments of the large intestine. The inferior mesenteric artery branches supply the left colonic structures and rectum. (Reused with permission from Buchberg BS, Mills SD. Surgical management of colon cancer. In: Bailey RH, Billingham RP, Stamos MJ, et al., eds. *Colorectal Surgery.* Philadelphia: Elsevier; 2013: F15-3.)

- Variant anatomy can lead to variant perfusion patterns. One must first be familiar with normal anatomy in order to identify abnormal anatomy. Variant anatomy is often seen when there has been previous arterial occlusion resulting in the formation of collateral arteries.

◎ LITERATURE REVIEW

A 1988 cadaveric study by Nelson and colleagues found that "normal" vascular anatomy of the celiac artery, SMA, and IMA was present only 22%, 24%, and 16% of the time, respectively.

Procedural Steps

- Two approaches for arterial access can be considered
  - Femoral artery—most common
  - Radial artery—involves an easier recovery for the patient but is often not the best option, given a longer path to the target vessels
1. After injecting lidocaine in the area, gain femoral artery access in the mid-CFA using ultrasound and a standard access kit.
2. Insert a J-wire up to the level of the iliac artery to ensure that you do not lose access.
3. Remove the needle and apply pressure to the artery to minimize blood loss as you insert a dilator over the guidewire.
4. Exchange the dilator for a 5-Fr sheath, and exchange the J-wire for a 0.035-inch guidewire.
5. Insert a floppy guidewire into the desired catheter, and advance it through the sheath under fluoroscopic guidance.
6. Remove the wire, and attach a contrast-filled syringe to the catheter, injecting under fluoroscopy in order to identify the desired aortic branch. Perform multiple runs until the anatomy is well visualized. Ensure visualization of both the SMA and IMA.
7. If you identify active extravasation, termed *blush*, proceed with superselection of the desired artery using a microcatheter. Fig. 7.8B shows active extravasation arising from a small branch of the right colic artery supplying the ascending colon. For comparison, Fig. 7.8A is a negative SMA angiogram.
8. Once the bleeding artery has been selected, embolize it according to operator preference.
9. Confirm stasis of the vessel with a final injection of contrast.
10. Remove the wire and catheter.
11. Remove the sheath and apply manual pressure for at least 15 minutes or use an arterial closure device.

Treatment Alternatives

- Conservative medical management such as blood transfusions, stopping/reversing anticoagulation
- Endoscopy/colonoscopy
- Surgical intervention, likely to result in a hemi- or total colectomy

Complications

- Nontarget embolization resulting in colonic ischemia
- Puncture-related complications
  - Retroperitoneal hemorrhage from an excessively high femoral artery puncture
  - Groin hematoma from suboptimal manual compression of femoral artery
  - Pseudoaneurysm of the femoral artery from a low puncture site
- Acute renal failure from contrast-induced nephropathy
- Allergic reaction to iodinated contrast

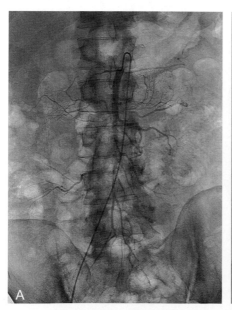 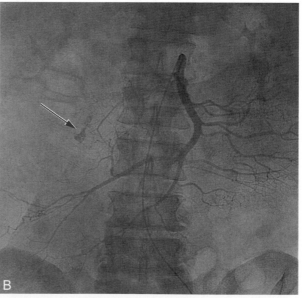

Fig. 7.8 Superior Mesenteric Artery Angiograms (A) Negative superior mesenteric artery (SMA) angiogram. (B) Positive SMA angiogram. (Courtesy Dr. James Walsh, Kings County Hospital, Brooklyn, NY.)

UPPER GASTROINTESTINAL BLEEDS

CASE PRESENTATION

A 53-year-old lawyer is brought to the emergency department after three episodes of hematemesis. His vital signs are stable. A gastroenterologist performs an endoscopy and places multiple hemoclips on an actively oozing duodenal ulcer, which results in stasis. The following day the patient has massive hematemesis, at which point IR is consulted for possible embolization.

- By definition, UGIBs arise anywhere proximal to the ligament of Treitz—namely, the esophagus, stomach, and portions of the duodenum.
- The most common cause of a UGIB is a duodenal ulcer. Other common etiologies include gastric ulcers and gastric/esophageal varices. Less common causes include, but are not limited to, Mallory-Weiss tears, esophagitis, angiodysplasias, and aortoenteric fistulas.
- UGIBs are five times more common than LGIBs.
- The goal of IR intervention in a UGIB is to isolate the site of active bleeding and embolize as proximal to the bleed as possible to avoid nontarget embolizations.
- As with LGIBs, the choice of embolic agents is multifactorial. The options for embolic agents are the same as those for LGIBs.

Indications

- A hemodynamically stable patient with a UGIB in which endoscopy was negative

- A patient with continued bleeding despite recent endoscopic intervention

Contraindications

- An acutely unstable patient
  - Aggressive resuscitation and/or surgery are appropriate options in such patients.
- The same relative contraindications as in LGIBs

Equipment

- The same equipment as in LGIBs

Anatomy

- The upper GI tract is fed by a well-collateralized blood supply from the celiac axis and SMA.
- Given the presence of extensive collaterals, embolization of the upper GI tract rarely results in ischemic injury. Conversely, embolization may fail secondary to this robust collateral network.

CLINICAL POINT

Upper gastrointestinal bleeds occurring proximal to the ampulla of Vater (union of the pancreatic and common bile ducts) can be visualized and potentially treated with upper endoscopy.

Celiac Axis Anatomy

- For a suspected UGIB, the celiac axis and SMA are the most important branches to investigate.
- The celiac trunk branches (Fig. 7.9) off the abdominal aorta at T12, just inferior to the diaphragm.

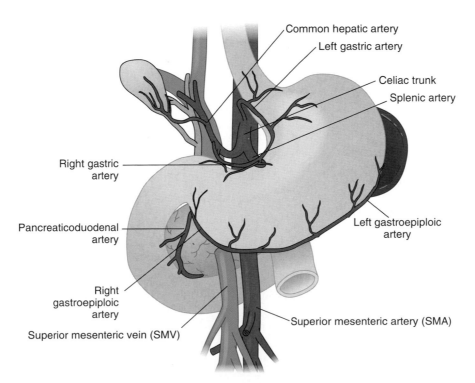

Fig. 7.9 The Blood Supply of the Stomach *SMA,* **Superior mesenteric artery**. (Reused with permission from Vikram R, Patnana M, Devine C, et al. *Gastric Carcinoma in Oncologic Imaging* (edited by Silverman PM). Philadelphia: Elsevier; 2012: F15-1.)

TABLE 7.2   Celiac Axis—Anatomy and Variants

Arterial Variant	Frequency (%)
"Normal" configuration—left gastric artery (LGA), common hepatic artery (CHA), and splenic artery (SA) originating off the celiac artery	85
LGA, CHA, SA, and dorsal pancreatic artery originating off the celiac artery	10
Only the LGA and SA originating off the celiac artery	3
LGA originating off the aorta	2

- The celiac artery typically branches into the left gastric, common hepatic, and splenic arteries, although variants in this branching pattern are common (Table 7.2).
  - The left gastric artery supplies the stomach.
  - Through collaterals, the gastroduodenal artery (GDA), which arises from the common hepatic artery, also supplies the stomach as well as the proximal duodenum.

Procedural Steps

1. Gain femoral or radial artery access.
2. Assuming femoral access, insert a J-wire up to the level of the iliac artery to ensure that you do not lose access.
3. Remove the needle and apply pressure to the artery to minimize blood loss as you insert a dilator over the guidewire.
4. Exchange the dilator for a 5-Fr sheath, and exchange the J-wire for a 0.035-inch guidewire.
5. Insert a floppy guidewire into the desired catheter, and advance it through the sheath under fluoroscopic guidance.
6. Remove the guidewire, and identify the desired aortic branch under fluoroscopy by injecting contrast. Perform multiple runs until the anatomy is well visualized. For UGIBs, ensure visualization of the left gastric artery, SMA, and GDA.
7. If you identify active extravasation, proceed with superselection of the artery using a microcatheter if needed.
8. Embolize the bleeder with your preferred embolic agent.
9. Confirm stasis of the vessel with a final contrast injection.
10. Remove all wires and catheters.
11. Remove the sheath and apply manual pressure for at least 15 minutes or use a closure device.

Treatment Alternatives

- Emergent surgery is indicated in an unstable patient.
- Conservative medical management, such as blood transfusions, and stopping/reversing anticoagulation.
- Endoscopy (clipping with or without cauterization).
- If the patient has extensive varices secondary to cirrhosis and portal hypertension, he or she might be a candidate for TIPS.

Complications

- Nontarget embolization resulting in organ ischemia; however, this is rare given the presence of collateral supply in the UGI vasculature.

SPLENIC ARTERY EMBOLIZATION

CASE PRESENTATION

A 19-year-old male who has been involved in a motor vehicle accident, though hemodynamically stable, is found to have a grade III splenic laceration on contrast-enhanced CT of the abdomen. IR is consulted for splenic artery embolization.

- The spleen, which is a highly vascular organ, is the most commonly injured organ in blunt force trauma.
- Salvatore Sclafani first reported gelatin foam embolization for splenic injuries in 1981 at Kings County Hospital in Brooklyn, New York. It has since become an important organ-saving nonoperative option in cases of splenic trauma.
- The goal of splenic artery embolization is to decrease the perfusion pressure of the spleen so as to help the body achieve stasis.
- In a hemodynamically stable patient, medical management is the gold standard.
  - However, if imaging shows a grade III or higher splenic injury, medical management often fails, and thus splenic artery embolization should be considered.

THE AMERICAN ASSOCIATION FOR THE SURGERY OF TRAUMA SPLENIC INJURY GRADING SYSTEM

- Grade I
  - Subcapsular hematoma less than 10% of total surface area
  - Capsular laceration less than 1 cm in depth
- Grade II
  - Subcapsular hematoma 10% to 50% of surface area
  - Intraparenchymal hematoma less than 5 cm in diameter
  - Laceration 1 to 3 cm in depth not involving trabecular vessels
- Grade III
  - Subcapsular hematoma greater than 50% of surface area or expanding
  - Intraparenchymal hematoma greater than 5 cm or expanding
  - Laceration greater than 3 cm in depth or involving trabecular vessels
  - Ruptured subcapsular or parenchymal hematoma
- Grade IV (Fig. 7.10)
  - Laceration involving segmental or hilar vessels with major devascularization (>25% of spleen)
- Grade V
  - Shattered spleen
  - Hilar vascular injury with devascularized spleen

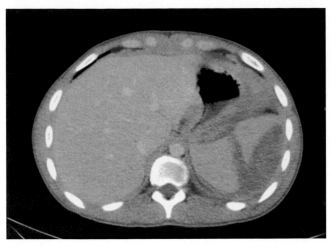

Fig. 7.10 Computed Tomography Angiogram of Grade IV Splenic Laceration (Courtesy Dr. James Walsh, Kings County Hospital, Brooklyn, NY.)

- The most common positive findings on splenic angiograms are active bleeding, pseudoaneurysms, and arteriovenous malformations.
- Currently, there is much debate on how to proceed when a splenic bleed is seen on CTA but angiography fails to elucidate the bleed. Protocols for such instances differ by institution.

Indications

- The indications for splenic artery embolization often differ by institution. Generally if imaging shows active extravasation from the splenic artery, a grade III (or higher) injury, or an active drop in hematocrit with suspected splenic artery etiology, then a splenic artery embolization may be indicated.

- If the decision to embolize is made, the location of embolization (distal versus proximal) is also a widely debated subject.
  - The potential drawback of proximal embolization is the inability to reembolize if a distal bleed recurs.
  - The potential drawbacks of distal embolization are splenic infarction and abscess formation.

◎ LITERATURE REVIEW

A meta-analysis performed by Schnüriger and colleagues in 2011 noted that "the available literature is inconclusive regarding whether proximal or distal embolization should be used to avoid significant rebleeding." This meta-analysis found that minor complications occur clinically and statistically more often with distal embolizations.

Contraindications

- Hemodynamically unstable patients (these are candidates for surgical splenectomy)
- Otherwise the same relative contraindications apply as in GIB.

Equipment

- Same equipment as in GIB

Anatomy

- The main artery supplying the spleen is the splenic artery, which is one of three main branches of the celiac trunk.
- There are also significant collateral pathways feeding the spleen, including the short gastric arteries, splenic capsular arteries, pancreatic arteries, and gastroepiploic arteries (Fig. 7.11).

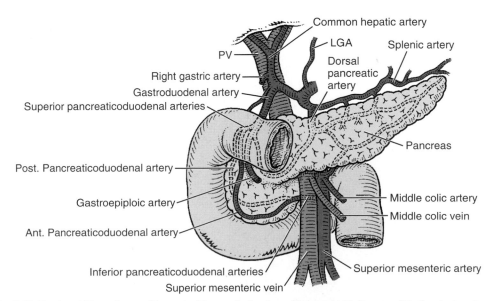

Fig. 7.11 Regional Vasculature (Reused with permission from Blumgart LH, Corvera CU. Surgical and radiologic anatomy. In: *Video Atlas: Liver, Biliary & Pancreatic Surgery.* Elsevier; 2011:F1-39).

Procedural Steps

1. Gain femoral or radial artery access.
2. Assuming femoral access, insert a J-wire up to the level of the iliac artery to ensure that you do not lose access.
3. Remove the needle, and apply pressure to the artery to minimize blood loss as you insert a dilator over the guidewire.
4. Exchange the dilator for a 5-Fr sheath, and exchange the J-wire for a 0.035-inch guidewire.
5. Flush the sheath with normal saline.
6. Use a curved (Cobra) or reversed curved (Simmons) catheter to select the celiac artery and perform a celiac angiogram. Evaluate both the splenic artery and the left gastric artery, as the latter is a common collateral artery to the spleen.
7. If extravasation is seen, the choice to perform a proximal or distal embolization is made.
   a. To perform a proximal embolization, advance the microcatheter just proximal to the main splenic artery, and insert detachable coils.
      i. This will rapidly decrease the perfusion pressure of the spleen, thus helping to stop the active bleeding, yet the uninjured spleen will continue to be well perfused by collateral pathways.
   b. To perform a distal embolization, advance the microcatheter as close to the site of active extravasation as possible, and insert detachable coils.
      i. This will result in the preservation of perfusion to a greater amount of splenic parenchyma. Fig. 7.12 shows a distal splenic artery embolization performed on a trauma patient with the subsequent cessation of the splenic bleed and eventual full recovery.
8. Confirm the absence of active extravasation with a final contrast injection.
9. Remove all wire and catheters.
10. Remove the sheath, and apply manual pressure for at least 15 minutes or use a closure device.

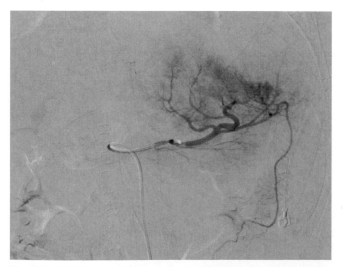

Fig. 7.12 Mid Proximal Splenic Embolization (Courtesy Dr. James Walsh, Kings County Hospital, Brooklyn, NY.)

Treatment Alternatives

- Splenectomy
- Conservative medical management

Complications

- *Splenic abscess formation* is more likely to result from distal embolizations.
- *Splenic infarction* can confer an increased risk of infection by encapsulated organisms.
- Rebleeding from the splenic artery.
- Typical puncture site complications.

PELVIC ANGIOGRAPHY IN SETTING OF TRAUMA

CASE PRESENTATION

A 22-year-old male with a gunshot wound to the abdomen is brought in by ambulance. He is hemodynamically unstable and is taken for emergent laparotomy; colectomy is performed and the pelvis packed. The patient, now hemodynamically stable, is sent for a CT of the abdomen/pelvis, which shows blush adjacent to the right internal iliac artery. IR is consulted for pelvic angiogram.

- The majority of vascular injuries in pelvic trauma are venous in nature and are thus not amenable to embolization; these venous bleeds can be managed conservatively with blood transfusions or by cauterizing and packing the pelvis in the operating room.
- The majority of pelvic arterial bleeds occur secondary to pelvic fractures. They have a high mortality rate if not treated immediately.
  - It takes great blunt force to cause pelvic fractures with arterial bleeds. The majority of such traumas occur in motor vehicle accidents, pedestrians struck by motor vehicles, motorcycle accidents, and falls from height.
  - A less common source of pelvic arterial injury is gunshot wounds, which can directly damage arteries leading to AVMs and/or pseudoaneurysms.

LITERATURE REVIEW

It was previously thought that the need for pelvic angiography could be predicted based on the type of pelvic fracture. However, Starr and colleagues showed in their 2002 article that there is no actual correlation between fracture type and subsequent need for angiogram/embolization.

- The majority of pelvic fractures that result in massive internal hemorrhage are due to injury to the internal iliac and/or superior gluteal arteries.
- When an angiogram is thought to be falsely negative (due to vasospasm, for example) but there is high clinical suspicion for internal iliac artery trauma, it is acceptable to

empirically embolize the bilateral internal iliac arteries. Alternatively, if angiography is negative but active hemorrhage is suspected (or was seen on CTA), the interventionalist may perform a *provocative angiogram* in which nitroglycerin is injected into the suspected artery in order to elicit a bleed, thus allowing for identification and treatment.

- Embolization agents in trauma include but are not limited to Gelfoam (temporary occlusion), microspheres (permanent embolization), and metallic coils (permanent embolization).

Indications
- In the acutely unstable trauma patient, emergent exploratory surgery is always the gold standard.

- If this patient stabilizes and is thought to have continued pelvic bleeding based on follow-up imaging or clinical suspicion, angiography with embolization becomes the gold standard.

Contraindications
- Acutely unstable patients with multiple traumatic injuries
- Same relative contraindications as in LGIB

Equipment
- Same equipment as in LGIB

Anatomy
- Fig. 7.13 shows a normal bilateral internal iliac arteriogram.

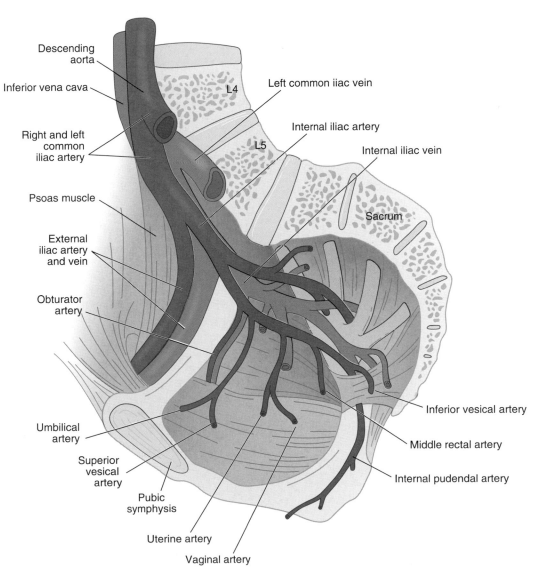

Fig. 7.13 Common Iliac Artery and Its Branches (Female) (Reused with permission from Rosenblum N, Nitti VW. Indications and Techniques for Vaginal Hysterectomy for Uterine Prolapse. In: Nitti VW, ed. *Vaginal Surgery for the Urologist.* Elsevier; 2012:F3.

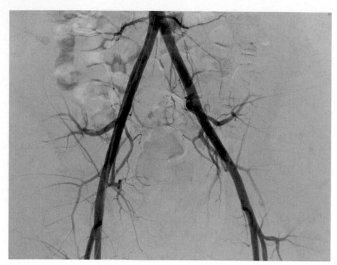

Fig. 7.14 Normal Bilateral Internal Iliac Arteriogram (Courtesy Dr. James Walsh, Kings County Hospital, Brooklyn, NY.)

- The majority of pelvic bleeds are secondary to injury to the anterior branches of the internal iliac artery or the superior gluteal artery (Fig. 7.14).

Procedural Steps

1. Gain femoral or radial artery access.
2. Assuming femoral access, insert a J-wire up to the level of the iliac artery to ensure that you do not lose access.
3. Remove needle, and apply pressure to the artery to minimize blood loss as you insert a dilator over the guidewire.
4. Exchange the dilator for a 5-Fr sheath, and exchange the J-wire for a 0.035-inch guidewire.
5. Flush the sheath with normal saline.
6. Insert a floppy guidewire into the desired catheter, and advance it through the sheath under fluoroscopic guidance into the distal abdominal aorta.
7. Perform a pelvic aortogram followed by bilateral internal iliac artery angiograms.
8. If you identify the site of active extravasation, proceed with superselection of the desired artery using a microcatheter if needed.
9. Once the bleeding artery has been selected, embolize it using your preference for embolic agent.

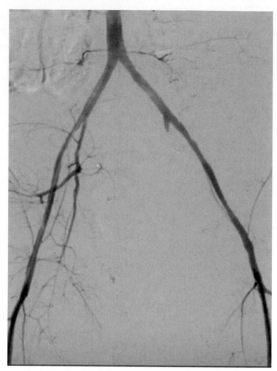

Fig. 7.15 Angiogram Status Post Left Internal Iliac Artery Embolization (Courtesy Dr. James Walsh, Kings County Hospital, Brooklyn, NY.)

10. Confirm stasis of the vessel with a final contrast injection. (Fig. 7.15 shows an angiogram status post left internal iliac artery embolization. Note the absence of flow distal to the coils.)
11. Remove all wires and catheters.
12. Remove the sheath, and apply manual pressure or use an arterial closure device.

Treatment Alternatives

- Exploratory laparoscopy/laparotomy in the acutely unstable patient

Complications

- Nontarget embolization
- Rebleeding
- Puncture site complications

TAKE-HOME POINTS

The Relationship Between Interventional Radiology and Vascular Surgery

- A large overlap exists between many of the arterial and venous disease processes treated by interventional radiology (IR) and vascular surgery.
- Proficiency in the physical examination of the vascular system is a must for both the interventional radiologist and the vascular surgeon.
- Angiography can be used for preprocedural planning for endovascular cases, presurgical planning, or solely for diagnostic purposes.
- Femoral cutdown and exposure by the vascular surgeon might become necessary in cases of heavily calcified vessels, small-caliber vessels, severely kinked vessels, excessive groin scarring, and/or obesity.
- Knowledge of the commonly used anticoagulants and antiplatelet agents encountered when a vascular patient is being managed is crucial.

Summary of Surgical Techniques in Solid Organ Transplantation

- Care of both transplant candidates and recipients is multidisciplinary and IR can offer numerous interventions for these patients.
- A sound knowledge of anatomy, surgical techniques, complications, and radiologic interventions is essential for the collaborating interventionist.

Trauma Surgery: Lower Gastrointestinal Bleeds

- Although not the first-line intervention for acute lower gastrointestinal bleed (LGIB), embolization does play a role in patients with continued and symptomatic LGIB.

- Even with a high clinical suspicion of an acute LGIB, angiograms are often negative owing to the intermittent nature of LGIBs.

Trauma Surgery: Upper GI Bleeds

- Although embolization is not the first-line treatment for upper gastrointestinal bleeds (UGIBs), patients with recurrent UGI bleeding after endoscopic intervention are often good candidates for endovascular intervention.
- When a patient is being assessed for a possible UGIB, it is essential to interrogate the superior mesenteric artery, left gastric artery, and gastroduodenal artery.
- A negative angiogram does not rule out a UGI source of bleeding given that UGIBs, as with LGIBs, are often intermittent.

Splenic Artery Embolization

- Splenic artery embolization is a well-accepted treatment option for splenic trauma.
- There are no universal indications to determine which patients will benefit most from the procedure.
- There is no universal technique, as choice of proximal versus distal embolization is left up to the interventionalist.

Pelvic Angiogram in Setting of Trauma

- Suspected pelvic hemorrhage secondary to trauma is often due to injury to the internal iliac and/or superior gluteal arteries.
- It is safe to empirically embolize the bilateral internal iliac arteries if there is a high clinical suspicion for internal iliac injury despite a negative diagnostic angiogram.
- A provocative angiogram uses nitroglycerin to elicit a bleed in cases of negative angiograms. This allows for the identification of blush and superselection prior to embolization.

REVIEW QUESTIONS

1. At which MELD score does a patient become a candidate for liver transplantation?
   a. 5
   b. 10
   c. 15
   d. 20

2. A 40-year-old female has a history of cirrhosis due to schistosomiasis and hepatic failure. The patient received a liver transplant 3 months earlier. She now presents with increased liver enzymes and general malaise. What is the best initial step in the management of this patient?
   a. Obtain an ultrasound.
   b. Obtain a CT angiogram.
   c. Obtain a transjugular liver biopsy.
   d. Obtain a percutaneous liver biopsy.

3. Which of the following is not an advantage of a piggyback anastomosis?
   a. Decrease in warm ischemia time
   b. Decrease in blood loss
   c. Minimization of hemodynamic disturbances
   d. Maintenance of the anatomic relationship between the hepatic vein and IVC

4. A 53-year-old male with no medical history presents with signs of liver failure. A CT of the abdomen was performed and a mass found in the liver. Biopsy was consistent with hepatocellular carcinoma. Which is not an indication for liver transplantation?
   a. A single lesion that is 4 cm in diameter with no extrahepatic spread
   b. Two lesions both 3 cm in diameter with no extrahepatic spread
   c. Three lesions that are each 2 cm in diameter with no extrahepatic spread
   d. A single lesion that is 6 cm in diameter with no extrahepatic spread

5. A 75-year-old male had a kidney transplant 3 months earlier for end-stage renal disease due to chronic hypertension. He presents with an increased creatinine, proteinuria, and a decrease in his urine output. He states that he has noticed increased swelling in his legs. What is the gold standard for diagnosis?
   a. Ultrasound
   b. CT scan
   c. Angiography
   d. Kidney biopsy

6. When femoral artery access is being performed, the target puncture site is where?
   a. The external iliac artery proximal to the inferior epigastric artery
   b. The easiest area to access
   c. At the common femoral artery over the femoral head
   d. Distal to the femoral artery bifurcation
7. Assuming normal anatomy, in order to rule out an active LGIB, which artery or arteries must be interrogated?
   a. Left gastric artery
   b. SMA and IMA
   c. Only the SMA
   d. Celiac trunk and SMA
8. Assuming normal anatomy, which arteries should be interrogated to rule out an active UGIB?
   a. SMA and IMA
   b. SMA, IMA, and left gastric artery
   c. SMA and GDA
   d. SMA, left gastric artery, and GDA

SUGGESTED READINGS

Ali M, Ul Haq T, Salam B, et al. Treatment of nonvariceal gastrointestinal hemorrhage by transcatheter embolization. *Radiol Res Pract.* 2013;2013:604328.

Bookstein JJ, Chlosta EM, Foley D, et al. Transcatheter hemostasis of gastrointestinal bleeding using modified autogenous clot. *Radiology.* 1974;113(2):277–285.

Gianturco C, Anderson JH, Wallace S. Mechanical devices for arterial occlusion. *Am J Roentgenol Radium Ther Nucl Med.* 1975;124(3):428–435.

Gomes AS. Radiological evaluation in transplantation. In: Busuttil RW, Klintmalm GBG, eds. *Transplantation of the Liver.* 3rd ed. Philadelphia: Elsevier; 2015:455–477.

Ingraham CR, Montenovo M. Interventional and surgical techniques in solid organ transplantation. *Radiol Clin North Am.* 2016;54 (2):267–280.

Nelson TM, Pollak R, Jonasson O, et al. Anatomic variants of the celiac, superior mesenteric and inferior mesenteric arteries and their clinical relevance. *Clin Anat.* 1988;1(2):75–91.

Rasmussen TE, Clouse WD, Tonnessen BH. *Handbook of Patient Care in Vascular Diseases.* 5th ed. Philadelphia: Wolters Kluwer; 2008.

Schnüriger B, Inaba K, Konstantinidis A, et al. Outcomes of proximal versus distal splenic artery embolization after trauma: a systematic review and meta-analysis. *J Trauma.* 2011;70 (1):252–260.

Sclafani SJ. The role of angiographic hemostasis in salvage of the injured spleen. *Radiology.* 1981;141(3):645–650.

Starr AJ, Griffin DR, Reinert CM, et al. Pelvic ring disruptions: prediction of associated injuries, transfusion requirement, pelvic arteriography, complications, and mortality. *J Orthop Trauma.* 2002;16(8):553–561.

Zurkiya O, Walker TG. Angiographic evaluation and management of nonvariceal gastrointestinal hemorrhage. *Am J Roentgenol.* 2015;205(4):753–763.

Obstetrics and Gynecology

Emily R. Ochmanek, Alexander Covington, Jennifer Wan, Kevin T. Williams

Interventional radiologists have a wide variety of skills and tools at their disposal, making our specialty a cornerstone of multidisciplinary patient care. One example is in the realm of women's health, where the practice plays a role in managing a variety of obstetric and gynecologic disorders ranging from life-threatening postpartum hemorrhage to minimally invasive approaches for treating benign conditions, such as infertility and uterine fibroids in the ambulatory setting. This chapter provides an overview of the most common interventional procedures employed in the management of obstetric and gynecologic conditions.

UTERINE ARTERY EMBOLIZATION

CASE PRESENTATION

A 42-year-old G2P2 female with no significant past medical history presents to her gynecologist for her annual well-woman examination. She reports increasing mass-like pelvic enlargement and pressure over the past 6 years, becoming more symptomatic of late, with recurrence of heavy periods after years of amenorrhea following the placement of a Mirena intrauterine device. Physical examination is notable for an approximate 20-week uterus. Ultrasound reveals an enlarged uterus, attributable to multiple fibroids, the largest of which measured over 9 cm in diameter. She undergoes pelvic magnetic resonance imaging, which confirms a heterogeneously enhancing fibroid measuring approximately 12 cm in greatest dimension. After weighing her treatment options, she elects to proceed with uterine artery embolization.

- Percutaneous transcatheter uterine artery embolization (UAE) has historically been employed for the treatment of uncontrollable obstetric or traumatic bleeding. However, application of the technique to treat symptomatic fibroids as an alternative to hysterectomy and myomectomy is a relatively recent development, introduced by J. H. Ravina in 1995.
- Uterine leiomyomas (i.e., fibroids or myomas) are benign smooth muscle neoplasms that occur in women of reproductive age (Fig. 8.1).
- They are the most common female pelvic tumor seen—nearly half of women over the age of 40 have fibroids, though less than 20% of these present with symptoms.

- African American women are two to three times more likely to develop uterine fibroids than women in the general population.
- The principle behind UAE is that embolic material is delivered via catheter into one or both uterine arteries to cause infarction of the fibroids without permanent damage to the remainder of the uterus, thereby maintaining fertility.
- UAE for symptomatic fibroids refractory to medical management is now a widely accepted alternative to surgical intervention. The American College of Obstetricians and Gynecologists endorses UAE as a safe and effective procedure for women who desire uterine preservation.
- Following UAE, leiomyomas typically decrease in volume by approximately 50% to 60%, with satisfactory clinical outcomes achieved in 85% to 90% of patients.

LITERATURE REVIEW

Two breakthrough trials—the uterine artery embolization (UAE) Versus Surgery for Symptomatic Uterine Fibroids (REST) trial and the Embolization Versus Hysterectomy (EMMY) trial—found that UAE was a viable alternative to surgery. Patients in both of these multicenter randomized controlled trials reported similar symptomatic relief, improvement in quality of life, and satisfaction in both treatment arms. The studies found that reintervention after UAE was often related to recurrent fibroids, a problem also seen with myomectomy and other uterine-sparing therapies.
- The EMMY trial
  - Compared UAE with total hysterectomy in 177 patients.
  - Found no difference in health-related quality-of-life measures between UAE and hysterectomy at 6- and 24-month follow-up.
  - Ten years after treatment, it was found that 24 out of the 77 patients who originally had successful UAE underwent secondary hysterectomy.
- The REST trial
  - Compared UAE with myomectomy/hysterectomy in 157 patients.
  - Found no difference in quality-of-life measures at 24-month and 5-year follow-up.
  - Found that patients who underwent UAE had a quicker recovery but required more reintervention than those who had surgery initially (13% at 12 months and 32% at 60 months). Treatments were cost neutral at 5 years.

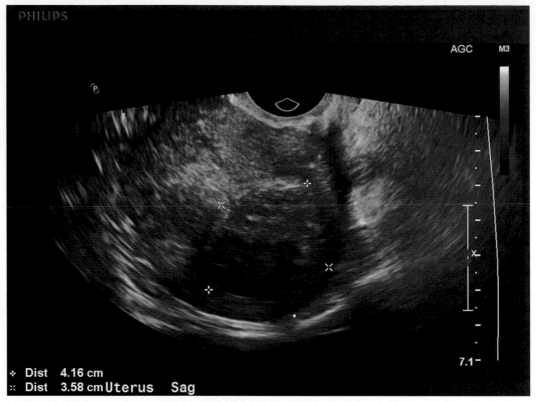

Fig. 8.1 Ultrasound image of a retroverted uterus containing multiple round hypoechoic and isoechoic foci, with a heterogeneous submucosal mass in the fundus (above) measuring up to 4.2 × 4.0 × 3.6 cm, most consistent with a leiomyoma.

Indications

- Patients with **symptomatic** fibroids who fail conservative treatment (e.g., hormonal therapy with a gonadotropin-releasing hormone agonist).
  - Qualifying symptoms include pelvic pain, menorrhagia, dyspareunia, or bulk symptoms such as pelvic pressure, urinary frequency, and/or constipation.

Contraindications

- Absolute
  - Viable pregnancy
  - Untreated genitourinary infection
  - Malignancy of the uterus, cervix, or adnexa
- Relative
  - Prior surgery or radiation that could alter pelvic arterial anatomy
  - Current use of gonadotropin-releasing agonist (vasospasm)
  - Enlarged uterus with volume greater than 20 to 24 weeks' gestation
  - Very large (>12 cm) fibroids
  - Pedunculated or large submucosal leiomyoma
  - Large hydrosalpinx, which can predispose a patient to infection after UAE
  - Extensive coexistent adenomyosis and/or endometriosis
  - Desire to maintain childbearing potential

- Coagulopathy, severe contrast allergy, or renal impairment

Equipment

- Pigtail catheter
- Angled 4- or 5-Fr catheter (e.g., Cobra, VCF flow, Rosch Inferior Mesenteric, Roberts Uterine or another curved catheter)
- Guidewire
- 3-Fr microcatheter/microwire
- Embolic particles in the 300- to 900-μm-diameter range
- Gelfoam

Anatomy

- See Fig. 8.2 and Table 8.1.
- The right and left common iliac arteries are the terminal branches of the abdominal aorta.
- The internal iliac arteries branch from the common iliac arteries anterior to the sacroiliac joint.
- The branching pattern of the internal iliac artery is variable, but it typically divides into anterior and posterior branches. The anterior branch typically gives off the **uterine artery**, which most commonly feeds fibroids, although collaterals are sometimes present (Figs. 8.3 and 8.4).
- (Box 8.1) Recall the branches of the internal iliac artery with the mnemonic "*I love going places in my very own underwear.*"

BOX 8.1 Branches of Internal Iliac Artery (Mnemonic)

I: iliolumbar artery
L: lateral sacral artery
G: gluteal (superior and inferior) arteries
P: (internal) pudendal artery
I: inferior vesical (vaginal in females) artery
M: middle rectal artery
V: vaginal artery (females only)
O: obturator artery
U: umbilical artery and uterine artery (females only)
  (The first three branches in the mnemonic (iliolumbar, lateral sacral and superior gluteal) are branches of the posterior division of the internal iliac artery, the remaining branches are of the anterior division.)

⟫ CLINICAL BOX

In 5% of patients, the ovarian arteries will additionally supply the uterus and will also require embolization.

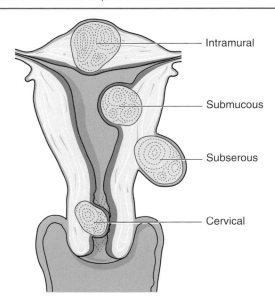

Fig. 8.2 Sites of Fibroids Throughout the Uterus (From Drife J, Magowan B. *Clinical Obstetrics and Gynaecology.* Edinburgh: WB Saunders; 2004.)

TABLE 8.1 Classification of Fibroids by Location

Location	Definition
Submucosal	Protruding into the endometrial cavity
Intramural	Within the myometrium
Subserosal	Based in the myometrium but covered by parietal peritoneum
Pedunculated	Attached to the uterus by a small stalk
Cervical	Located in the uterine cervix

From Kaufman JA. Abdominal aorta and pelvic arteries. In: Kaufman JA, Lee MJ, eds. *Vascular and Interventional Radiology: The Requisites.* 2nd ed. Philadelphia: Elsevier; 2014:199–228.

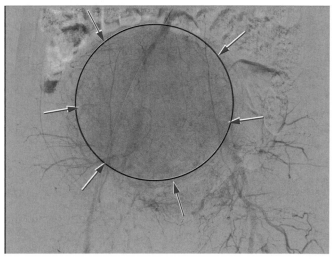

Fig. 8.4 Delayed image from a digital subtraction angiogram of the pelvis in the anteroposterior projection documenting the "blush" *(arrows)* of a large uterine fibroid supplied by the right and left uterine arteries.

Procedure

Preprocedural Orders

- Nil per os (NPO)
- Routine labs (complete blood count [CBC], creatinine, prothrombin time/international normalized ratio [PT/INR])
- Prophylactic antibiotics (e.g., 1 g cefazolin IV)

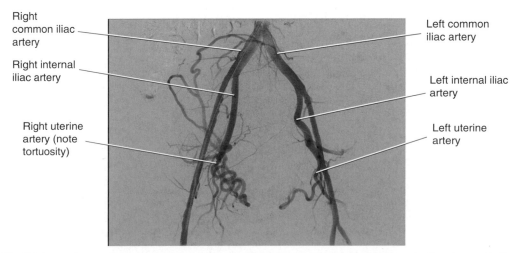

Fig. 8.3 Image from a digital subtraction angiogram of the pelvis in the anteroposterior projection demonstrating relevant female pelvic arterial anatomy, with catheter located at the aortic bifurcation.

- Foley catheter
- Periprocedural analgesia with both nonsteroidal antiinflammatory drugs (NSAIDs) (e.g., ketorolac) and narcotics (e.g., hydromorphone [Dilaudid] PCA (patient-controlled analgesia) in addition to the usual procedural sedation
- Antiemetic (e.g., ondansetron)

Procedural Steps

1. The right groin is prepped and draped in the usual sterile fashion; lidocaine 1% solution is used as a local anesthetic.
2. The common femoral artery is accessed using the Seldinger technique to allow placement of a 5-Fr hemostatic sheath.
3. A pigtail catheter is positioned within the distal abdominal aorta, and a pelvic angiogram is obtained to define the overall pelvic anatomy and identify the bilateral uterine arteries.
   a. Representative imaging shows tortuosity of the bilateral uterine arteries (Fig. 8.5) and heterogeneous perfusion (i.e., blush) (Fig. 8.6) throughout the uterus due to fibroids.
4. The guidewire is introduced into the contralateral external iliac artery to allow exchange of the pigtail catheter for a 4- or 5-Fr angled end-hole catheter. This catheter is then navigated into the internal iliac artery (Fig. 8.7), and a digital subtraction angiogram (DSA) is obtained in the anterior oblique projection to best display the uterine artery anatomy.
5. A 3-Fr microcatheter/microwire is inserted coaxially through the angled catheter in order to subselect the uterine artery (Figs. 8.8 and 8.9). The microcatheter is advanced beyond the dominant cervicovaginal branches to prevent nontarget embolization.

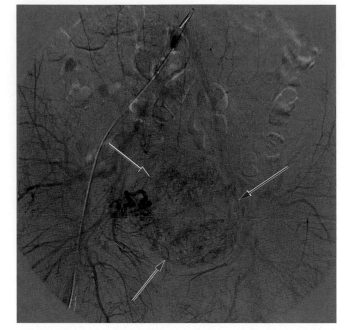

Fig. 8.6 Delayed pelvic angiogram showing heterogeneous blush *(arrows)* in the uterus representing the leiomyoma, with contributions from both the left and right uterine arteries.

6. Embolic particles are injected until there is near stasis of flow (approximately five heartbeats to carry away an injected contrast bolus).
7. The angled catheter is used to access the ipsilateral internal iliac artery by forming a redundant loop in the abdominal aorta and pulling the catheter into the desired vessel, called

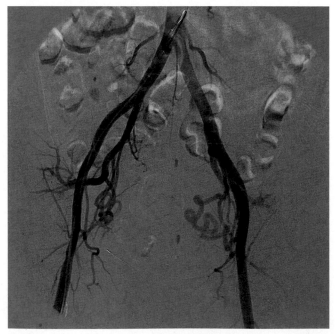

Fig. 8.5 Pelvic angiogram showing tortuous bilateral uterine arteries (left greater than right).

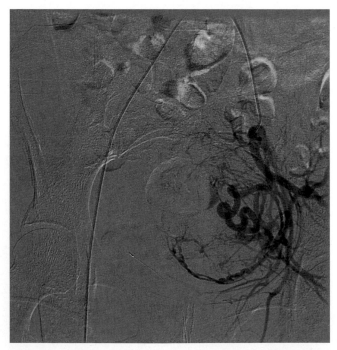

Fig. 8.7 Subselective digital subtraction angiogram of the anterior division of the left internal iliac artery in the right anterior oblique projection.

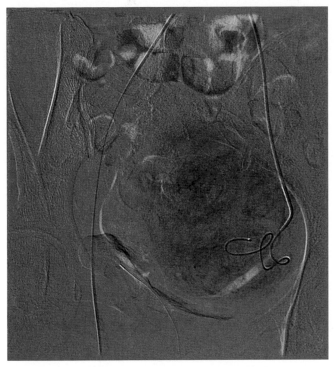

Fig. 8.8 Superselective left uterine artery angiogram demonstrating arterial blush of the fibroids.

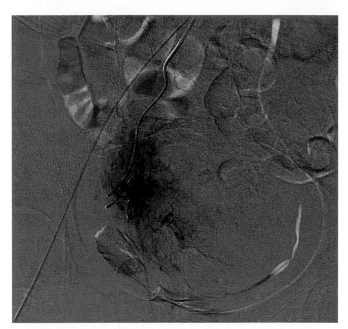

Fig. 8.10 Superselective right uterine artery angiogram demonstrating mild residual arterial blush of the fibroids.

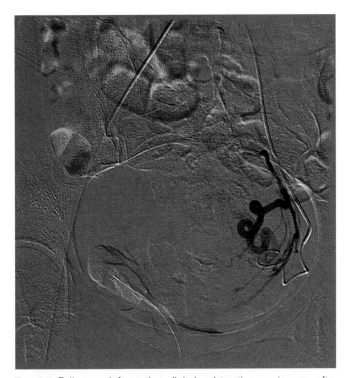

Fig. 8.9 Follow-up left uterine digital subtraction angiogram after embolization using two vials of 700- to 900-μm Embospheres demonstrates markedly decreased tumoral staining/fibroid blush.

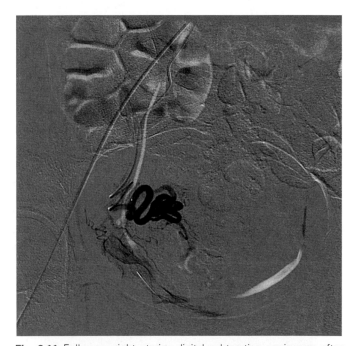

Fig. 8.11 Follow-up right uterine digital subtraction angiogram after embolization using nearly one vial of 700- to 900-μm Embospheres demonstrates no significant tumoral staining/fibroid blush.

the Waltman loop technique (Figs. 8.10 and 8.11). The procedure is then repeated step-for-step.

8. After reversing the Waltman loop, all equipment is removed, and a closure device is used or pressure is applied.

Postprocedural Care

- Most patients are admitted overnight for observation and pain management.
- Beginning about 2 to 6 hours after the procedure, the patient may experience up to 24 hours of moderate to severe cramping and pelvic pain. This will gradually diminish over the following week. Symptom severity generally correlates with the size of the fibroids treated, but it is still quite patient dependent.

- Postembolization syndrome is common; symptoms include fatigue, anorexia, low-grade fever, nausea, and vomiting.
- Initial inpatient pain management typically includes intravenous narcotics and NSAIDs (e.g., ketorolac). Oral narcotics and NSAIDs are continued on a staggered schedule following the patient's discharge. Stool softeners are also important, as narcotics tend to cause constipation.
- A follow-up interventional radiology (IR) clinic visit is recommended within 2 to 4 weeks to assess the appropriate management of pain and reaffirm the time line of expected symptom relief.
- A 6-month follow-up pelvic MRI scan with contrast with a contemporaneous clinic visit is also advised so that the findings may be reviewed with the patient (Figs. 8.12 and 8.13).

Alternative Treatments

- **Medical therapy** provides up to 75% of women with some level of symptomatic improvement, but long-term failure rates are high because of side effects. Options for medical therapy include the following:
  - Estrogen/progestin or progestin-only contraceptives
  - Levonorgestrel-releasing IUD
  - Gonadotropin-releasing hormone agonists
  - Gonadotropin-releasing hormone antagonists
- **Hysterectomy**: leiomyoma is the most common indication for hysterectomy, accounting for 30% to 50% of cases depending on the patient's race. This is the definitive treatment as it relieves existing symptoms and there is no chance of recurrence (Table 8.2).
- **Myomectomy** is the standard of care for patients who wish to preserve fertility. UAE is associated with an increased risk of abnormal placentation, spontaneous abortion,

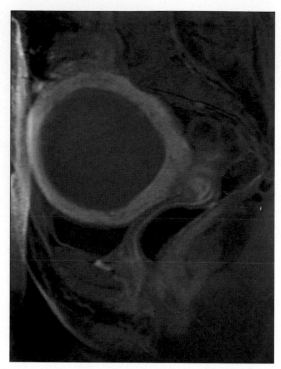

Fig. 8.13 Postembolization sagittal T1-weighted fat-saturated postcontrast image in the same patient demonstrating technical success, with marked reduction in size of the leiomyoma (now measuring 9 cm maximally), with central necrosis and no significant residual enhancement.

and preterm delivery. A hysteroscopic or laparoscopic approach may be used, depending on the location of the leiomyoma. There is a general recurrence rate of up to 60%, and up to 25% of patients require repeat intervention.
- **Myolysis** is the laparoscopic use of thermal, radiofrequency, or cryoablation to destroy leiomyoma tissue.
- **Uterine artery occlusion**: physical occlusion of uterine vessels, either laparoscopically or via a vaginally placed clamp.
- **MR-guided high-intensity focused ultrasound** is a noninvasive, essentially painless method of destroying fibroid tissue. Only a small area can be treated at a time, so this is not a good option for a large fibroid burden.

Complications

See Table 8.3.

SELECTIVE SALPINGOGRAPHY AND TRANSCERVICAL FALLOPIAN TUBE RECANALIZATION

CASE PRESENTATION

A 32-year-old otherwise healthy woman presents with her partner to her gynecologist to discuss their inability to conceive despite having discontinued contraception for more than the previous 12 months. She had a normal Pap smear and an unrevealing pelvic ultrasound. She was then referred for a hysterosalpingogram (HSG), which was abnormal, suggesting a proximal right tubal occlusion. An IR consultation was requested to pursue the option of diagnostic salpingography and potential tubal recanalization.

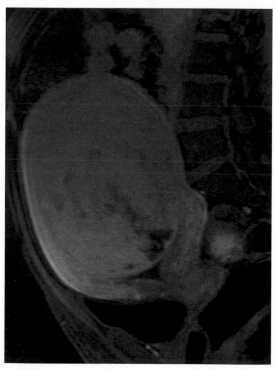

Fig. 8.12 Preembolization sagittal T1-weighted fat-saturated postcontrast image demonstrating a large enhancing fundal leiomyoma measuring up to approximately 16 cm.

TABLE 8.2   Complications of Surgery

	ABDOMINAL TRIAL		VAGINAL TRIAL	
	Abdominal Hysterectomy (*n* = 292)	Laparoscopic Hysterectomy (*n* = 584)	Vaginal Hysterectomy (*n* = 168)	Laparoscopic Hysterectomy (*n* = 336)
Major hemorrhage	7 (2.4)	27 (4.6)	5 (2.9)	17 (5.1)
Bowel injury	3 (1)	1 (0.2)	0	0
Ureteric injury	0	5 (0.9)	0	1 (0.3)
Bladder injury	3 (1)	12 (2.1)	2 (1.2)	3 (0.9)
Intraoperative conversion	1 (0.3)	23 (3.9)	7 (4.2)	9 (2.7)
Wound dehiscence	1 (0.3)	1 (0.2)	0	1 (0.3)
Hematoma	2 (0.7)	4 (0.7)	2 (1.2)	7 (2.1)
At least one major complication	18 (6.2)	65 (11.1)	16 (9.5)	33 (9.8)

From Garry R, Fountain J, Mason S, et al. The eVALuate study: two parallel randomized trials, one comparing laparoscopic with abdominal hysterectomy, the other comparing laparoscopic with vaginal hysterectomy. *BMJ.* 2004;328:129.

TABLE 8.3   Complications of Uterine Artery Embolization

Permanent amenorrhea (age < 45 years)	0%–3%
Permanent amenorrhea (age > 45 years)	20%–40%
Prolonged vaginal discharge	2%–17%
Transcervical leiomyoma expulsion	3%–15%
Septicemia	1%–3%
Deep venous thrombosis or pulmonary embolism	<1%
Nontarget embolization	<1%
Emergent hysterectomy	<1%
Death	<1%

Data from Stokes LS, Wallace MJ, Godwin RB. Quality improvement guidelines from uterine artery embolization for symptomatic leiomyomas. *J Vasc Interv Radiol.* 2010;21(8):1153–1163.

- Tubal occlusion is the most common etiology of female infertility (30%–40% of female infertility is related to tubal disease). Imaging workup typically begins with an HSG, which determines patency and depicts the course, size, and contour of the tubes. HSG may also detect peritubal abnormalities such as adhesions.
  - The differential diagnosis of tubal occlusion includes:
    - Common causes—spasm, infection, and prior surgery
    - Rare causes—granulomatous salpingitis due to TB, intraluminal endometriosis, parasitic infection, and congenital atresia
- Results of the HSG help the referring clinician and radiologist to determine the next steps in diagnosis and management. These could include
- *Selective salpingography,* a *diagnostic* test in which the fallopian tube is directly opacified by injecting contrast through a catheter placed in the tubal ostium.
- This precisely defines the anatomy of the tubes.
- *Fallopian tube recanalization* is a therapeutic procedure to open the tube by passing a guidewire and catheter through a proximal obstruction.

- It is a nonoperative alternative or adjunct to tubal surgery or assisted fertility procedures.
- It is associated with approximately 71% to 100% efficacy in the setting of idiopathic proximal tubal obstruction.
- It is also associated with 77% to 82% efficacy in the setting of salpinigitis isthmica nodosa, which is an idiopathic inflammatory process that results in subcentimeter protrusions from the isthmic portion of the tube.
- It has been shown to be 44% to 77% effective in the setting of occluded tubes after surgical reversal of previous tubal ligation.
- Approximately half of patients with bilateral proximal tubal obstruction are ideal candidates for recanalization because they present with focal tubal disease without pelvic adhesions.
- Postprocedure pregnancy success rates are highly variable, reflecting the multifactorial and diverse nature of the problem (including male factors).

Indications
Diagnostic Selective Salpingography
- Nonfilling of fallopian tube on HSG
- Differentiation of technically inadequate HSG or spasm from true obstruction or tubal disorder
- Discordance between HSG and laparoscopy
- Discordance between HSG and clinical diagnosis
- Patient not pregnant after surgical tubocornual anastomosis

Therapeutic Fallopian Tube Recanalization
- Infertility due to proximal fallopian tube occlusion
- Reocclusion after surgical reversal of tubal ligation

Contraindications
- Absolute
  - Active pelvic infection
- Relative

- Severe tubal or peritubal pathology not amenable to laparoscopic or surgical repair
- Distal tubal occlusion
- Severe intrauterine adhesions

Equipment

- Vaginal speculum with or without a tenaculum
- Catheters and guidewires (available in a prepackaged kit, the Thurmond-Rosch Recanalization set)
  - A larger multipurpose catheter, 4 or 5 Fr, for selective salpingography
  - A 3-Fr straight catheter and a 0.018-inch guidewire for recanalization

Anatomy (Fig. 8.14)

- Three segments of the fallopian tube should be visible at HSG (Fig. 8.15).
  - The *isthmus* courses within the broad ligament.
  - The *ampullary* portion curves over the ovary and is the most common site of fertilization.
  - The *infundibulum* is the terminal portion of the fallopian tube. It, along with the fimbriae, collects the oocyte after ovulation.

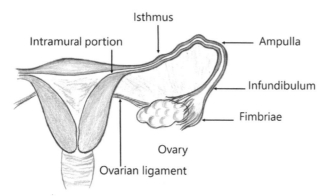

Fig. 8.14 Anatomy of the Fallopian Tube (From Srisajjakul S, Prapaisilp P, Bangchokdee S. Magnetic resonance imaging in tubal and nontubal ectopic pregnancy. *Eur J Radiol.* 2017;93:76–89.)

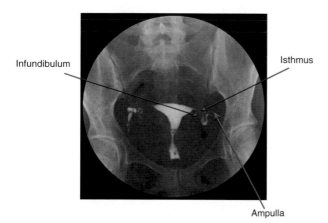

Fig. 8.15 Three segments of the tubes should be visible at hysterosalpingography.

Procedural Steps

Preprocedural Preparation

- Evaluation by an infertility specialist or gynecologist, including verification of unprotected intercourse for at least 6 months. The patient may have undergone an optional pelvic ultrasound and/or laparoscopy.
- Patient education and management of expectations, ideally performed with the patient's partner present.
- Schedule the procedure to occur in the first 5 days after the cessation of menstrual bleeding.
- Start prophylactic antibiotics (e.g., doxycycline 100 mg PO BID) on the evening prior or on the morning of the procedure, and continue for 5 days post procedure.
- Premedicate with lorazepam and fentanyl.

Procedural Steps

1. Place the patient in the lithotomy position.
2. Sterilely prep the perineum with betadine and place a drape.
3. Insert the vaginal speculum, and scrub the cervix with betadine.
4. Cannulate the cervix with a 5-Fr introducing catheter, and perform HSG if not previously done (Fig. 8.16).
5. If proximal tubal occlusion is confirmed on HSG, insert a multipurpose 4- or 5-Fr catheter coaxially through the introducing catheter, and selectively catheterize the ostium of the occluded tube.
6. Inject contrast into the occluded tube.
7. If proximal occlusion is confirmed by selective ostial injection, insert a 0.035-inch angled hydrophilic guidewire to gently probe and recanalize the occlusion. After the wire

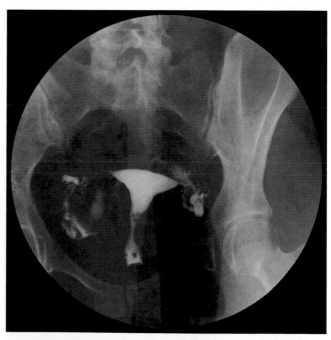

Fig. 8.16 Normal hysterosalpingogram: the endometrial cavity is normal in shape, size, and position. No intrauterine filling defects are visualized. There is synchronous filling of the fallopian tubes with free spillage of contrast into the pelvic cavity.

has been manipulated beyond the obstruction, it is removed and distal tubal patency is reassessed via ostial injection through the multipurpose catheter.

> » **CLINICAL POINT**
>
> To overcome common technical difficulties
> - Consider using a large metal speculum and/or a tenaculum to facilitate subsequent manipulations.
> - Apply firm cervical traction, and use a hydrophilic guidewire and/or preformed curved catheter to facilitate cannulation of the ostia.

8. Repeat the procedure on the contralateral side if occluded.
9. A final HSG is performed through the introducing catheter to document bilateral tubal patency.

Postprocedural Management

- Observe the patient for at least 1 hour. The patient may then be discharged if stable.
- Counsel the patient to expect spotting and cramping for 1 to 2 days.
- Instruct her to use pads rather than tampons as needed until her next cycle.
- Instruct her to avoid intercourse for 1 day post procedure.

Treatment Alternatives

- Surgical reconstruction
  - Alternative to in vitro fertilization (IVF) in patients with bilateral proximal or distal tubal occlusion
  - Poor success rate in patients with severe tubal disease or older women
- Fimbroplasty or neosalpingostomy
  - Alternative to IVF in patients with distal obstructions
  - Less effective than IVF
  - Up to a 15% risk of ectopic pregnancy
- Tubocornual anastomosis
  - Alternative to IVF in patients with proximal obstructions
  - Less effective than IVF
  - Up to a 30% risk of ectopic pregnancy
- Tubal reanastomosis
  - Alternative to IVF in young women with prior ring or clip sterilization who have a minimum of 4 cm of residual fallopian tube
- IVF
  - Has an approximately 30% live birth rate per cycle
  - Disadvantages include high cost, possible need for multiple cycles, increased rate of multiple gestations, requires use of fertility medicines that carry risks, and poses a slight increase in fetal complications.

Complications

- Reocclusion (25%)
  - Evaluation for repeat transcervical fallopian tube recanalization may be done if there is no pregnancy 6 months post procedure.

- Tubal perforation (2%–4%)
- Ectopic pregnancy (1%–5%)
  - For this reason, the patient should visit her gynecologist as soon as she has a positive pregnancy test.
- Pelvic infection (<1%)
- Radiation exposure is approximately 1 rad (10 mGy), the equivalent of a barium enema.

POSTPARTUM HEMORRHAGE

> **CASE PRESENTATION**
>
> A 34-year-old G3P2 female undergoes a seemingly uneventful vaginal twin delivery at 36 weeks 4 days. Following delivery of the two intact placentas, a large amount of blood is noted at the introitus. Despite uterine massage, the uterus remains large and boggy, and she has heavy, persistent bleeding. Visual inspection reveals no visible lacerations of the vagina or cervix. Two large-bore IVs are inserted for fluid resuscitation, and intravenous oxytocin is administered. The blood is typed and cross-matched. The uterus is packed with sponges. IR is consulted for emergent uterine artery embolization.

- **Postpartum hemorrhage** (PPH) is defined as blood loss greater than 500 mL after vaginal delivery, greater than 1000 mL after cesarean section, or any amount that if not replaced could lead to shock or death.
  - Some 4% of vaginal deliveries and 6% of cesarean sections are accompanied by excessive blood loss requiring transfusion.
- Worldwide, PPH accounts for 24% of maternal deaths, especially in underdeveloped countries).
- In the United States, PPH is a leading contributor to postpartum morbidity.
  - Shock can lead to renal failure and/or Sheehan syndrome.
  - Transfusion has associated risks.
  - Emergent hysterectomy means loss of future fertility.

Etiologies of Postpartum Hemorrhage (Box 8.2)

> **CLINICAL POINT**
>
> **Placental Accreta, Increta, and Percreta**
> - Early identification of abnormal placental implantation allows for predelivery planning and coordinated peripartum prophylactic intervention, both with the intent of preserving the uterus.
> - Invasive placentas place the patient at high risk of excessive bleeding during delivery (90% require blood transfusion) and maternal death (7% risk).
> - Internal iliac artery angiographic catheters or balloon occlusion catheters via a bilateral femoral artery approach are prophylactically placed before cesarean sections. Balloon catheter inflation immediately after delivery allows time for potential surgical management and, if necessary, emergent transarterial embolization. This decreases the need for transfusion as well as the risk for complications of bleeding.

BOX 8.2   Mnemonic

Etiology of PPH—the 4Ts:
Tone, Tissue, Trauma, Thrombin
- Tone
  - Uterine atony (most common cause)
  - Chorioamnionitis
  - Magnesium sulfate
  - Multiple gestations
  - Fetal macrosomia
  - Polyhydramnios
  - Prolonged labor
- Tissue
  - Retained products of conception
  - Infection
  - Placental implantation abnormalities (e.g., placenta accreta, increta, percreta)
- Trauma
  - Uterine rupture or inversion
  - Vaginal/cervical laceration
- Thrombin
  - Coagulopathy

- Management of PPH, depending on identification of the cause, can include:
  - Volume resuscitation
  - Pharmacologic vasopressors
  - Correction of coagulopathy
  - Oxytocin and uterine massage
  - Uterine balloon tamponade
  - Vaginal packing
- If primary management fails, transarterial embolization should be considered as an alternative to urgent hysterectomy.
- Embolization is 83% to 95% effective in controlling PPH.
  - Regardless of the cause, the goal of embolization is to stop bleeding before the onset of consumptive coagulopathy (~2–3 L of blood loss) or end-organ damage.
  - There is a need to ensure embolization of the collateral blood supply.
  - In cases of abnormal placentation, the success rate ranges from 20% to 100%.
  - The main predictor of failure is the development of disseminated intravascular coagulation (DIC).
  - Embolization does not preclude subsequent surgical intervention if still deemed necessary.

Indications
- Continued PPH after failure of primary measures

Contraindications
- No absolute contraindications for treatment of life-threatening hemorrhage

Equipment
- Gelfoam preferred as embolization agent
  - Can consider 3- to 10-mm coils if active extravasation is identified

- Less commonly used embolic agents include microspheres and PVA
- Possibly balloon occlusion catheters
- Guidewires (possibly including hydrophilic wires)
- 5- or 7-Fr hemostatic sheaths
- Selective 5-Fr catheters (Cobra, Sos, or Roberts Uterine Catheter)
- 3-Fr microcatheter and 0.018-inch wire

Anatomy
As previously described in the section on UAE
- The uterine artery is a branch of the anterior division of the internal iliac artery.
- It takes a classic course, passing through the cardinal ligament, over the ureter, and ending cephalad along the uterine body before anastomosing with the ovarian arteries.
- The ovarian arteries originate from the anterolateral aorta just below the renal arteries (20% come from renal arteries).
- In 1% of the population, the uterine artery originates from the ipsilateral ovarian artery.

Procedural Steps

▶▶ CLINICAL POINT
- Consider prophylactic preprocedural antibiotic with cefazolin 1 g IV.
- If multiple operators are available, consider bilateral access.

Unplanned Embolization in the Setting of Postpartum Hemorrhage
1. The common femoral artery is accessed using the Seldinger technique.
2. A 0.035-inch guidewire is advanced into the abdominal aorta under fluoroscopy.
3. A 5-Fr hemostatic sheath is inserted over the wire. The side arm may be connected to a heparinized saline infusion pressurized above arterial pressure.
4. A standard flush pigtail catheter is advanced to the level of the renal arteries. An aortogram is performed (Fig. 8.17) to include the pelvic floor within the field of view.
5. The pigtail catheter is exchanged for a 5-Fr Cobra catheter, and a guidewire is placed into the contralateral common femoral artery.
6. The Cobra catheter is exchanged for a Roberts uterine catheter to select the contralateral and ipsilateral internal iliac arteries. Alternatively, the Waltman loop technique may be used with other standard angiographic catheters to select the ipsilateral artery.
7. Selective angiogram (Fig. 8.18) of the internal iliac artery in contralateral oblique position allows for localization of the anterior divisional branch vessels.
8. Selective angiogram of the anterior division of the internal iliac artery for identification of the uterine artery.

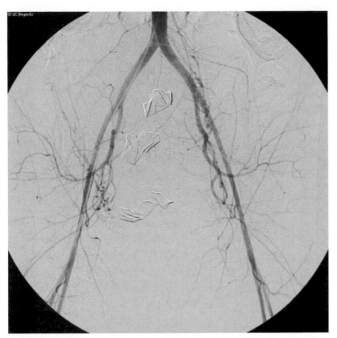

Fig. 8.17 Aortogram demonstrating surgical packing material within the uterus. No site of active contrast extravasation is identified.

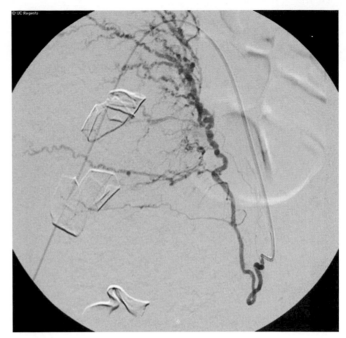

Fig. 8.19 Selective Catheterization and Angiogram of the Contralateral Left Uterine Artery.

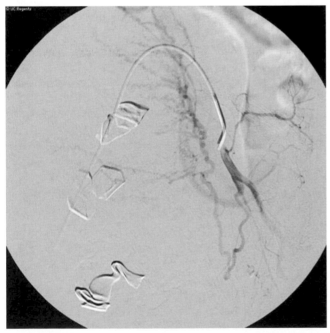

Fig. 8.18 Selective Angiogram of the Contralateral Left Internal Iliac Artery.

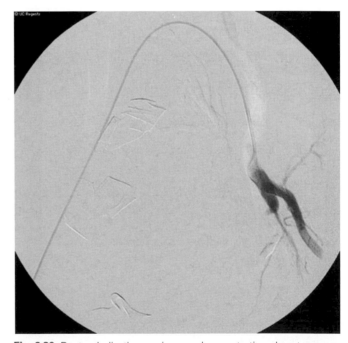

Fig. 8.20 Postembolization angiogram demonstrating abrupt nonopacification of the left uterine artery with stasis of contrast.

9. Selective catheterization of the uterine artery (Fig. 8.19) in the setting of vasospasm using a microcatheter.
    a. Use of a road map may be considered for superselective cannulation of smaller terminal branches if the site of extravasation is identified.
    b. Not seeing active extravasation (as in 42% of cases) does not preclude embolization.
10. Insertion of embolic material (Gelfoam cut into 1- to 3-mm pledgets or slurry):
    a. If extravasation is visualized—most likely in the uterine arteries—selective embolization (Fig. 8.20) should be performed.
    b. If no extravasation is visualized, nonselective empiric embolization is performed with the catheter (Fig. 8.21) positioned at the anterior division of the internal iliac artery.
11. Embolization is continued until there is a stagnant column of contrast, indicating complete stasis (Fig. 8.22).
12. A completion aortogram is performed.

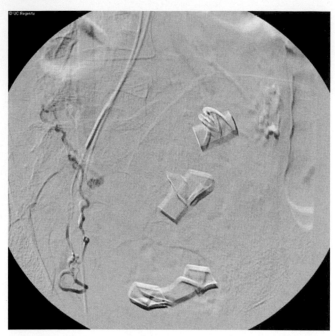

Fig. 8.21 Selective Angiogram of the Ipsilateral Right Internal Iliac Artery. Again, no extravasation is identified.

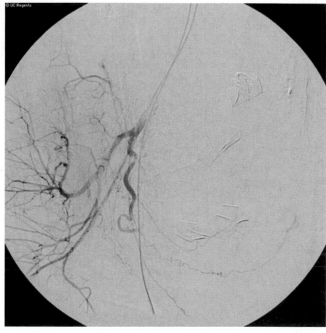

Fig. 8.22 Selective Catheterization and Angiogram of the Ipsilateral Right Uterine Artery.

Planned Embolization in the Setting of Abnormal Placentation

1. Ultrasound-guided predelivery access to both common femoral arteries is implemented.
2. A long angled 7-Fr sheath is inserted into each of the bilateral common femoral arteries.
3. Over a 0.035-inch Amplatz guidewire, a 5-Fr Cobra catheter is inserted into the contralateral internal iliac artery.
4. The 7-Fr guide sheaths are advanced over the iliac bifurcation into the contralateral common iliac artery.
5. Over a wire, an 80-cm flow-directed balloon catheter is positioned with the distal tip inserted in the contralateral internal iliac artery.
6. Insufflation is tested with diluted contrast to ensure adequate arterial occlusion. Once the precise volume that achieves sufficient occlusion has been determined, the balloon catheters are deflated.
7. The vascular sheath and coaxial system are secured to the patient via a sterile dressing.
8. Cesarean section performed by obstetrician colleagues.
9. If bleeding is evident and not immediately controlled following cesarean section, the balloon is immediately inflated.
10. If necessary, embolization through occlusion balloons can be performed, as previously described.

> ### ⟫ CLINICAL POINT
>
> Slurry is formed by rapidly mixing Gelfoam cubes with equal parts contrast and normal saline between two 10-mL syringes connected with a three-way stopock.

Alternative Treatments

- Exploratory laparotomy with surgical uterine artery ligation.
- Hysterectomy.

Complications

- Reported in less than 9% of cases:
  - Transient fever
  - Transient buttock numbness or ischemia
  - Foot ischemia
  - Uterine ischemia or necrosis
  - Uterine infection/abscess
- Fertility—retrospective anecdotal reports suggest higher pregnancy complications in patients who have undergone embolization.

TAKE-HOME POINTS

- **Uterine artery embolization** (UAE) is a widely accepted, safe alternative to surgery for the treatment of symptomatic fibroids and can be considered as a first-line treatment.
- Symptom relief is similar to that of surgery but with fewer major complications.
- UAE is not considered a first-line therapy for women with infertility due to fibroids who desire to become pregnant; however, successful pregnancy after UAE has frequently been reported. The patient's decision should be made in consultation with her gynecologist and interventional radiologist.
- Tubal occlusion is the most common etiology of female infertility (30%–40% of female infertility).
- **Tubal recanalization** is an efficacious procedure with a high technical success of 71% to 100% in the setting of idiopathic proximal tubal obstruction.

- The average reported pregnancy rate following tubal recanalization is 30%.
- Potential negatives to recanalization include a future 1% to 5% risk of ectopic pregnancy and a 25% risk of reocclusion within 6 months.
- **Postpartum hemorrhage** is a significant cause of morbidity and mortality in the United States and around the world. Uterine atony is the most common cause.
- For management of uncontrolled hemorrhage, transarterial embolization of the uterine arteries or internal iliac anterior division is a reasonable alternative to urgent hysterectomy, with a success rate of up to 95%.
- In the setting of known abnormal placentation (accreta, increta, or percreta), coordination with the obstetrician for pre-delivery placement of prophylactic occlusion balloons can help to decrease the associated morbidity and mortality.

REVIEW QUESTIONS

1. Which of the following would *not* be an appropriate candidate for UAE?
   a. A 33-year-old G1P1 with menorrhagia and several intramural leiomyomas measuring up to 8 cm in greatest dimension.
   b. A 52-year-old G2P2 postmenopausal female with multiple intramural leiomyomas and bleeding, though with a negative endometrial biopsy, who is a Jehovah's Witness.
   c. A 28-year-old G2P0 with difficulty conceiving and several small pedunculated submucosal leiomyomas with narrow stalks.
   d. A 40-year old G0P0 with poorly controlled uncontrolled diabetes, end-stage renal disease (on dialysis), and bulk symptoms related to a myomatous uterus.
2. The rate of permanent amenorrhea in a patient below 45 years of age is
   a. 0%.
   b. less than 5%.

   c. 5% to 10%.
   d. 20% to 40%.
3. Which of the following statements is inaccurate regarding embolization in the setting of postpartum hemorrhage?
   a. Success of the procedure is defined by the cessation of bleeding.
   b. Reported complications, such as transient fever or buttock pain, are less as compared with emergent laparotomy for the management of postpartum hemorrhage.
   c. Embolization for the management of postpartum hemorrhage precludes a patient from further surgical interventions.
   d. In the setting of known placenta percreta, predelivery occlusion balloons should be placed at the level of bilateral internal iliac arteries and immediately inflated following cesarean section if bleeding is identified and uncontrolled.

SUGGESTED READINGS

Bulman JC, Ascher SM, Spies JB. Current concepts in uterine fibroid embolization. *Radiographics*. 2012;32:1735–1750.

Fiori O, Deux JF, Kambale JC, et al. Impact of pelvic arterial embolization for intractable postpartum hemorrhage on fertility. *Am J Obstet Gynecol*. 2009;200(4):384.e1–384.e4.

Hehenkamp WJK, Volkers NA, Birnie E, et al. Symptomatic uterine fibroids: treatment with uterine artery embolization or hysterectomy—results from the randomized clinical embolisation versus hysterectomy (EMMY) trial. *Radiology*. 2008;246(3):823–832.

Josephs SC. Obstetric and gynecologic emergencies: a review of indications and interventional techniques. *Semin Intervent Radiol*. 2008;25(4):337–346.

Katz MD, Sugay SB, Walker DK, et al. Beyond hemostasis: spectrum of gynecologic and obstetric indications for transcatheter embolization. *Radiographics*. 2012;32(6):1713–1731.

Lee HY, Shin JH, Kim J, et al. Primary postpartum hemorrhage: outcome of pelvic arterial embolization in 251 patients at a single institution. *Radiology*. 2012;264(3):903–909.

Machan L. Selective salpingography and fallopian tube recanalization. In: Kandarpa K, Machan L, eds. *Handbook of Interventional Radiologic Procedures*. 4th ed. Philadelphia: Lippincott Williams and Wilkins; 2011:607–610.

Moss JG, Cooper KG, Khaund A, et al. Randomised comparison of uterine artery embolisation (UAE) with surgical treatment in patients with symptomatic uterine fibroids (REST trial): 5-year results. *BJOG.* 2011;118:936–944.

Smith M, Gipson M. Endovascular therapies for primary postpartum hemorrhage: techniques and outcomes. *Semin Intervent Radiol.* 2013;30(4):333–339.

Spies JB. Uterine fibroid embolization. In: Kandarpa K, Machan L, eds. *Handbook of Interventional Radiologic Procedures.* 4th ed. Philadelphia: Lippincott Williams and Wilkins; 2011:281–287.

Stokes LS, Wallace MJ, Godwin RB. Quality improvement guidelines from uterine artery embolization for symptomatic leiomyomas. *J Vasc Inter Radiol.* 2010;21:1153–1163.

van der Kooij SM, Hehenkamp WJ, Volkers NA, Birnie E, Ankum WM, Reekers JA. Uterine artery embolization vs hysterectomy in the treatment of symptomatic uterine fibroids: 5-year outcome from the randomized EMMY trial. *Am J Obstet Gynecol.* 2010;203:105e1.

Pediatrics

Rajat Chand, Bairbre Connolly

This chapter provides a brief overview of both the diagnostic and therapeutic aspects of image-guided procedures that are important in the pediatric population. The development of interventional radiology (IR) techniques in pediatrics necessitated modifications to available devices, development of new interventions, and tailoring of techniques to the younger population. Many pediatric applications in IR evolved from the modification of similar procedures and devices previously established in adults. Others originated in pediatrics and were subsequently applied to adults (e.g., cecostomy tube insertion). For some devices (e.g., inferior vena cava [IVC] filters), no pediatric-sized devices are as yet available.

As in traditional practice, IR for the pediatric population is a clinically oriented field of radiology that practices in a multidisciplinary model encompassing pre-, peri-, and postprocedural care. Such a multidisciplinary team includes trained nurses, medical radiation technologists, and interventional radiologists, all with experience in pediatrics. Additional valuable members of the team are pediatric anesthesiologists, child life specialists, and pediatricians. Closely involved staff must be fully trained in airway management and sedation pharmacology and ideally be certified in pediatric advanced life support (PALS). In this chapter, the most common pediatric IR procedures are briefly described, stressing features most pertinent to the pediatric population.

IMAGING MODALITIES

- Imaging equipment used in pediatric IR differs in specifications compared with that used in adults.
- There is greater emphasis on the use of ultrasound (rather than computed tomography [CT]) and on radiation safety.
- A wide range of patient sizes must be accommodated, from newborns to young adults.

Ultrasound

- Less body fat in the pediatric population and the lack of ionizing radiation make ultrasound an ideal imaging modality.
- Ultrasound is quick, provides multidirectional guidance in real time, shows visible vascularity, and is generally safe.
- The choice of probes is dictated by body size and indications are as follows:

- A 5- to 7-MHz curved probe for larger patient organ biopsies and drainages
- An 8-MHz vector probe for intercostal access, mediastinal approaches, infant nephrostomy, solid organ biopsies, and abdominal drainages
- A 10- to 12-MHz linear probe for neonatal percutaneous cholecystography, superficial pulmonary nodule localization and biopsy, and the detection of vascular anomalies
- A 15-MHz linear "hockey stick" for vascular access and joint/tendon injections
- An endocavitary probe (e.g., transrectal) for pelvic abscess drainage
- Portable ultrasound is invaluable for bedside procedures in neonatal and pediatric intensive care units (NICUs and PICUs).

X-Ray, Fluoroscopy, and Computed Tomography

- Low-dose pulsed fluoroscopy, last image hold, storing fluoroscopy runs, and electronic zoom are necessary functions.
- High-quality digital subtraction angiography (DSA) is employed only when necessary to evaluate high-resolution detail of small and large vessels in children.
- Biplane imaging is very important for the simultaneous acquisition of images in two planes, thus reducing the volume of contrast needed.
- Neonatal and pediatric protocols should be developed with assistance from the equipment manufacturers and on-site physicist (e.g., copper filtration, grids, air gap, reduced-dose protocols). The use of factory-set adult protocols should be avoided.
- CT is useful for deep lung lesions and certain bone procedures. CT fluoroscopy requires care to avoid high radiation exposure.
- The use of cone-beam CT can potentially reduce radiation dose while also providing the benefit of image-fusion software to aid in lesion localization.

Angiography

- Angiography is both diagnostic and therapeutic.
- Intracerebral vascular disease, renovascular hypertension, gastrointestinal (GI) vascular pathology, and trauma can all be evaluated.

- Procedures are often performed under general anesthesia; moderate sedation may be possible in older children and even in the very young.
- Vasculature in neonates and infants is generally superficial and more prone to vasospasm, thrombosis, and occlusion.
- Pediatric arterial access is a potentially challenging.
  - Access is usually obtained using ultrasound guidance. Palpation of arteries may be difficult in neonates, young infants, and obese children.
  - The umbilical artery can be used for up to 5 days after birth. Existing umbilical arterial lines can be converted for angiographic access.
  - Axillary access may be employed in patients with occluded femoral arteries or if the angle of approach to the required vessel is more favorable from above.
- Volume overload is problematic in smaller children, especially neonates. Careful attention must be paid to the volume of saline and contrast administered (maximum 3–6 mL/kg of contrast depending on length of procedure). The use of small syringes helps to minimize inadvertent administration of excessive fluids.
- Contrast injection rates vary depending on patient size and the vessel selected. Hand injections are usually acceptable in smaller patients, especially those weighing less than 15 kg.
- Closure devices are not usually employed or recommended in the pediatric population due to the smaller size of the arteries.
- Complications related to arterial access increase in patients who weigh less than 15 kg.
- Heparinization is usually employed to reduce thrombotic complications.
- Claudication or leg-length discrepancy following femoral occlusion occurs rarely.

Magnetic Resonance Imaging

- The use of MRI in pediatric IR is still limited.
- An emerging application is in treating specific bone lesions that are visible only on MRI.

Other Equipment

- A full range of suitable devices for children of all ages (neonates to 18 years) are required:
  - Blood pressure (BP) cuffs in a variety of sizes
  - Pulse oximeters
  - Temperature preserving and monitoring devices
  - A range of endotracheal tubes
  - A pediatric crash cart
- Additionally, distraction tools (music, DVDs, and games) can prove helpful.

PREPROCEDURAL CARE

Preprocedure Assessment

- Review the requested procedure to make sure that it is indicated.
- Evaluate the risk-versus-benefit ratio for the patient.
- Decide on the appropriate level of sedation or anesthesia.

- If other procedures are planned (e.g., surgical, endoscopic, or interventional), consideration should be given to coordinating them under the same period of anesthesia or sedation to reduce the number of anesthetic events required.

Benefits of a Preprocedural Outpatient Clinic Visit

- A full and detailed history and physical examination can be obtained.
- Patients and families are given the opportunity to meet members of the IR team.
- The intended procedure can be explained and alternatives discussed.
- A management plan can be created.
- Further consultations or preprocedural investigations can be organized if needed.
- Informed consent and patient assent can be obtained.

Consent

- Pediatric procedures require more time with substitute decision makers (parents/guardians) than with adults who can provide consent directly.
- The provision of sufficient time, quietness, and lack of distractions can help to shape a suitable environment within which to discuss informed consent.
- Common risks, rare but serious risks, and alternatives to treatment must be outlined.
- Information pamphlets, use of lay language, and diagrams can be helpful.

Laboratory Studies

- Not all procedures require preprocedural laboratory testing.
- For procedures that pose an inherent risk of bleeding (e.g., organ biopsy, insertion of a central venous access device, etc.), relevant laboratory results are ordered and reviewed.
- A review of electrolyte levels (to avoid arrhythmias) and creatinine (to avoid renal impairment) is important.
- It is important to know how normal laboratory values vary with patient age.

Choosing Anesthesia/Sedation

- Minor procedures (e.g., peripherally inserted central catheter [PICC]) can be performed using oral sucrose for neonates and infants below 6 months of age.
- Distraction techniques (videos, CDs, music, child life specialists, etc.) are very useful in engaging the pediatric patient and reducing the need for pharmacological agents.
- Nitrous oxide is a safe self-administered inhalational agent.
- Use of topical anesthetic creams and sprays reduces pain at the site of local anesthetic injection.
- Procedures that could typically be performed with local anesthesia or under minimal sedation in adults often demand deep sedation or general anesthesia in children.

- IR-administered sedation is usually limited to those patients considered healthy or have mild systemic disease, ASA I and II (a classification of the American Society of Anesthesiology). More complex patients usually require the presence of a pediatric anesthesiologist.
- Common agents:
  - Anxiolytics (oral/intranasal) are useful medications for calming.
    - Barbiturates have almost no analgesic effect in sedative doses and can, in fact, make children hypersensitive to environmental or physical stimuli.
  - Morphine and fentanyl are commonly used in combination.
    - Morphine requires 10 minutes to take effect and can provide analgesia for up to 2 hours. It is dosed at 0.05 mg/kg IV.
    - Fentanyl is given as a slow push in doses of 1 µg/kg IV safely fractionated in aliquots of 0.25 µg/kg IV. It takes effect within minutes with 100 times the potency of morphine, but it must be readministered every 30 to 60 minutes.
  - Ketamine can be administered at the precise time of acute pain (e.g., sclerotherapy, tract dilatation) and is used in combination with benzodiazepines to reduce adverse side effects of hallucinations, delusions, and nightmares.

Preparation for Anesthesia/Sedation

- Fasting requirements should be in line with institutional guidelines. For example,
  - Nothing by mouth for 6 to 8 hours after formula feed and solids
  - Nothing by mouth for 4 hours after breast milk
  - Nothing by mouth for 2 hours after clear liquids
- Maintenance intravenous fluids should be given preprocedure to avoid dehydration. This is especially important in patients receiving intravenous contrast. The rate is calculated with the 4:2:1 rule:
  - For the first 10 kg, 4 mL/kg per hour
  - For the next 10 kg, 2 mL/kg per hour
  - Thereafter, 1 mL/kg per hour for each kilogram

PROCEDURAL CARE

- Appropriate monitoring during the procedure is imperative, including attention to sedation, vital signs (heart rate [HR], respiratory rate [RR], pulse oximetry, BP, and temperature) and radiation exposure.

Temperature Control

- Children have limited ability to control their own temperature. Infants and young children rapidly lose body heat, especially from the head, and can become profoundly hypothermic.
- Monitoring of peripheral and/or core temperature is necessary for any child below 1 year of age and for older children undergoing a procedure for any significant length of time.

- Temperature-preserving equipment is vitally important, including warming blankets, cloth head covers or bonnets, plastic covers for the intubated child, warm air blowers, warm air mattresses, and chemical blankets for very low-birth weight patients (<1.5 kg).

Radiation Exposure

- Children are more sensitive to radiation exposure due to their greater cell turnover, smaller body sizes, and longer life expectancy in which to display adverse effects.
- When possible, imaging modalities not involving radiation (such as ultrasound) should be employed.
- It is important to protect vulnerable tissues (e.g., lens of the eye, gonads, red marrow, breast, intestinal mucosa, skin) from radiation exposure.
- Fluoroscopy
  - *Beam-on time* is kept to a minimum by stepping on the fluoroscopy pedal as infrequently and briefly as possible.
  - The lowest pulse rate adequate for the procedure is chosen (e.g., four per second).
  - The ability to review the last image avoids unnecessary additional fluoroscopy.
  - Strict collimation to area of interest limits unnecessary organ exposure.
  - True magnification is used judiciously.
  - Stored fluoroscopy runs are frequently adequate in lieu of new exposures.
- DSA
  - DSA is employed only when necessary or when a stored fluoroscopy run is inadequate for the needed purpose.
  - Careful planning prior to each DSA run ensures that all parameters—correct patient positioning, collimation, magnification minimized, lowest suitable frame rate (venous or arterial), contrast volume, and pump settings—are appropriate.
  - Children with faster HRs and greater cardiac output often necessitate higher frame rates.
- Rotational angiography
  - This offers potential contrast and radiation dose saving compared with repeating imaging in multiple different projections.
- CT
  - Low-dose pediatric protocols must be used if and when CT is required.

Antibiotics

- Routine use of antibiotics in the pediatric population is usually not indicated.
- Choice of antibiotics is procedure-dependent and based on drug uptake, excretion, and concentration used.

Contrast

- If iodinated contrast is needed, the amount is titrated according to the patient's weight and procedure duration.
  - 3 mL/kg is generally accepted and can be increased to 6 mL/kg for prolonged procedures.

- The incidence of allergic reactions to iodinated contrast is low in the pediatric population (0.2%–3.5%).
  - Minor reactions may be dose dependent and include the sensation of warmth and pain, nausea and vomiting, metallic taste, bradycardia, hypotension, and vasovagal reactions.
  - Premedication is required in known cases of contrast allergy.
  - Alternative contrast (CO_2, gadolinium) can be considered in known cases of contrast allergy.

POSTPROCEDURAL CARE

- Postprocedural care is an essential part of pediatric IR. It is determined by the nature of the procedure and its risks (e.g., evaluation for peritonitis after gastrostomy (G) tube insertion, following up hemoglobin after biopsy). Postprocedural care may be in the form of one or more of the following:
  - Ward visit for inpatients
  - Follow-up phone call for outpatients/day cases
  - Postprocedural visits to the IR clinic for evaluation
  - Online or printed material to supplement personal instructions for a fully informed discharge

COMMON PEDIATRIC PROCEDURES

Central Venous Access

- Indications include the need for total parenteral nutrition (TPN), medium- to long-term antibiotics, chemotherapy, frequent blood sampling, fluid replacement, dialysis or apheresis, and medical support in cases of severe illness.
- Access can be temporary or permanent, cuffed or uncuffed, tunneled or untunneled, and implanted or external.
- Options for vascular access include:
  - PICCs

- Central venous catheters (CVCs)
- Port-a-Caths (ports)
- The choice of device is based on indication, frequency of need, predicted duration, patient size, patient age, vessel patency, underlying illness, and somewhat on family, patient, or physician preference (Table 9.1).
- The tips of central lines placed in the upper venous system should be positioned at the distal superior vena cava/ entrance to the right atrium (cavoatrial junction). The tips of lines placed in the lower venous system are referred to as either short (in the infrarenal IVC) or long (above the renal veins at the diaphragm/lower right atrium).
- The most common general complications are infection and thrombosis.

Peripherally Inserted Central Catheters

- Most clinical indications in children can be met with a 3- or 4-Fr single-lumen PICC. Double-lumen lines are available but should only be used when needed.
- In neonates, a 1.9- or 3-Fr single-lumen or 2.6-Fr double-lumen PICC usually suffices.
- Prophylactic antibiotics are not routinely indicated.
- In infants and young children, total procedure time and total number of venipuncture attempts are important risk factors.
- PICC insertions are challenging in the very young. Resorting to a tunneled femoral or jugular venous line may be indicated if peripheral access cannot be achieved. It is prudent to prepare parents for this possibility.

Central Venous Catheters

- In small children, CVCs may be technically easier and faster to place than PICCs.
- The internal jugular vein is the most commonly used insertion site.
- Femoral CVCs are useful in children with occlusions in the upper venous systems, those with complex congenital

			Frequency	Common		
VAD	**Type**	**Duration of Need**	**of Use**	**Indications**	**Advantages**	**Disadvantages**
PICC	External (usually uncuffed)	Short- to medium-term (weeks)	Daily use	Antibiotics, TPN, medications	No needle is required for access. Insertion and removal are less invasive.	Dressing changes. External device with increased risk of dislodgment and infection.
CVC	External (both tunneled and untunneled, cuffed and uncuffed)	Short- to medium-term (months)	Daily or frequent use	Long-term TPN, dialysis, apheresis, chemotherapy, ICU support	No needle is required for access. Insertion and removal are less invasive.	Dressing changes. External device with increased risk of dislodgment and infection.
PORT	Fully internal	Medium- to long-term (months to years)	Intermittent	Chemotherapy	Minimal visibility. Less risk of infection.	A non-coring needle is needed for access. Insertion and removal are more invasive.

TABLE 9.1   Types and Features of Vascular Access Devices

CVC, Central venous catheter; *ICU,* intensive care unit; *PICC,* peripherally inserted central catheter; *TPN,* total parenteral nutrition; *VAD,* vascular access device; *Port-a-catheter.*

heart disease, and in cases of emergent indications (e.g., resuscitation, apheresis, acute hemodialysis).

- Infection and thrombosis are common risks with femoral CVCs in young children, especially in those who wear diapers.

Port

- Usually placed in the upper venous system, frequently in an infraclavicular subcutaneous pocket with the catheter placed through the internal jugular vein.
- A noncoring needle, to avoid damage to silicone septum, is used for access.
- Prophylactic antibiotics are not routinely indicated.

Percutaneous Biopsies

- Indicated to evaluate and diagnose medical diseases in a variety of solid organs (e.g., liver, kidney, bone, spleen, etc.).
- Unlike adults, pediatric patients may require general anesthesia.
- The diagnostic yield of percutaneous image-guided core biopsies is usually equivalent to that of surgical biopsies but with less associated morbidity.
  - Fine-needle aspiration (FNA) is most often used to assess infectious lesions, lymph node metastases, and thyroid lesions. As opposed to FNA, core needle biopsies yield more tissue and allow for more varied staining techniques, marker studies, and genetic analyses.
- Ultrasound is the most commonly used imaging modality for biopsies, as the needle can be seen in real time. The choice of probe depends on patient size and target tissue depth. CT-guided biopsies are also performed. MRI guidance is an emerging approach.
- The choice of biopsy needle varies according to the biopsy site, institutional and interventionalist preferences, and pathology requirements (most commonly 14–21 gauge).
- A prebiopsy assessment that includes a complete blood count and coagulation profile is usually required. Platelets should be greater than 50,000 and the international normalized ratio (INR) less than or equal to 1.5. Blood should be typed and screened in case blood products should be needed.
- The coaxial technique may be used for solid organ biopsies to reduce the risk of bleeding, leakage (air/bile), and/or tumor seeding.
  - An outer needle is passed through the organ capsule.
  - A finer biopsy needle is passed through the outer needle multiple times, obtaining cores in several different trajectories.
  - The tract can be sealed with a variety of plugging agents (Gelfoam, autologous clot, coils, glue, etc.) as the outer needle is removed.

Liver Biopsy

- Indications include assessment of liver diseases, assessment of liver lesions, and evaluation of potential transplant rejection.

- Ultrasound is the standard imaging modality.
- An intercostal approach (if biopsying the right lobe) or subxiphoid approach (if biopsying the left lobe) is taken.
- The main risk of percutaneous biopsy is bleeding secondary to capsular penetration; if large, this can be life threatening.
  - The coaxial technique may be performed to reduce bleeding in patients with minor derangements in the coagulation profile or for those requiring multiple core passes to reduce blood loss.
  - To avoid capsular penetration, transjugular liver biopsy can be performed in patients with severe ascites and/or uncorrected coagulopathy (see, hepatobiliary interventions).
- The creation of arteriovenous fistulas and hemobilia is uncommon.

Renal Biopsy

- Indications include assessment of generalized parenchymal renal diseases (e.g., nephritic or nephrotic syndrome), assessment of renal allographs for rejection, and diagnosis of focal lesions (e.g., renal tumors).
- Native kidneys are biopsied with the patient prone, and transplanted grafts are biopsied with the patient supine.
- The combination of moderate sedation and local anesthesia is usually adequate.
- The number of samples required is generally higher for the diagnosis of tumors than for the diagnosis of medical renal disease.
- Risks include hemorrhage, hematuria, and the creation of arteriovenous fistulas.

Spleen Biopsy

- Performed for the diagnosis of focal splenic lesions and diseases of the spleen.
- Ultrasound is the standard imaging modality.
- A normal coagulation profile is necessary, given the main risk of bleeding.

Bone Biopsy

- Choice of imaging modality depends on which best displays the target (fluoroscopy, CT, ultrasound, or MRI).
- General anesthesia is frequently required, as the procedure may be exquisitely painful.
- Common indications include the following:
  - Determining whether a lesion is benign or malignant
  - Determining the nature and extent of a systemic disease
  - Obtaining a specimen for microbiologic analysis of a suspected infection
- Sampling the soft tissue component of a musculoskeletal lesion may be preferable and easier than sampling the bone.
- The main risks include fracture, insufficient tissue sample, bleeding, and neurovascular injury.

Muscle Biopsy

- Indicated for the evaluation of primary lesions within the muscle (with or without associated bone lesions).

TABLE 9.2   Types and Features of Enteric Access

Tube Type	Indications	Advantages	Disadvantages
NG	Short-term feeding need (<3 months)	Placed in the patient's room. Minimally invasive.	Visible on face. Uncomfortable. Tube crossing the gastroesophageal (GE) junction may aggravate reflux.
NJ	Short-term feeding need in a patient with GERD (<3 months)	Minimally invasive.	May require imaging to place. Visible on face. Uncomfortable. Tube crossing the GE junction may aggravate reflux.
G	Long-term feeding need (>3 months)	Permits bolus feeds. Low-profile. Can be replaced at home.	Invasive procedure with inherent risk.
GJ	Long-term feeding need in a patient with GERD (>3 months)	Bypasses stomach, avoiding GERD issues. Convertible to G tube if reflux improves.	Invasive procedure with inherent risk. Requires imaging for tube changes.
Combined G and GJ tubes	Long-term feeding need and gastric venting (>3 months)	Permits decompressive venting of the stomach with simultaneous feeding into the jejunum.	Invasive procedure with inherent risk.

G, Gastrostomy; *GERD*, gastroesophageal reflux disease; *GJ*, gastrojejunostomy; *NG*, nasogastric; *NJ*, nasojejunostomy; *GE*, gastroesophageal.

- Sampling of suspected metabolic, mitochondrial, and genetic disorders requires large specimens aligned along the muscle fibers.
- The main risks include diagnostic failure due to misaligned biopsy orientation tangential to the muscle fibers, bleeding, and pseudoaneurysm formation.

Chest and Lung Biopsy

- A higher prevalence of non-squamous cell, sarcomatous lesions in the pediatric population necessitates core biopsy of suspected lesions.
  - FNA may be suitable for some infectious or metastatic diseases.
- Chest wall, mediastinal, and parenchymal lesions abutting the pleura are visible on ultrasound and are amenable to ultrasound-guided biopsy. Deeper parenchymal lesions are not visible on ultrasound because of overlying air and usually require CT guidance.
- The main risks include the development of pneumothoraces, hemothoraces, and hemoptysis.
  - Pneumothoraces occur less often in children than in adults, likely due to healthier lung tissue.
- IR also offers image-guided lung tattooing for lesions requiring excisional biopsy or in cases where thoracoscopic resection is planned.

Mediastinal Biopsy

- Anterior mediastinal lesions are frequently lymphomatous in etiology. Biopsy is indicated only if diagnosis is not possible from a pleural fluid sample or biopsy of a peripheral lymph node. Masses require multiple cores of tissue, usually accessible by ultrasound.
  - Airway compromise by anterior mediastinal masses may be life-threatening; therefore a pediatric anesthesiologist should be consulted prior to biopsy of such lesions. Biopsies may be obtained with the patient sitting rather than supine.

- Posterior mediastinal lesions may be amenable to ultrasound- or CT-guided biopsy and are frequently neurogenic in etiology (e.g., ganglioneuroma, neuroblastoma).
- The main risks are airway collapse (anterior lesions), bleeding, insufficient tissue sample, and pneumothoraces.

Gastrointestinal Interventions

- Adequate nutrition is essential for normal growth and development.
- When possible, enteral feeding (Table 9.2) is preferred to intravenous hyperalimentation.
- Gastrostomy (G) or Gastrojejunostomy (GJ) tubes are indicated in children who are unable to take in adequate calories or essential nutrients orally for a period of time, usually greater than 3 months.
- Common indications include neurologic disorders (e.g., cerebral palsy), cystic fibrosis, underlying malignancies, severe metabolic disease, congenital cardiac disease, and nutritional support for solid organ and bone marrow transplantation.
- In short-term cases (6 weeks or less) in children with functional GI tracts, temporizing measures such as a nasogastric (NG) or nasojejunostomy (NJ) tube may be sufficient.

Percutaneous Gastrostomy

- Different methods are available for placement of fluoroscopically guided G tubes:
  - The retrograde (also known as *push*) percutaneous approach through the abdominal wall into the stomach
  - The antegrade (also known as *pull*) approach, whereby the tube is pulled down through the esophagus and out the stomach and abdominal wall
    - Requires adequate esophageal caliber and the absence of esophageal pathology (e.g., stricture, epidermolysis bullosa)
- A push–pull technique is a hybrid of both.

- G tubes are typically easier to manage than GJ tubes.
- The main risk is peritonitis.

Percutaneous Gastrojejunostomy

- Indications include children who do not tolerate G-tube feeds and those with severe gastroesophageal reflux, poor gastric emptying, or risk of aspiration of gastric contents.
- A GJ tube is harder to manage for families, requires much more time for feeds (almost continuous), is more apt to clog, requires replacement under fluoroscopy, and can act as a lead point for intussusception.
- The insertion procedure is technically more difficult than that for a G tube.
- The main risk is peritonitis.

Cecostomy Tube (Fig. 9.1)

- A pigtail catheter is placed in the cecum (Fig. 9.1) to facilitate regular/controlled colonic washouts in children with fecal incontinence.
- It may be indicated in children with anal sphincter dysfunction (e.g., spina bifida or anorectal malformations).
- Placement is more challenging than that for a G or GJ tube.
- The main risks are fecal peritonitis and ventriculitis in children with ventriculoperitoneal shunts.
- Ongoing tube maintenance is required.

Esophageal Dilation (Fig. 9.2)

- Indications include postanastomotic stricture following tracheoesophageal repair, stricture following caustic ingestion, and epidermolysis bullosa.

- Performed antegrade through the mouth or nose or retrograde via a G tube, under sedation or general anesthesia. A guidewire and balloon are advanced to the area of the stricture and dilated under fluroscopy.
- The risks include esophageal perforation, bleeding, and recurrence.

Bowel Dilation

- Dilatation is indicated for benign anastomotic strictures or in cases of necrotizing enterocolitis within the colon, rectum, and duodenum, among other sites.
- The main risks include perforation, bleeding, and difficulty reaching the strictured site.

Hepatobiliary Interventions

- Indications for liver transplantation in pediatric patients include:
  - Intrahepatic or extrahepatic cholestasis
  - Cystic fibrosis
  - Metabolic diseases
  - Acute liver failure
  - Primary tumors
- Causes of cholestasis in pediatric patients include:
  - Biliary atresia
  - Congenital hepatic fibrosis
  - Neonatal hepatitis
  - Cystic fibrosis
  - α-1 antitrypsin deficiency
  - TPN cholestasis

Percutaneous Transhepatic Cholangiography (Fig. 9.3)

- Evaluates the biliary tree (e.g., biliary-enteric anastomosis in liver transplant patients) for complications such as leaks and strictures.

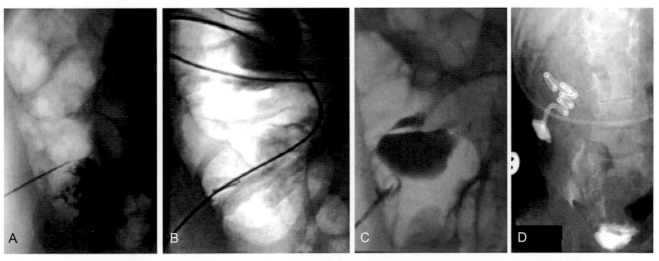

Fig. 9.1 Percutaneous Cecostomy. Series of fluoroscopic image-saves showing a gas filled ascending colon and cecum. The image-save technique is commonly used in pediatrics to reduce the amount of radiation directed at the patient. (A) After needle puncture of the cecum, injected contrast is seen within the cecal lumen. (B) Subsequently, a guidewire is advanced in the ascending colon and two metallic retention anchor sutures are deployed within the cecum. (C) Over the wire, a pigtail catheter is been formed in the cecum and the wire removed. (D) Final image shows the low-profile Trapdoor style cecostomy tube in a mature tract. (Courtesy of Bairbre Connolly.)

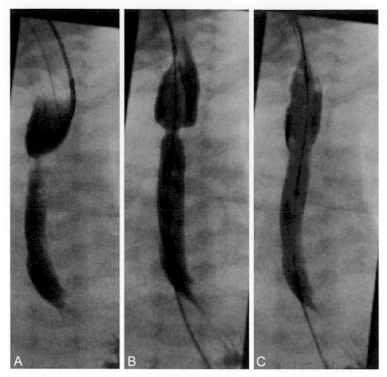

Fig. 9.2 Infant Several Months Following Tracheo-Esophageal Fistula Repair. Series of fluoroscopic image-saves, used to reduce the amount of radiation directed at the young patient. (A) The classic appearance of a tight upper esophageal anastamotic stricture with a catheter in the dilated upper pouch and contrast outlining the narrow stricture. Note that this infant is intubated for the procedure. (B) A guidewire is advanced across the stricture and balloon inflated to dilate the stricture. (C) A larger diameter balloon is placed across stricture for repeat dilatation. (Courtesy Bairbre Connolly.)

- An ultrasound-guided needle is used to access the biliary tree through the liver and is confirmed with subsequent opacification of the biliary system with radiopaque contrast.
- Ascites should be drained first to decrease the possibility of hemorrhage.
- If indicated, this procedure can be converted to drainage, dilatation, or stent placement.
- A variation of this procedure is ultrasound-guided access (25- or 27-gauge) directly into the gallbladder in patients with congenital anomalies (e.g., biliary atresia, biliary hypoplasia, Alagille syndrome, and TPN cholestasis).

Percutaneous Cholecystostomy

- This involves placement of a pigtail tube into the gallbladder.
- It is an uncommon therapeutic option for decompressing the gallbladder in acutely ill and severely compromised patients (e.g., in cases of acalculous or necrotizing cholecystitis).
  - It is a high-risk procedure in a high-risk patient population.

Hepatic Venography

- Useful in the evaluation of Budd-Chiari syndrome, veno-occlusive disease, transplant-associated venous strictures, and portal hypertension and as an indirect method of assessing portal venous pressures (sinusoidal)

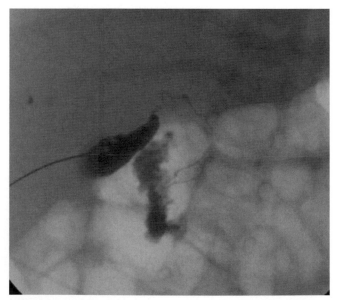

Fig. 9.3 Neonatal Cholangiogram. Neonatal cholangiogram through a 25G needle in the gallbladder (GB) shows a normal sized GB, patent but hypoplastic distal biliary tree, and lack of opacification of the intra-hepatic and common hepatic ducts. (Courtesy Bairbre Connolly.)

- In cases of reduced liver transplant grafts, the acute angle into the hepatic vein makes accessing the target vein difficult.
- It is the primary step in a transjugular liver biopsy, indicated in uncorrectable coagulopathy.

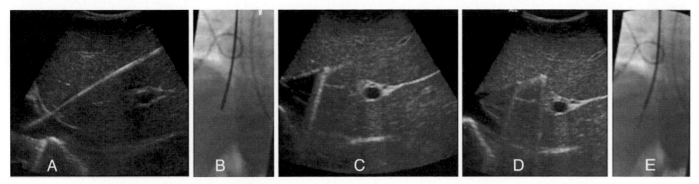

Fig. 9.4 Pediatric Transjugular Liver Biopsy. (A) Sagittal ultrasound image with catheter and wire seen in the right atrium, IVC, and hepatic vein. (B) Fluoroscopic image-save of the biopsy canula in the hepatic vein prior to throw of needle. The image-save technique reduces the amount of radiation directed at the patient. (C) Ultrasound image of the canula in the hepatic vein, planning a safe trajectory for the biopsy needle prior to firing. (D) Ultrasound monitoring in real time of the throw of the biopsy needle as it extends from the canula, ensuring a safe trajectory. (E) Fluoroscopic image-save of the needle in its fired position. (Courtesy Bairbre Connolly.)

- The right internal jugular vein is accessed → IVC → right hepatic vein.
- It allows reflux opacification of the portal venous anatomy for planning REX shunt surgery.

Transjugular Liver Biopsy (Fig. 9.4)

- As in adults, it is indicated to evaluate for severe liver disease in the presence of uncorrectable coagulopathy and severe ascites.
- The biopsy needle is advanced under image guidance through a catheter placed in the right hepatic vein.
- Biopsy is performed into the liver parenchyma without puncture of the liver capsule (as opposed to percutaneous liver biopsy, which by definition punctures the capsule).
- Termed *recirculation,* bleeding occurs back into the hepatic vein.
- In children, given the small size of the liver and the length of throw of the biopsy needle, careful biopsy using real-time ultrasound helps avoid capsular perforation.
- The main risks include bleeding, arrhythmia, and inadvertent capsule perforation.

Transjugular Intrahepatic Portosystemic Shunt

- Uncommonly performed in children.
- As in adults, this is a method to relieve portal hypertension frequently in children listed for liver transplant by shunting blood from the portal into the hepatic circulation, bypassing the liver parenchyma.
- Causes of portal hypertension in children include cirrhosis, biliary atresia, congenital hepatic fibrosis, hepatitis, cystic fibrosis, α-1 antitrypsin deficiency, and TPN cholestasis.
- The main risks are shunt occlusion, encephalopathy, and lack of suitably sized stents.

Thoracic Interventions
Drainage

- Placement of a pigtail catheter using ultrasound, CT, or fluoroscopic guidance

- Indications include evacuation of postoperative, spontaneous, or traumatic pneumothoraces or drainage of pleural fluid that has accumulated secondary to underlying diseases (e.g., pneumonia, chylous effusion, malignancy).
- Empyema (purulent or infected pleural fluid) contains fibrin and septae, often requiring subsequent fibrinolytics (e.g., tPA) administered through the chest tube.
- The main risks include air leak, bleeding, fluid shifts, and reperfusion pulmonary edema.

Intrathoracic Abscess Drainage

- An uncommon complication of pneumonia. Risk factors include congenital or acquired immune disorders, prematurity, endocarditis, cerebral palsy, poor oral hygiene, and congenital pulmonary abnormalities.
- Most common causative organisms are *Staphylococcus aureus* and *Haemophilus influenzae.*
- Not all abscesses require drainage, especially if the patient is asymptomatic.
- Differential diagnoses that should be considered include loculated empyema, infected congenital cystadenomatoid malformation, cavitary tuberculosis, pneumonia, hematoma, pulmonary infarction, foregut cysts, sequestration, and lymphangioma.
- The main risks of drainage include bleeding and aspiration of pus into the ipsi- and contralateral bronchial tree.

Tracheobronchial Stent Insertion

- Indications include tracheomalacia, tracheobronchomalacia, tracheal strictures, airway compression due to a mass, and vascular anomalies.
- Causes of bronchomalacia are multifold, including:
  - Congenital deficiency of cartilaginous rings, a primary cause.
  - Secondary causes such as external compression by an enlarged vessel, vascular ring, or a bronchogenic cyst.
  - Part of VACTERL syndrome from TE fistula or esophageal atresia.

- Using a stent that is at least 2 mm larger than the diameter of the narrowing is suggested in the pediatric population to allow for future growth.
- Limitations of stenting include lack of stent growth as the child grows, stent migration, stent ingrowth, and difficulty with stent removal.

Renal Interventions

- 1% to 5% of all children are hypertensive, and 5% to 25% of those have an arterial cause (e.g., stenosis).
- CT angiography is being increasingly employed, but renal arteriogram remains the gold standard in the diagnosis of renovascular hypertension.
- Intervention is indicated in those with medically refractory hypertension.
  - Dilatation of renal stenosis for hypertension is successful in approximately half of all cases, and half of these will be sustained after 1 year. Angioplasty can be repeated in those who restenose.
  - Main risks include dissection, artery rupture, thrombosis, restricture, and pseudoaneurysm formation.
- In very small infants under 18 months of age, the ability to treat a lesion with balloon angioplasty is challenging. It is preferred to wait until 2 or 3 years of age to do an arteriogram if the hypertension can be managed medically in the meantime.
- Occasionally, embolization of an ischemic vascular territory is undertaken (e.g., alcohol injection) to interrupt the hypertension-causing renin-angiotensin circuit.
- Etiologies for renovascular hypertension are numerous but include fibromuscular dysplasia (60%–80% of all causes), neurofibromatosis type I, midaortic syndrome, Williams syndrome, Takayasu arteritis, polyarteritis nodosa, and radiation therapy.

Pulmonary Vascular Interventions

- In pediatric IR, most pulmonary angiography is performed to
  1. Retrieve an embolized foreign body (e.g., catheter fragment)
  2. Treat pulmonary arteriovenous malformation (PAVM)
  3. Lyse a pulmonary embolism (PE)

Pulmonary Embolism in Pediatrics

- The incidence of PE in pediatric patients is 0.14/100,000 with a lower mortality compared to adults.
- About 84% of children with PE present with shortness of breath and/or chest pain. Approximately 15% of suspected PEs are confirmed on CT angiography.
- The leading cause of thrombosis and PE in children is the presence of a venous access device.

PAVMs in Pediatrics

- Pulmonary arteriovenous malformations (PAVM) are rare.
  - 70% to 95% of PAVMs occur in the setting of hereditary hemorrhagic telangiectasia (HHT). 25% of patients with HHT have PAVMs. Less than 5% of cases will present in childhood as most are not symptomatic until adulthood.

- About 10% of PAVMs are acquired from systemic diseases like hepatopulmonary syndrome.
- Embolization is performed to reduce right-to-left shunting and protect against cerebral abscess formation. It can be performed with coils, balloons, or plugs. Complexity of the lesions is based the anatomy and number of arterial segments feeding the AVM.
- The main risks include systemic embolization of the coil, stroke, and reopening of the PAVM.

Vascular Interventions

Treatment of Endovascular Thrombosis

- The treatment approach is tailored to the individual and depends on the severity and extent of the thrombosis, age of the clot, comorbidities, and whether limbs or organs are at risk.
- Treatment options range from anticoagulation (such as heparin), chemical thrombolysis (systemic tPA or catheter-directed tPA), mechanical thrombolysis (suction, clot disruption, and various thrombectomy devices), or a combination.
- Pediatric arterial thrombosis arises secondary to trauma, shock, dehydration, or iatrogenic causes.
  - Pediatric arteries are prone to spasm so concurrent treatment with a vasodilator, such as a calcium channel blocker, should be considered.
  - Can result in leg length discrepancy (chronic) or acutely as limb/organ loss
- Pediatric venous thrombosis usually occurs secondary to the presence of a CVC, anatomic abnormality (e.g., May Thurner syndrome, thoracic outlet syndrome), thrombophilia, or oral contraceptive use.
  - Deep venous thrombosis (DVT) leads to postthrombotic syndrome (PTS) in up to 26% of pediatric cases. This is partly due to age-related variations in levels of both coagulation factors and natural anticoagulants.
  - Placement of an IVC filter may be required to prevent dislodgement of a DVT into the pulmonary vasculature; however, no IVC filter specific for the small pediatric-sized patient has been designed.
- Vessel reocclusion is common following endovascular treatment in pediatric patients, and aggressive postprocedure anticoagulation is required.

Vascular Anomalies

- The International Society for the Study of Vascular Anomalies (ISSVA) divides vascular anomalies (Box 9.1) based on biology and clinical behavior and broadly classifies them as either vascular tumors or vascular malformations (high-flow or low-flow).
- IR plays a major role in treating patients with these anomalies, ideally as part of a multidisciplinary team that includes pediatric plastic surgeons, dermatologists, and hematologists.
- Although 80% to 90% of anomalies can be diagnosed through history and examination alone, ultrasound and MR help to further evaluate the nature and extent of tissue involvement.

BOX 9.1 ISSVA Classification of Vascular Anomalies

Vascular Tumors
- Infantile hemangioma
- Congenital hemangioma (RICH and NICH)
- Tufted angioma
- Kaposiform hemangioendothelioma
- Spindle cell hemangioendothelioma
- Other rare hemangioendotheliomas (epithelioid, composite, retiform, polymorphous, etc.)
- Dermatologic acquired vascular tumors (pyogenic granuloma, targetoid hemangioma, glomeruloid hemangioma, etc.)

Vascular Malformations
- Slow-flow
  - Capillary malformation (CM)
  - Venous malformation (VM)
  - Lymphatic malformation (LM)
- Fast-flow
  - Arterial malformation (AM)
  - Arteriovenous fistula (AVF)
  - Arteriovenous malformation (AVM)
- Complex combined
  - CVM, CLM, LVM, CLVM, AVM-LM, CM-AVM, etc.

Rapidly Involuting Congenital Hemangioma (RICH); Non-Involuting Congenital Hemangioma (NICH).

- Generally, low-flow lesions are treated with sclerotherapy, whereas high-flow lesions are treated with embolization.
  - Extensive sclerotherapy carries a risk of hemoglobinuria, requiring aggressive intravenous hydration and careful monitoring of urine output through a Foley catheter during and after the procedure.
  - Various sclerosants are available. Ethanol as a sclerosant carries a risk of cardiovascular collapse. Close communication between the radiologist and the anesthesiologist during the procedure is important.

- Risks of sclerosing include swelling, skin blistering/necrosis, hemoglobinuria, pain, and cardiovascular collapse.

Musculoskeletal Interventions

Osteoid Osteoma

- A benign, painful lesion in the cortex, medulla, or subperiosteum consisting of unmineralized osteoid and mineralized bone with loose fibrovascular tissue.
- Most common in males 10 to 35 years old.
- Long bones (e.g., femur, tibia) and the spine are commonly affected.
- Pain classically causes waking at night and occasional changes in gait. Pain is responsive to NSAIDs in most patients.
- X-ray or CT classically shows sclerotic bone with a central hypodense nidus.
- Bone lesions can be accessed with a coaxial needle system and then ablated (e.g., radiofrequency or laser) (Fig. 9.5). High-intensity focused ultrasound ablation is entirely noninvasive.
- The main risks of ablation include procedural failure, recurrence, pain, infection, and skin burn.

Aneurysmal Bone Cysts

- These are benign, locally aggressive, multiloculated cystic bone neoplasms that contain a fibroproliferative mesenchymal stroma with giant cell–like osteoclasts and vascular spaces.
- They have a "soap bubble" radiographic appearance (Fig. 9.6), and fluid-fluid levels are often demonstrated on CT and MRI. They are most commonly found in the femur, tibia, humerus, spine, and pelvis.
- Treatment is indicated to arrest expansion, improve stability, and decrease future fracture risk. Embolization of the arterial supply can be used as either a primary treatment or an adjunct prior to surgical resection. Sclerotherapy with various agents is an alternative treatment option.

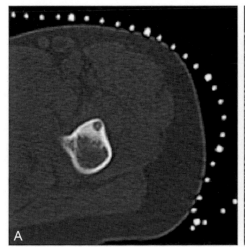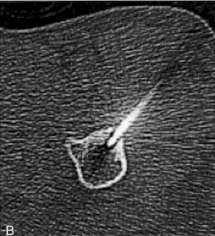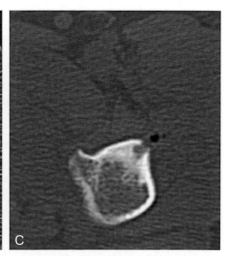

Fig. 9.5 Osteoid Osteoma. (A) Axial CT slice of the upper left femur showing an osteoid osteoma. Skin markers have been placed to plan approach. (B) CT fluoroscopy image of biopsy needle in the lesion, for sampling prior to ablation. (C) Cortical defect after lesional biopsy. (Courtesy Bairbre Connolly.)

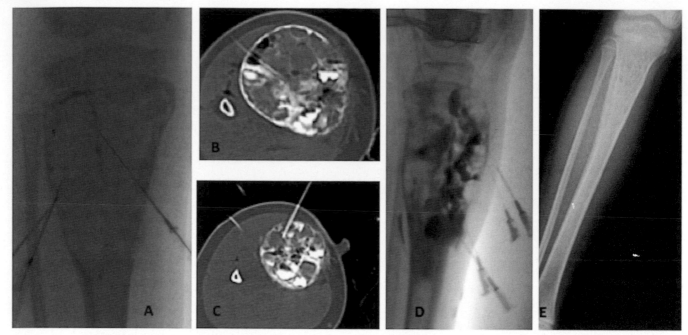

Fig. 9.6 Aneurysmal Bone Cyst of the Tibia. (A) Fluoroscopic image-save (a technique that reduced radiation directed at the patient) of the upper tibia of a young child with characteristic bubbly appearance of an aneurysmal bone cyst almost completely replacing the upper metaphysis. Several needles are in position during the first sclerotherapy treatment with sodium tetradecyl sulphate foam. (B and C) Two different axial images of the lesion with needles in situ and contrast already injected within the aneurysmal bone cyst. (D) Fluoroscopic image-save of the lesion with 4 needles in the lesion and contrast seen within the loculi of the bony lesion situ during sclertherapy treatment. (E) After three treatments and 2.5 years later, the tibia is almost completed healed. (Courtesy Bairbre Connolly.)

- The main risks of treatment include fracture, bleeding, recurrence, and premature growth plate fusion.

Steroid Injections

- Injection of the joint space or tendon sheath with corticosteroids is an efficacious treatment for juvenile arthritides and other inflammatory conditions.
- The accuracy of joint localization using clinical landmarks alone is less than 50%. Ultrasound-guided treatment (with or without fluoroscopy) increases injection accuracy, avoiding high systemic steroid doses while achieving high doses at the affected site.
- The main risks include infection, skin atrophy, crystal arthropathy, and a variable response to treatment.
  - Patients and parents should be educated on the signs and symptoms of septic arthritis, with instructions to contact their rheumatologist or interventional radiologist if signs of sepsis develop.

Botox Injections

- In pediatrics, Botox A (a neurotoxin produced by *Clostridium botulinum*) is used to treat muscle spasticity and drooling. The beneficial effects are temporary, typically lasting between 3 and 6 months.
- Ultrasound-guided intramuscular Botox injection into targeted muscles (Fig. 9.8) helps to reduce spasticity, improve gait and function, relieve pain, and reduce dystonia by targeting the neuromuscular junction.
  - Most commonly indicated in patients with cerebral palsy.

- Ultrasound-guided intrasalivary gland Botox injection (Fig. 9.7) is indicated in patients with sialorrhea.
  - Injections interrupt the parasympathetic innervation of the salivary glands, decreasing the amount of fluid and electrolytes in the saliva but leaving the sympathetic innervation, which is responsible for creating the proteinaceous and mucinous components of saliva that keep patient dentition intact.
- The main risks include systemic spread leading to botulism, neurovascular injury, and the formation of antibodies to Botox.

Genitourinary Interventions
Percutaneous Nephrostomy

- The most common causes of urinary tract obstruction in children are narrowing of the ureteropelvic junction (UPJ) and ureterovesical junction (UVJ).
- Common indications for percutaneous nephrostomy in children include the following:
  - Relief of obstruction (UPJ obstruction after pyeloplasty, UVJ obstruction after ureterovesical reimplantation)
  - Posterior urethral valves
  - Complex obstructive megaureter
  - As the initial step prior to nephrolithotripsy
- Percutaneous nephrostomy is technically challenging in neonates due to renal mobility.
- The main risks include urine leak, pelvic disruption, and bleeding.

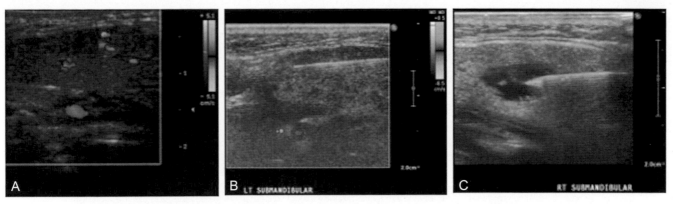

Fig. 9.7 Submandibular Gland Injection. (A) Ultrasound of the submandibular gland of a 5 year old child with severe drooling and cerebral palsy. Color doppler images shows vascularity of the gland and sites to be avoided during injection. (B) Needle seen within the submandibular gland of another child. (C) Needle slightly withdrawn to be well within the gland with bevel facing upwards, 0.25cc of injected Botox A (5 units/kg dissolved in sterile preservative free saline) is seen contained within the capsule of the gland. (Courtesy Bairbre Connolly.)

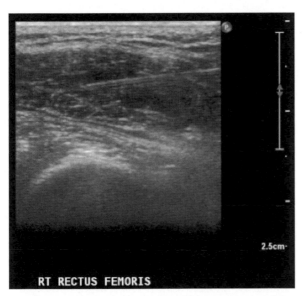

Fig. 9.8 Intramuscular Botox Injection. Ultrasound image of the rectus femoris muscle seen over the shaft of the femur in a child with severe spasticity. Needle in situ during the injection of the Botox A, which is injected into several sites within the muscle. Dosage calculated according to child's body weight, number of injection sites, and number of muscles to be treated. (Courtesy Bairbre Connolly.)

Varicocele Management

- Varicoceles are seen in around 1% of young boys; the incidence increases to 15% by late adolescence.
- Approximately 90% of varicoceles are unilateral and typically on the left side, whereas 10% are bilateral.
- The *nutcracker phenomenon* occurs when the left renal vein is compressed between the aorta and the superior mesenteric artery. The left gonadal vein enters the left renal vein at a sharp right angle and may be incompetent (absence of valves).
- Literature supports the hypothesis that varicoceles have a significant negative effect on the testis and future fertility and that varicocele repair can reverse or prevent this effect.
- Varicoceles are graded in various ways, clinically or by ultrasound, according to anatomy and degree of reflux.
- Transcatheter embolization of a varicocele is a feasible, safe, quick, and cost-effective procedure with minimal morbidity in children.
- The main risks include embolic escape, recurrence of varicocele, orchitis, and testicular ischemia.

Balloon Dilation of Ureteral Strictures and Ureteral Stent Insertion

- Strictures are congenital or acquired through ischemia, trauma, infection, postoperative changes, or malignancy.
- Stricture dilatation may be required prior to double-J stent insertion (one loop in the renal pelvis and one in the bladder).
- Stents are placed as a short-term intervention in. Stent exchanges are required to avoid stent encrustation.
- The main risks include infection, ureteral disruption, urine leak, hematuria, and bleeding.

⟫ CLINICAL POINT

Bähren Classification System (Fig. 9.9)
- Type 0—normal, no venous reflux
- Type I—single gonadal vein without duplication
- Type II—single gonadal vein with accessory veins (gonadal, lumbar, iliac veins, inferior vena cava)
- Type III—duplicated gonadal vein with a single trunk
- Type IV—competent renal/gonadal junction with reflux to collateral vessels
- Type V—gonadal vein that drains into a circumaortic renal vein

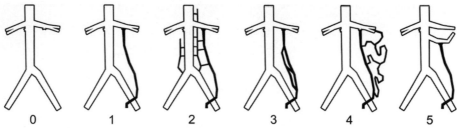

Fig. 9.9 The Bähren Classification System of Varicocele Anatomy. Type 0 anatomy shows no evidence of venous reflux on venography; type 1 anatomy shows reflux into a single gonadal vein without duplication. Type 2 anatomy shows reflux into a single gonadal vein that communicates with accessory gonadal, lumbar, and/or iliac veins or the vena cava. Type 3 anatomy shows reflux into a gonadal vein duplicated caudally, coalescing into a single trunk at the renal vein junction. Type 4 anatomy shows a competent valve at the renal/gonadal junction but with reflux into a renal hilar or capsular collateral vessel that communicates with the gonadal vein. Type 5 anatomy shows reflux into a gonadal vein that drains into a circumaortic renal vein. (Reused with permission from Sze DY, Kao JS, Frisoli JK, et al. Persistent and recurrent postsurgical varicoceles: venographic anatomy and treatment with *N*-butyl cyanoacrylate embolization. *J Vasc Interv Radiol.* 2008;19:539–545.)

🏠 TAKE-HOME POINTS

- Pediatric IR is an evolving field with broad clinical applications. Operating in this realm depends on a multidisciplinary team that incudes nurses and technologists trained in pediatrics, pediatric anesthesiologists, child life specialists, and pediatricians.
- Pediatric IR differs from IR in the adult population in several ways:
  - The types of procedures that are commonly performed
  - Indications for these procedures
  - Pathologies that are commonly encountered

- Ranges of patients, devices, and equipment
- Focus on minimally invasive and radiation-free techniques when possible
- Requirement for a family centered approach
- There is a greater reliance on the use of ultrasound in pediatric interventions as it is portable, provides images in real time, shows vascularity, and is generally safe. Most importantly, ultrasound, unlike both fluoroscopy and CT, is free of ionizing radiation.

REVIEW QUESTIONS

1. What is the most common complication after a percutaneous liver biopsy?
   a. Intraperitoneal bleeding
   b. Creation of an arteriovenous fistula
   c. Hemobilia
   d. Biloma formation
   e. Abscess formation

2. The failure of a muscle biopsy to yield a diagnostic tissue sample is most likely related to what cause?
   a. Small tissue sample
   b. Use of fine-needle aspiration rather than core biopsy
   c. Misalignment of the biopsy orientation
   d. Degradation of tissue sample
   e. All of the above

3. Compared with gastrostomy tubes, which of the following is true regarding GJ tubes?
   a. They are more likely to serve as a lead point in intussusception.
   b. They are less likely to become clogged.
   c. They pose more risk of aspiration of feeds.
   d. They are easier to replace.

SUGGESTED READINGS

Crowley JJ, Pereira JK, Harris LS, et al. Peripherally inserted central catheters: experience in 523 children. *Radiology.* 204:617–621.

Kaufman C, James C, Harned R, et al. Pediatric interventional radiology workforce survey: 10-year follow-up. *Pediatr Radiol.* 2017;47(6):649–650.

Krishnamurthy G, Keller MS. Vascular access in children. *Cardiovasc Intervent Radiol.* 2011;34:14–24.

Nelson O, Bailey P. Pediatric anesthesia considerations for interventional radiology. *Anesthesiol Clin.* 2017;35:701–714.

Roebuck DJ. Paediatric interventional radiology. *Imaging.* 2001;13:302–320.

Roebuck D, Hogan M, Connolly B, et al. Interventions in the chest in children. *Tech Vasc Interv Radiol.* 2011;14(1):8–15.

Rubenstein J, Zettel J, Lee E, et al. Pediatric interventional radiology clinic—how are we doing? *Pediatr Radiol.* 2016;46(8):1165–1172.

Frontiers of Interventional Radiology

Jeremy I. Kim, Thaddeus F. Sze, Pratik A. Shukla, Marcin K. Kolber, Kavi K. Devulapalli, Ari J. Isaacson, Eric M. Walser, Aaron Fischman, Maureen P. Kohi

The field of interventional radiology (IR) has been revolutionizing modern medicine for more than a half century, ever since the moment Dr. Charles Dotter ignored a surgeon's warning to *"VISUALIZE BUT DO NOT TRY TO FIX!!!"*—a request on a femoral angiogram. In the decades since, interventional radiology has expanded its reach into the diagnosis and treatment of diseases from head to toe, using minimally invasive techniques to reach some of the most inaccessible areas of the body. This chapter looks at the near future of interventional radiology, highlighting a few methods and procedures that are likely to impact medicine in the years to come.

PROSTATIC ARTERY EMBOLIZATION

CASE PRESENTATION

A 60-year-old male has lower urinary tract symptoms secondary to known benign prostatic hyperplasia. His prostate-specific antigen levels have ranged between 4.0 and 6.0, with prostate biopsies in the past showing no evidence of carcinoma. He has tried tamsulosin and finasteride but did not tolerate either. His international prostate symptom score is 20, with a quality-of-life score of 5; he was unhappy and therefore consulted his local IR clinic, expressing an interest in prostatic artery embolization.

- In the 1970s, internal iliac artery embolization was first described as a method of controlling massive hemorrhage after prostatectomy or prostate biopsy.
- In 2000, Demeritt et al. described the case of a patient with **benign prostatic hyperplasia** (BPH) who underwent selective prostate artery embolization for gross hematuria and was subsequently found to have shrinkage of his prostate with improvement in his urinary symptoms.
- In the early 2000s, treatment of BPH with prostatic artery embolization (PAE) was found to be safe in multiple animal models.
- Between 2010 and 2013, Dr. Francisco Carnevale of Brazil and Dr. Joao Pisco of Portugal published multiple case series on successful BPH treatments in humans.

- In 2014, Dr. Sandeep Bagla reported results from the first study in the United States describing the safety and efficacy of PAE. Since then, trials in the United Kingdom, France, Italy, Russia, Argentina, China, and Japan have all demonstrated PAE to be effective, with minimal complications.

▶▶ CLINICAL POINT

Benign prostatic hyperplasia becomes increasingly common as men age. Fifty percent of men over age 50 are affected by symptoms, including frequent urination, nocturia, hesitancy, urgency, urinary leakage, and a weak urinary stream. This increases the risk for urinary retention, recurrent urinary tract infections, bladder calculi, renal insufficiency, hematuria, and bladder decompensation.

- Medical therapy is the first-line treatment for moderate lower urinary tract symptoms, and surgical therapy is reserved for severe cases of BPH (further discussed under Alternative Treatments).
- PAE has been shown to provide significant improvement in clinical symptoms demonstrated by International Prostate Symptom Score (IPSS), quality-of-life (QOL), peak urinary flow, and postvoid residual volume with comparable results to **transurethral prostate resection** (TURP).
  - Compared with TURP, the advantages of PAE include:
    - A minimally invasive treatment option—typically an outpatient procedure with quicker recovery time.
    - Decreased risks of bleeding, sexual dysfunction, and urinary incontinence.
  - Compared with TURP, the disadvantages of PAE include:
    - A technically challenging procedure due to vessel tortuosity, atherosclerotic disease, and complex prostatic vascular supply that leads to an increased rate of technical failure.
    - Injury from nontarget embolization.
    - Less immediate improvement in symptoms compared with TURP.

International Prostate Symptom Score

- Scoring system used for screening, diagnosing, and trending patient symptoms as related to BPH.

- It asks seven questions, assessing:
  1. Bladder emptying
  2. Urinary frequency
  3. Intermittency
  4. Urgency
  5. Stream strength
  6. Straining
  7. Nocturia
- Score range from 0 to 35.
  - 1 to 7: mild symptomatology
  - 8 to 19: moderate symptomatology
  - 20 to 35: severe symptomatology

Quality-of-Life Score

- This evaluates a patient's feeling about his quality of life at the current level of urinary symptoms.

Indications

- Patients with BPH and moderate to severe chronic lower urinary tract symptoms
- Patients who have failed medical therapy
- Patient preference due to concern about potential side effects and complications from other therapies
- Patients with large prostates who cannot undergo prostatectomy under general anesthesia due to medical comorbidities

Contraindications

- Prostate malignancy—concern about causing cancer to become more aggressive in the setting of an ischemic environment
- Acute urinary retention—may first require decompression with bladder catheterization
- Acute renal insufficiency/injury—may first require percutaneous nephrostomy
- Neurogenic bladder—reducing prostate obstruction will not improve urinary tract symptoms in the setting of bladder weakness
- Severe uncorrectable coagulopathy

Equipment

- 4- or 5-Fr sheath
- 4- or 5-Fr diagnostic catheter
- 2.0- or 2.4-Fr microcatheter
- 0.014- or 0.018-inch guidewire
- Embolic agents (polyvinyl alcohol or spherical gelatin particle, size ranging from <100 μm to 300 μm)

Anatomy

Prostate Anatomy

- The normal prostate volume is less than 30 cm^3
- The prostate is located at the base of the bladder. The prostatic apex is caudal, and the base is cranial.
- The prostate, in combination with the vas deferens and seminal vesicles, contributes fluid to the ejaculate; this empties into the prostatic urethra.
- It is divided into three zones (Fig. 10.1):
  - Peripheral—70% of normal prostate gland volume
  - Central—25% of normal volume; most dense
  - Transitional—5% of normal volume; site of BPH

Arterial Anatomy

- The internal iliac artery branches from the common iliac artery and has two divisions:
  - The anterior division mostly supplies the pelvic viscera, including the prostate. Branches include the following arteries:
    - Inferior/middle rectal
    - Vesical
    - Prostatic (in males)
    - Uterine (in females)
    - Obturator
    - Inferior pudendal
    - Inferior gluteal
  - The posterior division mostly supplies the pelvic and gluteal musculature. Branches include the following arteries:
    - Lateral sacral
    - Iliolumbar
    - Superior gluteal

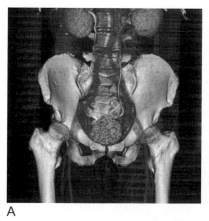
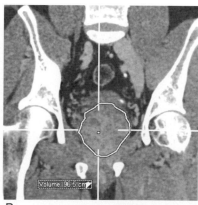
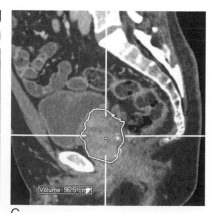

A   B   C

Fig. 10.1 Three-dimensional reconstruction (A) of an enlarged prostate from computed tomography volumetric measurements (B and C). (Courtesy Jeremy I. Kim.)

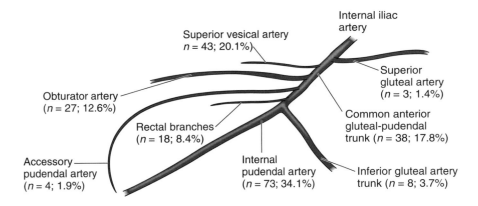

Fig. 10.2 High prostatic artery variability demonstrates different prostatic artery origins with the internal pudendal artery. (From Bilhim T, Pisco JM, Rio Tinto H, et al. Prostatic arterial supply: anatomic and imaging findings relevant for selective arterial embolization. *J Vasc Interv Radiol.* 2012;23[11]:1403–1415.)

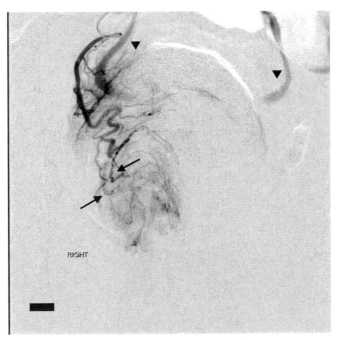

Fig. 10.3 Prostatic Arteries With a Corkscrew Appearance. (Courtesy Jeremy I. Kim.)

- Bilhim et al. (2012) showed that there is a high degree of variability in the origin of the prostatic artery (Fig. 10.2), with the **internal pudendal artery** being the most common origin.
  - They also showed that there can be multiple collateral vessels and/or shunts, which can create challenges with embolization and nontarget embolization, respectively.
- Prostatic arteries typically have a corkscrew appearance. (Fig. 10.3 is a digital subtraction angiogram [DSA] of the right prostatic artery—*arrows*. Contrast excretion via bilateral ureters into the bladder are also noted—*arrowheads*).

Procedural Steps
Preprocedural Evaluation
- **Prostate-specific antigen** (PSA) level
  - Free serum PSA level if PSA is elevated to further stratify cancer risk
- Uroflowmetry including peak urine flow and postvoid residual volume
- Urodynamics to evaluate bladder strength
- Prostate artery biopsy to exclude malignancy if suspected
- Computed tomography angiography (CTA) or magnetic resonance angiography (MRA) may be obtained for evaluation of the vascular and prostate anatomy.
  - Sites of origin and number of feeding arteries can be identified.
  - Obstruction due to atherosclerosis can be seen.
- Periprocedural medication protocols differ by institution and may include antibiotics, nonsteroidal antiinflammatory drugs (NSAIDs), analgesics, antiemetics, and antireflux medications.

Procedure
1. Local anesthetic with or without moderate sedation is used.
2. Vascular access is obtained via a common femoral artery approach.
3. A 4- or 5-Fr sheath is usually utilized with a 4- or 5-Fr catheter, which is introduced into the internal iliac artery.
4. Ipsilateral oblique angiography is performed to splay the branches of the internal iliac artery and identify the prostatic artery.
5. Prostatic artery vessels are selectively catheterized with a coaxial microcatheter.
   a. Contrasted cone-beam CT may be performed to verify correct microcatheter positioning.
6. Once positioning has been confirmed, the embolic material of choice is delivered until stasis.
   These steps are repeated on the other side.

Alternate Treatments

- Medical therapy is the first-line treatment for moderate lower urinary tract symptoms.
  - It is indicated for moderate symptomatology with no absolute indication for surgery.
  - Treatment options include α-adrenergic blockers, 5α-reductase inhibitors, and phosphodiesterase inhibitors.
- Surgery is reserved for severe cases of BPH where medical therapy has failed.
  - TURP is the most common surgical treatment, usually reserved for "smaller" prostates (<90 cm^3).
  - Prostatectomy or holmium laser enucleation of the prostate is appropriate for larger prostates (>90 cm^3).
  - Risks of surgery include bleeding, transurethral resection syndrome, urethral strictures, bladder neck contracture, retrograde ejaculation, erectile dysfunction, and incontinence.
- Other minimally invasive treatments include interstitial laser ablation, transurethral microwave ablation, and needle ablation.

Complications

- Nontarget embolization, most commonly of the bladder, rectum, and penis.
- Postembolization syndrome—nausea, vomiting, fever, and pain.
- Urinary retention, which is thought to be caused by urethral compression from prostate swelling/inflammation.
- Some consider postembolization syndrome and urinary retention as expected temporary side effects of treatment. Appropriate patient management can help alleviate symptoms.

MAGNETIC RESONANCE IMAGING-GUIDED BIOPSY AND ABLATION OF PROSTATE CANCER

CASE PRESENTATION

A 60-year-old male is found to have an elevated prostate-specific antigen at annual screening with his general practitioner. After referral to a urologist, a transperineal biopsy demonstrates an intermediate-grade peripheral zone tumor. He presents to the IR clinic in order to inquire about alternatives to radical prostatectomy.

- Prostate cancer is the most common malignancy among men in the United States, with an estimated prevalence of 15.9%.
- Serum PSA testing is the mainstay of screening, although there is controversy with regard to the overdiagnosis of cancers that would never have been clinically significant. PSA screening now carries a "D" rating (not recommended) from the US Preventative Services Task Force, yet it remains the screening method of choice. A high

PSA level is typically followed by a transrectal or transperineal biopsy, which may be followed by prostatectomy if the biopsy is positive.

- The negatives of this paradigm can potentially be alleviated by an MRI-based screening, biopsy, and treatment protocol, benefits of which include:
  - The ability to provide focal, rather than whole-gland, therapies
  - Less overtreatment of inconsequential low-risk prostate cancers
  - Fewer missed diagnoses of significant prostate cancers (as opposed to the blind biopsy technique)
  - Improved sensitivity for small tumors
  - Reduced cases of ciprofloxacin-resistant *Escherichia coli* sepsis (recent increasing incidence from 0.4% to 4.0% of all TRUS biopsies)
- Approval of 3 Tesla MRI in 2004, which enabled high-resolution imaging of the prostate with 85% sensitivity and near 100% specificity in detecting prostate malignancy.
  - Transrectal ultrasound is 50% sensitive and CT less so.
- In 2015, prostate MRI was the fastest growing area of MRI. It offers excellent visualization of surrounding vital structures such as the urethra and the periprostatic nerve bundle. Interventions with precise targeting and heat monitoring minimize the risk of inadvertent injury to these structures.
- Improvements both in imaging techniques and surface coils have enabled the development of transrectal devices for intervention and MR thermometry. Available technologies for tumor ablation include cryoablation, high-intensity focused ultrasound (HIFU), and focal laser ablation (discussed in detail further on).

Indications

- Low- to intermediate-risk prostate cancer (Gleason score of 6 or 7) in locations amenable to ablation. Tumor should be confined to the prostate. There should be no involvement of the seminal vesicles, nerve bundles, or surrounding tissues.

◎ KEY DEFINITION

The Gleason score (ranging from 2 to 10) is a grading system for prostate cancer.
Two samples are graded on a scale of 1 to 5, and those scores are added.
The lowest Gleason score of a cancer is 6, suggesting a well-differentiated, low-grade, less aggressive cancer.

Contraindications

- Contraindications to MRI include:
  - Certain metal implants, pacemakers/AICDs, and other metallic objects in the body
- Relative contraindications:
  - Previous abdominoperitoneal resection, although a transperineal approach is still possible
  - Bilateral hip prostheses—artifacts from these implants impact MR thermometry sequences

Equipment

- 3-Tesla MRI system
  - The room must be equipped with waveguides to bring laser light into the room.
- For biopsies:
  - Transrectal probe system such as DynaTRIM, stand for positioning the endorectal probe, and DynaLOC software for registering MRI images with the probe
- For focal ablation:
  - Cryoablation—Galil "ice-rod" and "ice-seed" cryoprobes
  - HIFU: transrectal probe currently in phase I trials
  - Laser: 980-nm diffusing tip Visualase laser system
    - Fiberoptics are contained within a cooling cannula connected to a saline pump to prevent overheating and charring of adjacent tissue.
    - Software used for image coregistration with MR thermometry data.

Anatomy

- For general anatomy, see the relevant section in the subchapter titled Prostate Artery Embolization.
- Most tumors (70%) occur in the peripheral zone.
- Attention must be paid to the urethra, periprostatic nerve bundles, and seminal vesicles.

Procedural Steps (Focal Laser Ablation)
Preprocedure
- Review previous imaging to plan the ideal approach.

Procedure
1. Patient is placed prone, head first in MR scanner.
2. The target lesion is reidentified.
3. The transrectal system is deployed.
4. Saline and lidocaine are injected through a 22-gauge Chiba needle through the rectal probe. This outlines the neurovascular bundle on T2 sequences and may provide thermal protection.
5. A cooling cannula is then advanced into target position, and the titanium stiffener is removed.
6. After the treatment plane has been selected, real-time thermometry of the treatment area begins.
7. A low-power test is performed (warmed tissue visible on thermometry display) to confirm placement and positioning of the fiber.
8. After adjustments are made, laser power is increased to ablative intensity.
9. The ablation zone as well as protected areas of interest (urethra and neurovascular bundles) are monitored continuously as treatment is performed.
   a. Typical burn lengths are 2 to 4 minutes at 15 to 20 W.
   b. Ablation will automatically stop if the temperature in regions of interest (ROIs) placed over the protected areas exceeds 50°C or if temperature in the center of the ablation zone exceeds 90°C (to prevent charring).
10. Laser fiber can be advanced or retracted in the cooling cannula to create overlapping ablation zones as necessary.
11. An ablation zone of 5 to 10 mm is maintained around the cancer to cover dendritic projections.

Follow-up

- The normal appearance of a postablative prostate is a "flat tire" morphology due to focal atrophy with fibrotic tissue. MRI signal is dark at the site of the ablation. Cystic degeneration at the ablation site is also a normal appearance with tissue replaced by fluid in the ablation cavity.
- Repeat PSA and multiparametric MRI at a 6-month follow-up appointment. This time gap allows for resolution of potentially confusing postprocedural inflammation.
  - Generally PSA decreases by approximately 50% in this interval.
- Postprocedural assessments with Sexual Health Inventory in Men (SHIM) and IPSS scores.

Alternate Treatments

- Androgen deprivation—hormonal therapy meant to decrease signals for tumor growth
- Prostatectomy—surgical alternative associated with significant morbidity, longer recovery time, and complications including impotence
- Radiation—beam therapy or brachytherapy (radioactive beads) used to shrink the prostate gland and tumor

Complications

- Failure to fully ablate tumor, with recurrence necessitating repeat biopsy and ablation
- Creation of a rectal fistula or sinus tract, associated with an increased risk of infection
- Spermatocele

TRANSRADIAL ARTERY ACCESS FOR NONCORONARY INTERVENTIONS

CASE PRESENTATION

A 40-year-old premenopausal female with no significant past medical history presents to her gynecologist for menorrhagia with symptomatic anemia. Her hemoglobin was found to be 9 mg/dL, down from a baseline of 14 mg/dL. Ultrasound demonstrates a large submucosal leiomyoma with isoechoic fluid in the endometrial canal suggestive of blood. Pelvic magnetic resonance imaging demonstrates a T2-weighted bright uterine fibroid that does not appear to be necrotic. She is referred to the outpatient IR clinic to discuss uterine artery embolization (UAE) as a less invasive treatment option compared with hysterectomy. She states that her friend underwent a UAE procedure and experienced significant pain and discomfort post procedure. Physical examination is unremarkable except for a body mass index of 40. A radial artery approach is discussed with the patient, as femoral access can prove difficult in an obese patient; additionally, the radial approach would allow her to obtain a more comfortable position to deal with postprocedural pain.

- Arterial access is necessary for many noninvasive interventional procedures; the common femoral artery has been the mainstay for arterial access for patients requiring catheter-directed arterial interventions.

- Manual compression is used to achieve postprocedural hemostasis in patients who have undergone transfemoral arterial access (TFA). Arterial closure devices have been developed to help achieve hemostasis, but these are associated with unique complications including arterial thrombosis, infection, and deployment failure, which may necessitate open surgical repair.
- Other general complications related to TFA include hematomas, retroperitoneal hemorrhage, and pseudoaneurysm formation.
- **Transradial access** (TRA) has been well established for coronary interventions, although its use in interventional radiology has been historically limited. TRA has recently gained popularity in noncoronary interventions; a large single-institution study by Posham et al. in 2016 demonstrated the safety and efficacy of TRA for peripheral applications.
- Comparing both approaches, the potential benefits of a TRA approach include:
  - Decreased bleeding
  - Decreased potential access-site complications
  - Shorter postprocedure monitoring time
  - Easier to achieve hemostasis using radial artery compression devices
  - Increased postprocedural comfort
  - Earlier postprocedural ambulation

Indications

- Although there are no definite indications for TRA, it may prove beneficial in many different situations, including those involving:
  - Obese patients where the common femoral artery is very deep to the skin
  - Patients with prior groin surgery
  - Patients with femoral stents
  - Incapacitated patients who are unlikely to keep their lower extremity flat for the required time post procedure
  - Patients with a particular arterial anatomy

Contraindications

- Absolute contraindications:
  - **Barbeau D waveform** on the preprocedural evaluation
  - Prior TRA resulting in symptomatic or asymptomatic radial artery occlusion
- Relative contraindication:
  - Small radial artery size (<2 mm) due to inability to introduce a standard 6-Fr sheath

Equipment

- High-resolution 5- to 7-Hz linear transducer for preprocedural evaluation of the radial artery and for precise intraprocedural needle entry visualization
- Specialized short 5- to 7-Fr vascular sheath
- Catheters designed for a cranial approach to peripheral interventions; these must be longer than catheters used in TFA to reach the same target vessels. For example,
  - Long vertebral catheters (100–150 cm in length) are typically used for UAE.

- A Sarah Radial OPTITORQUE diagnostic catheter is used or hepatic interventions.
- TRA for iliofemoral treatments has been investigated; these procedures, however, require longer sheaths, catheters, and treatment devices (balloons and/or stents) that have yet to be developed.
- Long microcatheters
- Radial artery arteriotomy compression devices (i.e., TR Band, Bengal Band, Hemoband, RadStat, RadiStop, etc.)

Anatomy

- Radial artery access is technically feasible, as not many anatomic variations exist.
  - High radial origin is a common variant that usually does not affect TRA.
- A radial artery loop (Fig. 10.4) poses some technical difficulties, although techniques have been described to pass through the loop.
- Important to note—patients with dialysis access may have altered radial artery hemodynamics.

Transradial Access Technique
Preprocedure

1. Physical examination should include radial and ulnar pulse checks.
2. During the preprocedural consultation, the **Barbeau test** is performed as follows:
   a. Pulse oximeter is placed on the patient's thumb, producing a waveform of perfusion.
   b. After analyzing the initial waveform, the radial artery is compressed, and the new waveform is analyzed.
   c. Barbeau waveform D is a contraindication to TRA (Table 10.1 and Fig. 10.5).

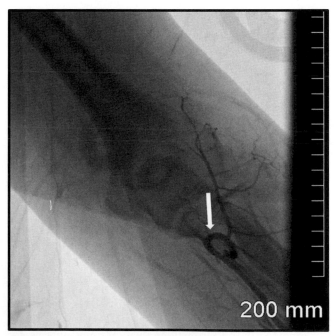

Fig. 10.4 A radial artery loop (arrow) has been described; it poses some technical difficulties, although techniques have been described to pass through the loop. (Courtesy Jeremy I. Kim.)

TABLE 10.1	Barbeau Waveform Classification	
Barbeau	**Waveform Palmar Patency (TRA Implication)**
A	No change in initial waveform after compression of the radial artery (can proceed)
B	Persistent but dampened waveform after compression of the radial artery (can proceed)
C	Initial dampening of waveform after compression of the radial artery with recovery within 2 min of compression (can proceed)
D	Dampening of waveform after compression of the radial artery without recovery within 2 min of compression (contraindicated)

TRA, Transradial access.
From Barbeau GR, Arsenault F, Dugas L, et al. Evaluation of the ulnopalmar arterial arches with pulse oximetry and plethysmography: comparison with the Allen's test in 1010 patients. *Am Heart J.* 2004;147(3):489–493.

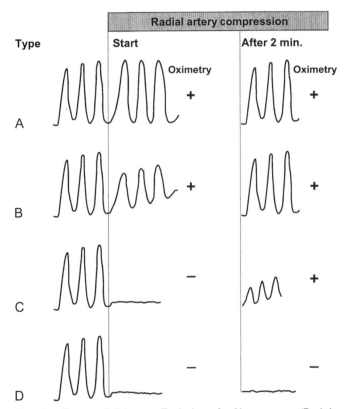

Fig. 10.5 Transradial Access Technique for Noncoronary/Peripheral Applications. (From Barbeau GR, Arsenault F, Dugas L, et al. Evaluation of the ulnopalmar arterial arches with pulse oximetry and plethysmography: comparison with the Allen's test in 1010 patients. *Am Heart J.* 2004;147[3]:489–493.)

3. The radial artery is interrogated under ultrasound to ensure patency, measure size, and evaluate for anatomic variations.
4. On the day of the procedure, the Barbeau test and sonographic evaluation are repeated.
5. Preprocedural medications are provided as appropriate for each individual procedure (i.e., antibiotics, sedation, etc.).

A nitroglycerin and lidocaine paste can be applied to the wrist in the preprocedural waiting area for dilatation of the radial artery and local anesthetic effects, respectively.

Procedure

1. The patient's left wrist is prepped and draped in sterile fashion.
   a. A left-sided approach is favored over a right-sided one to prevent catheters from positioning across the great vessels. Stroke has been reported in the cardiac literature with right-sided approaches.
2. Subcutaneous 1% lidocaine is administered at the skin entry site to provide local anesthesia.
3. Under ultrasound guidance, radial artery access is achieved using a short 21-gauge micropuncture needle through the anterior wall of the distal radial artery (Fig. 10.6).
4. A specialized vascular sheath is then inserted. A cocktail of 3000 IU heparin, 2.5 mg of verapamil (calcium channel blocker), and 200 μg nitrate is administered through the sheath to prevent radial artery occlusion/vasospasm.
5. As previously described, long catheters and coaxial microcatheters are necessary to carry out the intended procedure. A cranial approach to uterine artery embolization is shown in Fig. 10.7.
6. After conclusion of the procedure, a radial artery compression (e.g., TR band [Fig. 10.8]) device is placed over the arteriotomy site and is overinflated with 11 to 12 mL of air. After the vascular sheath has been removed, air is removed from the compression device until a small flash of arterial blood is seen under the band, after which 1 mL of air is readded to the device. This technique allows for adequate pressure to achieve hemostasis without risking radial artery occlusion.

Postprocedure

1. Patients are moved to the IR recovery suite after completion of the procedure.
2. The TR band is removed 1 to 1.5 hours post procedure by slowly removing air.
   a. If a flash of blood is seen, the TR band is reinflated for continued pressure.
3. Patients are monitored for access-related complications for up to 1 hour after removal of the compression device.
4. Patients are seen in clinic 1 to 2 weeks post procedure to be evaluated for access- and procedure-related complications with a thorough physical and ultrasound examination.

Alternate Techniques

- TRA has gained popularity in IR in recent years. However, TFA remains the mainstay of catheter-directed arterial therapies.
- Transbrachial access (TBA) has also been described.
  - As in TFA, manual compression is necessary to achieve hemostasis.
  - Higher risks of nerve injury and bleeding are reported with TBA compared with TRA.

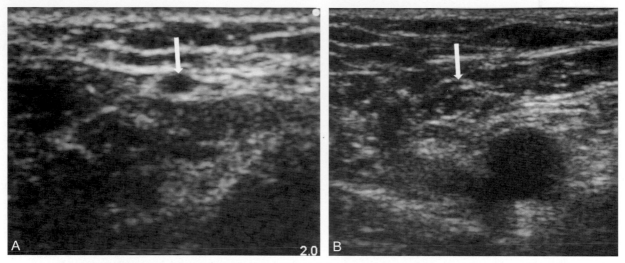

Fig. 10.6 (A) Radial artery (arrow) visualization with a high-frequency high-resolution linear transducer; (B) radial artery accessed with the micropuncture needle under ultrasound guidance *(arrow)*. (Courtesy Jeremy I. Kim.)

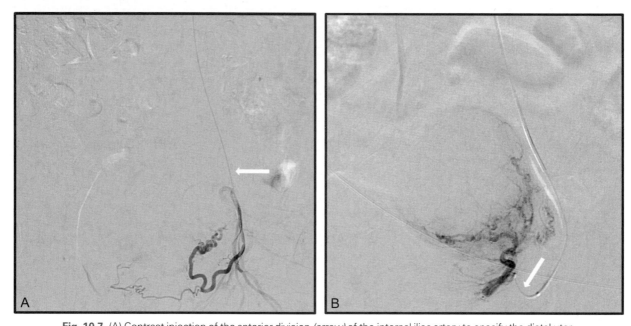

Fig. 10.7 (A) Contrast injection of the anterior division *(arrow)* of the internal iliac artery to opacify the distal uterine artery. (B) Injection of a uterine artery in a different patient using a coaxial microcatheter *(arrow)*. Note: Both the diagnostic catheter and microcatheter enter the left iliac artery in a craniocaudal fashion via a transradial access approach (vs. a transfemoral arterial access). (Courtesy Jeremy I. Kim.)

- Currently available TRA catheters are not long enough to perform lower extremity procedures. The ability to torque the distal end of these long catheters has been questioned as well. TFA is still generally preferred in these patients, although TRA has been reported to be effective in the treatment of aortoiliac disease.
- Retrograde pedal access has been used in conjunction with TFA to treat difficult-to-transverse cases of lower extremity occlusion. Recently TRA has been used in combination with retrograde pedal access for the treatment of these lesions.
- Dialysis access interventions have traditionally been treated with a TBA or TFA approach, but recent studies have reported the TRA approach as well.

Outcomes/Complications

- Major
  - Pseudoaneurysm formation
  - Seizure
- Minor
  - Bleeding resulting in hematoma
  - Infection
  - Asymptomatic radial artery occlusion
  - Arm pain
  - Radial artery spasm
- In the largest series to date, Posham et al. (2016) analyzed 1500 cases of peripheral arterial intervention using TRA. They reported a technical success rate of 98.2%, with only 1.2% of patients requiring crossover to TFA.

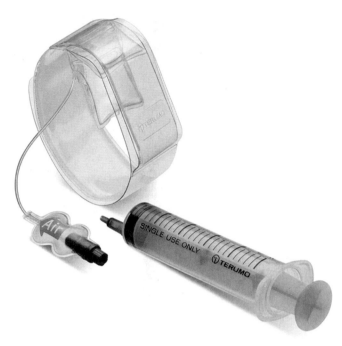

Fig. 10.8 TR Band Radial Artery Compression Device. (Courtesy TERUMO Corp., Tokyo, Japan.)

- An additional complication described in the cardiology literature is stroke, although this complication is not seen in Posham's study.
  - Of note, using an approach via a left upper extremity rather than a right upper extremity decreases the frequency of wires and catheters being placed across the origin of the great vessels (i.e., common carotid artery) and theoretically lessens the chances of stroke.

BARIATRIC ARTERY EMBOLIZATION

CASE PRESENTATION

A 55-year-old female with morbid obesity (body mass index of 45), type 2 diabetes, coronary artery disease, and obstructive sleep apnea is referred to interventional radiology after lifestyle modifications (therapy, nutrition, and exercise) failed to elicit significant weight loss. She is a poor surgical candidate, and her bariatric surgeon is interested in enrolling her in a clinical trial evaluating the safety and efficacy of bariatric artery embolization in the treatment of her obesity.

- Obesity and obesity-related health conditions are increasing. Two-thirds of Americans are classified as overweight, obese, or morbidly obese.
- Surgical intervention for obesity results in greater weight loss as compared with nonsurgical interventions. A frequent dramatic effect of bariatric surgery is reversal of type 2 diabetes within days of surgery, before any effective weight loss, suggesting a metabolic component in the efficacy of surgery.
- The gastrointestinal tract is regulated by a variety of neuroendocrine feedback mechanisms. Several hormones are associated with appetite and satiety (Table 10.2).
  - The only known appetite-stimulating hormone is **ghrelin**, a 28-amino acid peptide primarily secreted by X/A cells in the gastric fundus, where almost three-quarters of the body's ghrelin is produced. Plasma levels of ghrelin are known to increase significantly before meals and decrease after meals.
- Preclinical investigation of embolization of the gastric fundus via the **left gastric artery** (LGA) in animal models demonstrated significant decreases in plasma ghrelin levels as well as decreased weight gain/increased weight loss compared with sham controls. Significantly higher levels of GLP-1 were also noted.
- Early clinical investigations in humans are promising for (1) decreasing ghrelin levels and (2) leading to weight loss in patients treated with LGA embolization.
- Clinical trials investigating bariatric artery embolization (BAE) are under way, and standardized protocols are in development.
- As in bariatric surgery, a multidisciplinary approach utilizing a team of clinicians in endocrinology, nutrition, psychology, physical therapy, surgery, and interventional radiology will ultimately be required for effective long-term weight loss.

Indications
- Specific indications for BAE have yet to be defined. Indications may be analogous to those for bariatric surgery:
  - BMI greater than 40 kg/m^2.
  - BMI greater than 35 kg/m^2 with an obesity-related comorbid condition for which more conservative measures have failed.

TABLE 10.2 Neuroendocrine Regulation of Appetite and Satiety		
Hormone	**Source in GI tract**	**Effects**
Ghrelin	Gastric fundus (majority)	Stimulates appetite
		Increases GI motility
	Duodenum, pituitary gland (minority)	Decreases insulin
GLP-1	Ileum and colon	Promotes satiety
		Slows gastric emptying
		Decreases glucagon
CCK	Proximal small bowel	Slows gastric emptying
		Gallbladder contraction
Leptin	Adipose cells throughout the body	Promotes satiety
PYY	Ileum and colon	Slows gastric emptying
		Inhibits gastric acid

- An additional proposed indication is the use of BAE as a bridge to bariatric surgery for poor surgical candidates with obesity-related comorbid conditions.

Contraindications

- Absolute:
  - Vascular anatomy of the celiac axis that, in the opinion of the interventional radiologist, is not amenable to BAE. This may be evaluated on a preprocedural CTA.
- Relative:
  - Renal failure, iodinated contrast allergy.

Equipment

- Micropuncture set
- 5-Fr sheath and J-wire
- Multiple catheter options and a variety of microcatheters
- 5-Fr catheter, 2.4- or 2.8-Fr microcatheter
- 0.035-in guidewire, 0.014-in or 0.018-in microwire
- Lengths of equipment depends on transradial versus transfemoral approaches
- Embolic agent (current clinical trials employ calibrated microspheres)

Anatomy

- The celiac artery (celiac axis) arises anteriorly from the abdominal aorta at the level of T12.
- The LGA is the first and smallest branch of the celiac artery, coursing superiorly along the lesser curvature of the stomach before anastomosing with the right gastric artery.
  - Branches extend over the gastric fundus to anastomose with the short gastric arteries.
- The target of embolization in BAE is the gastric fundus, the superior portion of the stomach between the gastric cardia and body that forms the upper curvature of the stomach (Fig. 10.9).
- The interventional radiologist should be aware of anatomic variants related to the LGA:
  - Replaced left hepatic artery arising from the LGA (4%–11%)

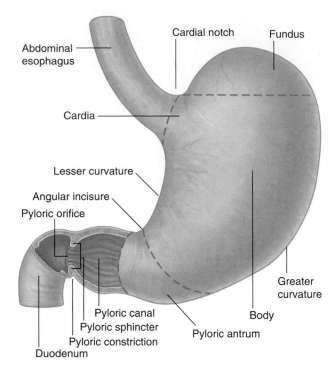

Fig. 10.9 Stomach and Duodenum. (Reused with permission from Rake R, Vogl AW, Mithcell AWM, et al. *Gray's Anatomy for Students.* 3rd ed. Philadelphia: Elsevier; 253–420, 2015, F4-61).

- Anomalous origin of the LGA directly off of the aorta (2%–3%)
- Replaced common hepatic artery arising from the LGA (0.5%)
- Gastromesenteric, gastrosplenic, and hepatogastric trunks (extremely rare)

Procedural Steps

Clinical trials investigating best practice are under way.

1. Arterial access is obtained. The TRA should be considered due to the patient's body habitus and potential for access site complications if a femoral approach is used.
2. A 4- or 5-Fr catheter is advanced to the celiac axis and parked at the origin of the LGA (Fig. 10.10A).

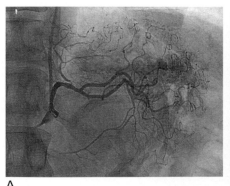
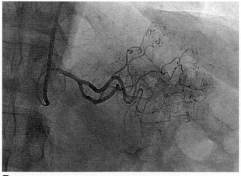
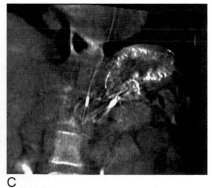

Fig. 10.10 Bariatric Artery Embolization. The catheter is introduced into the left gastric artery and angiography is performed. (A) Branches to the cardia, fundus, and body, with right gastric artery anastomosis visualized inferiorly. The catheter is advanced into the fundal branches, and angiography is performed, with anastomosis no longer visualized. (B) Cone-beam computed tomography during injection of the fundal branches. (C) Isolated enhancement of the gastric fundus without uptake of nontarget contrast. (Courtesy Aaron Fischman.)

3. A microcatheter is advanced up the LGA to the level of the gastric fundus (see Fig. 10.10B).
4. Contrast injection is timed with cone-beam CT (CBCT) imaging (see Fig. 10.10C) to localize the expected distribution of embolic material, identify vascular collaterals not apparent on angiography, and avoid nontarget embolization.
5. Embolic microspheres are injected slowly under fluoroscopic guidance until flow to the fundus is visibly decreased.
6. Postembolization DSA and CBCT are repeated.
7. Postprocedural follow-up at regular intervals should include serum ghrelin levels and trending of body weight.

Treatment Alternatives

- Roux-en-Y gastric bypass, sleeve gastrectomy, and adjustable gastric banding are the most popular surgical interventions performed for bariatric indications.
- Surgical interventions result in greater weight loss and improvements in obesity-related conditions than nonsurgical (lifestyle) modifications, with the tradeoff of increased surgical complications like perianastomotic leak, gallstones, and need for operative revisions.

Complications

- Major
  - Porcine models have shown the development of superficial fundal ulcers with subsequent gastric perforation when large-volume embolics have been used.
  - Nontarget embolization
    - The complicated vascular anatomy of the stomach with its rich collateralization network makes this an important complication to avoid, requiring preprocedural assessment of the celiac access with cross-sectional angiography.
- Minor:
  - Epigastric discomfort, experienced in 3 of 5 patients who underwent BAE in the only reported prospective trial to date (Kipshidze, 2013)

MAGNETIC RESONANCE–GUIDED FOCUSED ULTRASOUND

CASE PRESENTATION

A 45-year-old female presents to the interventional radiology clinic with a history of menorrhagia. Ultrasound and magnetic resonance imaging demonstrate a large anterior intramural fibroid. Her uterine fibroid symptom and health-related quality-of-life questionnaire is 60. She has tried oral contraceptives yet found little relief of her symptoms. She seeks a minimally invasive treatment for uterine fibroids and presents for possible magnetic resonance–guided focused ultrasound (MRgFUS) treatment.

- Uterine leiomyomas (or fibroids) are common smooth muscle tumors affecting up to 60% of women by age 45.

- Fibroids can vary with regard to size and location and can result in a variety of symptoms including menorrhagia, pelvic pressure and pain, urinary frequency, constipation, dyspareunia, and infertility.
- Treatment of fibroids varies depending on patient preference and extent of symptoms, with medical, surgical, and minimally invasive options available.

▶ CLINICAL POINT

Uterine Fibroid Symptom and Health-Related Quality-of-Life Questionnaire
- Validated instrument to quantify bleeding, bulk, and other fibroid-related symptoms.
- Consists of an 8-item symptom severity scale and 29-item health-related quality-of-life questionnaire related to concern, activities, energy, mood, control, self-consciousness, and sexual function.
- Items are scored on a 5-point scale with a raw symptom severity score ranging from 8 to 40.
- The symptom severity score is converted to a 0- to 100-point scale using the equation *transformed score = total raw score − 8/32 × 100.*
- A symptom severity score of 41 or greater was used as a cutoff for entry into the first major multicenter trial of MRgFUS for treatment of fibroids.
- Rigid adherence to the UFS-QOL may not be appropriate in all clinical circumstances.
- Assessment of symptoms in the context of fibroid size and location must be considered prior to proceeding with medical or surgical treatment.

- HIFU generates heat in tissues resulting in coagulative necrosis.
- Historically, implementation of HIFU as a form of ablative therapy has been slow due to difficulty in finding an appropriate imaging modality that could both guide treatment and provide real-time thermal feedback.
- The concept of MRI guidance was introduced in 1993 and was first shown possible in animal models in 1995.
- Early systems had drawbacks including long treatment times and lack of thermal feedback, which increased risk of inadequate treatment and thermal injury to surrounding tissues. Newer MRgFUS systems allow for safer and more efficient treatment by lessening treatment time and providing adequate thermal feedback prior to preventable tissue damage.
- In 2004, the ExAblate MRgFUS system, having shown its ability to significantly improve both bulk and bleeding symptoms related to fibroids, was approved by the US Food and Drug Administration (FDA) for the treatment of symptomatic uterine fibroids.
- Advantages of MRgFUS include:
  - Noninvasive treatment without ionizing radiation
  - Accurate lesion targeting by MRI guidance and real-time evaluation of treatment response through thermal imaging
  - Outpatient procedure

- Disadvantages of MRgFUS include:
  - Patients with large fibroids, who are less likely to respond to treatment and may be better served with uterine artery embolization or hysterectomy.
  - Time-consuming process, with the typical treatment lasting between 3 and 5 hours.
  - Difficulty for some patients in lying prone for an extended period of time.
  - Risks including skin injury, bladder and bowel injury, and back/leg pain secondary to nerve stimulation.

Indications

- Patients with clinically significant symptoms related to uterine fibroids such as menorrhagia, pelvic pressure, pelvic pain, and urinary symptoms
- The following imaging characteristics are optimal for treatment by MRgFUS:
  - T2 hypointesity
    - T2 hyperintense fibroids may be more difficult to treat; however, newer HIFU technology may overcome this limitation.
  - Homogeneous fibroid with postgadolinium enhancement
  - Location within 12 cm of the anterior abdominal wall
    - Posterior fibroids may be inadequately treated secondary to limitations in ultrasound beam range.
  - Small total fibroid burden
    - Multiple treatment sessions or fibroid volume reduction with GnRH agonists prior to MRgFUS treatment may be necessary to treat large-volume fibroids.
  - Noncalcified fibroids
    - Calcifications will reflect the ultrasound beam, resulting in inadequate treatment and nontarget tissue heating.

Contraindications

- Patients with any general contraindication to undergoing 3-Tesla MRI or receiving gadolinium contrast
  - Most commonly, patients with ferromagnetic objects such as intracranial aneurysm clips or embedded metallic foreign bodies
- Patients weighing greater than 250 lb for the ExAblate system or 310 lb for the Sonalleve system
- Any circumstance in which nontarget tissue heating may occur
  - Dermal scars or skin irregularities in the path of the ultrasound beam are prone to burns.
  - Bowel and bones must not be in the direct path of the ultrasound beam to avoid potential tissue damage.
  - Foreign objects in the path of the beam, such as an intrauterine device or surgical clips, must be avoided to prevent nontarget heating.

Equipment

- MRgHIFU uses a modified MRI table (Fig. 10.11) that contains a phased-array ultrasound transducer.
  - The transducer is enclosed in a bath containing degassed water and a Mylar membrane.

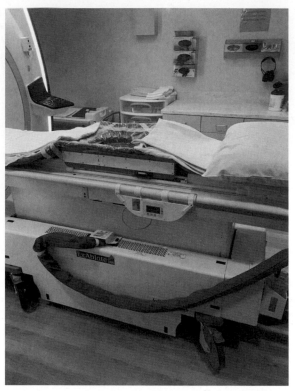

Fig. 10.11 Setup of the MRgFUS treatment table with the probe, on which the patient will lie prone during therapy in the MRI scanner. (Courtesy ExAblate O.R. © 2018 General Electric Company.)

- Ultrasound coupling gel and pelvic gel pads are applied to allow for transduction of the ultrasound beam to the patient (*acoustic coupling*).
- Pelvic MRI coil optimizes image quality.

Anatomy

- Key features of the uterus (Fig. 10.12) on MRI include:
  - Myometrium (*white arrow* in Fig. 10.12)
  - Junctional zone (*black arrow* in Fig. 10.12)
    - Normal thickness less than 8 mm
  - Endometrial canal (white star)

Procedural Steps
Preprocedure

- Moderate sedation is used.
- An indwelling urinary catheter is placed given the potential for long treatment time and the need to empty or fill the bladder to achieve adequate positioning of the uterus.
- Similarly, a rectal catheter may be needed for rectal filling in order to displace the bladder out of the beam path or to move the uterus more anteriorly.

Procedure

1. Patient is placed prone on table.
2. Patient's abdomen must be inspected and shaved free of hair.
3. Additional care must be taken to remove air bubbles between the ultrasound gel and the patient's skin in order to avoid skin burns and achieve adequate target visualization.

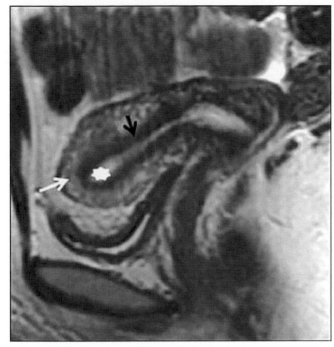

Fig. 10.12 Normal Appearance of the Uterus on Sagittal T2-Weighted Imaging. (Courtesy Maureen P. Kohi.)

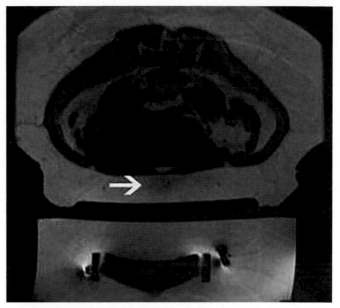

Fig. 10.13 Example of Thermal Injury. (Courtesy Maureen P. Kohi.)

4. Multiplaner localizing images are taken to allow proper positioning of the uterus directly anterior to the transducer.
5. Initial T2 fast spin echo images in the axial, coronal, and sagittal plane are acquired.
6. Images are then sent to the MRgHIFU workstation where treatment planning and lesion targeting are performed.
7. Individual focused ultrasound pulses known as sonication are then delivered onto points in the fibroid.
8. The ultrasound beam path is overlaid with MRI anatomic images. This allows for the beam to be adjusted as necessary in order to ensure optimal treatment and avoid nontarget tissue heating.
9. Thermal maps and dose estimates superimposed on MRI anatomic images allow for real-time monitoring of tissue heating during the procedure.

Complications
- Complications from MRgFUS are largely attributed to the effects of high focused ultrasound along the beam trajectory. These can be divided into three categories based on location—those occurring anterior to the target lesion, those occurring at the level of the target lesion, and those occurring beyond the target lesion.
- Near-field complications largely consist of thermal burns to the skin, due to either targeting a site too close to the skin surface or improper coupling due to scars or skin folds.
  - Thermal injuries attributable to improper coupling due to the presence of hair can be prevented by proper cleansing and shaving prior to treatment.
  - Certain scars can be marked during treatment planning, thereby preventing heating during therapy.
  - Fig. 10.13 shows an example of thermal injury as manifested by T1 hypointensity in the anterior subcutaneous tissue.

- At the level of the target lesion itself, complications include (Fig. 10.14):
  - Transient pain and uterine cramping from sonication
    - Patients are placed under moderate sedation during the procedure to lessen this sensation.
    - As an additional safe measure, patients can selectively stop the current sonication with a provided stop button.
  - Nontarget sonication of adjacent bowel or bladder
    - Adjunct maneuvers, including filling or emptying of the bladder via an indwelling catheter and/or filling of the rectum via a rectal tube, can be performed to prevent bowel and bladder injury.
- Complications occurring beyond the target site include:
  - Leg and back pain secondary to sonication extending to the level of exiting nerve roots at the lumbosacral junction.
    - Sonication of pelvic bones that may also indirectly result in nerve injury.

Alternate Treatments
- Medical management
  - Oral contraceptive pills
    - Commonly prescribed, especially for patients with menorrhagia
  - GnRH agonists
    - Result in rapid reduction in fibroid size by decreasing tumor vascularity
    - Side effects resulting from hypoestrogenism—hot flashes, vaginal dryness, and osteoporosis—may make this form of treatment intolerable for some patients.
    - Use of GnRH agonists is not recommended for more than 6 months.
- Surgical treatment
  - Options include hysterectomy, myomectomy, and laparoscopic radiofrequency ablation.
  - Hysterectomy is a definitive therapy but is not without complications, including pelvic floor dysfunction, sexual dysfunction, and long-term urinary incontinence.

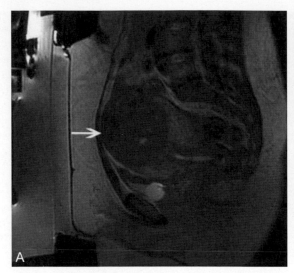 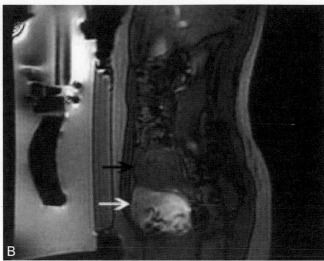

Fig. 10.14 (A) Localizes sequence before MRgFUS treatment. Note the small bowel anterior to the uterus with a decompressed bladder. (B) After bladder fill of 200 to 300 mL saline through the Foley catheter, the bowel is moved out of the beam path. (Courtesy Maureen P. Kohi.)

- Myomectomy—which can be performed hysteroscopically, laparoscopically, or via laparotomy—is less invasive than hysterectomy, but fibroids may recur.
- Laparoscopic ablation utilizes thermal energy to induce fibroid necrosis.
- Uterine artery embolization

- Minimally invasive treatment option performed by interventional radiologists
- Disadvantages include utilization of ionizing radiation and potential to result in premature menopause.
- Further discussed in Chapter 8, Obstetrics and Gynecology

🏠 TAKE-HOME POINTS

Prostatic Artery Embolization
- Prostatic artery embolization (PAE) for the treatment of benign prostatic hypertrophy and associated lower urinary tract symptoms is an effective minimally invasive treatment option.
- Compared with transurethral prostate resection (TURP), PAE has a less immediate effect but similar late improvement in symptomatology. PAE has a shorter postprocedural hospital stay and overall recovery time.
- Unlike with TURP, there is little to no chance of sexual dysfunction or urinary incontinence after PAE.
- Clinical and technical failure after PAE can usually be attributed to vessel tortuosity, severe atherosclerotic disease, and generally hypovascular prostates. Additional treatment sessions may be required.

Magnetic Resonance–Guided Ablation of Prostate Cancer
- In cases of prostate cancer, focal therapies such as magnetic resonance–guided focal laser ablation are emerging as alternative to whole-gland treatments. Complications such as impotence are lessened due to the ability to precisely target treatment with MRI guidance.

Transradial Artery Access
- Transradial access is a safe and effective alternative to transfemoral access for catheter-directed arterial therapies.
- Preprocedural evaluation with the Barbeau test is crucial for evaluating the patient's palmar arch tolerability for the procedure.
- Patients do not need to be kept immobile after a TRA approach, which is beneficial for postembolization patients who may find more comfort assuming a fetal position.

- Obese patients may benefit from TRA due to the deep position of the common femoral artery, which would make initial femoral access and postprocedural hemostasis more difficult in this subset.
- Major complications with TRA are rare; minor complications related to TRA have been reported to be less frequent than with transfemoral arterial access.

Bariatric Artery Embolization
- Ghrelin, produced primarily by cells in the gastric fundus, is the primary hormone implicated in appetite stimulation.
- Transarterial embolization of the left gastric artery has been shown to decrease serum ghrelin levels and induce weight loss in animal models, with clinical human trials currently under way.
- The rich collateral supply to the gastric fundus and variations in arterial anatomy represent possible pitfalls to the procedure. Preprocedural mapping of arterial anatomy with a computed tomography angiography is recommended to avoid nontarget embolization and potential organ ischemia.

Magnetic Resonance–Guided Focused Ultrasound
- MRgFUS is a novel noninvasive treatment for symptomatic uterine fibroids.
- It can be performed on an outpatient basis with a shorter postprocedure recovery time compared with uterine artery embolization or surgical alternatives.
- Further research is needed to establish its long-term and comparative efficacy.

REVIEW QUESTIONS

1. Which of the following statements is *false* regarding prostatic artery anatomy?
   a. There is high anatomic variability.
   b. There are most typically two main prostatic arteries on each side.
   c. Prostatic arteries typically have a "corkscrew" appearance.
   d. The prostatic artery is a branch of the posterior division of the internal iliac artery.

2. Which of the following statements is *false*?
   a. Normal prostate volume is less than 30 cm^3.
   b. The transitional zone is the site of BPH and target area for TURP.
   c. TURP is the first line of therapy for BPH.
   d. Some 50% of men over the age of 50 have BPH.

3. Which of the following is an absolute contraindication to TRA?
   a. Barbeau A
   b. Barbeau B
   c. Barbeau C
   d. Barbeau D

4. Which of the following should be administered via the TRA sheath immediately after its placement into the radial artery to prevent radial artery vasospasm/occlusion?
   a. Normal saline or lactated Ringer solution flush
   b. Iodinated contrast
   c. A cocktail of heparin, calcium channel blockers, and nitrates
   d. A cocktail of warfarin, beta blockers, and nitrates
   e. None of the above

5. Hemostasis after TRA is usually achieved by
   a. Manual compression for up to 15 minutes
   b. Access-site closure devices
   c. Compression band applied over the wrist within seconds
   d. Surgical closure for patients undergoing TRA

6. Which of the following is the most common variant anatomy associated with the left gastric artery?
   a. Anomalous origin of the left gastric artery
   b. Gastromesenteric trunk
   c. Replaced common hepatic artery
   d. Replaced left hepatic artery

SUGGESTED READINGS

Barbeau GR, Arsenault F, Dugas L, et al. MM. Evaluation of the ulnopalmar arterial arches with pulse oximetry and plethysmography: comparison with the Allen's test in 1010 patients. *Am Heart J*. 2004;147:489–493.

Carnevale FC, Antunes AA, da Motta Leal Filho JM, et al. Prostatic artery embolization as a primary treatment for benign prostatic hyperplasia: preliminary results in two patients. *Cardiovasc Intervent Radiol*. 2010;33(2):355–361.

Coakley FV, Foster BR, Farsad K, et al. Pelvic applications of MR-guided high intensity focused ultrasound. *Abdom Imaging*. 2013;38(5):1120–1129.

DeMeritt JS, Elmasri FF, Esposito MP, Rosenberg GS, et al. Relief of benign prostatic hyperplasia-related bladder outlet obstruction after transarterial polyvinyl alcohol prostate embolization. *J Vasc Interv Radiol*. 2000;11(6):767–770.

Fischman AM, Swinburne NC, Patel RS. A technical guide describing the use of transradial access technique for endovascular interventions. *Tech Vasc Interv Radiol*. 2015;18(2):58–65.

Gunn AJ, Oklu R. A preliminary observation of weight loss following left gastric artery embolization in humans. *J Obes*. 2014;2014:185349.

Isaacson AJ, Fischman AM, Burke CT. Technical feasibility of prostatic artery embolization from a transradial approach. *AJR Am J Roentgenol*. 2016;206(2):442–444.

Kipshidze N, Archvadze A, Kantaria M. First-in-man study of left gastric artery embolization for weight loss. In: *Presented at the 62nd Annual Scientific Meeting of the American College of Cardiology*; Mar 10 2013. San Francisco, CA.

Oto A, Sethi I, Karczmar G, et al. MR imaging-guided focal laser ablation for prostate cancer: phase I trial. *Radiology*. 2013;267(3):932–940.

Pisco J, Campos Pinheiro L, Bilhim T, et al. Prostatic arterial embolization for benign prostatic hyperplasia: short- and intermediate-term results. *Radiology*. 2013;266(2):668–677.

Pisco JM, Pinheiro LC, Bilhim T, et al. Prostatic arterial embolization to treat benign prostatic hyperplasia. *J Vasc Interv Radiol*. 2011;22(1):11–19.

Posham R, Biederman DM, Patel RS, et al. Transradial approach for noncoronary interventions: a single-center review of safety and feasibility in the first 1,500 cases. *J Vasc Interv Radiol*. 2016;27(2):159–166.

Weiss CR, Gunn AJ, Kim CY, et al. Bariatric embolization of the gastric arteries for the treatment of obesity. *J Vasc Interv Radiol*. 2015;26(5):613–624.

11

Adrenal Venous Sampling

James J. Morrison, Frederick S. Keller

CASE PRESENTATION

A 50-year-old female presents with hypertension refractory to multiple medications, having previously tried furosemide, hydralazine, prazosin, and verapamil. She is found to be hypokalemic, for which she is prescribed supplements. Her aldosterone-to-renin ratio is elevated, prompting a referral to endocrinology for suspicion of hyperaldosteronism. During workup, abdominal computed tomography reveals a low-density 1.2-cm left adrenal nodule. The patient is referred to interventional radiology (IR) for adrenal venous sampling.

- **Adrenal venous sampling** (AVS) is the gold standard in identifying a subtype of primary aldosteronism (whether hypersecretion is unilateral or bilateral).
  - In AVS, blood samples are obtained from the veins draining each adrenal gland as well as from the peripheral circulation to compare the levels of **cortisol** and **aldosterone**.
- Computed tomography (CT) evaluation of the adrenal glands is insufficient for diagnosis and subtyping.
  - Subcentimeter aldosterone-producing adenomas may escape detection.
  - Even if a nodule is detected, its presence is not indicative of hypersecretion owing to the prevalence of non-functioning cortical adenomas.
- Preprocedural abdominal CT with intravenous contrast can assist in identifying the position of the right and left adrenal veins and evaluating for variants such as retro- or circumaortic left renal veins.
- **Primary aldosteronism** is a potentially curable cause of hypertension; it is seen in 5% to 10% of hypertensive patients.
- **Bilateral adrenal hyperplasia** is the most common cause of primary aldosteronism and is treated with mineralocorticoid receptor antagonists.
- Unilateral adrenalectomy is performed in patients with aldosterone-producing adenomas, thus alleviating symptoms of hypokalemia and hypertension in nearly all cases and completely curing patients in up to 80% of cases.

INDICATIONS

- Distinguishing between aldosterone-secreting adenomas (microscopic or macroscopic), nonsecreting adenomas, and bilateral adrenal hyperplasia
- Sampling of adrenal hormones (i.e., norepinephrine, epinephrine)
- Workup of hypersecretory adrenal diseases including pheochromocytoma (where the tumor is not evident on any other imaging modality), Cushing disease, and syndromes of androgen excess

CONTRAINDICATIONS

- No absolute contraindications.
- Relative contraindications include severe renal impairment and iodinated contrast allergy.

KEY EQUIPMENT

- Micropuncture access kit
- Ultrasound
- 6-Fr sheath
- 0.035-inch J-wire, hydrophilic guidewire
- Two 5.5-Fr straight catheters (preformed catheters may be used, depending on operator preference; Fig. 11.1).
- Hole punch
- 10-mL syringes for sample collection
- Steam

ANATOMY

The venous drainage of the adrenal glands is primarily through a single central vein on each side (Fig. 11.2).

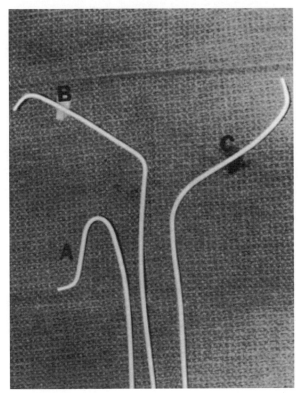

Fig. 11.1 **Common Catheter Shapes.** (A) Reverse-curve catheter. (B) Double-curve catheter. (C) Left-adrenal catheter. (Courtesy Frederick Keller.)

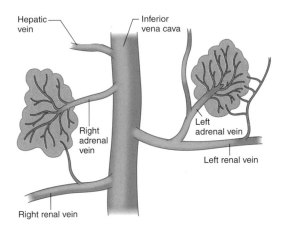

Fig. 11.2 Standard Anatomy for the Adrenal Veins.

Right Adrenal Gland (Fig. 11.3)

- The right adrenal gland is often the more difficult gland to sample as the central right adrenal vein empties directly into the inferior vena cava (IVC).
- The vein is most commonly found along the right posterolateral aspect of the IVC. The inferior emissary vein can be

a reassuring finding when one is searching for the right adrenal vein.
- Variant venous drainage can be seen, including:
  - Draining into the left posterolateral aspect of the IVC
  - Draining into a short hepatic vein

Left Adrenal Gland (Fig. 11.4)

- The left adrenal vein empties into the superior portion of the left renal vein.
- The left adrenal vein and left inferior phrenic vein often connect before reaching the left renal vein.
- It is important to be aware of left renal vein variants, such as retro- or circumaortic left renal veins, as these variations can increase the difficulty of finding and sampling the left adrenal vein.

Adenomas (Fig. 11.5)

- Tumors are not often visualized but can be very characteristic when seen.

PROCEDURAL STEPS

- Procedural protocols for AVS vary by institution. The main differences in institutional protocols are related to:
  - Sequential versus simultaneous sampling
  - Sampling with or without the use of adrenocorticotropic hormone stimulation.
- Electrolyte imbalances (commonly hypokalemia) should be corrected before performing the procedure.

Protocol for Sequential Adrenal Vein Sampling (With Adrenal Stimulation)

1. Shape the catheters with steam to the desired shape.
2. Create a hole with the hole punch near the tip of the catheter to facilitate sample acquisition. This technique prevents collapse of the adrenal vein when a sample is being drawn.
3. Administer cosyntropin (ACTH) 0.25 mg IV.
4. Obtain ultrasound-guided micropuncture access of the right femoral vein.
5. Administer heparin (70–100 U/kg), typically heparin 1000 U IV.
6. Upsize to a 0.035-inch guidewire, and advance the guidewire to the IVC.
7. Place a sheath.
8. Advance the right adrenal catheter to the level of the right adrenal gland, and then remove the guidewire.
9. Probe with the catheter tip along the IVC (in the general region of the right adrenal vein as seen on CT).
10. Catheterize the right adrenal vein.
11. Gently hand-inject contrast to confirm selection of the right adrenal vein.
12. Collect a blood sample (8–10 mL) from the right adrenal vein. This should be done at least 15 minutes after the dose of cosyntropin.
13. Disengage the catheter from the right adrenal vein, rotate it to the left, and pull it inferiorly.

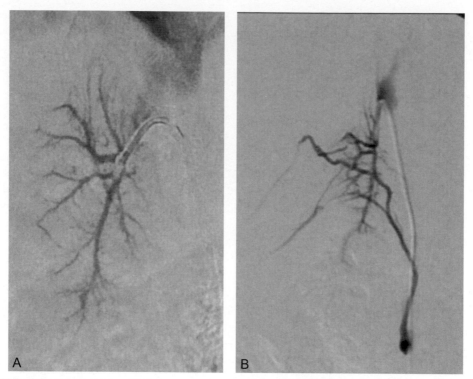

Fig. 11.3 Right Adrenal Veins. (A) Common appearance of the right adrenal vein arising from the right postero-lateral inferior vena cava. (B) Catheter tip in the right adrenal vein with contrast opacification of the inferior emissary vein extending inferiorly to the right renal vein. (Courtesy Frederick Keller.)

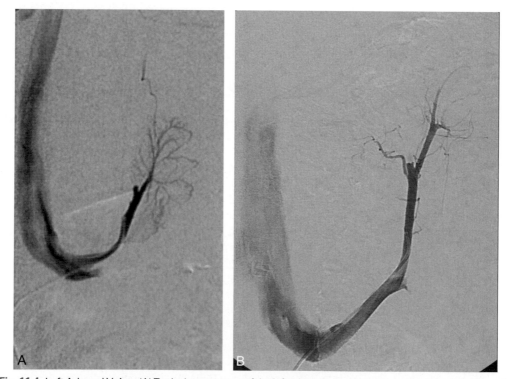

Fig. 11.4 Left Adrenal Veins. (A) Typical appearance of the left adrenal vein. The origin of the left inferior phrenic can be seen along the medial aspect of the left adrenal vein as it exits the gland. (B) Left adrenal vein originating from a retroaortic left renal vein. (Courtesy Frederick Keller.)

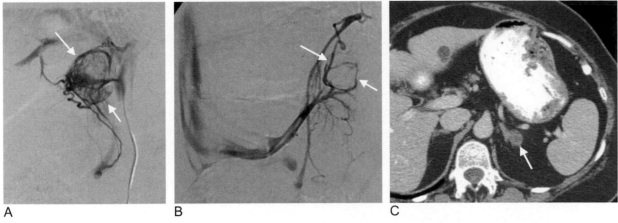

Fig. 11.5 Adrenal Adenomas. (A) Right adrenal adenoma (arrows). (B) Left adrenal adenoma (arrows). (C) Left adrenal adenoma (arrow) seen on computed tomography, corresponding to the adenoma seen on venography in (B). (Courtesy Frederick Keller.)

14. Catheterize the left renal vein with assistance of a hydrophilic guidewire.
15. Exchange the current catheter for a left adrenal vein catheter over the guidewire.
16. Slowly retract the left adrenal vein catheter until the superiorly oriented tip engages with the left adrenal vein.
17. Gently hand-inject contrast to confirm selection of the left adrenal vein.
18. Collect a blood sample (8–10 mL) from the left adrenal vein.
19. Remove the catheter.
20. Collect a peripheral blood sample from the sheath.
21. Remove the sheath.
22. Compress the insertion site manually until hemostasis is achieved.

> ## CLINICAL POINT
>
> **Interpretation of Results**
> - Blood samples from AVS are sent for aldosterone and cortisol assay. The results are used to confirm successful catheterization of each adrenal vein as well as to determine the presence of bilateral or unilateral disease.
> - To confirm successful catheterization of the adrenal veins, the ratio of adrenal vein cortisol to peripheral blood cortisol is calculated for each side. This is known as the *selectivity index* (Table 11.1).
>   - A selectivity index greater than 5 confirms adrenal vein catheterization.
> - To determine if there is unilateral or bilateral disease, the aldosterone/cortisol ratio is calculated. This is known as the *lateralization index* (Table 11.2).
>   - A lateralization index greater than 4 indicates unilateral disease.

TABLE 11.1	Selectivity Index
≤5	Adrenal vein probably not selected
≥5	Successful adrenal vein sampling

TABLE 11.2	Lateralization Index
≥4	Unilateral aldosterone-producing adenoma
2–4	Borderline
≤2	Bilateral adrenal hyperplasia

TREATMENT ALTERNATIVES

- AVS is the gold standard for both differentiation of aldosterone-secreting adenomas from bilateral adrenal hyperplasia as well as lateralization of the aldosterone-secreting tumor. There is no diagnostic alternative.
- CT evaluation and laboratory analysis alone are not sufficient to identify the side requiring treatment.
- There is an alternative AVS technique that involves simultaneous rather than sequential (as described earlier) sampling of both adrenal veins.
  - Simultaneous sampling protocols involve catheterization of both adrenal veins before sampling (either through unilateral or bilateral femoral vein sheaths).
  - Samples are drawn in parallel once the catheters are in place. A peripheral blood sample is drawn from the sheath.
  - Simultaneous sampling may be performed with or without the use of cosyntropin; however, cutoff values of selectivity and lateralization indices will vary with the protocol used.
  - Cone-beam CT (Fig. 11.6) can be used in difficult cases to confirm catheter positioning.

COMPLICATIONS

- Complications as a result of AVS are rare. As related to venous sampling, they include:
  - Thrombosis of the adrenal vein
  - Dissection of the adrenal vein
  - Adrenal hemorrhage
- Typical access site–related complications

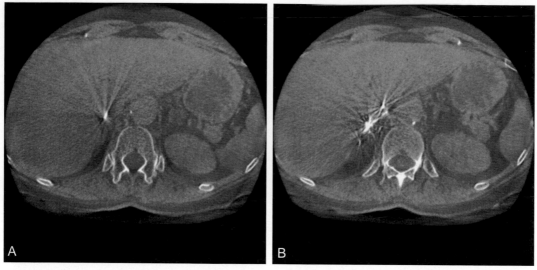

Fig. 11.6 Cone-beam computed tomographic confirmation of catheterization of the right adrenal vein with gentle hand injection of contrast material. Injected contrast is seen opacifying the right adrenal vein (A) and gland (B). (Courtesy Frederick Keller.)

 TAKE-HOME POINTS

- Adrenal vein sampling is the gold standard for distinguishing between bilateral and unilateral aldosterone hypersecretion and for lateralizing aldosterone-secreting adenomas.

- Primary aldosteronism from a unilateral hypersecreting adenoma accounts for a subset of hypertensive patients whose condition can be improved and even cured with intervention.

REVIEW QUESTIONS

1. The ratio of adrenal vein cortisol to peripheral vein cortisol is known as the
   a. selectivity index.
   b. lateralization index.
   c. sensitivity index.
   d. specificity index.

2. The comparison of right adrenal vein aldosterone/cortisol ratio to left adrenal vein aldosterone/cortisol ratio is known as the
   a. selectivity index.
   b. lateralization index.
   c. sensitivity index.
   d. specificity index.

3. Why is a side hole added to the end of the catheter at the start of the case?
   a. To make manipulation of the catheter in finding the adrenal veins easier.
   b. To increase the rate of flow of contrast material during hand injection.
   c. To prevent collapse of the adrenal vein during sample acquisition.
   d. To avoid damaging the wall of the IVC.

SUGGESTED READINGS

Carr CE, Cope C, Cohen DL, et al. Comparison of sequential versus simultaneous methods of adrenal venous sampling. *J Vasc Interv Radiol.* 2004;15(11):1245–1250.

Daunt N. Adrenal vein sampling: how to make it quick, easy, and successful. *Radiographics.* 2005;25(suppl 1):S143–S158.

Kahn SL, Angle JF. Adrenal vein sampling. *Tech Vasc Interv Radiol.* 2010;13(2):110–125.

Rossi GP, Auchus RJ, Brown M, et al. An expert consensus statement on use of adrenal vein sampling for the subtyping of primary aldosteronism. *Hypertension.* 2014;63(1):151–160.

Arteriovenous Fistulas and Grafts

Ryan Trojan, Chad Thompson

CASE PRESENTATION

A 54-year-old male with end-stage renal disease (ESRD), hypertension (HTN), and diabetes mellitus (DM) presents with increased bleeding from a left brachiocephalic fistula following dialysis. The patient receives dialysis on Mondays, Wednesdays, and Fridays; he underwent a full session yesterday. His nephrologist orders a fistulogram to be performed before the patient's next dialysis session.

HISTORY

- In 1924, Georg Haas performed the first hemodialysis (HD) session on a human in Germany.
- In 1943, Willem Kolff completed the first modern dialysis session with a drum dialyzer.
- In 1965, the first **arteriovenous fistula** (AVF) was surgically created. The following year, the paper "Chronic Hemodialysis Using Venipuncture and a Surgically Created Arteriovenous Fistula," by Michael Brescia, James Cimino, Kenneth Appel, and Baruch Hurwich, was published in the *New England Journal of Medicine*.
  - At this same time, Charles Dotter and colleagues were performing the first angioplasty procedure with a newly developed balloon angioplasty catheter.
- In 1982, David H. Gordon and Sidney Glanz presented on the results of treating 16 stenotic AVFs with balloon angioplasty.

PATHOPHYSIOLOGY

- Patients in renal failure require an access point to receive hemodialysis (HD).
- Venous dialysis catheters can be placed in the acute setting. They are not, however, optimal for long-term use because they carry risks of central venous stenosis, central line infection, thrombosis, and general catheter malfunction.
- An AVF is a surgically created connection between a native artery and vein. An **arteriovenous graft** (AVG) is a surgically created connection between an artery and vein using a synthetic graft. Both are used for long-term dialysis access.
- Interventional radiologists play a central role in preserving and maintaining these valuable access sites. Minimally invasive interventional radiology (IR) techniques have replaced surgical revision as the treatment of choice for failing or thrombosed fistulas and grafts.
  - **Angioplasty** and **thrombectomy** are the most common interventions performed.
- Common problems with AVFs and grafts include failure to mature, thrombosis, and outflow stenosis.
- Vascular access problems in renal failure patients continue to be a leading cause of morbidity and hospitalization in this patient population.
- Vascular access failure is estimated to cost more than one billion dollars annually in the United States.

KEY DEFINITIONS

Primary failure is seen in an AVF/graft that is never usable or fails within the first 3 months of use.
Primary patency describes a patent fistula without revision.
Secondary patency describes a patent fistula following revision.

INDICATIONS

- Decrease in AVF flow to <500 mL/min or drop of >20% from baseline
- Decrease in AV graft flow to <650 mL/min or drop of >20% from baseline
- Increased venous pressures
- Thrombosis
- Failure to mature
- Any sign of dysfunction
- Indications for placing a stent:
  - Venous rupture after angioplasty that fails balloon tamponade
  - Venous stenosis that does not respond to balloon angioplasty
  - Central stenosis that recurs within 3 months of successful balloon angioplasty

CONTRAINDICATIONS

- Absolute
  - Access site infection
  - Uncorrectable coagulopathy

- Relative
  - Contrast allergy
  - Hyperkalemia
  - If the serum potassium is >6.0 mEq/L, a temporary femoral dialysis catheter is placed and the patient goes to dialysis immediately. The fistulogram is done following dialysis.
- Contraindications specific to thrombectomy
  - Presence of a right-to-left shunt, as in a patent foramen ovale
  - Severe pulmonary hypertension or right-sided heart failure
  - Steal phenomenon in the ipsilateral extremity
- Contraindications specific to pharmacologic thrombolysis
  - Major surgery within the previous 3 weeks
  - Internal bleeding in the previous 6 weeks
  - Intracranial tumor
  - Brain surgery within the previous 6 months
  - History of hemorrhagic stroke
  - Transient ischemic attack (TIA) or stroke within the previous 3 months

EQUIPMENT

- Micropuncture kit for access
- Flow switch
- Wire options—Bentson, Glidewire, or Roadrunner
- Catheter options—5-Fr 40-cm Berenstein or a 5-Fr 40-cm straight
- Introducer sheaths—5- to 9-Fr in 4-cm length (6- and 7-Fr sheaths are most commonly used)
- Angioplasty balloons (Table 12.1) and inflation device
- 5-Fr Fogarty catheter
- Stents
  - Almost all stents used in dialysis access are self-expanding. Balloon-mounted stents can be used in cases of central stenosis.
- Thrombectomy device options—AngioJet, Cleaner, or Trerotola
  - Angiojet (Boston Scientific, Marlborough, MA, USA; Arrow, Wayne, PA, USA; Argon, Frisco, Tx, USA)—pharmacomechanical thrombectomy device that aspirates thrombus and sprays a tPA solution

- Cleaner XT (Argon)—mechanical rotational thrombectomy system
- Arrow-Trerotola PTD (Arrow)—mechanical thrombectomy device

> ## ◎ KEY DEFINITION
>
> **Nominal pressure (NP)** is the inflation pressure required for the balloon to reach the specified diameter.
> **Rated burst pressure (RBP)** is the inflation pressure at which 99.9% of balloons will survive with 95% confidence.

ANATOMY

Arterial Anatomy of the Upper Extremity (Fig. 12.1)

- Subclavian artery
  - The right subclavian artery takes off at the brachiocephalic trunk and ends at the lateral border of the right first rib.
  - The left subclavian artery takes off at the aortic arch and ends at the lateral border of the left first rib.
- The axillary artery takes off at the lateral margin of the first rib and ends at the inferior border of the teres major.
- The brachial artery takes off at the inferior border of the teres major and ends at the division of the radial and ulnar arteries.
- The radial artery courses along the radial aspect of the forearm and terminates into the superficial and palmar arches.
- The ulnar artery courses along the ulnar side of the forearm and terminates into the superficial and palmar arches.
  - The common interosseous artery is a branch of the ulnar artery.

Venous Anatomy of the Upper Extremity (Fig. 12.2)

- Superficial venous anatomy
  - The basilic vein travels along the medial aspect of the upper extremity, joining the brachial vein to form the axillary vein.
  - The cephalic vein courses along the anterolateral aspect of the upper extremity before joining the axillary vein.

TABLE 12.1	Examples of Different Types of Angioplasty Balloons						
Trade Name	**Type**	**Diameter**	**Length**	**Cost**	**NP**	**RBP**	**Wire**
Ultraverse (Bard)	Standard pressure	3–12 mm	20–300 mm	$80–$85	6–8 atm	9–21 atm	0.035-in
Dorado (Bard)	Standard pressure	3–10 mm	20–200 mm	$160–$170	8 atm	20–24 atm	0.035-in
Atlas (Bard)	Standard pressure	12–26 mm	20–60 mm	$260–$465	4–7 atm	12–18 atm	0.035-in
Mustang (Boston Scientific)	Standard pressure	3–12 mm	12–200 mm	$370–$380	8–10 atm	14–24 atm	0.035-in
Conquest (Bard)	Standard pressure	5–12 mm	20–80 mm	$150–155	6–8 atm	20–30 atm	0.035-in
Peripheral Cutting (Boston Scientific)	High pressure	2–8 mm	15–20 mm	$820–$830	4–6 atm	8–12 atm	0.014–.018-in

NP, Nominal pressure; *RBP,* rated burst pressure.

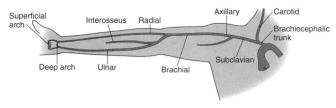

Fig. 12.1 Arterial Anatomy of the Upper Extremity. (Courtesy Ryan Trojan and Chad Thompson.)

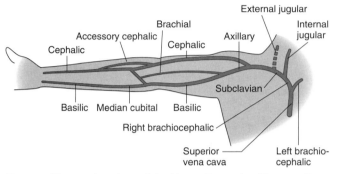

Fig. 12.2 Venous Anatomy of the Upper Extremity. (Courtesy Ryan Trojan and Chad Thompson.)

- Deep venous anatomy
  - The radial, ulnar, brachial, axillary, and subclavian veins follow the courses of their paired arteries.

Types of Arteriovenous Fistulas

- Lower arm: radial artery → cephalic vein
- Upper arm: brachial artery → cephalic vein or brachial artery → basilic vein

Arteriovenous Graft Types

- Lower arm: brachial artery → cephalic vein (looped) (Fig. 12.3)

- Upper arm: brachial artery → axillary vein (straight) or axillary artery → axillary vein (looped)
- Lower extremity: femoral artery → femoral vein (looped)

> ### ◎ LITERATURE REVIEW
>
> **2006 National Kidney Foundation Kidney Disease Outcomes Quality Initiative (KDOQI) Clinical Practice Guidelines**
> - Order of preference for dialysis access creation:
>   1. Radiocephalic AVF
>   2. Brachiocephalic AVF
>   3. Transposed brachiobasilic AVF
>   4. Arteriovenous graft
> - Criteria for adequate fistula maturation at 6 weeks (*Rule of 6s*):
>   - 6 mm or less from the skin surface
>   - 6-mm diameter
>   - 6-cm straight segment for cannulation
>   - 600-mL/min blood flow

Determining Fistula Versus Graft

- Fistulas are generally preferred over grafts, given their improved long-term patency and fewer overall complications.
- AVGs are indicated in patients with shorter life expectancies, since grafts have shorter maturation times and lower primary failure rates. These general differences are summarized in Table 12.2.

> ### ◎ LITERATURE REVIEW
>
> Young et al. (2002) found that grafts are three times more likely to require an access intervention and more than three times more likely to require a thrombectomy as compared with native fistulas.

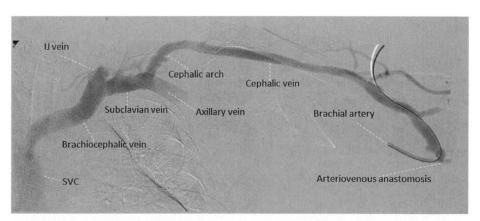

Fig. 12.3 Anatomy of a Normal Left Brachiocephalic Fistula. *SVC,* Superior vena cava. (Courtesy Ryan Trojan and Chad Thompson.)

TABLE 12.2   Arteriovenous Fistula Versus Arteriovenous Graft

	Arteriovenous Fistula	Arteriovenous Graft
Median time to use	4 weeks to 1 year	1–3 weeks
Primary failure	9%–36%	<15%
1-year secondary patency, excluding primary failure	82%	67%
2-year secondary patency, excluding primary failure	73%	50%
Composition	Native vessel	PTFE
Diameter	Variable	4–8 mm
Average infection risk	2%–5%	10%

PTFE, Polytetrafluoroethylene.

PROCEDURAL STEPS

Physical Exam (Table 12.3)

- Inspect the ipsilateral hand of the vascular access site for signs of necrosis.
- Evaluate the skin overlying the access site for signs of infection.
- Palpate the fistula/graft to assess for a thrill and auscultate for a bruit.
- Determine the direction of flow within the fistula. If this is not obvious, compress the fistula with the tip of your finger, and feel for a pulse on either side. The side without a pulse is the outflow side.

▶▶ CLINICAL POINT

What's the difference between a *thrill* and a *bruit*? A thrill is a vibration felt by palpation. A bruit is a sound generated by turbulent flow in a vessel that is heard by auscultation.

Preprocedural Optimization

- Labs: complete blood count (CBC), basic metabolic panel (BMP)
  - If serum potassium is >6.0 mEq/L, place a femoral temporary dialysis catheter and dialyze the patient.

TABLE 12.3   Physical Exam Findings

Venous Outflow Stenosis	Arterial Stenosis	Central Venous Stenosis
Hyperpulsatile fistula	Flat fistula	Ipsilateral arm/facial edema
Prolonged bleeding after dialysis	Reduced pulse	Collateral veins over the shoulder and upper chest
Ipsilateral arm edema	Ecchymosis of the extremity due to failed cannulation	

- If the international normalized ratio (INR) is >2.0, consider correction.
- If platelets are below 50K, transfuse.
- Do not stop Plavix or aspirin, but hold low-molecular-weight heparin for 1 day prior to the planned procedure.
- Moderate sedation: yes
- Antibiotics: not routinely

Procedural Planning

- Review previous fistulogram studies and, if available, initial an operative report for the fistula.
- Using the patient's chief complaint, physical exam findings, and ultrasound findings, determine if there is an inflow (juxta-anastomotic stenosis or arterial anastomosis stenosis) or outflow (outflow or central vein stenosis) problem. Fistulas often suffer from both inflow and outflow issues and will subsequently require two access points for complete treatment.
  - **Inflow problem:** the needle should be placed in the outflow vein at least 7 to 10 cm away from the arteriovenous anastomosis, with the needle directed toward the inflow.
  - **Outflow problem:** the needle should be placed in the outflow vein within 4 to 6 cm of the arteriovenous anastomosis, with the needle directed toward the outflow.
  - **Problem site unknown:** the catheter should be placed in the outflow vein toward the arteriovenous anastomosis and navigated into the afferent brachial artery using a Glidewire and Berenstein catheter combination. A diagnostic fistulogram should be performed through the catheter prior to placing a sheath.
- Examine the skin over the fistula looking for signs of infection. Check distal pulses in the same limb.

Procedural Steps—Fistulogram

1. Position the patient supine with the access site arm abducted 60 to 90 degrees and the palm up.
2. Prep and drape the skin overlying the expected access site or sites in a sterile fashion.
3. Administer lidocaine at each access site.
4. Access can be obtained with a standard micropuncture set and use of ultrasound.
5. In the setting of outflow/central stenosis, a 22-gauge needle is inserted into the fistula vein in antegrade fashion (i.e., toward the central veins).
6. A 0.018-inch guidewire is passed into the fistula.
7. The needle is removed and exchanged for a coaxial dilator.
8. The wire and inner dilator are removed, leaving the outer sheath in the fistula.
9. A diagnostic fistulogram can be performed through the outer sheath of the micropuncture set. Contrast is injected to evaluate for stenosis of the outflow or central vein. A complete fistulogram includes evaluation of the arterial anastomosis, outflow vein, and central veins. A single antegrade access may not allow for a complete fistulogram; thus retrograde access (i.e., toward the arterial anastomosis) may also be required.

10. If an intervention is planned, exchange the outer sheath of the micropuncture kit set with a vascular sheath, which will allow for passage of wires, balloons, thrombectomy devices, or stents. If no intervention is planned, remove the catheter and compress.

 CLINICAL POINT

Access site hemostasis is achieved with manual compression at a rate of 2 minutes per French size for venous access and 3 minutes per French size for arterial access.

Treating a Stenosis

> **CLINICAL POINT**
>
> A functionally significant stenosis is defined as a reduction of >50% of normal vessel diameter accompanied by hemodynamic or clinical abnormality.
>
> Failed angioplasty is a >30% residual stenosis following angioplasty.
>
> A 50% stenosis results in a >75% reduction in cross-sectional area of the vessel.

1. Cross the stenosis with a guidewire such as a 0.035-inch Bentson wire. A tight stenosis may have to be crossed with a catheter and Glidewire.
2. Measure the vein adjacent to the stenosis, and select a balloon that is 10% to 20% larger than the diameter of the native vessel. If the stenosis is severe, consider serial dilation with an intermediate-sized balloon prior to reaching the target diameter.
3. Insert the balloon over the guidewire, and center it over the stenosis, using a reference image for guidance.
4. Using an inflation device with a 1:1 mixture of contrast/saline, slowly inflate the balloon under fluoroscopy.
5. Once the stenosis has been dilated, leave the balloon inflated for 1 to 2 minutes.
6. Deflate and remove the balloon while maintaining wire access across the stenosis.
7. Perform a postdilation fistulogram by injecting contrast through the sheath to determine if there is residual stenosis or vein injury.

Treating a Clot

1. Access a thrombosed fistula in the same fashion as described earlier for a nonthrombosed fistula. If it is a thrombosed loop graft, entry requires accessing both the venous limb and the arterial limb with a 6- or 7-Fr short sheath near the apex of the graft (*crossed-catheter technique* with one catheter directed toward the arterial anastomosis and another directed toward the venous anastomosis) (Fig. 12.4).
2. Administer 3000 to 5000 units of intravenous heparin.
3. Use a 5-Fr Berenstein catheter and guidewire to navigate into the central veins.
4. Perform angiography of the central vein past the venous anastomosis to document patency.

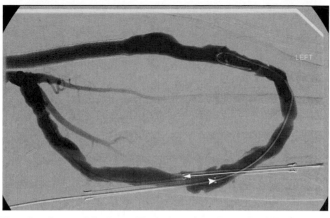

Fig. 12.4 Crossed Catheter Technique for a Loop Graft Thrombectomy. A 6-Fr sheath *(white arrow)* is directed toward the arterial anastomosis, and a 7-Fr sheath *(white arrowhead)* is directed toward the venous outflow. (Courtesy Ryan Trojan and Chad Thompson.)

5. Remove the catheter over the wire while maintaining the tip of the wire within the superior vena cava (SVC) or inferior vena cava (IVC).
6. With a Berenstein catheter and hydrophilic guidewire, place a wire in the afferent artery.
7. Thrombolysis is performed with an Angiojet (or other device, depending on preference) first in the venous outflow and then in the inflow segment of the graft or fistula.
8. Via an over-the-wire technique, advance a 5-Fr Fogarty catheter into the afferent artery, and inflate the balloon gently.
9. Pull the inflated balloon across the arterial anastomosis, dragging the thrombus into the venous outflow. Deflate the balloon, and repeat two to three times.
10. Once most of the thrombus has been removed, dilate any residual stenosis with an appropriately sized balloon.
11. The fistula should have a continuous thrill. A completion fistulogram can confirm and document successful treatment.

Placing a Stent

1. Gain wire access across the stenosis.
2. Size the stent 1 to 2 mm larger than the vessel to be treated. The stent should be long enough to treat the diseased vessel and should not cover more than 10 mm of normal vessel on either side of the stenosis.
3. Advance the stent over the wire to the region of interest.
4. Deploy the stent by slow retraction, allowing it to expand fully. Stents will sometimes migrate forward during deployment, and the delivery catheter will have to be retracted under fluoroscopy during deployment to ensure accurate placement.

Collateral Vessel Embolization

- Collaterals can be treated with coil placement or surgical ligation.
- Treatment of collaterals is operator dependent and is mostly indicated in fistulas presenting with failure to mature.

ALTERNATE TREATMENTS

- Catheter-based interventions have replaced surgical revision as the treatment of choice for failing or thrombosed fistulas and grafts.
- Indications for surgical referral
  - Infected graft pseudoaneurysm
  - Vascular access steal syndrome

COMPLICATIONS

- Vascular stenosis (Figs. 12.5–12.9)
  - Pathway: endothelium injury → release inflammatory mediators → induction of smooth muscle cell migration and proliferation → neointimal hyperplasia that results in stenosis
  - Causes of endothelial injury include puncture-induced injury, turbulent flow, intimal hyperplasia at valve sites, and central venous catheter trauma.
- Thrombosed fistula
  - Usually secondary to an underlying stenosis
  - The thrombus has to be removed and the stenosis treated.
- Failure to mature
  - Describes an AVF/graft that is never usable or fails within the first 3 months of use

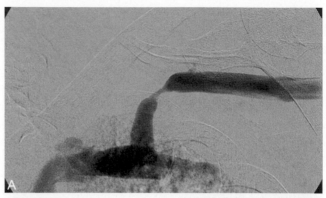
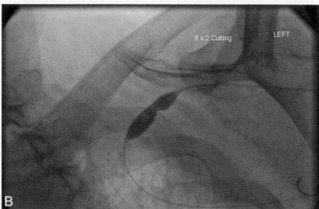
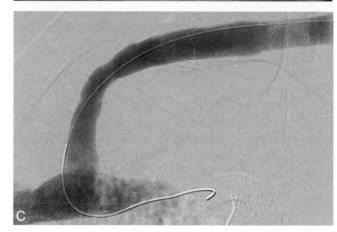

Fig. 12.6 Brachiocephalic fistula with cephalic arch stenosis (A) pre-angioplasty, (B) during balloon angioplasty with an 8 mm x 2 cm cutting balloon, and (C) post-angioplasty. (Courtesy Ryan Trojan and Chad Thompson.)

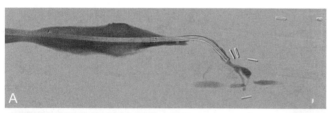
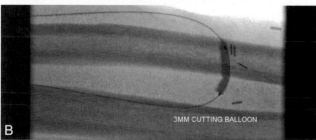
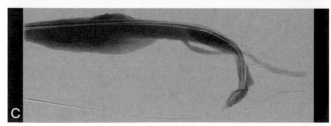

Fig. 12.5 Radiocephalic fistula with a juxta-anastomotic stenosis (A) pre-angioplasty, (B) during balloon angioplasty with a 3 mm cutting balloon, and (C) post-angioplasty. (Courtesy Ryan Trojan and Chad Thompson.)

- Causes of failure to mature include inflow artery stenosis, focal venous stenosis, diffuse venous stenosis, and the presence of accessory (collateral) veins.
- Pseudoaneurysm
  - Pseudoaneurysms are prone to develop in grafts and are at risk for infection.
  - Cannulation of a graft or fistula can predispose to pseudoaneurysm formation.
  - If there are signs of infection, surgical referral is warranted.

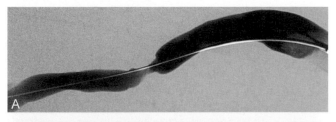

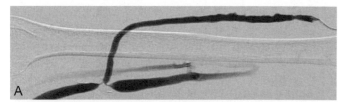

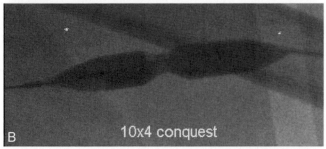

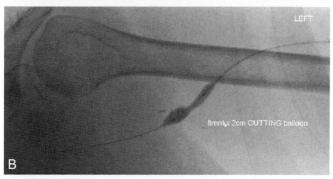

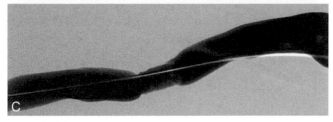

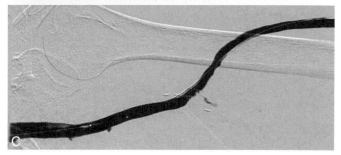

Fig. 12.7 Brachiobasilic fistula with stenosis of the outflow basilic vein (A) pre-angioplasty, (B) during balloon angioplasty with a 10 mm x 4 cm Conquest balloon, and (C) post-angioplasty. (Courtesy Ryan Trojan and Chad Thompson.)

Fig. 12.8 Brachioaxillary straight graft with a venous anastomotic stenosis (A) pre-angioplasty, (B) during angioplasty, and (C) post-angioplasty. (Courtesy Ryan Trojan and Chad Thompson.)

- Aneurysm (Fig. 12.10)
  - Defined as abnormal dilation of segments of the outflow vein >150% of the normal diameter of the vessel.
  - Most vascular access aneurysms have a benign course, and a fistulogram should be performed to evaluate for underlying stenosis, which would predispose to aneurysm formation.
  - If the aneurysm increases dramatically in size or there is infection/degeneration of the overlying skin, the fistula is at risk for spontaneous rupture, and a surgical consult is warranted.

> ### ▶ CLINICAL POINT
>
> **Law of Laplace:** Wall tension *(T)* = internal pressure *(P)* × radius *(R)*. As the radius increases, so does the tension. This principle makes rupture inevitable for a rapidly enlarging vascular access aneurysm and demands prompt surgical referral for possible surgical ligation.

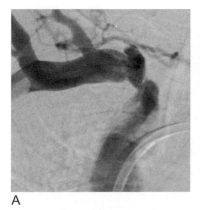

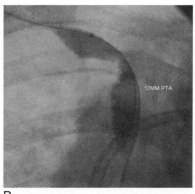

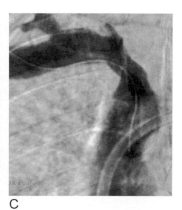

A   B   C

Fig. 12.9 Brachiocephalic stenosis (A) pre-angioplasty, (B) during angioplasty, and (C) post-angioplasty. There are multiple collaterals on the pre-angioplasty angiogram; these are no longer seen following angioplasty. The patient had a history of a right internal jugular tunneled dialysis catheter. (Courtesy Ryan Trojan and Chad Thompson.)

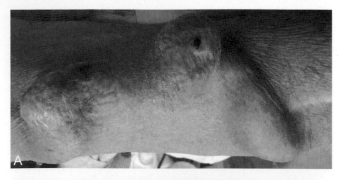

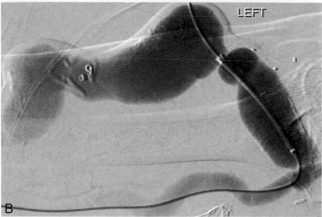

Fig. 12.10 Fistula Complications (A) Aneurysmal dilation of a left brachiobasilic fistula. The patient presented with heart failure attributable to the arteriovenous fistula, which is a rare complication of arteriovenous fistula placement. (B) The stenosis in the outflow basilic vein was not treated. The fistula was surgically removed, and a straight brachioaxillary graft was placed. (Courtesy Ryan Trojan and Chad Thompson.)

- Infection
  - Accounts for 20% of vascular access loss and is the most likely source of bacteremia in a HD patient
  - Graft infections should generate a surgical referral for possible intervention.
  - Fistula infections are treated with a 6-week course of intravenous antibiotics. If septic emboli are present, excision of the fistula is recommended.
- Hand ischemia
  - Vascular access–related steal syndrome results from vascular insufficiency due to arterial flow through an upstream AVF or graft.
  - Physical exam signs include skin necrosis, decreased arterial pulses, hand pain, and pallor of skin distal to the vascular access site.

- Treatment options include surgical revision/ligation or banding. Treat a vascular access–related stenosis in a patient with signs of steal syndrome with caution, as it can exacerbate the symptoms of steal syndrome.
- Venous rupture following angioplasty
  - Occurs in 2% to 3% of dilations
  - Treatment algorithm
    1. With a wire across the site of rupture, immediately place the balloon in the region of rupture, and keep it inflated for 5 minutes.
    2. Following balloon tamponade, repeat the fistulogram.
    3. If active extravasation is still seen, consider covered stent placement.
    4. If the rupture is in the region of the arteriovenous anastomosis, consider placement of an occluding Fogarty balloon in the brachial artery and urgent vascular surgical consultation.
- Embolization during thrombectomy
  - Occurs in 5% of thrombectomy procedures
  - Treatment algorithm
    1. Advance a soft wire such as a Bentson past the thrombus.
    2. Advance a 5-Fr Fogarty balloon on the wire past the thrombus. Inflate and retract the thrombus into the graft/fistula using the balloon.
    3. Use a suction catheter device to remove the embolus.
- Symptomatic Pulmonary embolism
  - Stop the procedure and proceed with medical/interventional management as indicated.

🏠 TAKE-HOME POINTS

- The number of patients in need of renal replacement therapy continues to increase. AVFs and grafts are the ideal means for permanent dialysis access.
- Interventional radiologists are key to the continued maintenance of AVFs and grafts.
- Common procedures performed by the interventional radiologist on AVFs/AVGs are angioplasty, thrombolysis, angioplasty, and stent placement.
- Fistula and graft dysfunction and postplacement complications are common. The most commonly seen issues are stenosis and thrombosis of the fistula/graft, failure of the AVG/AVF to mature, and aneurysm formation. Severe intraprocedural complications include vascular rupture and arterial embolization.

REVIEW QUESTIONS

1. A patient presents with painful arm swelling and facial edema. The fistula is very pulsatile. What is the most likely diagnosis?
   a. Outflow vein stenosis
   b. Juxta-anastomotic stenosis
   c. Central vein stenosis
   d. Thrombosed fistula

2. The patient is a 73-year-old male with a right brachiocephalic fistula and reported difficult access at HD. HD occurs on Mondays, Wednesdays, and Fridays, with the last full session having been completed 4 days prior. Labs: Na, 145; K, 6.1; Creat, 8.4; INR, 1.5; Plt, 75 K. An ultrasound is performed, showing that the fistula is thrombosed. What is the next best step in management?
   a. Proceed with the fistulogram
   b. Place a right, internal jugular, tunneled dialysis catheter for access, and proceed to HD.
   c. Give systemic thrombolytics.
   d. Place a femoral TDC and proceed to HD.
   e. Obtain an electrocardiogram prior to starting the fistulogram.

SUGGESTED READINGS

Aruny JE, Lewis CA, Cardella JF, et al. Quality improvement guidelines for percutaneous management of the thrombosed or dysfunctional dialysis access. *J Vasc Interv Radiol.* 1999;10 (4):491–498.

National Kidney Foundation. KDOQI clinical practice guidelines and clinical practice recommendations for 2006 updates: hemodialysis adequacy, peritoneal dialysis adequacy and vascular access. *Am J Kidney Dis.* 2006;48:S1–S322.

Oliver M, Woo K, Beathard G. Overview of chronic hemodialysis vascular access. In: Collins K, Motwani S, eds. *UpToDate.* Waltham, MA: UpToDate Inc. https://www.uptodate.com/contents/overview-of-chronic-hemodialysis-vascular-access.

Turmel-Rodrigues L, Renaud CJ. *Diagnostic and Interventional Radiology of Arteriovenous Accesses for Hemodialysis.* Dordrecht, The Netherlands: Springer; 2013.

Young EW, Dykstra DM, Goodwin DA, et al. Hemodialysis vascular access preferences and outcomes in the Dialysis Outcomes and Practice Patterns Study (DOPPS). *Kidney Int.* 2002;61(6): 2266–2271.

Woo K. Arteriovenous fistula creation for hemodialysis and its complications. In: Collins K, Lam A, eds. *UpToDate.* Waltham, MA: UpToDate Inc. https://www.uptodate.com/contents/arteriovenous-fistula-creation-for-hemodialysis-and-its-complications.

13

Arteriovenous Malformations

Jeffrey A. Brown, Luke A. Lennard, Gustavo Elias, Malcolm K. Sydnor

CASE PRESENTATION

A 16-year-old female is referred to the interventional radiology clinic for evaluation of right lower extremity swelling. She reports worsening right leg swelling with a faint bluish discoloration that has developed over the course of several years. She states there is pain when she walks or stands over long periods, relieved by rest and lying flat. Physical exam reveals tenderness to palpation over a palpable mass along the medial aspect of the right calf. You have been consulted for possible embolization of a vascular malformation. Ultrasound reveals a high-flow arteriovenous malformation (AVM), confirmed on CT angiography (CTA) imaging. Patient undergoes successful embolization of this AVM with a combination of coils and glue.

HISTORY

- First descriptions of vascular malformations came from the Papyrus Ebers, an Egyptian hieratic script, dated 1550 BC. The text contained descriptions of hemorrhoids, skin tumors, varicose veins, and aneurysms.
- Earliest attempts in vascular surgery to repair AV fistulas created from penetrating injuries with bloodletting occurred over 200 years ago.
- AVMs were first described in the 1800s by Drs. Luschka (1854) and Virchow (1863).
- Early surgical attempts at AVM repair centered around ligation of the feeding artery (*skeletonization*) or extirpation. These procedures often resulted in gangrene distally and hemorrhage, respectively.
- First endovascular embolization of an AVM was performed by Drs. Luessenhop and Spence in 1960.
- First percutaneous endovascular ablation of a spinal AVM was performed by neuroradiologists Drs. John Doppman and Thomas Newton in the late 1960s.
- Advancements in technique and embolic agents during the late 1970s and early 1980s helped transcatheter embolization assume a primary role in the treatment of congenital vascular malformations.
- A 1982 article published by Drs. Mulliken and Glowacki proposed a vascular anomaly classification system based on endothelial cell characteristics.

- In 1993, Jackson et al. proposed a complementary classification system based on flow characteristics (high-flow versus low-flow malformations).
- The International Society for the Study of Vascular Anomalies (ISSVA) developed a Mulliken-based consensus classification system in 1996 that continues to provide the current framework for the classification of AVMs.

PATHOPHYSIOLOGY

- Vascular malformations are congenital anomalies resulting from aberrant vessel formation in utero, generally between weeks 4 and 10.
- Direct connections are formed between arteries, veins, or lymphatics without intervening capillary beds.
- The point of aberrant vascular connection is termed the *nidus*. In AVMs, blood is shunted across the nidus from the high-pressure arterial circulation to the low-pressure venous circulation. One malformation may contain multiple nidi.
- An important distinction of vascular malformations is that they are lined with mature endothelial cells and tend to grow at the same rate as the individual.
- The majority of vascular malformations are isolated occurrences in otherwise healthy individuals. However, a few notable syndromes associated with vascular malformations are:
  - **AVMs**
    - **Hereditary hemorrhagic telangiectasia** (HHT, also known as Osler-Weber-Rendu syndrome)
    - Parkes-Weber syndrome
  - **Venous malformations (VMs)**
    - Klippel-Trenaunay syndrome
    - Blue rubber bleb nevus syndrome

> ## CLINICAL POINT
>
> Elevated D-dimer is highly specific for VMs and can help distinguish between lymphatic malformations and slow-flow Klippel-Trenaunay syndrome from high-flow Parkes-Weber syndrome.

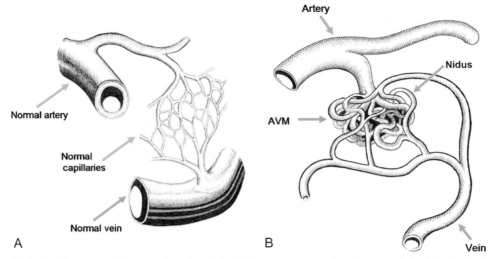

Fig. 13.1 Arteriovenous Malformations (AVMs). (A) Diagram representing the normal physiologic arteri and venous anatomy. (B) An AVM with multiple draining veins. (From McCafferty IJ, Jones RG. Imaging and management of vascular malformations. *Clin Radiol.* 2011;66[12]:1208–1218.)

ANATOMY

Classification of Vascular Anomalies (Fig. 13.1)

- ISSVA developed a classification system based upon that proposed by Mulliken and Glowacki, which utilized endothelial cell characteristics (Box 13.1).
- A complementary system based on flow characteristics was introduced by Jackson et al. and is often used as well in describing vascular malformations.
  - **High flow:** AVMs, AV fistulas
  - **Low flow:** VMs, lymphatic malformations
- Low-flow lesions usually present with swelling and pain due to partial thrombosis.
- Vascular malformations are further classified based on their morphology at angiography or ultrasound, which dictates the specific approach to treatment.
  - AVMs (Fig. 13.2)
    - Type I (arteriovenous): no more than three separate arteries shunt to the initial part of a single venous component
    - Type II (arteriolovenous): multiple arterioles shunt to the initial part of a single venous component
      - Arteriole components demonstrate a plexiform appearance at angiography
    - Type IIIa (arteriolovenous, non-dilated): multiple shunts are present between arterioles and venules
      - Appear as blush or fine striation at angiography
    - Type IIIb (arteriolovenous, dilated): multiple arteriole-venule shunts are present and are dilated
      - Appear as complex vascular network at angiography
  - VMs (Fig. 13.3)
    - Type I: sequestered VM with minimal venous drainage (see Fig. 13.3A)

BOX 13.1 Vascular Anomaly Classification System of International Society for the Study of Vascular Anomalies

Vascular Tumors
- Benign
  - Infantile hemangioma
  - Congenital hemangioma
  - Tufted angioma
- Locally aggressive
  - Kaposiform hemangioendothelioma
  - Retiform hemangioendothelioma
  - Kaposi sarcoma
- Malignant
  - Angiosarcoma
  - Epithelioid hemangioendothelioma

Vascular Malformations
Simple
- Capillary malformations
- Lymphatic malformations
- Venous malformations
- Arteriovenous malformations[a]
- Arteriovenous fistulas[a]

Combined
- Capillary venous malformation, capillary lymphatic malformation
- Lymphatic venous malformation, capillary lymphatic venous malformation
- Capillary arteriovenous malformation[a]
- Capillary lymphatic arteriovenous malformation[a]

[a] High-flow lesion.

From International Society for the Study of Vascular Anomalies: ISSVA classification for vascular anomalies (Approved at the 20th ISSVA Workshop, Melbourne, April 2014). Available at http://www.issva.org/classification. Accessed June 6, 2018.

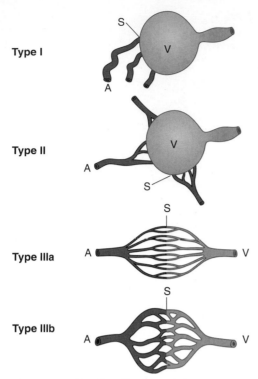

Type I

Type II

Type IIIa

Type IIIb

Fig. 13.2 Arteriographic Classification of Arteriovenous Malformations Used for Preoperative Planning. *A,* Artery; *S,* shunt; *V,* vein. (From Markovic JN, Shortell CE. Multidisciplinary treatment of extremity arteriovenous malformations. *J Vasc Surg Venous Lymphat Disord.* 2015;3[2]:209–218, Fig. 9.)

- Type II: combination of VM with drainage into normal veins and VMs with slow drainage (see Fig. 13.3B)
- Type III: combination of VMs with drainage into dysplastic veins and VMs with rapid venous drainage (see Fig. 13.3C)
- Type IV: VMs composed of dysplastic veins (see Fig. 13.3D)
- Lymphatic malformations are further characterized by ultrasound as either macrocystic (>2 cm) or microcystic (<2 cm).

CLINICAL FEATURES

- While present at birth, vascular malformations can have a variable presentation based on location and rate of growth. Superficial and extremity lesions may be readily evident on physical examination while deep lesions may be clinically silent.
- Tend to grow slowly at a rate proportional to the individual, which further acts to delay detection, particularly if deep in location.
  - Rate of growth may be accelerated during times of hormonal fluctuation (pregnancy, puberty) or following failed attempts at intervention.
- Malformations may be single, multiple, focal, or infiltrate across multiple soft tissue planes.
- VMs
  - 40% located in head and neck, 40% in extremities, and 20% in trunk

- Presents with pain and swelling related to:
  - Mass effect on adjacent structures
  - Hemorrhage
  - Venous engorgement related to activity or stasis
  - Thrombosis
  - Regional muscular dysfunction
- Physical exam findings include:
  - Soft/rubbery, serpiginous, ecchymotic/faintly blue lesions that can engorge with dependent positioning or Valsalva
- Lymphatic malformations
  - Presents in a similar fashion to VMs. May rapidly expand with intralesional hemorrhage or infection.
  - Physical exam findings include changes related to aberrant lymphatic drainage and may include skin texture changes, discoloration, hyperkeratosis, or lymphedema.
- AVMs
  - Primarily occur in the extremities and pelvis.
  - 40% are detectable at birth.
  - Generally present as a pulsatile, non-tender mass. If left untreated, AVMs may follow a progressive clinical course with clinical presentation dependent upon stage:
    - Stage I (quiescence): cutaneous blush, skin warmth
    - Stage II (expansion): darkening blush, pulsation, thrill/bruit
    - Stage III (destruction): steal, pain, dystrophic skin changes, distal ischemia, ulceration, necrosis (Figs. 13.4 and 13.5)
    - Stage IV (decompensation): high-output cardiac failure
  - Conservative treatment is usually all that is needed. AVMs are notoriously difficult to treat, and recurrence/failure of treatment is common.

Imaging Features

- Vascular malformation may be strongly suspected based on physical examination findings, but imaging plays an essential role in the diagnosis, classification, and treatment of these diseases.
- A methodical approach to imaging is required to avoid excessive workup and delays in diagnosis and treatment. Patients will often have already had varying degrees of diagnostic imaging prior to presentation.
- Initial imaging should consist of gray scale and Doppler ultrasound. This will distinguish low- versus high-flow lesions and venous versus lymphatic malformations.
- MRI/MRA is the modality of choice for confirmation, characterization, and further differentiation of vascular malformations. This modality provides detailed information on surrounding structures as well as an objective means of post-therapy follow-up.
- Angiography and phlebography (direct puncture of the nidus) is rarely used for diagnostic purposes alone but is essential for vascular intervention.

Arteriovenous Malformations

- Ultrasound/Doppler
  - Well-defined anechoic structures (Fig. 13.6)

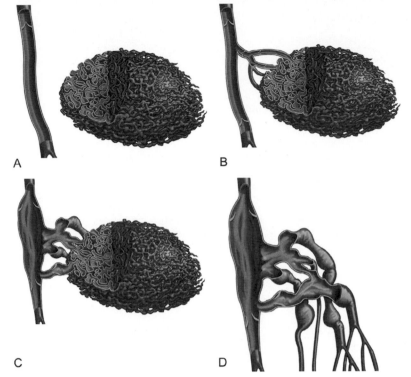

A

B

C

D

Fig. 13.3 Classification of Venous Malformations Based on Venous Drainage Pattern. (A) Type I VM shows negligible venous drainage into normal venous circulation. (B) Type II VM anatomy reveals normal venous outflow into general venous circulation. (C) Type III anatomy demonstrates drainage from the VM by way of abnormally ectatic or dysplastic veins. (D) Type IV lesions are composed entirely of ectatic or dysplastic veins. (From Legiehn GM, Heran MK. Venous malformations: classification, development, diagnosis, and interventional radiologic management. *Radiol Clin North Am.* 2008;46[3]:545–597.)

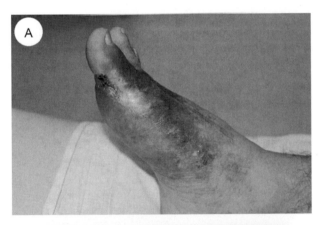

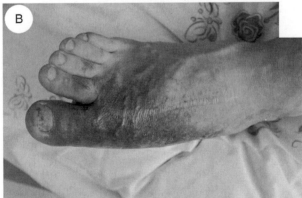

Fig. 13.4 Dystrophic Skin, Ulcerative, and Necrotic Changes Associated with Clinical Stage III Arteriovenous Malformation. (A) Lateral and (B) AP views of the right foot demonstrating dystrophic skin, ulceration, and necrotic changes associated with clinical stage III AVM. (From Rosen RJ, Nassiri N, Drury JE. Interventional management of high-flow vascular malformations. *Tech Vasc Interv Radiol.* 2013;16[1]:22–38.)

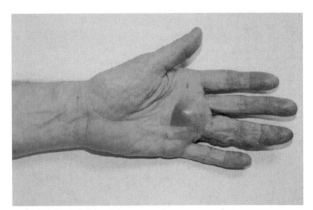

Fig. 13.5 Mass Associated with Arteriovenous Malformation in the Palm. Notice distal skin changes and vascular engorgement in the 4th digit. (From Rosen RJ, Nassiri N, Drury JE. Interventional management of high-flow vascular malformations. *Tech Vasc Interv Radiol.* 2013;16[1]:22–38.)

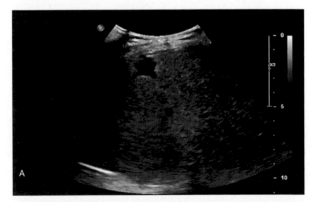

Fig. 13.6 Hepatic AVM (arteriovenous malformation). Grayscale ultrasound of the liver demonstrates a well circumscribed, well-defined anechoic structure. (Courtesy Jeff Brown, Virginia Commonwealth University.)

- Feeding and draining flow patterns on color Doppler imaging. The nidus will demonstrate a mixed appearance on color Doppler.
- Pulsatile flow can be seen in the draining veins, indicating lack of intervening capillary bed.
- **MRI/MRA** (Fig. 13.7)
  - T1- and T2-weighted images demonstrate hypointense flow voids representing hypertrophied arterial feeders and dilated draining veins with linear connections.

- No soft tissue component (MRI is excellent for detecting involvement of adjacent structures or across soft tissue planes).
- Increased signal within the vascular channels on gradient echo sequences and following gadolinium contrast.
- **Angiography** (Figs. 13.8 and 13.9)
  - Multiple enlarged feeding arteries with rapid shunting into dilated draining veins.

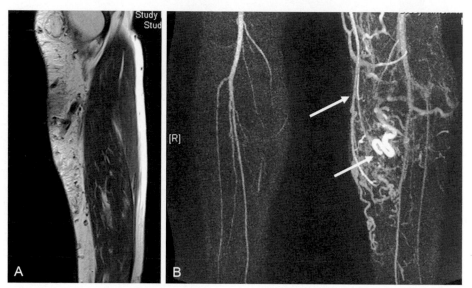

Fig. 13.7 MR Imaging of an Arteriovenous Malformation. (A) T2 sagittal image of patient with subcutaneous high flow AVM with dilated veins seen as multiple flow voids within the subcutaneous fat. (B) Maximum Intensity Projection (MIP) of MR angiography on same patient demonstrating early filling within tortuous dilated venous structures *(arrow)*. (From McCafferty IJ, Jones RG. Imaging and management of vascular malformations. *Clin Radiol.* 2011;66[12]:1208–1218.)

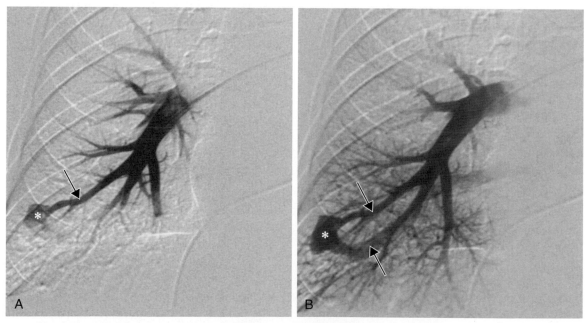

Fig. 13.8 (A) Early-phase angiography shows arterial filling *(arrow)* of a pulmonary arteriovenous malformation nidus *(asterisk)*. (B) Later phase angiography with opacification of the feeding artery *(long arrow)*, nidus *(asterisks)*, and draining vein *(short arrow)*. (From Valji K, ed. Pulmonary and bronchial arteries. In: *The Practice of Interventional Radiology With Online Cases & Videos.* Philadelphia: Elsevier; 2012: 443–475.)

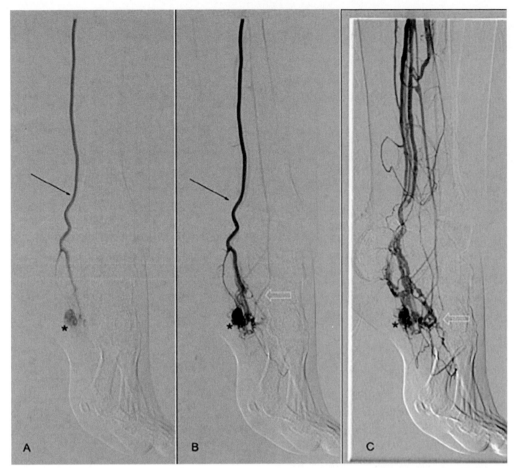

Fig. 13.9 (A) Arterial angiography demonstrates a lower extremity arteriovenous malformation with opacification of the primary feeding artery *(arrow)* and nidus *(asterisk)*. (B) Later phase angiography with arterial feeder *(thin arrow)*, nidus *(asterisk)*, and early venous filling *(open arrow)*. (C) Further delayed imaging demonstrates further venous shunting *(open arrow)* and nidus *(asterisk)*. (Courtesy Jeff Brown, Virginia Commonwealth University.)

- The nidus is the point at which the draining veins are first opacified by the feeding arteries.
- CT/CTA (Figs. 13.10 and 13.11)
  - Enlarged feeding arteries with rapid shunting into draining veins without intervening tissue enhancement.
  - This modality is generally reserved for assessment of bleeding or compression of adjacent structure. May be useful in the setting of an equivocal MRI.
- Radiography
  - Limited role in evaluation of AVMs; may show osseous sequelae such as local destruction, bony overgrowth, or pathologic fracture.

Venous Malformations

- Ultrasound/Doppler
  - Generally hypoechoic (82%) with a heterogeneous echotexture.
  - 84% will show monophasic or biphasic flow, and 16% will show no flow on Doppler imaging.
- MRI/MRA (Figs. 13.12 to 13.14)
  - Can appear as single or multilobulated, cavitary, or serpiginous masses.

- Typically isointense or hypointense on T1-weighted imaging and hyperintense on T2.
- Low signal areas on gradient echo may represent calcification (phlebolith), hemosiderin, or thrombosis.
- Homogeneous or heterogeneous enhancement following contrast.
- Angiography
  - Useful in morphologic characterization and assessing patency of deep venous system prior to treatment.
  - Determining volume of contrast required to fill the malformation is important in deciding volume of sclerosant to use for treatment.
- CT/CTA
  - Hypodense to heterogeneous on non-contrast imaging, depending on degree of fat present. Gradual peripheral enhancement following contrast administration.
  - May see dystrophic calcifications.
  - Good for assessing involvement of adjacent osseous structures.
- Radiography
  - Limited utility; may see phleboliths or adjacent osseous destruction.

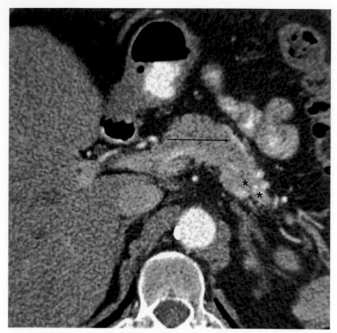

Fig. 13.10 CT angiography of the abdomen demonstrates a linear hyperdensity leading up to multiple hyperdense foci within the pancreas. Initial differential considerations include neuroendocrine tumor and arteriovenous malformation. Subsequent angiography showed a pancreatic arteriovenous malformation. The linear density is a feeding artery *(long arrow)* arising from the celiac axis and extending into the nidus *(asterisk)*. (Courtesy Jeff Brown, Virginia Commonwealth University.)

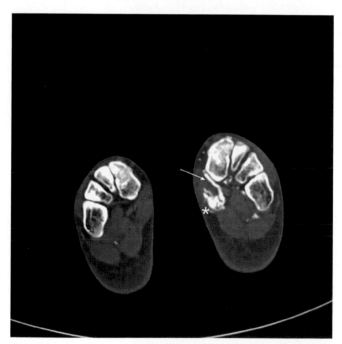

Fig. 13.11 Lower extremity CT angiography demonstrating arteriovenous malformation nidus *(asterisks)* and aberrant feeding artery *(arrow)*. (Courtesy Jeff Brown, Virginia Commonwealth University.)

Lymphatic Malformations

- Ultrasound/Doppler (Fig. 13.15)
  - Macrocystic LMs will have variably sized cystic anechoic spaces with internal septations and debris,

differentiating them from VMs. The spaces will not demonstrate flow on Doppler imaging, but septations may.
  - Microcystic LMs will appear hyperechoic without detectable flow, making them difficult to distinguish from the VMs that appear hyperechoic and without flow.
- **MRI** (Fig. 13.16)
  - Appear as fluid-filled, multiloculated cystic masses. Variable septations and fatty elements.
  - Low signal on T1 and high signal on T2. Postcontrast enhancement most evident in prominent septae.
  - Macrocystic and microcystic components are easily distinguishable.
- **CT**
  - Limited role, usually reserved for evaluation of enlargement or compression of adjacent structures.
  - Low-density, fluid-filled masses. May have fluid-fluid levels if internal hemorrhage has occurred.
  - May see enhancement of the peripheral walls following contrast.

INDICATIONS

Absolute Indications

- Hemorrhage
- Impending high-output congestive heart failure
  - An extremely rare occurrence that is usually associated with high-flow pelvic or renal AVMs
- Lesions located at a life- and/or limb-threatening region (e.g., proximity to airway)
- Lesions threatening vital functions (e.g., seeing, hearing, eating, or breathing)
- In the case of pulmonary AVMs, all lesions with a feeding artery at least 3 mm in diameter, as this appears to be a threshold size for nearly all bland thromboemboli that can result in stroke.

Relative Indications

- The decision to treat a vascular malformation is based on the potential improvement in the patient's quality of life weighed against the complication risk. In most cases, conservative management is recommended; however, the following are some relative indications that may prompt treatment:
  - Recurrent or worsening pain and swelling
  - Ischemic changes (e.g., atrophy or ulceration)
  - Sequelae of venous hypertension (e.g., skin thickening, hyperpigmentation, or ulceration)
  - Deformity (e.g., limb length discrepancy, usually by overgrowth)
  - Thromboembolic complications
  - Causing gait disturbance or interfering with physical activity
  - Lesions located in a region with high complication risk (e.g., hemarthrosis, deep vein thrombosis)
  - Lesions causing recurrent infection or sepsis

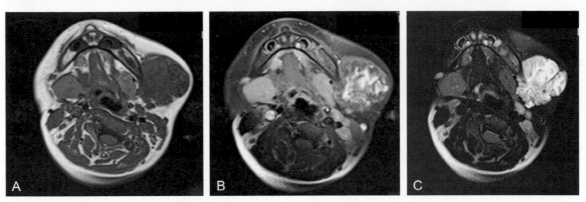

Fig. 13.12 (A) Precontrast T1 axial MRI shows a lobulated mass that is isointense to muscle. (B) Postcontrast axial T1 sequence reveals heterogeneous enhancement. (C) Hyperintense signal is demonstrated on T2 imaging. Findings are compatible with a venous malformation. (From McCafferty IJ, Jones RG. Imaging and management of vascular malformations. *Clin Radiol.* 2011;66[12]:1208–1218.)

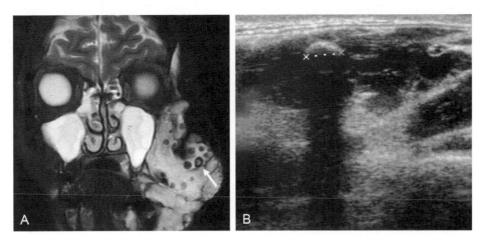

Fig. 13.13 (A) Coronal T2 MRI demonstrates a high-intensity venous malformation in the left face. Multiple low-signal foci internally representative of phleboliths and pathognomonic for venous malformation. (B) Gray scale ultrasound of the venous malformation shows an echogenic focus with posterior acoustic shadowing compatible with phlebolith. (From McCafferty IJ, Jones RG. Imaging and management of vascular malformations. *Clin Radiol.* 2011;66[12]:1208–1218.)

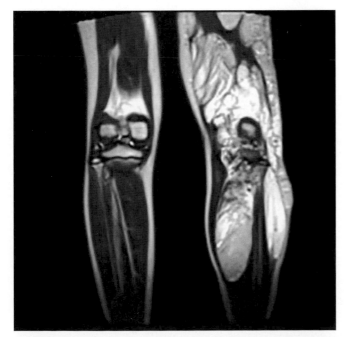

Fig. 13.14 T2 Coronal MRI of the Lower Extremities. Large, polylobulated, hyperintense lesion of the left leg with typical imaging characteristics of a venous malformation. (Courtesy Jeff Brown, Virginia Commonwealth University.)

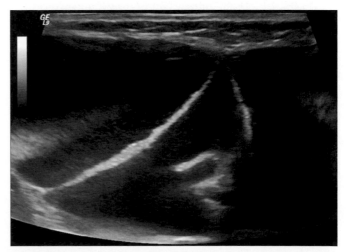

Fig. 13.15 Gray Scale Ultrasound. Macrocystic lymphatic malformation of the neck with large anechoic spaces, thick internal septae, and low-level internal echoes suggestive of debris. (From McCafferty IJ, Jones RG. Imaging and management of vascular malformations. *Clin Radiol.* 2011;66[12]:1208–1218.)

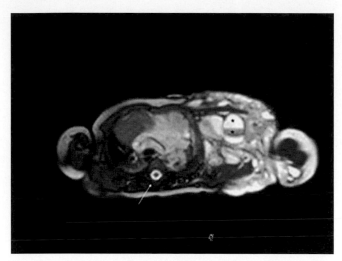

Fig. 13.16 Axial T2 MRI of the Thorax. Pediatric patient with an extensive T2 hyperintense lymphatic malformation involving a large portion of the left thorax and axilla. For reference, the spinal canal is located medially *(white arrow)*. Notice the cystic structure with fluid-fluid level *(asterisks)*, compatible with internal hemorrhage. (Courtesy Jeff Brown, Virginia Commonwealth University.)

- Hormonal changes (growth spurts, puberty, menarche, and pregnancy) can often cause the enlargement of existing channels and the recruitment of new collaterals, and treatment may be warranted at these times or even prior to these events in anticipation of clinical worsening.

CONTRAINDICATIONS

- There are no absolute contraindications to treatment. Treatment is usually indicated when patients become symptomatic. Some relative contraindications include:
  - Coagulopathy, which can usually be addressed by giving FFP, cryoprecipitate, or deficient factors as needed
  - Proximity of the vascular lesion to major nerve trunks, especially in the presence of preexisting neuropathy
  - Lesions involving or near the airway or orbit
  - VMs with extensive cutaneous involvement
  - VMs involving deep veins of the lower extremities
  - Known patent foramen ovale with history of right-to-left shunt
  - Chronic pulmonary embolic disease with decreased reserve
  - Renal impairment
  - Limited access to the lesion due to prior embolotherapy

EQUIPMENT

- Basic micropuncture set, coaxial microcatheter system
- 0.035-inch guidewire (Amplatz, Bentson, or hydrophilic guidewire)
- 5-Fr catheter
- Occlusion device per operator preference. Choices include:
  - Mechanical

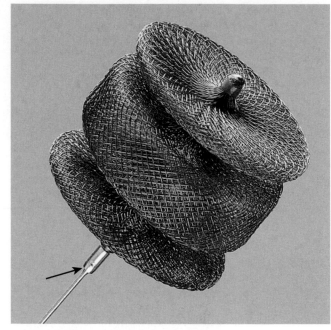

Fig. 13.17 Amplatzer II Vascular Plug With Three Lobes and Delivery Wire *(Arrow)*. (Courtesy AGA Medical, Plymouth, MN.)

  - Embolization coil or occlusive plug (Amplatzer) (Fig. 13.17)
- Chemical (Table 13.1)

PROCEDURE STEPS

Periprocedural Considerations

- Low-molecular-weight heparin is recommended for 2 weeks prior to the procedure for patients with extensive VMs and low fibrinogen. Cryoprecipitate transfusion is given if fibrinogen is still low on the day of the procedure.
- Prophylactic antibiotics can be given preprocedure.
- Intraarterial vasodilators (e.g., nitroglycerin) are administered to reduce the risk of vessel thrombosis and spasm during the procedure.
- Heparinized saline can be infused through a peripheral IV placed in the affected limb during sclerotherapy to reduce risk of secondary thrombosis. Confirmation of deep vein patency can be performed before and after sclerotherapy.
- Systemic anticoagulation is monitored during the procedure with activated clotting time.
- Pre- and post-procedure chest radiographs and lung function tests are recommended if using bleomycin.
- Pulmonary artery and peripheral artery pressure monitoring is recommended if using absolute alcohol.

Arteriovenous (High-Flow) Malformation
Endovascular Access

1. Usually performed under general anesthesia for patient comfort, physiologic monitoring, and respiratory control. Local anesthesia is administered as well.
2. Vascular access is acquired under ultrasound guidance using standard Seldinger technique and utilizing a

TABLE 13.1 Comparison of Different Embolics

Embolic	Mechanism of Action	Advantages	Disadvantages
Absolute alcohol	Causes protein denaturation and dehydration of endothelial cells with instant platelet adhesion and thrombosis. Causes a pronounced inflammatory response.	• Readily available • Inexpensive • Very potent with high efficacy • Can be added to ethiodized oil to improve visualization, increase viscosity, and increase efficacy.	• High local and systemic toxicity and therefore less favorable in the treatment of superficial/mucosal lesions or those in close proximity to major nerves. • May cause hemoglobinuria, oliguria, acute kidney injury, respiratory depression, cardiac arrhythmias, pulmonary artery hypertension, seizures, hyperthermia, and rhabdomyolysis. • Radiolucent
STS	An ionic surfactant that incites endothelial cell inflammation, sludging of erythrocytes, and thrombosis of vessel, which leads to eventual fibrosis and luminal collapse.	• Detergent properties create microbubbles that reduce egress and increase endothelial contact time • Less toxic (than ethanol) • Can form a relatively stable foam that has a more potent sclerosing effect	• Not as permanent as alcohol
Polidocanol	A detergent sclerosant	• Has a local anesthetic effect • Good efficacy • Low local and systemic complication rates	• Exerts a lesser endothelial-cidal effect. • Bradyarrhythmias and reversible cardiac arrest are rare complications
n-BCA	Permanent liquid embolic and tissue adhesive that rapidly polymerizes on contact with blood and forms a cast of the vascular bed.	• No acute or long-term tissue toxicity	• Recanalization of the AVM nidus • Pulmonary embolism • Inadvertent catheter adhesion and formation of subcutaneous or intramuscular glue masses that can subsequently be a source of infection, tissue erosion, or muscular dysfunction.
Onyx	Mixture of EVOH and DMSO that precipitates as the DMSO diffuses into blood and forms a cast of the vascular bed.	• Low viscosity • Decreased risk of catheter adhesion	• Expensive
Bleomycin	Cytotoxic anti-neoplastic antibiotic that induces single- and double-stranded DNA breaks and is an endothelial sclerosant.	• Low inflammatory response makes it useful for treating intramuscular, orbital, or airway lesions where edema may normally impair function	• Pulmonary fibrosis is a feared, though rare, complication, • Cutaneous pigmentation
Doxycycline	Induces an inflammatory reaction resulting in fibrin and collagen deposition. Inhibits matrix metalloproteinase and suppresses VEGF, which promotes angiogenesis	• Fewer neurotoxic effects • Less local skin reaction • Effective at treating microcystic LMs	• Hemolytic anemia • Hypoglycemia with metabolic acidosis
OK-432 (Picibanil)	A lyophilized powder that induces apoptosis of lymphatic endothelium and causes a local cellular inflammatory reaction	• Good response rates with macrocystic LMs	• Severe delayed swelling can occur leading to airway obstruction • Use is contraindicated in patients with penicillin allergy

AVM, Arteriovenous malformation; *LM*, lymphatic malformation.

microaccess system: a 21-gauge needle is used to introduce a 0.018-inch microwire, a 5-Fr coaxial micropuncture catheter is placed over the microwire, the inner dilator and microwire are removed, and a standard 0.035-inch guidewire is introduced through the outer catheter. The access site is dependent upon location of the AVM.

3. A catheter is advanced over the guidewire to a position proximal to the AVM. Choice of catheter is dependent upon location of the AVM, and exchange of multiple catheters may be necessary in navigating to the desired location.

4. Selective angiography is performed to delineate anatomy of the feeding arteries, draining veins, local collateral vessels, and normal regional vasculature.

5. The 0.035-inch guidewire is removed and a 2- to 3-Fr microcatheter with compatible 0.010- to 0.018-inch guidewire is advanced through the standard catheter to a position as close to the nidus of the AVM as possible.

6. Superselective angiography is performed to help determine the appropriate volume of sclerosant.

7. Embolic material is then deployed via the microcatheter. The selection of embolic agent is multifactorial, and no single agent is considered ideal. Often, multiple embolic agents are required to achieve the desired therapeutic effect.

8. Repeat angiography is performed with additional embolization as necessary.

9. The patient is monitored over several hours with frequent skin and neurovascular checks.

10. Patient may be discharged the same day, barring complications.

Percutaneous Access

1. If endovascular access of the nidus is not reasonably achievable, then direct puncture may be an effective alternative.

2. Using ultrasonographic guidance, a 21-gauge needle is placed into the nidus. Needle is exchanged for an appropriate sheath set over a microwire.

3. Angiography is performed to determine the appropriate volume of sclerosant.

4. An embolic agent is then inserted into the nidus followed by repeat angiography.

5. Embolization and angiography are repeated until the desired effect is achieved.

6. Equipment is removed with application of pressure at the site of arterial access. Use of a closure device may be beneficial.

ALTERNATIVE TREATMENTS

- Surgical resection
- Thermal ablation
- Depending on the severity of symptoms and expendability of the tissue, the involved organ may be resected (e.g., renal AVM).

COMPLICATIONS

- Infection
- Bleeding
- Tissue necrosis
- Nerve injury
- Deep vein thrombosis
- Acute renal failure
  - Sclerosants cause hemolysis, so hemoglobinuria, along with the intravenous contrast that is used, may lead to ARF.
- Distal/paradoxical emboli
- Persistence, reperfusion, or recanalization of the malformation
  - Especially worrisome for high-flow lesions
  - Future treatments are made more difficult if the access point has been occluded by a prior treatment.
- Postembolization syndrome: nausea, pain, fever, and leukocytosis
- Pleurisy (after treatment of pulmonary AVMs)

🏠 TAKE-HOME POINTS

- AVMs consist of dysplastic arteries that shunt into arterialized veins, creating a vascular nidus without a normal intervening capillary network. Destruction of the nidus is critical for effective treatment.
- High-flow AVMs usually present in childhood. Rapid growth is usually seen during growth spurts, pregnancy, and puberty.
- Notable syndromes associated with AVMs include hemorrhagic hereditary telangiectasia and Parkes-Weber syndrome.
- Pulmonary AVMs with feeding arteries greater than 3 mm in adults should be treated.

REVIEW QUESTIONS

1. Which of the following is NOT a benign vascular lesion?
   a. Infantile hemangioma
   b. Angiosarcoma
   c. Tufted angioma
   d. Congenital hemangioma

2. Postoperative complications of sclerotherapy include which of the following?
   a. Infection
   b. Tissue necrosis
   c. Bleeding
   d. Deep venous thrombosis
   e. All of the above

3. Regarding AVMs, pulsatile flow can be seen in draining veins on ultrasound, which indicates lack of an intervening capillary bed.
   a. True
   b. False

SUGGESTED READINGS

Burrows PE. Endovascular treatment of slow-flow vascular malformations. *Tech Vasc Interv Radiol.* 2013;16(1):12–21.

Cahill AM, Nijs EL. Pediatric vascular malformations: pathophysiology, diagnosis, and the role of interventional radiology. *Cardiovasc Intervent Radiol.* 2011;34(4): 691–704.

Greben CR, Setton A, Putterman D, et al. Pulmonary arteriovenous malformation embolization: how we do it. *Tech Vasc Interv Radiol.* 2013;16(1):39–44.

Legiehn GM, Heran MK. A step-by-step practical approach to imaging diagnosis and interventional radiologic therapy in vascular malformations. *Semin Intervent Radiol.* 2010;27(2): 209–231.

Madani H, Farrant J, Chhaya N, et al. Peripheral limb vascular malformations: an update of appropriate imaging and treatment options of a challenging condition. *Br J Radiol.* 2015;88(1047). 20140406.

Pimpalwar S. Vascular malformations: approach by an interventional radiologist. *Semin Plast Surg.* 2014;28(2):91–103.

Pollak JS, White Jr. RI. Pulmonary arteriovenous malformations. In: Baum S, Pentecost MJ, eds. *Abrams' Angiography: Interventional Radiology.* 2nd ed. Philadelphia: Lippincott Williams & Wilkins; 2006.

Rosen RJ, Nassiri N, Drury JE. Interventional management of high-flow vascular malformations. *Tech Vasc Interv Radiol.* 2013;16(1):22–38.

Balloon-Assisted Retrograde Transvenous Obliteration

Alicia L. Eubanks, Edward W. Lee

CASE PRESENTATION

A 53-year-old male with a history of alcoholic cirrhosis with prior episodes of esophageal variceal bleeding presents to the hepatology clinic with ascites and stage II hepatic encephalopathy. His esophageal varices have been successfully managed with banding and treatment with propranolol, but previous esophagogastroduodenoscopy also revealed large fundal varices. The patient has presented to the emergency room several times within the past 2 years with episodes of abdominal pain, hepatic hydrothorax, and hepatic encephalopathy, but he has not been considered a good candidate for transjugular intrahepatic portosystemic shunt (TIPS) placement. Contrast-enhanced abdominal CT demonstrates cirrhosis, minimal ascites, and extensive gastric varices with a spontaneous gastrorenal shunt and a widely patent splenic vein. The patient is referred to interventional radiology for possible treatment of his gastric varices with balloon-assisted retrograde transvenous obliteration (BRTO).

◎ LITERATURE REVIEW

Park et al. (2014) reviewed 24 studies on BRTO totaling 1016 patients and concluded that BRTO is a safe and efficacious therapy for patients with gastric varices. Overall technical success rate was 96.4%, and clinical success rate—defined as no recurrence or re-bleeding of gastric varices or complete obliteration of varices on follow-up imaging—was 97.3%.

INDICATIONS

- Primary indications (good evidence of technical and clinical success) include:
  - Gastric varices that have previously bled
  - Actively bleeding gastric varices
  - Prophylactic treatment of gastric varices that are likely to bleed
  - Gastric varices in a patient with hepatic encephalopathy refractory to medical management
- Secondary indications (less supportive evidence and subject to ongoing research) include:
  - Esophageal varices
  - Hepatic encephalopathy in the presence of a gastrorenal shunt

CONTRAINDICATIONS

- Contraindications to BRTO are relatively few, as the primary indication, active gastric variceal bleeding, is associated with a high rate of mortality.
- Contraindications that have been suggested include:
  - Hepatocellular carcinoma >5 cm in diameter
  - Large-volume intractable ascites
  - **Portal vein thrombosis**
    - In the presence of chronic portal vein thrombosis, the gastrorenal shunt may be the only venous outflow tract, and thus BRTO may pose a serious risk.
  - Splenic vein thrombosis
  - Presence of high-risk esophageal varices
- Relative contraindications of severe coagulopathy and iodinated contrast allergy should be managed accordingly.

- **Balloon-assisted retrograde transvenous obliteration (BRTO)** is a minimally invasive therapy for both emergent and prophylactic treatment of gastric variceal bleeding. The procedure involves the insertion of an occlusion balloon into the outflow vein of a spontaneous portosystemic shunt (most commonly, a **gastrorenal shunt**) to completely occlude blood flow followed by catheter-directed injection of a sclerosing agent into the varix.
- BRTO is a relatively new procedure that first gained popularity in Asia as an effective alternative to endoscopic management of gastric varices.
- Along with its established safety and efficacy, BRTO avoids some of the complications (hepatic encephalopathy, fulminant liver failure) associated with TIPS in the management of variceal bleeding secondary to portal hypertension.
- The clinical aim of BRTO is to completely obliterate gastric varices, to stop any ongoing gastric bleeding, and to prevent re-bleeding.
- Preprocedural contrast-enhanced MRI or CT is important for planning the procedural approach (Fig. 14.1).

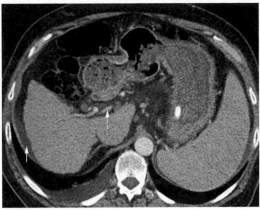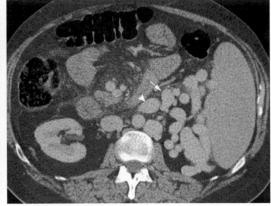

Fig. 14.1 Pre-procedural CT. (A) Axial contrast-enhanced CT demonstrates diminutive portal vein *(dotted arrow)* and minimal perihepatic ascites *(white arrow)*. (B) Axial CT demonstrates enlarged spleen with multiple perisplenic collateral vessels. A large splenorenal shunt *(arrowhead)* is seen arising from a dilated left renal vein *(white arrowhead)*. (From Park JK, Cho SK, Kee S, et al. Vascular plug-assisted retrograde transvenous obliteration of portosystemic shunts for refractory hepatic encephalopathy: a case report. *Case Rep Radiol.* 2014;2014:391–420.)

EQUIPMENT

- Sonography and fluoroscopy equipment
- Micropuncture set
- 0.035-inch guidewires (Bentson or SuperStiff Amplatzer; Glidewire; Rosen wire)
- 8- or 14-Fr reinforced vascular sheath
- 4- or 5-Fr selection catheter such as a Glide catheter or C2 catheter
- Occlusion balloon, sized appropriately for the patient's anatomy
- Sclerosant (ethanolamine oleate, sodium tetradecyl sulfate foam, polidocanol foam, or Gelfoam)

ANATOMY (Fig. 14.2)

- It is important to understand the normal portosystemic anatomy and to compare this to the individual patient's portosystemic collaterals as seen in preprocedural imaging.
  - Patients undergoing this procedure will have a great deal of variation in their venous anatomy.
- Shunts that can be occluded with BRTO include:
  - Gastrorenal (most common)
  - Splenorenal
  - Gastrosplenorenal
  - Gastrocaval
  - Gastrophrenic
  - Gastropericardial
  - Plexus-like systems

> ### ⏩ CLINICAL POINT
>
> BRTO is less commonly used for gastric varices without a gastrorenal shunt, except in the hands of experienced operators. In these cases, it may be prudent to consider alternative treatment options.

- There are a number of classification systems that can be used to describe the anatomy and hemodynamics of these portosystemic shunts, including:
  - The **Kiyosue system** classifies variant anatomy with reference to the afferent portal veins and the resultant hemodynamics that may impact the procedure. By using this system to plan the procedural approach, the interventional radiologist considers how to attain a pressure equilibrium within the particular portal venous feeders and gastric veins so that stasis occurs and there is no spillover of sclerosant.
  - The **Saad modification** of the Kiyosue classification system classifies variant anatomy with reference to the efferent, systemic draining veins. This is a strictly anatomic classification and may also be used to predict potential sites of sclerosant spillage.

PROCEDURAL STEPS

Preoperative Preparation

- Review the patient's chart, laboratory tests, and imaging studies. CBC, platelet count, and coagulation profile are vital in the management of an acutely bleeding patient.
- Coordinate with all teams involved in the patient's care. If the patient is hemodynamically unstable, the anesthesia team should be present to manage the patient throughout the procedure.

Procedural Steps

1. Upon review of the preprocedural imaging, select an access site (transjugular or transfemoral) that will allow the operator to approach the portosystemic shunt from the systemic side. Most commonly, the shunt is entered through the **left renal vein**.
2. The vein is accessed via the Seldinger technique with the standard micropuncture set.

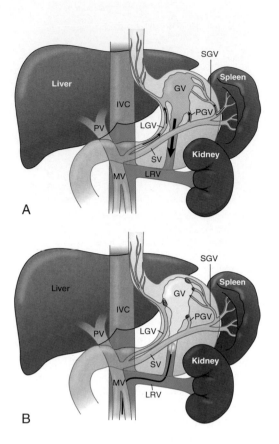

Fig. 14.2 (A) Basic portosystemic venous anatomy of gastric vein *(GV)* with the classic gastrorenal or splenorenal shunts. (B) Conventional BRTO procedure through transfemoral approach with balloon in the gastrorenal shunt. *IVC,* Inferior vena cava; *LGV,* left gastric vein; *LRV,* left renal vein; *MV,* mesenteric vein; *PGV,* posterior gastric vein(s); *PV,* main portal vein; *SGV,* short gastric vein(s); *SV,* splenic vein. Afferent vein *(thin arrows).* Drainage vein *(thick arrow).* (From Garcia-Pagán JC, Barrufet M, Cardenas A, et al. Management of gastric varices. *Clin Gastroenterol Hepatol.* 2014;12[6]:919–928.e1.)

3. While maintaining wire access, replace the access needle with an 8- or 14-Fr reinforced vascular sheath that is advanced over the guidewire into the inferior vena cava.
4. Replace the guidewire with a 0.035-inch Glidewire.
5. Thread a 4- or 5-Fr Glide catheter or C2 catheter over the Glidewire, and use the catheter to select the left renal vein/left gonadal vein/duplicated IVC, depending on the anatomic target.
6. Select the shunt, and advance the selection catheter into the efferent shunt.
7. Once the desired position has been attained with the 5-Fr selection catheter, exchange the catheter for an occlusion balloon over an anchoring wire.
8. Once the balloon delivery catheter is in place, inflate the balloon to completely occlude the shunt.
9. Remove the guidewire, and perform a venography though the balloon catheter at this point to evaluate for potential sources of sclerosant escape (Fig. 14.3).

10. If there is contrast runoff, either reposition the balloon by advancing it closer to the gastric varices or deal with the sources of escape in one of the following ways:
    a. Inject small volumes of sclerosant to selectively fill the non-target veins.
    b. Coil embolize or balloon-occlude the runoff veins.
11. Once assured that the sclerosant will be trapped in the shunt, inject sclerosant (± liquid embolic agent) through the balloon catheter until stasis is achieved and the entire varix is treated (see Fig. 14.3).
12. Leave the balloon inflated for 4 to 48 hours (generally 6–12 hours) to allow the indwelling sclerosant to work in place. Maintain the patient on bed rest during this time.
13. Upon returning to the IR suite, deflate the occlusive balloon under fluoroscopy, and check for obliteration of the varix by performing venography by observing for complete stasis of flow and no sclerosant migration (see Fig. 14.3).
14. Remove the balloon/sheath system while applying pressure to the access site to achieve hemostasis. Once hemostasis is achieved, clean the area and dress the access site.

> ### ➢➢ CLINICAL POINT
>
> Why is sclerosant injected distal to the occlusive balloon?
>   The pressure of antegrade flow through the varix will prevent migration of the sclerosant material, causing it to abut the occlusive balloon and become static.

Postprocedural Care

- Patients should be admitted for overnight observation following the conclusion of the procedure, being carefully watched for signs of hemodynamic instability and bleeding with vital sign checks and periodic CBC draws.
- Monitor liver function tests and ammonia level for postprocedural elevation. If elevation does occur, this is usually transient.
- Schedule a triple-phase contrast-enhanced abdominal CT within 2 to 3 days post procedure to assess whether the varices were completely obliterated and to identify any immediate complications or potential sources of future bleeding.
- Upon discharge, follow up routinely at 1, 3, and 6 months with triple-phase CTs and/or upper GI endoscopy (Fig. 14.4).

ALTERNATE TREATMENTS

- Endoscopic banding and ligation
  - Efficacious and well established in the management of esophageal varices but relatively less effective in the management of gastric varices
- TIPS
  - Procedure performed by interventional radiologists, discussed further in its dedicated chapter.
  - Can relieve the source of portal hypertension causing variceal bleeding but is contraindicated in patients with poor hepatic function and/or hepatic encephalopathy.

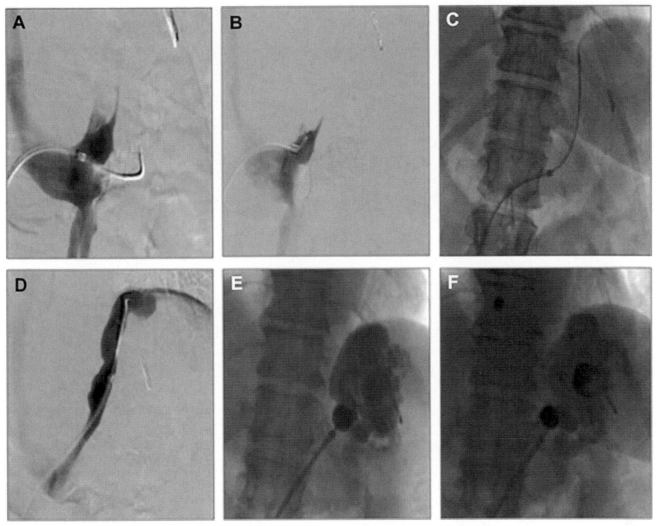

Fig. 14.3 Balloon-Assisted Retrograde Transvenous Obliteration Procedural Steps. (A) Left renal venogram via sheath with catheter tip at the renal hilum. Gonadal veins are incidentally filling inferiorly. (B) Inferior phrenic and/or adrenal vein confluence is catheterized. (C) A catheter is carefully advanced into the gastrorenal shunt for support. (D) Variceal outflow is delineated with digital subtraction contrast injection. (E) With occlusion balloon catheter inflated, the entirety of the gastrorenal shunt and gastric vein (GV) are delineated back to the splenic vein origin. (F) Mixed density from the sclerosant foam injection throughout the shunt and/or variceal complex. (Reused with permission from Basseri S, Lightfoot CB. Balloon-occluded retrograde transvenous obliteration for treatment of bleeding gastric varices: case report and review of literature. *Radiol Case Rep.* 2016;11[4]:365–369.)

⟩⟩ CLINICAL POINT: TECHNICAL VARIANTS

Coil-Assisted Retrograde Transvenous Obliteration
- Uses vascular coils and Gelfoam rather than an indwelling balloon and sclerosant to embolize gastric varices.
- This eliminates the need for an indwelling balloon and avoids complications related to the use of sclerosant.
- After the balloon-occluded venogram step of BRTO, a double microcatheter system is used. A Renegade Hi-flow catheter is advanced distally, and a Renegade STC catheter is placed proximally. Detachable coils are deployed through the proximal catheter, and Gelfoam is pushed through the distal catheter (Fig. 14.5).

Vascular Plug-Assisted Retrograde Transvenous Obliteration
- Similar to Coil-Assisted Retrograde Transvenous Obliteration (CARTO) except a vascular plug is deployed proximally rather than coils.
- Use of a vascular plug eliminates the complications associated with sclerosant but is best suited for smaller gastrorenal shunts, as the vascular plug is only available in sizes up to 22 mm (blocks shunts up to 18 mm) (Fig. 14.6). Coils can block shunts larger in size.

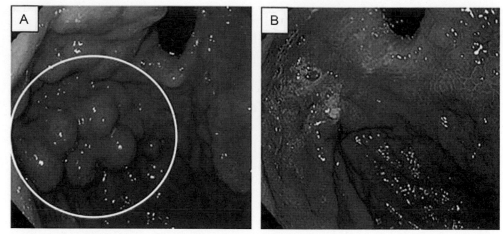

Fig. 14.4 Endoscopy Before and After CARTO. (A) Preprocedure image demonstrating massive gastric varices *(circle)* and (B) 6-month post-procedure upper GI demonstrating complete resolution of previously seen gastric varices (GVs). (From Lee EW, Saab S, Gomes AS, et al. Coil-assisted retrograde transvenous obliteration (CARTO) for the treatment of portal hypertensive variceal bleeding: preliminary results. *Clin Transl Gastroenterol.* 2014;5:e61, Fig. 4.)

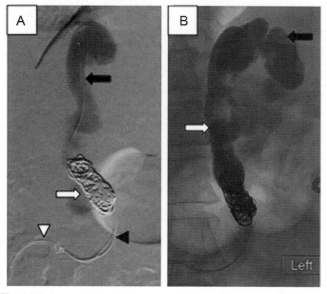

Fig. 14.5 Fluoroscopic Images of Coil-Assisted Retrograde Transvenous Obliteration (CARTO). (A) A double microcatheter system with the proximal microcatheter *(black arrowhead)* used for coil deployment, and the distal microcatheter *(black arrow)* used for Gelfoam injection. Multiple detachable coils *(white arrow)* are in position (B) Technically successful CARTO demonstrating complete stasis and opacification of gastrorenal shunt *(white arrow)* and gastric varices *(black arrow)*. (From Lee EW, Saab S, Gomes AS, et al. Coil-assisted retrograde transvenous obliteration (CARTO) for the treatment of portal hypertensive variceal bleeding: preliminary results. *Clin Transl Gastroenterol.* 2014;5:e61.)

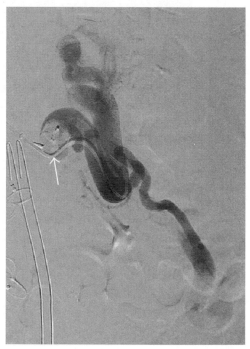

Fig. 14.6 Venogram After Deployment of Amplatzer Vascular Plug *(Arrow)* Within Splenorenal Shunt. (From Park JK, Cho SK, Kee S, et al. Vascular plug-assisted retrograde transvenous obliteration of portosystemic shunts for refractory hepatic encephalopathy: a case report. *Case Rep Radiol.* 2014;2014:391–420.)

COMPLICATIONS

Immediate

- Hematuria
  - Ethanolamine oleate, a commonly used sclerosant, has hemolytic properties. This side effect may be minimized by using an alternate sclerosant.

- Pulmonary embolism
- Cardiac arrhythmia
- Anaphylaxis
- Fever
- Premature balloon rupture
  - May result in the potentially dangerous migration of sclerosant or embolic material

Long Term

- Encephalopathy
- Portal hypertensive gastropathy
- Post-BRTO gastropathy

- Worsening esophageal or duodenal varices
- Ascites
- Infection

🏠 TAKE-HOME POINTS

- Consider BRTO as a potential first-line therapy in patients with actively bleeding gastric varices, particularly when TIPS is contraindicated due to poor hepatic function or the presence of hepatic encephalopathy.
- Carefully plan approach using preprocedural imaging.

- Ensure that the shunt is completely occluded and that sclerosant cannot escape by alternate pathways.
- Postprocedure monitoring with vital sign checks, trending of CBC, and a repeat contrast-enhanced abdominal CT is warranted.

REVIEW QUESTIONS

1. A 58-year-old male presents to the emergency room with a 2-week history of hematemesis and melena. His wife explains that although he recently has decreased his drinking, he had a 20-year history of heavy alcohol use and was diagnosed with alcoholic cirrhosis decompensated by hepatic encephalopathy 1 year ago. At the time of his diagnosis, the man underwent esophagogastroduodenoscopy, which demonstrated stable, isolated large fundic varices without esophageal involvement. At the time, endoscopic treatment was deferred and the patient was asked to return for routine follow-ups, but he reports that he has been too busy with work to return to the doctor. The patient is admitted and sent for an abdominal CT scan, which demonstrates extensive gastric varices with active bleeding. At this time, which treatments would be appropriate to consider?
   a. Endoscopic ligation and banding only
   b. TIPS and BRTO
   c. Endoscopic therapy or BRTO
   d. TIPS only

2. A 63-year-old female underwent a BRTO at your institution approximately 3 hours ago, with an uneventful procedural course. The final postprocedure venography showed good occlusion of the selected varix with no collateral escape of sclerosant. The patient's nurse calls you with concern that the patient has become hypotensive and tachycardic and that her hemoglobin and hematocrit have dropped precipitously within the past hour. Which of the following complications is a likely cause of the change in the patient's condition?
   a. Anaphylactic reaction to the iodinated contrast used during the procedure
   b. Rupture of the occlusive balloon
   c. Bleeding of esophageal varices
   d. Hemolysis due to the use of ethanolamine oleate as a sclerosant

---

SUGGESTED READINGS

Chang MY, Kim MD, Kim T, et al. Plug-assisted retrograde transvenous obliteration for the treatment of gastric variceal hemorrhage. *Korean J Radiol*. 2016;17(2):230–238.

Lee EW, Saab S, Gomes AS, et al. Coil-assisted retrograde transvenous obliteration (CARTO) for the treatment of portal hypertensive variceal bleeding: preliminary results. *Clin Transl Gastroenterol*. 2014;5:e61.

McCarty TR, Bakhit M, Rustagi T. Isolated gastric varices and use of balloon-occlusive retrograde transvenous obliteration: a case report and literature review. *J Gastrointestin Liver Dis*. 2016; 25(1):115–117.

Park JK, Cho SK, Kee S, et al. Vascular plug-assisted retrograde transvenous obliteration of portosystemic shunts for refractory hepatic encephalopathy: a case report. *Case Rep Radiol*. 2014;2014:391–420.

Park JK, Saab S, Kee ST, et al. Balloon-occluded retrograde transvenous obliteration (BRTO) for treatment of gastric varices: review and meta-analysis. *Dig Dis Sci*. 2015;60(6):1543–1553.

15

Bronchial Artery Embolization

Clayton W. Commander, Charles T. Burke

CASE PRESENTATION

A 21-year-old male with cystic fibrosis (CF) hospitalized for an exacerbation develops sudden-onset hemoptysis and hypoxemia. Over the next 8 hours, he vomits 500 mL of bright red blood and is transferred to the intensive care unit (ICU). A chest x-ray reveals a new opacity in the right mid-lung. Bronchoscopy confirms active hemorrhage into the airway. A thoracic surgery consult is placed; however, given the patient's underlying lung disease and poor pulmonary reserves, he is deemed a poor surgical candidate. An interventional radiology consult for bronchial artery embolization is then recommended.

OVERVIEW

- **Bronchial artery embolization** (BAE) for controlling massive hemoptysis was first introduced in 1973 by Remy et al.
  - BAE offered a minimally invasive, targeted treatment for achieving rapid control of hemorrhage from a bronchial artery source.
  - Placing the patient under general anesthesia was not a requirement, though it was an option particularly if there was concern that the patient's airway could become compromised from the active extravasation.
- Prior to this innovation, surgery, which was associated with substantial morbidity and mortality, was the only definitive treatment for hemoptysis.
- BAE is now considered a **first-line therapy** for patients with massive hemoptysis.
- Generally, patients with diseases resulting in chronic pulmonary inflammation are at the greatest risk of having hemoptysis requiring BAE. The suggested pathophysiologic pathway is:
  - Chronic inflammation results in local tissue hypoxia and decreased pulmonary arterial blood flow.
  - To compensate for this, multiple angiogenic proteins are released, causing recruitment of systemic vessels and hypertrophy of the bronchial arteries.
  - This results in a relative increase in blood pressure in these neovessels, making them prone to pseudoaneurysm formation and rupture. These collateral vessels tend to have thinner walls than native vessels, making them more prone to rupture.

- In the setting of malignancy, angiogenesis and recruitment of neighboring vessels is commonplace, which can lead to pulmonary hemorrhage and hemoptysis.
- A common indication for BAE is hemorrhage in the setting of **cystic fibrosis**.
  - Cystic fibrosis, the most common fatal autosomal recessive disease occurring in 1 out of 3000 Caucasian births, is caused by mutations in the CFTR gene. CFTR is a chloride ion transport protein that, when defective, results in thickened pulmonary secretions and impaired mucociliary clearance. This creates a cycle of thickened secretions that results in pulmonary inflammation and infection, leading to worsening lung function.
  - Approximately 1% of all patients with cystic fibrosis will have at least one episode of major hemoptysis per year.

> ## CLINICAL POINT
>
> Think global, act local: while cystic fibrosis is the most common indication for BAE in developed countries, the most common cause of hemoptysis worldwide remains **tuberculosis**.

- Other conditions that result in impaired mucociliary clearance that can lead to hemoptysis requiring interventional radiology (IR) intervention include:
  - Primary ciliary dyskinesia
  - Bronchiectasis
  - Chronic obstructive pulmonary disease (COPD)
  - Sarcoidosis
  - Chronic granulomatous disease
  - Mycobacterial disease
  - Fungal infections
  - Bronchial artery aneurysms
  - Pulmonary arteriovenous malformations (such as in the setting of hereditary hemorrhagic telangiectasia)

> ## CLINICAL POINT
>
> What is the most common cause of death in a patient with massive hemoptysis?
> Asphyxiation (not exsanguination)! Blood fills the airways, *drowning* the patient.

INDICATIONS

- Massive hemoptysis, defined as 200 to 300 mL of expectorated blood within a 24-hour period
- Moderate hemoptysis, defined as at least 100 mL of expectorated blood per day occurring at least 3 times within 1 week
- Mild hemoptysis, defined as chronic, small-volume (<100 mL) expectorated blood
- Palliation of recurrent or debilitating hemoptysis
- Embolization of a bronchial artery aneurysm

CONTRAINDICATIONS

- Nonbronchial artery sources of hemorrhage including upper GI bleeds, upper airway bleeds, systemic collateral artery bleeds, and pulmonary artery hemorrhage.
- Concern that potential nontarget embolization could affect the nearby spinal artery, causing spinal cord ischemia.

EQUIPMENT

- Micropuncture kit
- Catheters:
  - 5- or 6-Fr pigtail catheter (for the aortogram)
  - Reverse-curved catheter—Michaelson, Shepherd's Crook, or Simmons I
  - Forward-looking catheter—Cobra, H1H, or RC
- Guidewires
- Microcatheters (help to prevent nontarget embolization)
- Embolic agents:
  - **Particles** (preferred)—polyvinyl alcohol (PVA) with particle size 300 and 500 µm
  - Coils (for emergent embolization)
    - Coils are not favored in BAE, as they prevent future access to the embolized artery in the event of recurrent hemoptysis, which commonly occurs. Therefore, if coils are used, it will not be possible to get a catheter distal to that site to repeat embolization.
  - Gelfoam (for temporary embolization; delivered as a slurry)

ANATOMY

- The bronchial arteries usually arise from the aorta at the T5/6 level (Fig. 15.1A). The left mainstem bronchus serves as a useful fluoroscopic landmark.
- Up to 20% of patients have an anomalous origin of the bronchial arteries. Takeoff sites include, but are not limited to, the subclavian artery (see Fig. 15.1B), intercostal arteries, and the inferior phrenic artery.
- The most common variant is having one left and two right bronchial arteries, where the left arises from the aorta and the rights arise from the common intercostobronchial trunk.
- The arterial supply to the spinal cord must be evaluated prior to or during the procedure.

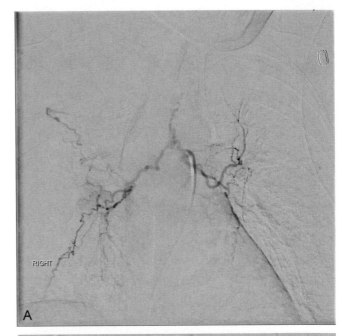

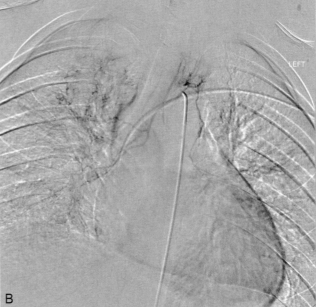

Fig. 15.1 Bronchial Artery Angiography. (A) Selective angiography with both bronchial arteries arising from a common trunk off the aorta. (B) Anomalous origin off the left subclavian artery.

- The **anterior spinal artery**, which is fed by multiple medullary arteries, is the dominant artery supplying the cord. In most cases, the medullary artery supplying the anterior spinal artery arises from an intercostal artery in the low to mid-thoracic spine.
- However, in some cases, the dominant medullary artery arises from the intercostobronchial trunk. Nontarget embolization of this branch has been associated with transverse myelitis, or inflammation of the spinal cord.

⏩ CLINICAL POINT

Which is the name of the dominant branch of the anterior spinal artery supplying the lower two-thirds of the spinal cord?
Artery of Ademkiewicz.

PROCEDURAL STEPS

Pre-op

- Perform a targeted neurologic examination to establish the patient's baseline.
- Review chest x-ray or chest CT to rule out a foreign body and possibly localize the site of bleeding.

Procedural Steps

1. Access the common femoral artery via the Seldinger technique.
2. A thoracic aortogram (Fig. 15.2) is performed for planning purposes.

3. Engage the suspected bronchial artery with a 5- or 6-Fr catheter (Fig. 15.3A).
4. Introduce a microcatheter into the selected artery, and perform bronchial arteriography (see Fig. 15.3B).
5. Carefully scrutinize the selective angiography for:
   a. Verification that it is a bronchial artery, which courses along the mainstem bronchus while the intercostals run between ribs.
   b. Contributions from the anterior spinal artery.
   c. Evidence of bleeding—extravasation, hypertrophy, tortuosity, bronchial-to-pulmonary shunt (Fig. 15.4).
6. Perform embolization. Following injection, stasis of flow should be documented (see Fig. 15.3C).

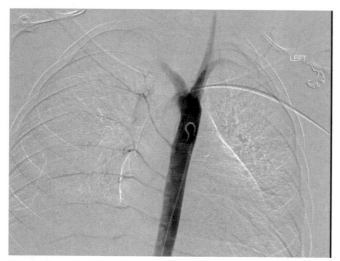

Fig. 15.2 Thoracic aortogram reveals the great vessels and several intercostal arteries. Note the left upper extremity peripherally inserted central catheter (PICC).

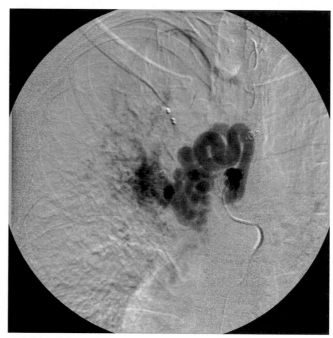

Fig. 15.4 Markedly Dilated and Tortuous Right Bronchial Artery With Active Extravasation.

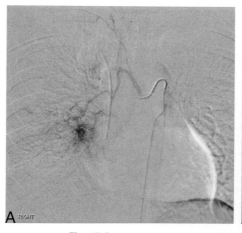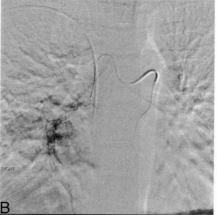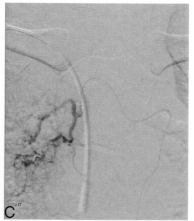

Fig. 15.3 (A) Selective arteriography of the right bronchial artery with extravasation. (B) Superselection of the bleeding branch with a microcatheter. (C) Postembolization arteriogram with no residual hemorrhage.

CLINICAL POINT

What structure serves as a fluoroscopic landmark for the general location of the bronchial arteries? The left mainstem bronchus.

ALTERNATIVE TREATMENTS

- Surgery
  - The only definitive treatment for patients with hemoptysis from a bronchial arterial source.
  - Underlying comorbidities and the emergent nature make surgery a dangerous option. Mortality rates range from 18% to 40% in patients with massive hemoptysis.
  - Compared with **lobectomy**, BAE has the advantage of preserving lung function. What is not known is the degree to which BAE negatively impacts lung function, particularly in CF patients. This is an active area of research.
- **Bronchoscopy**
  - Can be both diagnostic and therapeutic. However, it fails to localize the site of bleeding in up to 50% of cases.
  - Has been shown that bronchoscopy adds no additional benefit in the treatment of hemoptysis for patients who are candidates for BAE.
- Medical management
  - The "wait and watch" approach has reported mortality rates of at least 50%.

COMPLICATIONS

- **Spinal cord ischemia and transverse myelitis**
  - The most feared complications of BAE.
  - Sequelae of transverse myelitis include spastic diplegia and weakness in the lower extremities.
  - The near universal use of nonionic contrast agents and superselective microcatheterization have effectively eliminated the risk of transverse myelitis.
- Recurrent hemorrhage
  - Commonly seen with rates ranging from 10% to 55%.
  - The typical BAE patient has chronic pulmonary inflammatory disease. Recruitment of neovascularity continues despite successful BAE, so the cycle of repeat hemoptysis requiring repeat BAE will tend to recur.
  - In patients with recurrent hemoptysis, repeat embolization is appropriate and effective, with success rates approaching those of the initial BAE (near 90%).
- Chest pain
  - Most common complication, with a reported incidence of 24% to 91%.
  - Generally a self-limiting condition that tends to resolve within the first postprocedure week.

- Risk can be reduced by adhering to superselective embolization.
- Dysphagia
  - Occurs in approximately 20% of cases as a result of nontarget embolization of esophageal arteries.
  - Generally a self-limiting condition that tends to resolve within the first postprocedure week.
  - Risk can be reduced by adhering to superselective embolization.
- Additional rare but reported complications include:
  - Bronchial necrosis
  - Bronchioesophageal fistula
  - Lower extremity neurologic deficits

TAKE-HOME POINTS

- BAE is a highly effective first-line therapy for control of hemoptysis. Immediate control of massive hemoptysis is achieved in a reported 75% to 98% of cases.
- Common indications include the emergent treatment of patients with mild, moderate, or massive hemoptysis including as palliative treatment in the setting of hemorrhagic malignancy.
- Diseases resulting in chronic pulmonary inflammation are generally implicated in most cases of hemoptysis. Worldwide, tuberculosis is the most common cause, though cystic fibrosis is the most common in developed countries.
- Prior to treatment, a detailed review of available radiologic studies should be undertaken in an attempt to both localize the site of bleeding and develop an understanding of the patient's anatomy, as variations in bronchial arterial anatomy are common. Digital subtraction aortography is useful for localizing the origin of the bronchial arteries, the anterior spinal artery, and the artery of Adamkiewicz.
  - In approximately 70% of patients, the bronchial arteries arise from descending thoracic aorta at the level of T5 to T6.
  - In 10% of patients, the bronchial arteries arise from the aorta at other levels.
  - In the remaining 20% of patients, the bronchial arteries arise as a second order branch from various vessels (brachiocephalic, subclavian, etc.) originating from the aorta.
  - The artery of Adamkiewicz typically arises from an intercostal artery between T8 and L1.
- PVA particles are the preferred embolic agent though coils may be used in emergent situations. Temporary embolic agents (Gelfoam) usually lead to rapid recanalization and recurrent hemorrhage. The use of coils prevents future access to the embolized artery in the event that recanalization occurs resulting in recurrent hemorrhage necessitating repeat BAE. However, in the case of life-threatening hemoptysis or a pseudoaneurysm, coils are a useful tool.
- Success rates are high (>90%), though recurrent hemorrhage is not uncommon with certain underlying pathologies (up to 55%). BAE may be repeated in the setting of recurrent hemorrhage.

REVIEW QUESTIONS

1. Bronchial arteries usually arise from the aorta at what level?
   a. T3 to T4
   b. T4 to T5
   c. T5 to T6
   d. T6 to T7

2. Massive hemoptysis is defined as how many mL of expectorated blood in 24 hours?
   a. 100
   b. 250
   c. 300
   d. 500
   e. 1000

3. What is the preferred embolization agent in cases of bronchial artery embolization?
   a. Onyx
   b. Gelfoam
   c. PVA particles
   d. Embolization coils

SUGGESTED READINGS

Brinson GM, Noone PG, Mauro MA, et al. Bronchial artery embolization for the treatment of hemoptysis in patients with cystic fibrosis. *Am J Respir Crit Care Med.* 1998; 157(6):1951–1958.

Burke CT, Dixon RG. *High yield imaging: interventional.* Philadelphia: Elsevier; 2010:236–238.

Burke CT, Mauro MA. Bronchial artery embolization. *Semin Intervent Radiol.* 2004;21(1):43–48.

Lorenz J, Sheth D, Patel J. Bronchial artery embolization. *Semin Intervent Radiol.* 2012;29(3):155–160.

Sopko DR, Smith TP. Bronchial artery embolization for hemoptysis. *Semin Intervent Radiol.* 2011;28(1):48–62.

Deep Vein Thrombosis

Manu K. Singh, Muhammad Umer Nisar, Stuart E. Braverman

CASE PRESENTATION

A 25-year-old female presents to the emergency room (ER) with left thigh pain and swelling for three days. On physical examination, there is tenderness, warmth, erythema, and superficial venous dilation. Deep venous thrombosis (DVT) was suspected and confirmed via lower extremity Doppler examination. A contrast-enhanced CT of her abdomen and pelvis was positive for May-Thurner syndrome, and interventional radiology was consulted.

- In 1271, the first case of a DVT was reported by Henri de Perche in a 20-year-old cobbler who developed unilateral pain and swelling of his right calf.
- In the 1700s, an increase in the incidence of DVT was noted in women after childbirth.
- In 1856, German pathologist Rudolf Virchow published about the Virchow triad, which explained the pathophysiology of the disease.
- In the 1940s, oral anticoagulants were first used to treat DVTs.
- In 1957, May and Thurner described an anatomic variant of the iliac vasculature—**compression of the left common iliac vein by the crossing right common iliac artery**—which was found to predispose patients to developing DVTs (Fig. 16.1).
- In the 1990s, the first catheter-directed thrombolysis was performed.
- Signs and symptoms of having a DVT include:
  - Pain, swelling, warmth, and redness
  - Increased extremity size compared to the unaffected side
  - Palpable cord, representing the dilated, thrombosed vein
- Risk factors for the development of a DVT include:
  - Recent prolonged immobilization (flight) or hospitalization
  - Recent surgery
  - Malignancy
  - Previous DVT
  - Lower extremity trauma
  - Use of oral contraceptives or hormone replacement therapy
  - Pregnancy or postpartum status

- **Wells score** is used to check for the pretest probability of having a DVT (Table 16.1).
- **D-dimer** is a degradation product of cross-linked fibrin. D-dimer levels are increased to >500 ng/mL when acute DVTs are present. It is a sensitive laboratory test that lacks specificity, so a low D-dimer level (i.e., <500 ng/mL) can essentially exclude an acute DVT.
- Duplex ultrasound is commonly used to confirm the diagnosis. An echogenic thrombus may be seen; however, more reliable sonographic findings include:
  - Loss of compressibility
  - Loss of phasic flow
  - Absent color flow (if completely occlusive)
  - Lack of flow augmentation (during calf squeeze)

▶ CLINICAL POINT

Virchow triad describes the factors behind clot formation in the vessel, the combination of (1) hypercoagulability, (2) stasis, and (3) endothelial injury.

INDICATIONS

- General indications for medical therapy of acute DVTs include:
  - Threatened limb viability
  - Extensive thrombosis with high risk of progressing to a **pulmonary embolism**
  - Recent onset of symptoms (<14 days)
  - Proximal DVT in the iliofemoral or femoral veins
  - Underlying predisposing anatomic anomaly
  - Good physiologic reserve (18–75 years old)
  - Life expectancy >6 months
- **Catheter-directed thrombolysis** (CDT) may be performed to treat DVTs as an adjunct to medical therapy.
  - Advantages of this combined approach include more rapid clot lysis with better long-term vessel patency rates and less risk of postthrombotic syndrome.
  - Disadvantages include an increased risk of bleeding—intracranial hemorrhages, retroperitoneal hematomas, and gastrointestinal bleeds, most commonly.

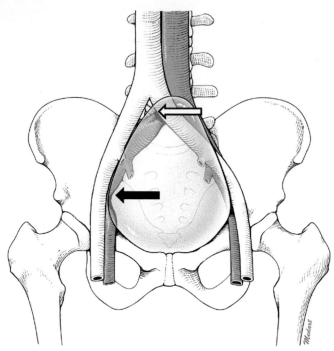

Fig. 16.1 May-Thurner Syndrome. Compression of the left common iliac vein by the right common iliac artery-causes a DVT to form. Schematic figure shows, the left common iliac artery crossing anterior to the right common iliac vein. Two focal sites of compression are also shown, one at the right external iliac vein *(black arrow)* and the other, proximally, at the right common iliac vein *(white arrow)*. (Reused with permission from Im S, Lim SH, Chun HJ, et al. Leg edema with deep venous thrombosis-like symptoms as an unusual complication of occult bladder distension and right May-Thurner syndrome in a stroke patient: a case report. *Arch Phys Med Rehabil.* 2009;90[5]:886–890, Copyright © 2009 American Congress of Rehabilitation Medicine, Elsevier, Fig. 3.)

TABLE 16.1 **Wells Score**	
Clinical Feature	**Score**
Paralysis, paresis, or recent plaster immobilization of lower extremities	1
Recently bedridden for more than 3 days or major surgery within 4 wk	1
Localized tenderness along the distribution of the deep venous system	1
Entire leg swollen	1
Calf swelling >3 cm compared to asymptomatic leg	1
Pitting edema	1
Collateral superficial veins	1
Active cancer	1
Alternative diagnosis likely	–2

3 or more ➜ high probability of having a DVT.
1 or 2 ➜ moderate probability of having a DVT.
0 ➜ low probability of having a DVT.
DVT, Deep venous thrombosis.

CONTRAINDICATIONS

- Absolute contraindications to catheter-directed thrombolysis include:
  - Active internal bleeding
  - Disseminated intravascular coagulation

- Recent (<3 months) neurosurgery, cerebrovascular event, or intracranial trauma
  - Any absolute contraindication to anticoagulation
- Relative contraindications to catheter-directed thrombolysis include:
  - Bleeding diathesis/thrombocytopenia
  - Organ-specific bleeding risk (e.g., recent myocardial infarction, cerebrovascular accident, gastrointestinal bleed, surgery, or trauma)
  - Renal or hepatic failure
  - Malignancy (i.e., brain metastasis)
  - Pregnant or lactating patient
  - Severe uncontrolled hypertension

ANATOMY (FIG. 16.2)

- The deep veins of the lower extremities follow the course of the corresponding arteries.
- The deep veins of the calf include the (1) anterior tibial, (2) posterior tibial, and (3) peroneal (or fibular) vein.
  - The **anterior tibial vein** receives blood from the dorsal pedal vein. It runs in the anterior compartment of the leg in front of the interosseous membrane between the tibia and the fibula.
  - The **posterior tibial vein** drains the plantar surface of the foot and the posterior compartment of the leg. As its name suggests, it is found posterior to the tibia.
  - The **peroneal vein** runs along the posteromedial aspect of the fibula before joining the posterior tibial vein.
- The anterior and posterior tibial veins join to form the tibioperoneal trunk and **popliteal vein**. The popliteal vein ascends along the posterior aspect of the knee and anteromedial thigh. It is medial to the popliteal artery in the lower knee, superficial to the artery in the posterior compartment, and lateral to the artery above the knee.
- The popliteal vein becomes the **superficial femoral vein** at the adductor hiatus. In the lower thigh, it lies lateral to the femoral artery, and in the upper thigh, it lies medial to the artery. It joins the deep femoral vein to form the **common femoral vein**.
- At the inguinal ligament, the common femoral vein becomes the **external iliac vein**.

EQUIPMENT

- Basic angiography set
- 6- and 8-Fr sheaths
- Hydrophilic guidewire
- Infusion catheter system ± mechanical thrombectomy device

PROCEDURAL STEPS

1. Using a 21-gauge micropuncture set, ultrasound-guided access is achieved in the popliteal vein.

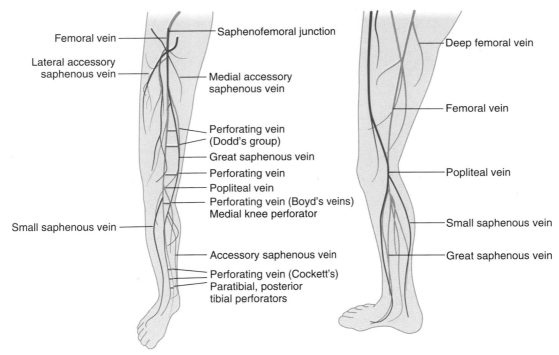

Fig. 16.2 Lower Extremity Venous Anatomy. (Reused with permission from Creager M, Beckman J, Loscalzo J. *Vascular Medicine.* 2nd ed. Elsevier; 2012:F54–F51.)

>> **CLINICAL POINT**

Depending on the location of the DVT, US-guided access via the popliteal vein is typically the chosen approach. Approaches through the tibial, jugular, or contralateral femoral veins have been described as well.

2. A micropuncture catheter is placed over the microwire.
3. Micropuncture catheter and wire are exchanged for a 6-Fr sheath.
4. A venogram is performed to evaluate extent of the thrombus (Fig. 16.3).

5. The thrombus is then crossed with a hydrophilic guidewire.
6. An infusion catheter with multiple sideholes is placed across the thrombosed segment to deliver thrombolytics along the entire clot (Fig. 16.4).
7. Multiple passes are made with a mechanical thrombectomy device (e.g., Angiojet catheter) to aspirate any residual thrombus (Fig. 16.5).

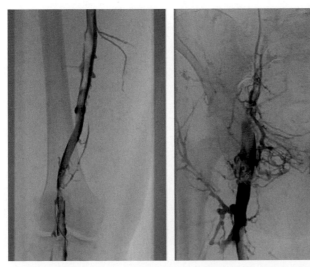

Fig. 16.3 Venography Demonstrates Extent of Deep Venous Thrombosis. (Courtesy Stuart E. Braverman.)

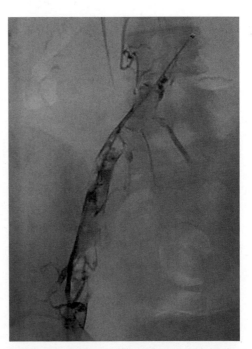

Fig. 16.4 An Infusion Catheter Is Placed Across the Iliofemoral Clot. (Courtesy Stuart E. Braverman.)

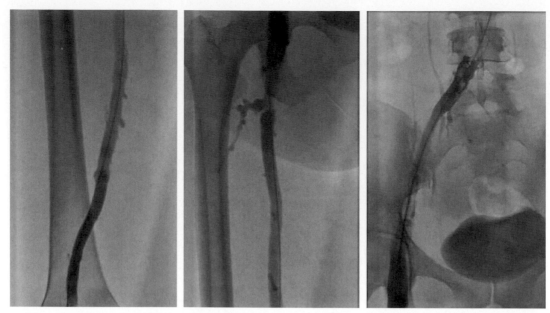

Fig. 16.5 Status Post Power Pulse With AngioJet and Tissue Plasminogen Activator (TPA). (Courtesy Stuart E. Braverman.)

8. Any observed potential causes of the DVT are appropriately treated. Here an iliac vein "spur" is balloon dilated (Fig. 16.6). A stent can be placed across the lesion.
9. Final venogram demonstrates patent vasculature (Fig. 16.7).

> ▷ **CLINICAL POINT**
>
> Should I place an IVC filter? Filters are not indicated in the management of uncomplicated DVT unless the patient cannot be anticoagulated, has a low cardiopulmonary reserve, or has had a previous massive PE.

ALTERNATE TREATMENTS

- EkoSonic Endovascular system (EkoS)
  - Uses ultrasonographic waves, the acoustic pulses of which effectively make the fibrin clot more porous,

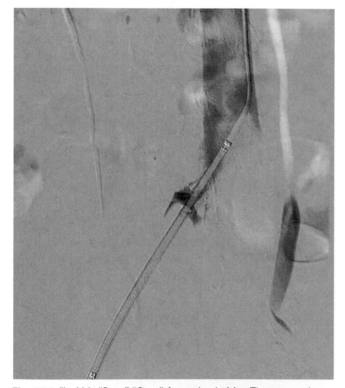

Fig. 16.6 Iliac Vein "Spur." "Spur" formation in May-Thurner syndrome is thought to be secondary to chronic pulsations/trauma from the overriding right iliac artery. This results in accumulation of elastin and collagen causing "spur" formation. (Courtesy Stuart E. Braverman.)

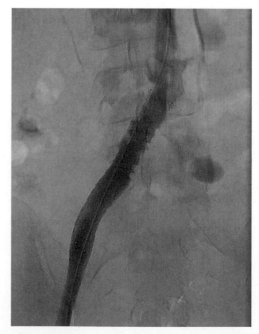

Fig. 16.7 Patent Right Iliac Vein After Stenting. (Courtesy Stuart E. Braverman.)

along with simultaneous administration of clot-dissolving drugs for enzymatic thrombolysis in order to speed up time-to-clot dissolution.
- Commonly used in the endovascular treatment of pulmonary emboli.
- Consider this case of a 27-year-old professional weight lifter with 2 weeks of right upper extremity swelling and tingling (Fig. 16.8) successfully treated with EkoS.
- Pharmacologic treatment
  - The mainstay of DVT treatment is medical therapy via anticoagulation. The goal of anticoagulation is to reduce the likelihood of pulmonary embolism by limiting clot propagation and promoting endogenous lysis.
  - Medications

- Parenteral anticoagulation includes:
  - Low-molecular-weight heparin (preferred)
  - Unfractionated heparin (used in renal failure)

> **CLINICAL POINT**
>
> When treating patients with renal failure (CrCl <30), unfractionated heparin with a bridge to warfarin is recommended as low molecular-weight-heparin and NOACs are contraindicated.

- Long-term anticoagulation considerations include:
  - Warfarin (Coumadin), a vitamin K antagonist (VKA) oral anticoagulant

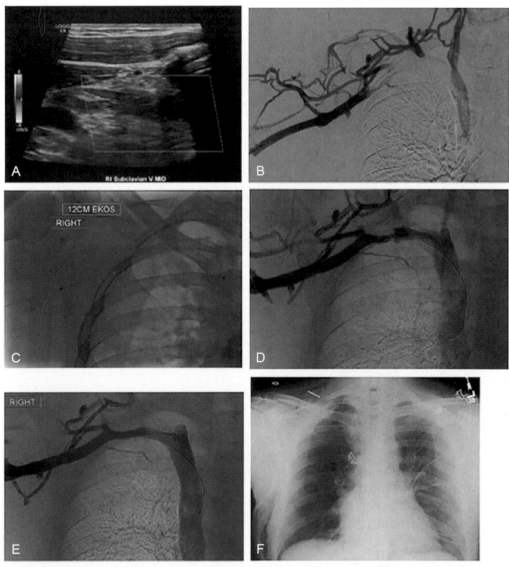

Fig. 16.8 Initial upper extremity Doppler was performed, which demonstrated (A) occlusive echogenic clot within the subclavian vein that was (B) confirmed on venography. (C) A 12-cm EkoS catheter was placed across the occlusion, and infusion was initiated for a period of 24 hours. Follow-up run demonstrates (D) resolution of the thrombus but with residual stenosis and possible web formation. Angioplasty was performed, and (E) repeat venography demonstrated no residual stenosis. Surgical decompression was performed in this patient with **Paget-Schrötter syndrome**. Postoperative radiograph demonstrates (F) postsurgical changes of the right hemithorax status post removal of the right first rib *(white arrow)*. (Courtesy Stuart E. Braverman.)

- Non-vitamin K antagonist oral anticoagulants (NOACs) such as rivaroxaban (Xarelto), apixaban (Eliquis), dabigatran (Pradaxa), and edoxaban (Savaysa)
- The 10th edition of the antithrombotic guidelines recommends NOACs over warfarin for initial and long-term treatment of venous thromboembolism in patients without cancer.
  - For long-term treatment of "cancer-associated thrombosis," LMWH is recommended
- Initial parenteral anticoagulation is given before dabigatran and edoxaban, is not given before rivaroxaban and apixaban, and is overlapped with VKA therapy.
- Duration of treatment for a *minimum* of 3 months is recommended in nearly all scenarios (Table 16.2).

COMPLICATIONS

- Asymptomatic pulmonary embolism
- Paradoxical embolism to the brain due to atrial septal anomalies

TABLE 16.2	Duration of Treatment
Situation	**Duration of Treatment**
Patients with reversible risk factor(s) (surgery, trauma, prolonged bed rest)	Minimum of 3 months or until risk factor(s) has resolved
Unprovoked DVT (with low/moderate risk of bleeding)	Extended/indefinite therapy is discussed with health care provider after an initial 3–6 months of therapy.
Unprovoked DVT (with high risk of bleeding)	3 months is recommended in most cases
DVTs associated with active cancer	Indefinite therapy for as long as cancer treatment is ongoing (minimum of 3 months)
Two or more episodes of DVT or if a risk factor is permanently present	Consider lifelong therapy

DVT, Deep venous thrombosis.

- Postthrombotic syndrome
  - Venous hypertension due to the thrombus and valvular insufficiency/reflux results in edema, skin pigmentation, venous ulcers, and venous dilation.
- Major bleeding

◎ LITERATURE REVIEW

Vedantham et al. (2005) reported major bleeding as the most frequent major complication, with a rate of 2.8% in their review of 30 studies.

- Access site–related issues
- Rare but with high morbidity/mortality:
  - Symptomatic pulmonary emboli, intracranial hemorrhage, and death

🏠 TAKE-HOME POINTS

- In patients presenting with acute DVTs, the cornerstone of treatment is anticoagulation. NOACs are generally recommended over VKAs for long-term anticoagulation. Consult the latest anti-thrombotic guidelines for more specific recommendations.
- The prime indication for venous thrombolysis is threatened limb due to DVT (*Phegmasia Ceruleans Dolan*)
- In functional patients with reasonable life expectancy, thrombolysis may be considered in cases of:
  - Acute iliofemoral DVT <21 days from onset of symptoms
  - Clinical failure of conventional anticoagulation therapy
  - Prevention of postphlebitic syndrome
- Thought process for catheter-directed interventions:
  - New thrombi usually undergo lysis the fastest
  - Use a catheter length that will allow you to infuse over the entire clot
- Try establishing flow as quickly as possibly by considering pharmacomechanical thrombectomy before simple thrombolysis
- Consider venous stenting for obstructive regions in the iliac vein

REVIEW QUESTIONS

1. Which of the following does NOT increase the risk of thromboembolism?
   a. Recent surgery
   b. Malignancy
   c. Previous history of DVT
   d. Exercise
   e. Pregnancy
2. Which of the following is NOT included in Wells criteria to check for pretest probability of DVT?
   a. Active cancer
   b. Pitting edema
   c. Immobilization
   d. Calf swelling >1 cm compared to asymptomatic leg
   e. Recent surgery
3. Medical treatment for DVT may include all the following EXCEPT:
   a. Low-molecular-weight heparin
   b. Unfractionated heparin
   c. Warfarin
   d. Rivaroxaban
   e. Clopidogrel

SUGGESTED READINGS

Kaufman J, Lee M. *Vascular and Interventional Radiology: The Requisites*. 2nd ed. Philadelphia: Elsevier; 2014.

Kearon C, Akl EA, Omelas J, et al. Antithrombotic therapy for VTE disease: CHEST guideline and expert panel report. *Chest*. 2016; 149(2):315–352.

Patterson BO, Hinchliffe R, Loftus IM, et al. Indications for catheter-directed thrombolysis in the management of acute proximal deep venous thrombosis. *Arterioscler Thromb Vasc Biol*. 2010;30(4):669–674.

Valji K. *Vascular and Interventional Radiology*. 2nd ed. Philadelphia: Elsevier; 2007.

Vedantham S, Padginton C. Percutaneous options for acute deep vein thrombosis. *Semin Intervent Radiol*. 2005; 22(3):195–203.

Endovascular Aneurysm Repair

Eric C. King, Eric C. Kim, Cuong (Ken) Lam

CASE PRESENTATION

A 65-year-old Caucasian male with hypertension, hyperlipidemia, and a 30–pack year smoking history presents to the emergency department with abdominal and back pain. Physical examination showed hemodynamically stable vitals, a pulsatile abdominal mass, and weakened distal pulses. Abdominal CT revealed a nonruptured abdominal aortic aneurysm with a diameter of 5.9 cm. Patient was sent for urgent endovascular repair of his **abdominal aortic aneurysm** (AAA).

- Although initially introduced for patients who were poor candidates for open surgical repair, **endovascular aneurysm repair (EVAR)** is now considered the gold standard treatment of AAA.
  - As a less invasive technique with no open exposure of the aorta or need for aortic clamping, perioperative mortality has significantly decreased with EVAR.
  - Since EVAR can be performed on patients with contraindications to open surgical repair, the incidence of ruptured AAAs and its associated morbidity and mortality has decreased in the United States.
- AAAs are a common vascular disease in the elderly. Age-related aortic wall weakening causes focal fusiform or saccular enlargement of the aorta.
  - Aneurysmal dilation is defined as a portion of the aorta at least 1.5 times greater in diameter than the normal aorta, or any portion of the abdominal aorta >3 cm in diameter (Fig. 17.1).
  - AAAs are most commonly located in the infrarenal position (>80%). A minority of them are in the juxtarenal or suprarenal position.
  - **Fusiform** morphology is more commonly seen. Saccular aneurysms only represent 1% to 2% of aneurysms and are theorized to have higher rupture rates, although the natural history is unclear.
  - While there are many causes of AAA, atherosclerotic change is the most common culprit.
  - Common risk factors for AAA include increased age, male gender, atherosclerosis, hypertension, family history, and smoking status.
  - The most feared complication of AAA is rupture, with the risk of rupture being proportional to the diameter of the aneurysm (Table 17.1).

- EVAR is performed by inserting a compressed graft within a catheter and sheath through an access vessel, most often the common femoral artery. Upon advancement into the abdominal aorta, the endograft is deployed and expanded to contact the aortic wall proximally and iliac vessels distally to exclude the aortic aneurysm sac from systemic circulation.

INDICATIONS

- EVAR is indicated in patients with:
  - Symptomatic AAAs (abdominal or back pain/tenderness, signs of rupture, or evidence of embolization)
  - AAAs ≥5.5 cm in diameter in men or ≥5 cm in women
  - Known AAAs with diameter growth of >5 mm in a 6-month period
  - Contained ruptured AAAs
  - Inflammatory AAAs
- To optimize success of EVAR, an appropriate seal where the endograft attaches to the arterial wall is paramount. This is especially important since endografts do not rely on active surgical anastomosis. Because of this, patients must also match **anatomic inclusion criteria** (see Imaging Evaluation under Procedural Steps).

CONTRAINDICATIONS

- Exclusion criteria (see Imaging Evaluation under Procedural Steps):
  - Adverse proximal neck anatomy
  - Adverse iliac artery anatomy
  - Circumferential aortic calcification
  - Extensive tortuosity
- Allergy to iodinated contrast medium
- Mycotic aneurysms—if the patient is a surgical candidate, that method is preferred
- Severe uncorrectable iliac occlusive disease
- Marfan or Ehlers-Danlos syndrome

EQUIPMENT

Stent Grafts (Fig. 17.2)

- Grafts are either polyester (trade name—Dacron) or polytetrafluoroethylene (PTFE)

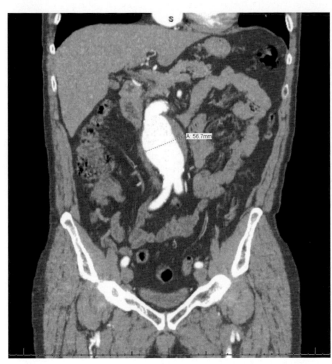

Fig. 17.1 Patient A: Coronal Computed Tomography Angiogram (CTA). A 5.7-cm infrarenal abdominal aortic aneurysm. (Courtesy Dr. Cuong [Ken] Lam, Kaiser Permanente Los Angeles Medical Center.)

TABLE 17.1   Aneurysmal Diameter and Annual Risk of Rupture

Diameter	Risk of Rupture (%)
<4.0 cm	<0.5
4.0–4.9 cm	0.5–5
5.0–5.9 cm	3–15
6.0–6.9 cm	10–20
7.0–7.9 cm	20–40
≥8.0 cm	30–50

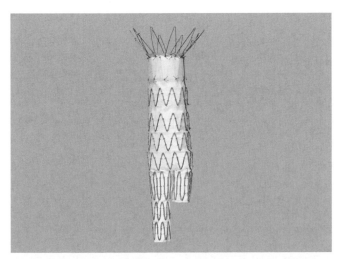

Fig. 17.2 Zenith Flex Abdominal Aortic Aneurysm Endovascular Graft Bifurcated Main Body Graft. (Courtesy Cook Medical.)

- Stents are MR-compatible alloys (nitinol or eligiloy) or MR-incompatible ferromagnetic alloy (steel)
- Stent grafts are typically sized 10% to 20% larger than the diameter of the proximal neck to appose the aortic wall without causing folds in the graft that could lead to turbulent flow and thrombosis.
- Stent grafts exist both as off-the-shelf or custom-made models for the specific patient.
- Common variations include:
  - *Bifurcated* stent grafts extend from the proximal abdominal aorta to both common iliac arteries.
  - *Aorto uni-iliac* stent grafts extend from the abdominal aorta into a single common iliac artery. This method requires occlusion of the contralateral common iliac artery and subsequent fem-fem bypass.
  - *Fenestrated* stent grafts are custom-made with prefabricated reinforced holes for aortic branch vessels. This custom-made technique allows for greater contact with the aortic wall.
  - *Branched* stent grafts are similar to fenestrated grafts, with the addition of branching arms that insert into aortic branches that are in the zone of the aneurysm.
- Major aortic branch vessels must be preserved by surgical conduits or stents.
  - A second stent graft adjacent to the main endograft can be used in emergent procedures or as a bailout technique if a main aortic branch is accidentally covered by the endograft, termed the *snorkel* or *chimney* technique.

> ### ▶▶ CLINICAL POINT
>
> Fenestrated and branched grafts take 2–4 weeks to custom make, and therefore use of these is not possible in an urgent or emergent setting.

Arterial Closure Devices

- Traditionally, vascular access for EVAR required surgical cutdown to accommodate large delivery systems measuring up to 21 Fr.
- Vascular closure devices now allow for percutaneous closure of arterial access sites.
  - Most closure devices can close up to 8-Fr arteriotomies.
  - Angioseal, a commonly used device, deploys a collagen plug.
  - Perclose, a suture-mediated device, can close up to 24-Fr arteriotomies.

ANATOMY

- The **abdominal aorta** begins at the diaphragmatic hiatus (T12) and ends at the bifurcation of the common iliac arteries (varies from L3 to L5).
  - Major aortic branch arteries include the phrenic, celiac, superior mesenteric, adrenal, renal, gonadal, inferior mesenteric, lumbar, and middle sacral arteries.

- Common iliac artery aneurysms are seen in 20% of patients with AAA.
- The common iliac artery bifurcates into the internal iliac and external iliac arteries.
  - The external iliac artery becomes the common femoral artery at the inguinal ligament. Since the inguinal ligament is not visible under fluoroscopy, the corresponding angiographic landmarks are the circumflex iliac artery (laterally) and inferior epigastric artery (medially).

PROCEDURAL STEPS

Imaging Evaluation

- Pre- and postcontrast CTA is the preferred modality, but MRA can be used if indicated.
- Conventional angiogram is not preferred as it only provides luminal diameters without accounting for mural thrombus.
- For accurate measurement of vessel length, width, and angulation, 3D reconstructions that are aligned perpendicular to the lumen (center-line reconstruction) should be used (Fig. 17.3). Coronal and sagittal reformatted images should be reviewed as well.
- Check all vessels for patency, tortuosity, atherosclerotic burden, and size. The access site, most commonly the common femoral arteries, must be able to accommodate sheaths between 18 and 28 Fr in size.
- Evaluate for aberrant aortic branch vessels.
- Evaluate for popliteal and common iliac artery aneurysms.
- Review the device indications for use (IFU) to ensure suitable anatomy.

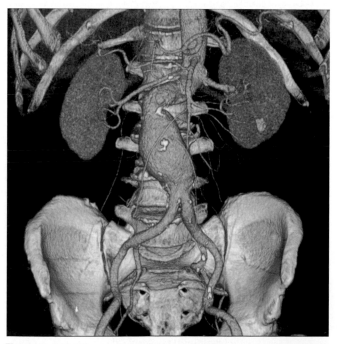

Fig. 17.3 CTA 3D volume rendering showing a large infrarenal abdominal aortic aneurysm with an angled proximal neck. (Courtesy Dr. Cuong [Ken] Lam, Kaiser Permanente Los Angeles Medical Center.)

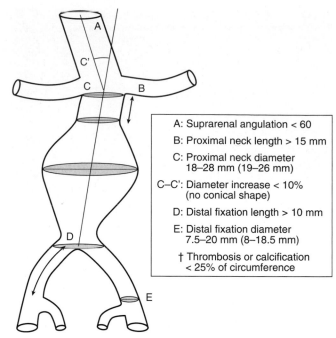

A: Suprarenal angulation < 60

B: Proximal neck length > 15 mm

C: Proximal neck diameter 18–28 mm (19–26 mm)

C–C': Diameter increase < 10% (no conical shape)

D: Distal fixation length > 10 mm

E: Distal fixation diameter 7.5–20 mm (8–18.5 mm)

† Thrombosis or calcification < 25% of circumference

Fig. 17.4 Favorable Anatomy of an Abdominal Aortic Aneurysm for Treatment With Endovascular Aneurysm Repair. (Courtesy Dr. Cuong [Ken] Lam, Kaiser Permanente Los Angeles Medical Center.)

- Although each device manufacturer has different criteria for EVAR deployment suitability, approximately one-third of patients will have friendly anatomy, one-third will have difficult anatomy, and one-third will have anatomy that contraindicates EVAR.
- Favorable anatomy (Fig. 17.4):
  - Proximal landing zone length >10 to 15 mm
    - Measured from the takeoff of the most inferior renal artery to the most superior aspect of the aneurysm
  - Distal landing zone length >30 mm
  - Proximal angulation <60 degrees
  - Aortic bifurcation angulation <90 degrees
- Difficult anatomy:
  - Proximal landing zone <10 mm
  - Proximal angulation >60 degrees
  - Conical neck (>3-mm difference in diameter of the proximal and distal necks)
  - Maximal diameter of landing zone >22 to 30 mm
  - Stenotic aortic bifurcation
  - Aneurysmal common iliac artery
    - Can consider preprocedural internal iliac artery embolization and extending the distal graft into the external iliac artery (Fig. 17.5)

Patient Preparation

- Review the stent-graft design including the location of all radiopaque markers. Consult with the manufacturer representative and device website as needed.
- Determine whether general anesthesia is needed or if locoregional anesthesia with moderate sedation would suffice.

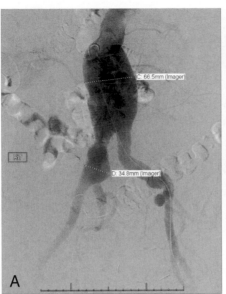
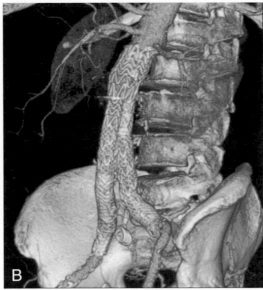

Fig. 17.5 (A) Conventional angiogram in the coronal oblique projection. Note the aneurysmal right common iliac artery. (B) CTA 3D volume rendering with a vascular occlusion device at the right internal iliac artery, which was deployed 2 weeks prior to endovascular aneurysm repair. This allowed endograft extension into the right external iliac artery to treat the aneurysmal right common iliac artery. (Courtesy Dr. Cuong [Ken] Lam, Kaiser Permanente Los Angeles Medical Center.)

- Start prophylactic antibiotics (e.g., cefazolin) to cover *Staphylococcus aureus*, *Staphylococcus epidermidis*, and enteric gram-negative rods.
- Arrange for clinic visits and follow-up imaging at 1 month, 6 months, and then yearly thereafter.

Procedural Steps

1. Access the common femoral arteries either percutaneously or via surgical cutdown.
2. Insert a 5- or 6-Fr sheath into both common femoral arteries.
3. Infuse 80 to 100 IU/kg heparin through the sheath, and check activated clotting time at baseline, 3 minutes after heparin, and every 30 minutes thereafter (goal of 2–2.5 times the baseline).
4. Use the contralateral common femoral artery (CFA) to perform a diagnostic angiogram using a pigtail catheter.
   a. Locate the renal artery ostia and note the location of the most inferior artery (Fig. 17.6).
   b. Lock the table position, and mark the lowest ostium on the screen.
5. Use the ipsilateral CFA to deliver the endograft delivery system to the infrarenal aorta over a super-stiff guidewire.
   a. Line up the proximal radiopaque markers, and angle the fluoroscope to remove parallax.
   b. Slowly deploy the stent immediately caudal to the lowest renal artery.
   c. Deploy the graft until the ipsilateral limb of the endograft is fully extended (Fig. 17.7).
   d. Retract the nose cone of the delivery device.
6. Use the contralateral CFA to cannulate the contralateral limb of the endograft (Fig. 17.8).

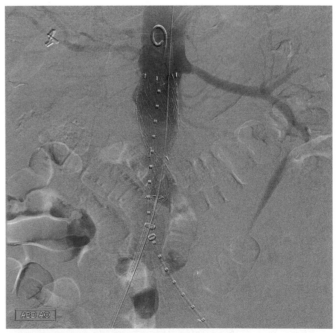

Fig. 17.6 Conventional Angiogram in the Coronal Oblique Projection. The proximal endograft is being deployed below the left renal artery. (Courtesy Dr. Cuong [Ken] Lam, Kaiser Permanente Los Angeles Medical Center.)

7. When the pigtail catheter is in the graft neck, spin the catheter to ensure it is within the graft.
8. Perform an angiogram to identify the internal iliac artery ostium, and mark its location on the screen.
9. Insert the contralateral limb stent-graft deployment system, and deploy the device, ensuring sufficient overlap with the main graft.

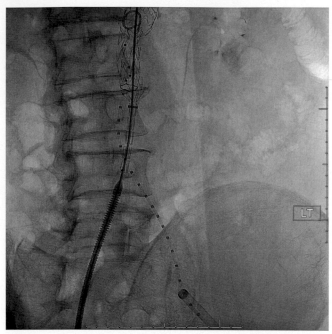

Fig. 17.7 Conventional Angiogram in the Coronal Oblique Projection. The endograft is deployed until the contralateral gate is released. Note the radiopaque marker of the contralateral gate. (Courtesy Dr. Cuong [Ken] Lam, Kaiser Permanente Los Angeles Medical Center.)

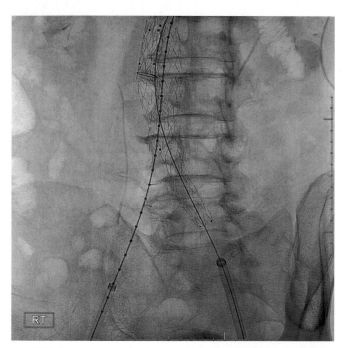

Fig. 17.8 Conventional Angiogram in the Coronal Oblique Projection. The endograft has been extended into the contralateral common iliac artery. Note the radiopaque marker of the contralateral gate. (Courtesy Dr. Cuong [Ken] Lam, Kaiser Permanente Los Angeles Medical Center.)

10. Use a compliant, low-pressure balloon at the points of graft overlap/attachment to mold the graft and ensure a good seal.
11. Insert a pigtail catheter above the main aortic graft, and perform an angiogram in multiple obliquities to evaluate for graft position, endoleak, and aortic branch vessel patency.

12. Close the access artery either with suture or with a vascular closure device.

ALTERNATIVE TREATMENTS

Open Surgical Repair of Abdominal Aortic Aneurysms

- Open surgical repair involves opening the aneurysm sac, removing thrombus from the aorta, and suturing a graft into the aorta proximally and distally.
- Complication rate is 11% after open repair and 3% after EVAR.
  - Reintervention rate for EVAR is 20% to 30% during the subsequent 8 years.
    - Majority of reinterventions are for endoleaks.
  - Only 2% to 4% of complications after EVAR require open surgical intervention.
- 30-day mortality rate is 4% after open repair and 1% after EVAR.
  - Mortality with EVAR increases with renal failure, age >80, lower limb ischemia, and congestive heart failure.
  - Mortality rates become equivalent after 2 years of follow-up. Initial cost savings are lost after these 2 years due to more frequent reintervention seen with EVAR.
- Open surgical repair may be preferred in younger patients who have a low or average perioperative risk. EVAR is most appropriate in patients with favorable anatomy who are at a high perioperative risk.

COMPLICATIONS

- **Endoleaks** (Table 17.2 and Fig. 17.9)
  - Occurs in 20% to 40% of cases

TABLE 17.2 **Types of Endoleak and Treatment**		
Type	**Description**	**Treatment**
1A/B	Incomplete seal of the stent graft to the native vessel proximally (IA) or distally (IB)	Immediate treatment, usually with extension of the stent graft
2	Retrograde filling of the aneurysm sac by collateral vessels	Treat if the sac continues to enlarge, usually with permanent embolization
3	Inadequate seal between modular stent-graft components or graft defects	Immediate treatment, usually with additional devices within the stent graft
4	Porous stent-graft material	Usually self-limited upon discontinuation of periprocedural anticoagulation
5	Endotension (sac expansion without clear evidence)	Treat if sac continues to enlarge, usually with a combination of methods

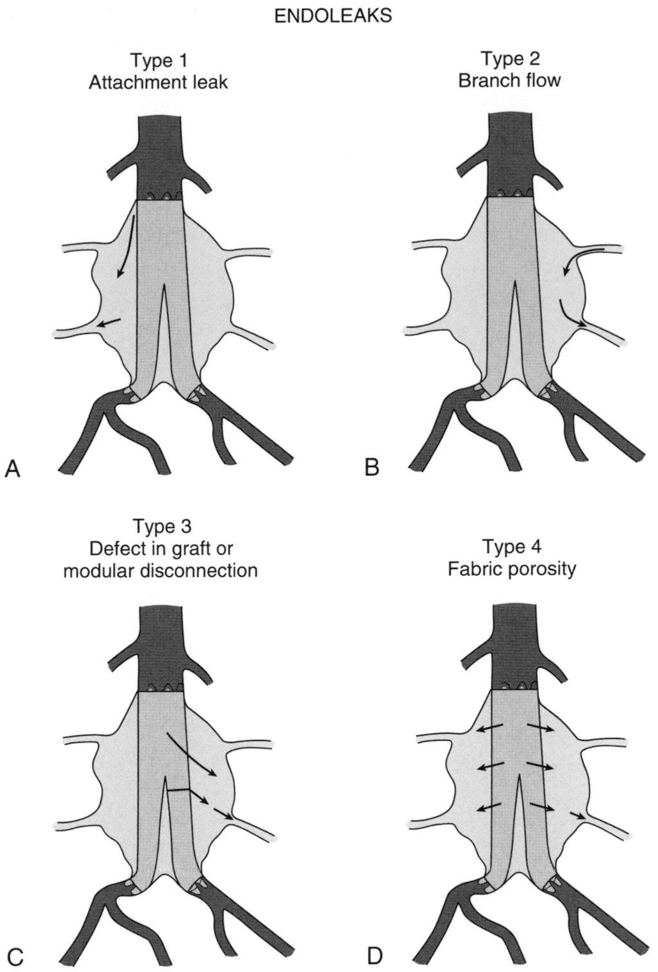

ENDOLEAKS

Type 1
Attachment leak

Type 2
Branch flow

Type 3
Defect in graft or
modular disconnection

Type 4
Fabric porosity

A   B   C   D

Fig. 17.9 Endoleaks of Abdominal Aortic Aneurysm After Endo-luminal Graft (ELG) Repair. (A) Type 1 leak (attachment leak). Blood continues to enter the aneurysm sac at one of the three ends of the bifurcated ELG, the points where the ELG should be tightly affixed to the arterial wall. Egress, as with all endoleaks, is through branches of the aorta that remain patent. Treatment of type 1 leaks is indicated. (B) Type 2 leak (branch artery leak). Blood enters the aneurysm sac through a patent branch artery. This type of leak can be self-limited and may be only observed. Treatment is indicated if the aneurysm enlarges. (C) Type 3 leak (loss of integrity of ELG). Either the modules of the ELG have become separated or a rent has formed in the fabric of the ELG. Blood enters the sac from the ELG lumen through the site of loss of ELG integrity. Treatment is indicated. (D) Type 4 leak (fabric porosity). Blood enters the sac from the ELG lumen through intact cloth of the ELG. (From Bertino RE, et al. *Diagnostic Ultrasound*. Philadelphia: Elsevier; 2011:Fig. 12.10.)

- Type 2 is the most common endoleak.
  - Collateral feeding vessel is typically the lumbar or inferior mesenteric arteries.
  - Up to 40% will spontaneously thrombose, but embolization of the culprit vessel is indicated with sac enlargement.
- Types 1 and 3 should be treated immediately by performing angioplasty of the graft attachment sites, extending the graft, or deploying a balloon-expandable bare metal stent within the graft.

- Postimplantation syndrome
  - Common, benign, self-limited sequelae of fever and leukocytosis resembling sepsis.
  - Consider reducing risk with preprocedural methyl-prednisone
- Contrast-induced nephropathy
  - Perioperative hydration will reduce risk.
  - Use of intravascular ultrasound can reduce the dependence on fluoroscopy and thereby decrease contrast load.
- Buttock claudication
  - 30% to 50% risk of transient claudication due to embolization of the internal iliac artery.
  - Increased risk in younger patients and in those with left ventricular dysfunction.
- Thrombosis
  - 5% risk, usually occurring in the first 2 months post procedure
  - No role for routine anticoagulation
- Graft migration
  - 3.6% risk at 1 year
  - Becomes clinically significant if >5-mm migration.
- Graft kinking
  - Attempt salvage with angioplasty or stenting
- Graft rupture
  - 5% to 6% risk in the endovascular cases versus 1% to 2% in the surgical cases
- Spinal cord ischemia
  - The artery of Adamkiewicz supplies the anterior spinal artery. It typically originates between T9 and T12 but can originate anywhere between T5 and L3.
  - There is increased risk with extensive coverage of the abdominal aorta or prior repair due to coverage of arteries supplying the thoracic and lumbar spine.
  - Consider perioperative lumbar drain placement to reduce this risk.
- Infection
  - Risk is reduced with use of perioperative antibiotics.

TAKE-HOME POINTS

- AAAs are most commonly due to atherosclerosis and are defined as either luminal diameter >3 cm or >1.5 times the patient's normal diameter.
- Indications to treat include size >5.5 cm in men or >5.0 cm in women, growth >1 cm in a year, or the presence of symptoms.
- Decision for open surgical versus endovascular repair with a stent graft depends on patient age, comorbidities, surgical risk, and individual anatomic factors.
- A common complication of EVAR is endoleak, which accounts for a reintervention rate that is more than four times that seen with open surgical repair.
- The 30-day mortality rate and average length of hospitalization are lower in EVAR versus open repair. Mortality rates eventually reach equipoise, and initial cost savings with endovascular intervention are lost beyond 2 years due to the more frequent reintervention.

REVIEW QUESTIONS

1. Which is true regarding abdominal aortic aneurysms?
   a. They are most often discovered during the investigation of other conditions.
   b. They are infrarenal in 75% of cases.
   c. Their incidence of rupture increases with aneurysm size.
   d. They should be repaired when diameter exceeds 4 cm.
2. There is a 20% to 40% risk of an endoleak status post endovascular aneurysm repair. Which type of endoleak requires immediate correction?
   a. Type I, due to incomplete seal of the stent graft to the vessel
   b. Type II, due to retrograde filling from collateral vessels
   c. Type III, due to inadequate seal between modular stent-graft components or graft defects
   d. a and b
   e. a and c
3. The annual risk of rupture of a 6.0-cm aneurysm is approximately what percent? Aneurysms expand at an average rate of how many centimeters a year?
   a. 5; 0.4
   b. 5; 1
   c. 15; 0.4
   d. 15; 1

SUGGESTED READINGS

Blankensteijn JD, de Jong SECA, Prinssen M, et al. Two-year outcomes after conventional or endovascular repair of abdominal aortic aneurysms. *N Engl J Med.* 2005;352:2398–2405.

Bryce Y, Rogoff P, Romanelli D, et al. Endovascular repair of abdominal aortic aneurysms: vascular anatomy, device selection, procedure, and procedure-specific complications. *Radio Graph.* 2015;35:593–615.

Trial Participants EVAR. Endovascular aneurysm repair versus open repair in patients with abdominal aortic aneurysm (EVAR trial 1): randomized controlled trial. *Lancet.* 2005; 365:2179–2186.

Kothandan H, Haw Chieh GL, Khan SA, et al. Anesthetic considerations for endovascular abdominal aortic aneurysm repair. *Ann Card Anaesth.* 2016;19:132–141.

Lederle FA, Wilson SE, Johnson GR, et al. Immediate repair compared with surveillance of small abdominal aortic aneurysms. *N Engl J Med.* 2002;346:1437–1444.

Powell JT. Final 12-year follow-up of surgery versus surveillance in the UK Small Aneurysm Trial. *Br J Surg.* 2007;94:702–708.

Schermerhorn ML, Buck DB, O'Malley AJ, et al. Long-term outcomes of abdominal aortic aneurysm in the Medicare population. *N Engl J Med.* 2015;373:328–338.

Stavropoulos SW, Charagundla SR. Imaging techniques for detection and management of endoleaks after endovascular aortic aneurysm repair. *Radiology.* 2007;243:641–655.

Walker TG, Kalva SP, Yeddula K, et al. Clinical practice guidelines for endovascular abdominal aortic aneurysm repair. *J Vasc Interv Radiol.* 2010;21:1632–1655.

Foreign Body Retrieval

Shantanu Warhadpande, Pranav Moudgil, Monte L. Harvill

CASE PRESENTATION

A 43-year-old woman with breast cancer presents to the emergency department with sudden-onset chest discomfort and palpitations. She had a Port-a-Cath placed 1 day prior in her right chest. A chest x-ray visualizes the port in the right upper thorax; the catheter, however, is no longer secured to the port and has instead migrated to the heart and has become lodged in the tricuspid valve—half of the catheter in the right atrium and the other half in the right ventricle. With each heartbeat, the tricuspid closes onto the midshaft of the catheter, visibly kinking it. The immediate fear is that the catheter may drift farther into the pulmonary arteries and cause a pulmonary embolism. Treatment options include open heart surgery or an attempt at endovascular retrieval. An interventional radiologist is urgently consulted to review imaging and determine the viability of an endovascular attempt at catheter retrieval.

- John Thomas described the first endovascular retrieval of an **intravascular foreign body** (IFB) in 1964.
- Since then, percutaneous retrieval of intravascular foreign bodies has surpassed open surgical retrievals as the preferred initial approach.
- The increased number of endovascular procedures and increased use of therapeutic intravascular foreign bodies in patients (inferior vena cava [IVC] filters, stents, coils, catheters, etc...) has resulted in an increase in dislodged/separated/broken/malpositioned IFBs. IFB retrieval is, in most cases, feasible and safe.
- Common IFBs include:
  - Catheter fragments (most common)
  - Guidewires
  - IVC filters/broken legs
  - Stents
  - Embolization coils
- Many IFBs are preventable and result from operator inexperience.
- **Venous IFBs** usually result from device fracture or separation of one module from the rest of the device (i.e., catheter separating from mediport or IVC filter leg breaking off from the rest of the filter).
- **Arterial IFBs** usually result from improper deployment (i.e., malpositioned embolization coil).

- Venous foreign bodies travel centrally toward the heart while arterial foreign bodies travel distally toward the periphery.
  - Major concerns for venous foreign bodies, therefore, are **heart perforation** and **pulmonary embolism**.
  - Major concerns for arterial IFB include **arterial perforation** and **arterial occlusion**.
- Various devices are specifically available to assist these cases, but in many situations, the interventionalist must adapt and use endovascular tools not originally intended for IFB retrieval.
- The interventionalist must first determine whether retrieval is necessary or not. The next consideration is whether the IFB can be retrieved endovascularly. At times, a multidisciplinary approach is necessary to weigh the risks and benefits between an endovascular versus a surgical approach.
  - The major advantage of endovascular IFB retrieval is that it avoids a surgical procedure, which is associated with higher morbidity.
  - Literature has demonstrated a very high serious complication rate for indwelling IFBs. Success rate of endovascular IFB retrieval, in indicated cases, is as high as 94%.
  - However, there are situations, after taking the procedural risks/feasibility, IFB location, imaging findings, and patient's symptoms into consideration, where it may be prudent to simply leave the IFB alone.
- Historically, IFBs have been approached aggressively with prompt attempts at retrieval given the high rate of serious complications and symptoms secondary to indwelling IFBs.
- IFB-induced symptoms vary and are determined by the location of the foreign body.
  - Table 18.1 details some of the most commonly seen symptoms.
  - Important to note that many patients have absolutely no symptoms secondary to the IFB.

TABLE 18.1 Commonly Seen Symptoms With Intravascular Foreign Body

Due to Arterial IFB	Due to Venous IFB
Claudication	Localized chest pain
Limb ischemia	Ventricular tachycardia
Limb swelling	Pulmonary embolism

IFB, Intravascular foreign body.

INDICATIONS

- Prompt removal of an IFB is indicated when:
  - Patient is symptomatic.
  - There is concern for migration to the heart or pulmonary arteries (typical of venous IFBs).
  - There is concern for arterial occlusion.

CONTRAINDICATIONS

- Each patient with an IFB must be approached on a case-by-case basis.
  - Leaving an IFB in situ in an asymptomatic patient is a viable option and must be considered, especially in a terminally ill patient with a clinically insignificant IFB.
- Absolute contraindications:
  - Large IFBs that cannot be retrieved endovascularly
  - Unstable patients with possible impending clinical deterioration
- Relative contraindications:
  - Difficult-to-access IFB site
  - Vascular perforation secondary to the IFB

ANATOMY

- Because of the multitude of presentations, it is not feasible to isolate any given aspect of anatomy for a comprehensive discussion. A general understanding of vascular anatomy and vessel distribution is essential to guiding therapy.
- One must consider the location of an IFB relative to potential sites of embolization and know the vascular pathway of each potential course of embolization.
- Also important is to relate the anatomy of the vascular access site to the site of the foreign body as this will dictate the geographic path of the retrieval process.

EQUIPMENT

- Basic angiography set
- 8-Fr sheath
- 0.035-in hydrophilic guidewire
- 5-Fr guide catheter
- Snare (Fig. 18.1)
  - Amplatz gooseneck snare
  - En Snare
  - Double-looped guidewire within catheter snare
  - Basket snare
- Flexible grasping forceps

PROCEDURAL STEPS

Preprocedural

- Review of previous imaging is paramount to the planning and success of any IFB retrieval (Figs. 18.2 and 18.3).

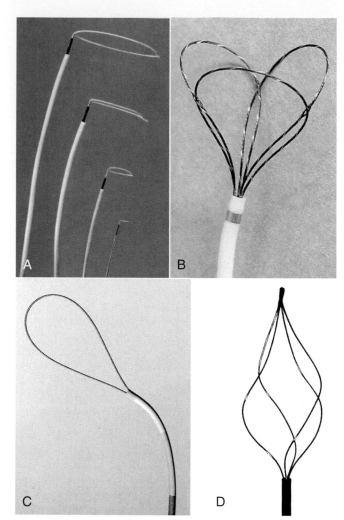

Fig. 18.1 Different Snare Retrieval Devices. (A) Amplatz gooseneck snares. (B) En Snare. (C) Snare formed by looping a guidewire through a catheter. (D) Basket. (A, ©2018 Medtronic. All rights reserved. Used with the permission of Medtronic.; B, courtesy Merit Medical Systems Inc., South Jordan, Utah; C and D from Kaufman JA: *Vascular and Interventional Radiology: The Requisites.* Philadelphia: Elsevier; 2014, Figure 4-51.)

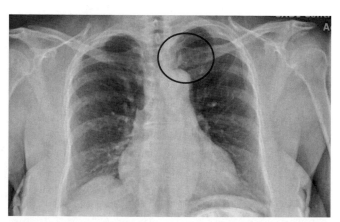

Fig. 18.2 Anteroposterior Chest X-ray Displaying a Retained Portion of Guidewire in the Left Chest. Intravascular guidewire (circle) is faintly visualized. (Reused with permission from Segal M, Krauthamer A, Hall B, et al. Endovascular retrieval of foreign body in persistent left-sided superior vena cava. *Radiology Case Reports.* 2017;12[4]:768–771.)

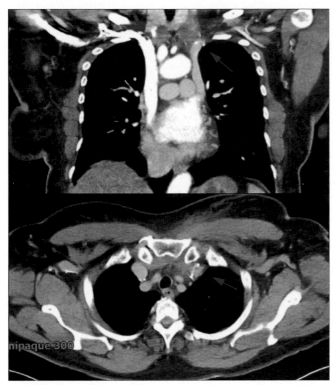

Fig. 18.3 Foreign Body in the Left Brachiocephalic Vein. Computed tomography (CT) chest with intravenous contrast with 3-mm helical axial imaging and coronal reformation displaying rudimentary left superior vena cava (SVC) with retained guidewire at the left brachiobasilic junction (arrow). (Reused with permission from Segal M, Krauthamer A, Hall B, et al. Endovascular retrieval of foreign body in persistent left-sided superior vena cava. *Radiology Case Reports.* 2017;12[4]: 768–771.)

- Open discussion with anesthesia personnel is also essential to ensure appropriate level of patient sedation.
- Fully informed consent should be acquired from the patient/DPOA where all potential sequences of events, complications, risks, benefits, and alternatives are outlined thoroughly.

Procedural Steps

1. Vascular access is achieved usually via the common femoral artery, common femoral vein, or the jugular veins with an 18-gauge needle.
2. A 0.035-inch access microwire is advanced, and the needle is removed, establishing the Seldinger technique.
3. An appropriately sized sheath that will be able to encompass the foreign body is implanted next. A common diameter is 8 to 10 Fr. At this point, the access wire can be switched for a hydrophobic guidewire.
4. A 6- to 7- Fr guiding catheter is introduced over the wire.
5. Through this guidecath, an extraction device, most commonly a loop snare (Amplatz gooseneck), is introduced and positioned adjacent to the foreign body.
6. The guidewire can be removed, and the snare is manipulated to grasp the foreign body (Fig. 18.4A).
7. At this point, the snare is retracted and the foreign body removed while maintaining tension on the loop snare (see Fig. 18.4B).
   a. If the loop snare is unsuccessful in grasping the foreign body, triple-loop snares (EN Snare) or Dormia baskets (Gemini) have been shown to be effective in these instances. As a last resort, flexible grasping forceps (Cook Urological) or tip-deflecting wires have also been shown to be useful adjuncts.

TREATMENT ALTERNATIVES

- Surgical retrieval
  - Accounts for 6% to 10% of IFB cases
  - Often uses invasive and open procedures to remove the foreign body.
  - Considered only when endovascular removal attempts have failed or foreign bodies have been otherwise deemed irretrievable.

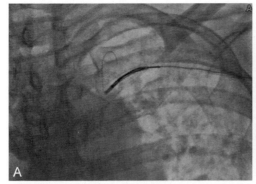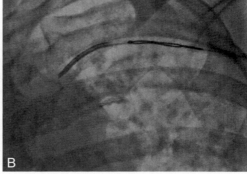

Fig. 18.4 Fluoroscopic imaging of endovascular retrieval of a foreign body located in a persistent left superior vena cava using a 15-mm Amplatz Gooseneck snare and a 6-Fr Multipurpose-A (MPA) catheter (Covidien Medtronic HQ, Minneapolis, MN). Imaging displays initial snare of the foreign body (A) and the foreign body being removed with no retained element (B). (Reused with permission from Segal M, Krauthamer A, Hall B, et al. Endovascular retrieval of foreign body in persistent left-sided superior vena cava. *Radiology Case Reports.* 2017;12[4]:768–771.)

- No intervention
  - Close observation and follow-up with no attempt at retrieval, typically in cases where a procedure would be deemed excessively risky and potentially fruitless
  - This option is most common in moribund patients and the terminally ill.

COMPLICATIONS

- Complications largely depend on the location of the IFB and the strategy undertaken to retrieve it.
  - This can include arrhythmias, valvular/myocardial damage, endocarditis, thrombophlebitis, sepsis, and ischemia.
  - Thromboembolism in association with the indwelling foreign body or prolonged procedure time can be seen.
  - Perforation or vessel wall damage secondary to endovascular manipulation is possible.
  - A worrisome potential is the distal embolization of the foreign body, especially to a location that makes it irretrievable endovascularly.

- Typical access site–related complications:
  - Access site hematoma is the most common complication overall.

🏠 TAKE-HOME POINTS

- Intravascular foreign bodies can be subdivided into arterial or venous IFBs. Arterial IFBs travel distally and can cause arterial occlusion while venous IFBs travel centrally and can lead to pulmonary emboli.
- When facing an IFB, the first question to answer is whether the IFB merits removal. IFBs that are causing symptoms or are at high risk for causing arterial occlusion/PE need to be retrieved promptly. Asymptomatic or morbidly ill patients may simply be observed.
- Foreign body retrieval relies on many of the basic needles, catheters, and guidewires used in general practice. Special snares are the only equipment unique to this procedure.
- The complication rate of IFB retrieval is very low, with the most common complication being access-site hematoma. Current literature includes several reports of 0% complication rate. Severe but rare complications include sepsis and arrhythmia.

REVIEW QUESTIONS

1. An absolute indication for IFB retrieval includes:
   a. The IFB is in the venous system
   b. The IFB is in the arterial system
   c. Patient is symptomatic
   d. Patient is terminal
   e. IFBs are always removed
2. Which of the following are possible complications of IFBs?
   a. Sepsis
   b. Distal embolization
   c. Arrhythmia
   d. Vessel perforation
   e. All of the above
3. Which part of the equipment set is unique to foreign body retrieval?
   a. 18-gauge needle
   b. IVC filter
   c. Dormia basket
   d. Fogarty catheter
   e. C-arm

SUGGESTED READINGS

Motta Leal Filho JM, et al. Endovascular techniques and procedures, methods for removal of intravascular foreign bodies. *Rev Bras Cir Cardiovasc.* 2010;25(2):202–208.

Schechter MA, O'Brien PJ, Cox MW. Retrieval of iatrogenic intravascular foreign bodies. *J Vasc Surg.* 2013;57(1):276–281.

Woodhouse JB, Uberoi R. Techniques for intravascular foreign body retrieval. *Cardiovasc Intervent Radiol.* 2013;36:888–897.

Inferior Vena Cava Filter

Jeffrey H. Savin, Andrew Kesselman, Ryan M. Kiefer, Andrew S. Niekamp, Michael A. Savin

CASE PRESENTATION

A 56-year-old male suffers bilateral femur fractures following a motor vehicle accident. Open reduction internal fixation is scheduled for tomorrow. The trauma team cannot anticoagulate the patient due to the planned operation, so interventional radiology places a retrievable inferior vena cava (IVC) filter. Three months later, the patient is ambulating and returns to the interventional radiology clinic to discuss IVC filter retrieval.

- The incidence of pulmonary embolism in the United States is about 600,000 per year.
- The mortality of an untreated pulmonary embolus is between 18% and 38%.
- Anticoagulation is the first-line treatment for the prevention of pulmonary emboli (PE).
  - IVC filters are used to prevent PE in those who have recurrent PE on therapeutic anticoagulation or in whom anticoagulation is contraindicated.
- History of IVC filter innovation
  - In 1893, IVC ligation was first performed to prevent pulmonary emboli.
  - In 1943, the first modern reports of IVC ligation showed that IVC thrombosis was a frequent complication of this operation.
  - In 1957, IVC fenestration was first used to prevent PE. Sutures were initially used, followed by clips in 1959 and staples in 1964. IVC thrombosis continued to be an issue.
  - In 1960, the first (and only) randomized control trial conducted in 35 patients positively demonstrated that anticoagulation decreased the risk of recurrent PE.
  - In 1968, the first percutaneous IVC interruption with a Mobin-Uddin umbrella was performed. This was a device with multiple holes placed in the IVC in an attempt to prevent IVC occlusion.
  - In 1969, a spring-like filtration device was used.
  - In 1972, the Greenfield IVC filter was introduced. This would become the predecessor of the modern-day filter.
  - In 2003, the first retrievable IVC filter was approved by the US Food and Drug Administration (FDA).

INDICATIONS

- The following indications apply to all filter types; however, retrievable filters should be considered when the filter is only needed for a short-term basis (up to 1 year).

> ### ▶ CLINICAL POINT
>
> A large prospective 20-year follow-up study of the Greenfield filter found the rate of recurrent PE to be 4%, the rate of caval occlusion to be 4%, and that significant filter movement did not occur.

Indications for Placement

- Patients with **venous thromboembolic disease** (VTE = PE and/or DVT) and one of the following:
  - Absolute or relative contraindication to anticoagulation
  - Complication from anticoagulation
  - Failure of anticoagulation
    - Recurrent PE despite adequate therapy
    - Propagation/progression of deep venous thrombosis (DVT) during therapeutic anticoagulation
  - Inability to achieve or maintain adequate anticoagulation
  - Limited pulmonary reserve or severe cardiopulmonary disease and residual DVT
  - Free-floating iliofemoral or IVC thrombus
- **Prophylactic placement** in patients who are at high risk for developing thromboembolic disease but who cannot be anticoagulated. Such situations include:
  - Severe trauma
    - Closed head or spinal cord injury
    - Multiple long bone or pelvic fractures
  - Prophylaxis prior to surgery

Indications for Retrieval

- Adequate primary (pharmacologic) therapy of VTE
- Patient no longer at risk for developing a PE
- Filter is the source of major morbidity that would be relieved by retrieval (e.g., unmanageable pain secondary to limb perforation)
- Filter is no longer protective as a result of a change in position or loss of structural integrity

CONTRAINDICATIONS

Contraindications for Placement

- Absolute contraindications:
  - Complete IVC thrombosis
  - Inability to gain access or image during filter placement
  - IVC too large to accommodate a filter (Bird's Nest filter can be placed in IVCs up to 40 mm in size)
  - Severe uncorrectable allergy to a filter component
- Relative contraindications:
  - Severe uncorrectable coagulopathy
  - Bacteremia or untreated infection

Contraindications for Retrieval

- Continued indication for vena caval filtration
- Significant retained thrombus within the filter
- Anticipated return to a high-risk state for developing PE in the future
- Life expectancy of less than 6 months
- Lack of vascular access for retrieval

EQUIPMENT

Placement Equipment

- Basic angiography set
- 5-Fr sheath
- Pigtail catheter (marked pigtail can help determine IVC width)
- Guidewire
- Filter (Figs. 19.1 and 19.2)
  - Filter kit typically contains the IVC filter, sheath, loading cartridge, and pusher.

Retrieval Equipment

- Basic angiography set, introducer needle, dilator, and coaxial retrieval sheath system
- Retrieval options include:
  - Retrieval snare
  - Snare-cone
  - In expected difficult/complex retrieval cases:

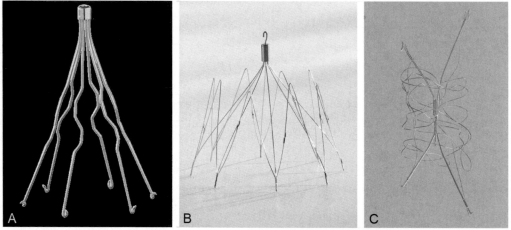

Fig. 19.1 Permanent Inferior Vena Cava Filters. (A) Greenfield™ Stainless Steel Vena Cava Filter. (Courtesy of Boston Scientific.) (B) VenaTech© Convertible™. (Courtesy B. Braun Interventional Systems Inc.) (C) Bird's Nest® Vena Cava Filter. (The use of any of the retrieval options other than the "retrieval snare" is not promoted or marketed by Cook Medical for use with our devices shown here).

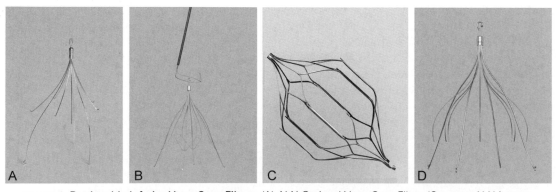

Fig. 19.2 Retrievable Inferior Vena Cava Filters. (A) ALN Optional Vena Cava Filter. (Courtesy ALN International Inc.) (B) Günther Tulip® Vena Cava Filter. (The use of any of the retrieval options other than the "retrieval snare" are not promoted or marketed by Cook Medical for use with our devices shown here) (C) OPTEASE® Vena Cava Filter. (Courtesy Cordis.) (D) Celect™ Platinum Vena Cava Filter. (The use of any of the retrieval options other than the "retrieval snare" is not promoted or marketed by Cook Medical for use with our devices shown here.)

- Rigid endobronchial forceps
- Laser-assisted system (ex. CVX-300 excimer XeCl laser system)

ANATOMY

- Blood from the lower extremities returns to the heart via the **inferior vena cava**, the largest vein in the body. Blood goes to the right atrium of the heart, where it is pumped into the right ventricle and then into the pulmonary arteries. The main pulmonary artery trunk divides into the left and right pulmonary arteries, which further divide into segmental and subsegmental arteries throughout the lungs. Lower extremity DVTs can propagate along this pathway before depositing in the lungs, causing a PE.
- The IVC is the favored site of filtration, given ease of access, physical properties (long and straight), and low venous blood pressure, which makes filter migration and displacement less likely.
- The average width of the IVC is 19 to 20 mm, and most filters are approved for use in IVCs up to 28 to 30 mm in size.
- In 2% to 3% of patients, the width is greater than 28 mm, termed *mega cava*. This can be secondary to elevated right heart pressure leading to backup in and distention of the IVC. The Bird's Nest filter can be used in IVCs up to 40 mm in size. Alternatively, filters may be placed in the bilateral common iliac arteries.
- Anatomic variants involving the IVC are rare but can sometimes necessitate altering the treatment approach. Variants include:
  - Left-sided IVC, which is found in less than 1% of patients
  - **Duplicated IVC**, found in 1% of patients
    - May require placing a filter in each IVC
  - **Circumaortic renal vein**, found in up to 11% of patients
    - Important to be aware of this variant, as the retro-aortic vein drains into the IVC lower than it typically does, usually at the L3 level.

PROCEDURAL STEPS

Inferior Vena Cava Placement

1. Access either the right internal jugular (IJ) or common femoral veins (FV) via the Seldinger technique.
   a. Advantages of femoral access:
      i. Air embolus is less likely than with jugular access
      ii. Does not require passage through the right atrium, decreasing the risk of arrhythmia
      iii. Less chance of misplacement into a gonadal vein
   b. Advantages of jugular access:
      i. Avoids the possibility that an iliofemoral thrombus is obstructing access into the IVC
      ii. Less risk of postinsertion thrombosis
2. Perform an IVC venogram to determine caval patency and size and identify congenital variants (Fig. 19.3).

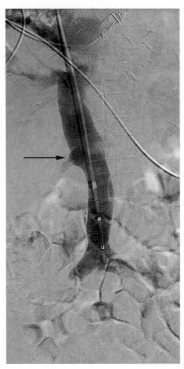

Fig. 19.3 Normal Inferior Vena Cava Venogram. Access was via the right internal jugular vein, so that a temporary central line could be placed concurrently. Injection into the distal abdominal aorta. The lowest renal vein was identified *(arrow)*. (Courtesy Justin Shafa, MD.)

   a. For the rare mega cava, a Bird's Nest filter may be placed or filters may be placed in the bilateral common iliac veins.
   b. For a circumaortic renal left renal vein, the filter should be placed below this vein.
   c. For duplicated IVC, filters may be placed in both IVCs.
3. . Position a pigtail catheter at the confluence of the common iliac veins for cavography. A marked pigtail may be used to measure IVC width.
4. Cavography can be performed using digital subtraction angiography at 4 to 6 frames per second using an injection rate of iodinated contrast at 15 to 20 mL/s for 2 seconds.
5. Reinsert a guidewire into the pigtail under fluoroscopic guidance, and remove the pigtail while keeping the guidewire in place.
6. Deploy the filter according to the manufacturer's instructions, usually over the guidewire. Proper filter location in the infrarenal IVC is vital.
   a. Ideally, the upper tip of the filter should be at the most inferior renal vein.
   b. Suprarenal IVC filter placement can be considered in situations where there is:
      i. Infrarenal thrombus preventing infrarenal filter placement
      ii. Thrombus extending from a previous infrarenal IVC filter
      iii. Extrinsic compression of the infrarenal IVC (e.g., large abdominal mass or pregnant patient)

iv. Gonadal vein thrombosis

v. Need to preserve surgical candidacy for patients being considered for operative IVC mobilization

7. Postdeployment venogram.

8. Equipment is removed, and pressure is held over the access site.

>> **CLINICAL POINT**

The filter is deployed at or below the lowest renal vein so that, in the uncommon event that the filter becomes occluded, renal vein blood flow will be preserved.

Filter Retrieval

- After placement of a retrievable IVC filter, routine monitoring and timely retrieval are pivotal aspects of patient care.

- For retrievable filters, the length of internal dwell time is directly related to the incidence of complications such as filter tilt, malposition, caval penetration, device fracture, and caval occlusion. This has spurred greater emphasis on filter retrieval as advocated by the American College of Radiology and the Society of Interventional Radiology.

- The vast majority of retrievable IVC filters are designed with a hook at the apex, making them amenable to retrieval via jugular access. However, even filters without hooks can be removed with a variety of methods as described later.

Standard Method

1. After standard right IJ access, short sheath insertion, and wire/catheter placement beyond the IVC filter, an appropriate snare device is selected. A snare-cone can be used to engage the filter apex when a hook is absent.

2. The hook at the apex of the IVC filter is snared (Fig. 19.4).

3. A telescoping sheath is then advanced over the filter to collapse it.

4. The entire filter is then removed *en bloc* from the body.

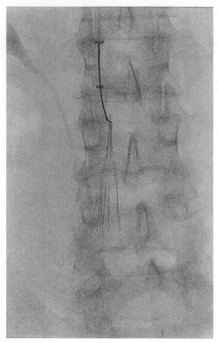

Fig. 19.4 Filter Retrieval. Hook of the filter is snared, and the snare is pulled back to provide slight tension, before the telescoping sheath can be advanced over the filter. (Courtesy Justin Shafa, MD.)

5. Equipment is removed, and pressure is held over the access site.

Advanced Retrieval Methods

- Filter position variations (secondary to caval penetration, malposition, and tilt) may render the standard retrieval technique ineffective. In these cases, advanced techniques have been developed that have an overall retrieval rate of greater than 95%.

- Filter realignment and repositioning
  - Severely tilted or malpositioned filters can be repositioned using stiff wires or balloons (Fig. 19.5).

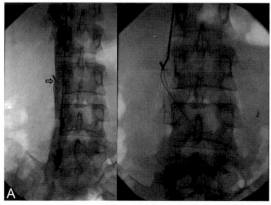
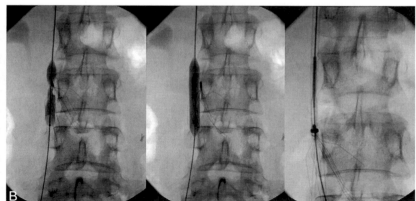

Fig. 19.5 (A) Venogram shows a small opening *(arrow)* between the filter tip and inferior vena cava wall that was cannulated with a wire. (B) Balloon angioplasty with a 8 × 30-mm Dorado balloon successfully displaced the filter from the wall, allowing for subsequent removal via the standard techniques. (Reused with permission from Lynch FC. Balloon-assisted removal of tilted inferior vena cava filters with embedded tips. *J Vasc Intervent Radiol.* 2009;20(9):1210–1214; Elsevier, Fig. 1BC.)

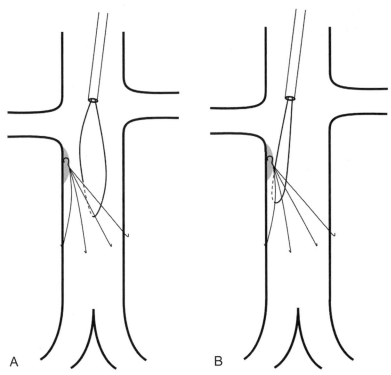

Fig. 19.6 Schematic representation of an inferior vena cava (IVC) containing a tilted conical-type filter with an embedded hook secondary to a fibrous capsule *(gray shading)*. Comparison of the (A) loop-snare technique with the wire between the filter struts with the (B) hangman technique with the wire between the filter neck and IVC wall just beneath the embedded hook. (From Al-Hakim R, McWilliams JP, Derry W, et al. The hangman technique: a modified loop-snare technique for the retrieval of inferior vena cava filters with embedded hooks. *J Vasc Interv Radiol.* 2015;26:107–110, Fig. 1.)

- Repositioning can allow for successful removal of the filter with the traditional snare technique.
- **Loop-snare technique** (Fig. 19.6A)
  - In this technique, a guidewire is first passed beyond the filter apex from a transjugular approach. The wire is then redirected cephalad by using a curved catheter. The free end of the wire is grasped by a snare and pulled out the jugular vein sheath so that both ends of the wire exit the patient with the wire looped around the filter apex. A telescoping sheath is then inserted over both ends of wire and over the filter, and the system is removed.
- **Hangman technique** (Fig. 19.6B)
  - A popular method for advanced filter retrieval, this is a slight modification of the loop-snare technique. Rather than creating a loop around the filter legs, the loop-snare creates a wire loop between the filter neck and IVC wall (Fig. 19.7). This technique may fail in cases with an embedded hook.
- Forceps retrieval
  - Endobronchial forceps may be utilized when traditional snares fail in order to get a firmer grasp of the filter apex (Fig. 19.8).
- Excimer laser sheath (Fig. 19.9)

- The filter apex is engaged utilizing a standard snare. The laser sheath is then used to free the embedded portions of the filter from the caval wall, allowing collapse and retrieval.

ALTERNATIVE TREATMENTS

- Pharmacologic anticoagulation
  - First-line therapy for VTE prevention and, if a DVT is already present, treatment
    - Over the past few decades, options were heparin, warfarin, Lovenox, and their analogs.
    - Novel oral anticoagulation agents have been developed, including:
      - Dabigatran (Pradaxa)
      - Rivaroxaban (Xarelto)
      - Apixaban (Eliquis)
  - For patients who cannot receive anticoagulation, there are few alternatives to IVC filter placement.
- Nonpharmacologic prophylaxis
  - Compression stockings and sequential compression devices (SCDs)

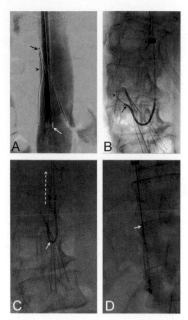

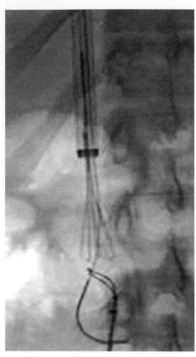

Fig. 19.7 (A) Venogram obtained before retrieval via a 14-F sheath *(white arrow)* demonstrated an Option retrievable filter with significant lateral tilt and an embedded filter hook *(black arrow)*. Note the contrast opacified space between the filter neck and inferior vena cava (IVC) wall *(arrowhead)*. (B) A reverse curve catheter was placed adjacent to the filter with the leading end at the level of the filter neck *(arrow)*, and an angled 0.035-inch Glidewire was directed between the filter neck and IVC wall *(arrowhead)*. (C) The leading end of the wire was snared and withdrawn through the sheath, creating a loop around the filter neck *(solid arrow)*. The reverse curve catheter was withdrawn, and tension was applied cranially *(dashed arrow)*. (C) The embedded hook was released and snared *(arrow)*, followed by sheathing of the filter for removal. (From Al-Hakim R, McWilliams JP, Derry W, et al. The hangman technique: a modified loop snare technique for the retrieval of inferior vena cava filters with embedded hooks. *J Vasc Interv Radiol.* 2015;26:107–110, Fig. 2.)

Fig. 19.9 The laser sheath is then used to free the embedded portions of the filter from the caval wall, allowing collapse and retrieval. (Courtesy Andrew Niekamp.)

- Patient mobilization is also a key aspect of VTE prevention, as this decreases venous stasis, one of Virchow's triad.
- Surgical and endovascular treatment
  - Massive or submassive life-threatening acute PEs (such as a saddle embolus) can be treated with surgical thrombectomy/embolectomy or endovascular thrombectomy/thrombolysis.
  - There are several different types of pharmacomechanical thrombolysis/thrombectomy methods available to interventionalists, including:
    - Conventional thrombolysis
    - Ultrasound-accelerated thrombolysis
    - Suction/aspiration thrombectomy
    - Rheolytic thrombectomy
    - Mechanical thrombectomy

COMPLICATIONS

- While the use of IVC filters is generally safe, complications may occur.
- As with any endovascular procedure, the general risks of venous access and endovascular intervention apply, including bleeding, hematoma, AV fistula, infection, allergic reaction to contrast, and renal toxicity from contrast, among others.
- Potential long-term complications from having a filter include:
  - IVC thrombosis
  - Filter migration (Figs. 19.10–19.12)

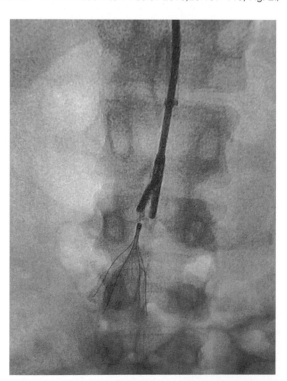

Fig. 19.8 Endobronchial Forceps During Complicated Inferior Vena Cava Filter Retrieval. (Courtesy James Walsh, MD, and Andrew Kesselman, MD, Brooklyn, NY.)

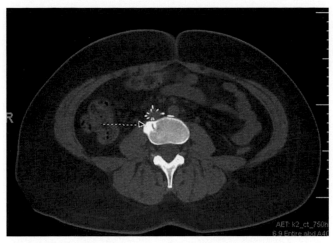

Fig. 19.10 Leftward-directed study struts project posterior to the abdominal aorta at the level of the bifurcation. (Courtesy Andrew Niekamp.)

- Filter fracture
- IVC perforation, which is usually asymptomatic but can potentially cause aortic injury, small bowel injury, adhesions, bowel obstruction, and peritonitis
- Filter tilt
- Permanent and retrievable filters are both approved for permanent use. However, the complication rate for retrievable filters is higher than it is with permanent filters. Therefore, if a filter is not expected to be retrieved at some point in the future, a permanent one should be placed.

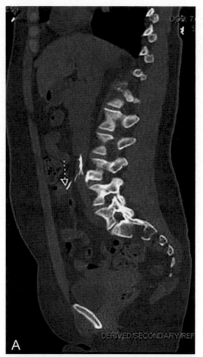

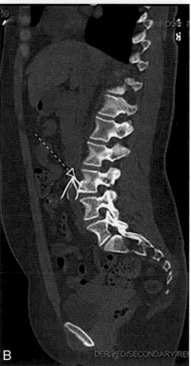

Fig. 19.11 (A,B) Anterior prongs extend outside the inferior vena cava wall adjacent to a loop of small bowel with loss of the fat plane. This likely extends into the bowel wall; however, there is no surrounding inflammatory change or abnormal fluid collection. (Courtesy Andrew Niekamp.)

🏠 TAKE-HOME POINTS

- Inferior vena cava (IVC) filters are embolic protection devices for patients at risk for having a pulmonary embolus (PE) who cannot be anticoagulated or for whom anticoagulation has failed.
- Contraindications to filter placement are rare and include thrombosis of the IVC and the inability to access or image the IVC.
- IVC cavography is performed prior to filter placement to determine caval patency, size, and identify congenital variants. Anatomic variants can change the approach/location/number of filters placed.
- Retrievable IVC filters allow for protection from PE in patients who are only at temporary risk of having one. When no longer needed, filter removal should be performed to limit potential long-term complications.

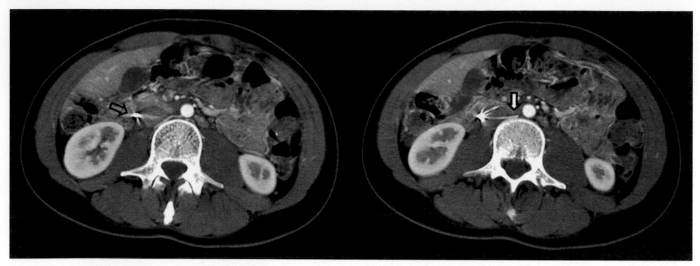

Fig. 19.12 Computed tomography performed 34 days after the prophylactic placement of a filter following multiple long bone fractures shows the filter apex appearing to be outside the cava *(open arrow)* and several filter legs perforating the cava medially *(solid arrow)*. (Reused with permission from Lynch FC. Balloon-assisted removal of tilted inferior vena cava filters with embedded tips. *J Vasc Intervent Radiol.* 2009;20(9):1210–1214, Fig. 1A.)

REVIEW QUESTIONS

1. Which of the following filter types is not designed to be retrievable?
   a. Celect
   b. Option
   c. Greenfield
   d. Tulip

2. Which of the following statements about IVC filters is true?
   a. IVC filters are only indicated for permanent filtration
   b. IVC filters are ideally placed superior to the renal veins
   c. Bird's Nest filters are only indicated with caval diameters <28 mm
   d. IVC filter retrieval is contraindicated if significant thrombus exists within the filter

3. Which of the following is an advantage of jugular access for IVC filter placement?
   a. Decreased risk of arrhythmia
   b. Decreased risk of air embolus
   c. Decreased risk of thrombosis
   d. Decreased risk of misplacement

SUGGESTED READINGS

Angel LF, Tapson V, Galgon RE, et al. Systematic review of the use of retrievable inferior vena cava filters. *J Vasc Interv Radiol.* 2011;22(11):1522–1530. e3.

Caplin DM, Nikolic B, Kalva SP, et al. Quality improvement guidelines for the performance of inferior vena cava filter placement for the prevention of pulmonary embolism. *J Vasc Interv Radiol.* 2011;22(11):1499–1506. https://doi.org/10.1016/j.jvir.2011.07.012.

Decousus H, Leizorovicz A, Parent F, et al. A clinical trial of vena caval filters in the prevention of pulmonary embolism in patients with proximal deep-vein thrombosis. *N Engl J Med.* 1998;338(7):409–416.

Greenfield LJ, McCurdy JR, Brown PP, et al. A new intracaval filter permitting continued flow and resolution of emboli. *Surgery* 1972;73:599–606.

Greenfield LJ, Proctor MC. Twenty-year clinical experience with the Greenfield Filter. *Cardiovas Surg.* 1995;3:199–205.

Kuo WT, Cupp JS. The excimer laser sheath technique for embedded inferior vena cava filter removal. *JVIR* 2010;21:1896–1899.

Mismetti P, Laporte S, Pellerin O, et al. Effect of a retrievable inferior vena cava filter plus anticoagulation vs anticoagulation alone on risk of recurrent pulmonary embolism: a randomized clinical trial. *JAMA.* 2015;313(16):1627–1635. https://doi.org/10.1001/jama.2015.3780.

Niekamp A, Majdalany B, Dittmar K. *Advanced Retrieval Techniques for Inferior Vena Cava Filters. American Roengten Ray Society.* Electronic Educational Exhibit: Toronto, Canada; 2015.

Savin MA, Shlansky-Goldberg RD. Greenfield filter fixation in large venae cavae. *JVIR* 1998;9:75–80.

Stavropoulos SW, Ge BH, Mondschein JI, et al. Retrieval of tip-embedded inferior vena cava filters by using the endobronchial forceps technique: experience at a single institution. *Radiology* 2015;275:900–907.

Peripheral Arterial Disease

Brandon P. Olivieri, Stephen Seedial, Larry E. Mathias, Keith Pereira

CASE PRESENTATION

A 73-year-old male with a history of diabetes, hypertension, hyperlipidemia, and 60-pack-year smoking history presents with severe lifestyle-limiting lower thigh and calf claudication after ambulating only one block with symptoms refractory to maximum medical therapy. Ankle-brachial indices (ABI), pulse volume recordings, and ultrasound examination demonstrate a suspected high-grade right superficial femoral artery stenosis. Because of the ongoing symptoms despite adherence to maximal medical therapy, the decision is made to revascularize.

- In 1964, Charles Dotter performed the first percutaneous angioplasty by dilating a superficial femoral artery stenosis with coaxial catheters. In 1969, he introduced the transluminally placed "coil spring endarterial tube graft," initiating the era of endovascular stenting.
- In 1974, German cardiologist Andreas Grüntzig introduced the first balloon catheter.
- In 1985, Julio Palmaz introduced his balloon-expandable stent.
- The Centers for Disease Control and Prevention (CDC) estimates that there are approximately 8 million people with **peripheral artery disease (PAD)/critical limb ischemia (CLI)** in the United States, with 12% to 20% of those age 60 or older.

LITERATURE REVIEW

Hirsch 2001, PARTNERS (Peripheral Artery Disease [PAD] Awareness, Risk, and Treatment: New Resources for Survival) study
- 6979 patients age 70 and older (or 50–69 with a smoking history) were screened for PAD. Ankle-brachial indices (ABI) of ≤0.9, documented PAD history, or history of lower extremity revascularization were considered diagnostic of PAD.
    - 29% (1865 patients) were diagnosed with PAD.
        - 55% of these diagnoses were new diagnoses of PAD alone.
        - 35% of these diagnoses were newly diagnosed PAD and coronary artery disease (CAD).
- In those patients with a documented history consistent with PAD, only 83% of them and 49% of their primary care doctors were aware of the PAD diagnosis.
- This suggests that, despite its high prevalence, PAD may be underdiagnosed and undertreated due to poor patient and physician awareness.

CLINICAL PRESENTATION

- Clinical presentation of PAD (Table 20.1)
    - 20% to 50% of patients are asymptomatic at presentation, with functional impairment only on diagnostic testing.
    - 10% to 35% initially present with lower extremity claudication. Claudication is reproducible, occurring after a definite distance traveled/level of exertion and relieved after rest. Caused by reversible muscle ischemia, claudication symptoms include:
        - Pain
        - Discomfort
        - Aching
        - Heaviness
        - Fatigue
        - Tightness/cramping
        - Burning
    - 40% to 50% of patients present with atypical leg pain, broadly defined as lower extremity discomfort with exertion that is not consistent and may require prolonged rest for recovery.
    - 1% to 2% of patients presents with critical limb ischemia. This includes:
        - Pain at rest (Rutherford Class 4)
        - Ischemic ulceration (Rutherford Class 5)
        - Gangrene (Rutherford Class 6)

RISK FACTORS

- Risk factors in the development of PAD (Fig. 20.1) are multifactorial.
    - Atherosclerosis is a systemic disease process, and cardiovascular risk factor modification is of paramount importance in patients with PAD and CLI (Fig. 20.2). The majority of deaths in patients with PAD and CLI are from cardiovascular disease.
    - Patients with PAD have a 15% to 30% mortality rate at 5-year follow-up; 75% of deaths can be attributed to cardiovascular disease (myocardial infarction [MI] and stroke).
    - 25% of patients with CLI will die of cardiovascular disease within 1 year.

TABLE 20.1　Rutherford-Baker and Fontaine Classification of Peripheral Arterial Disease Severity

Symptom	Rutherford-Baker Classification	Fontaine Classification
Asymptomatic	Stage 0	Stage I
Mild claudication	Stage 1	Stage IIA (symptoms with >200 m walking)
Moderate claudication	Stage 2	Stage IIB (symptoms with <200 m walking)
Severe claudication	Stage 3	
Rest pain	Stage 4	Stage III
Ischemic ulceration	Stage 5	Stage IV
Severe ischemic ulceration or gangrene	Stage 6	

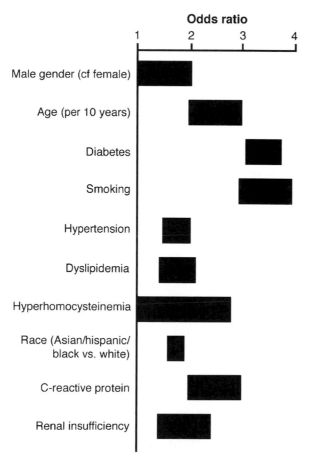

Fig. 20.1 Approximate range of odds ratios for risk factors for symptomatic peripheral arterial disease. (Reused with permission from Norgren L, Hiatt WR, Dormandy JA, et al. Fowkes. Inter-Society Consensus for the Management of Peripheral Arterial Disease (TASC II). *J Vasc Surg.* 2007;45(1 suppl):S5–S67, FA2.)

MANAGEMENT PRINCIPLES

- Principles behind PAD/CLI treatment are to decrease all-cause cardiovascular morbidity and mortality and offer simultaneous improvement in quality of life.
- For PAD, the goal is to treat occlusive/subocclusive disease for long-term patency and prevent progression to limb ischemia.
- For CLI, the goal is to prevent limb loss/major amputation and improve flow of nutrient-rich blood to:
  - Promote healing of either existing wounds (Rutherford 5 and 6)
  - Increase the chance of healing after surgical debridement and/or minor amputation
- Reduce **cardiovascular risk factors**—namely, by counseling on smoking cessation, promoting dietary changes, and supervising an exercise regimen.
  - Smoking is the strongest risk factor for progression of PAD, promotes disease progression, reduces revascularization patency rates, and increases amputation rates.
  - Exercise should be initiated for all symptomatic patients. It increases blood flow, endothelial response, and angiogenesis and reduces local inflammation.
  - If the patient has diabetes, attain goal of hemoglobin A1C < 7.0.

Medical Management (Table 20.2)

- Lipid-lowering high-dose statin therapy
  - Goal LDL < 70 mg/dL
  - Benefits include slowing disease progression, increasing activity tolerance, reducing systemic cardiovascular events, and lowering amputation rate.
  - Mechanism of action involves reducing inflammation, stabilizing plaque, improving endothelial function, and possibly supporting pro-angiogenic effects.
- Antiplatelet therapy (aspirin, clopidogrel [Plavix], ticlopidine)
  - Benefits include decreased risk of MI, cerebrovascular accident (CVA), and vascular death.
- Antihypertensives
  - Goal BP <140/90 in non-diabetics and <130/80 in diabetics
  - Angiotensin Converting Enzyme (ACE) inhibitor is the favored initial treatment. It reduces the risk of MI, CVA, and cardiovascular death in patients with PAD.
  - β-blockers offer cardioprotective effects.
- Anti-claudication medication
  - Cilostazol
    - Benefits include increased exercise tolerance and decreased pain noted as early as 4 weeks post initiation.
    - Mechanism of action: phosphodiesterase III inhibitor, antiplatelet effects, vasodilatory properties, and vascular smooth muscle cell inhibition.
  - Pentoxifylline—overall efficacy data is limited as is use

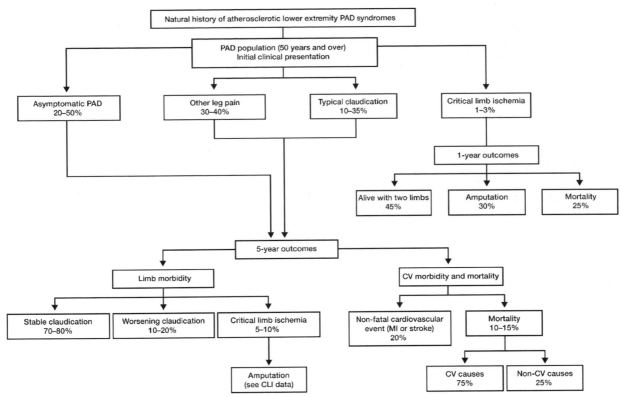

Fig. 20.2 Fate of the Claudicant Over 5 Years (adapted from ACC/AHA guidelines 5). *CLI*, Critical limb ische-mia; *CV*, cardiovascular; *MI*, myocardial infarction; *PAD*, peripheral arterial disease. (Reused with permission from Hirsch AT, et al. *J Am Coll Cardiol*. 2006;47:1239–1312.)

TABLE 20.2 Medical Management of Claudication/Peripheral Arterial Disease

Treatment	Benefit
Antiplatelet therapy	Confers no to little symptomatic improvement, but it decreases the risk of myocardial infarction, CVA, and vascular death in PAD/CLI patients.
Lipid-lowering therapy	Offers symptomatic improvement including disease regression, increased activity tolerance, reduction in cardiovascular events, and lower amputation rate. Current American College of Cardiology/American Heart Association (ACC-AHA) guidelines give a class 1a recommendation to the use of high-intensity statin therapy (40–80 mg atorvastatin PO or 20–40 mg rosuvastatin PO daily) in patients with PAD/CLI.
Diabetic glucose control	Aggressive control of blood glucose and maintaining hemoglobin A1C at 7.0 is recommended for all diabetic patients with the purpose of prevented progression of atherosclerotic disease. For some patients (elderly, those with comorbidities), less stringent goals may be discussed.
Smoking cessation	Smoking is the strongest risk factor for progression of PAD. It promotes disease progression, reduces revascularization patency rates, increases amputation rates, and increases cardiovascular death rates. Smoking cessation is associated with a more than one-third reduction in 10-year death rates. Consider referral to smoking cessation program and/or use of adjunctive pharmacotherapy.
Blood pressure management	ACE inhibitors reduce the risk of MI, CVA, and cardiovascular death in patients with PAD. β-Blocker use is encouraged due to cardioprotective effects.
Exercise regimen	Symptomatic improvement is achievable through several proposed mechanisms (increased blood flow, increased endothelial response, reduced local inflammation, increased angiogenesis). Referral to exercise therapy or initiation of an exercise regimen should be the initial treatment for all symptomatic patients.
Cilostazol	Phosphodiesterase III inhibitor that is direct vasodilator and has anti-platelet aggregation properties. Increased exercise tolerance and decreased pain can be seen as early as 4 weeks post initiation.
Pentoxifylline	Xanthine derivative (indirect phosphodiesterase inhibitor) whose use improves symptomatic disease but is not to replace a more definitive therapy. Slightly lesser effect than pentoxifylline.
Investigational drugs	Therapies currently under investigation include anti-chlamydial treatments, antioxidants (glutathione), bosentan, hemodilution, stem cell therapy, therapeutic angiogenesis, hyperbaric oxygen therapy, and spinal cord stimulation.

CLI, Critical limb ischemia; *CVA*, cerebrovascular accident; *MI*, myocardial infarction; *PAD*, peripheral arterial disease.

Surgical Treatment

- **Revascularization** is elective for claudication patients. Goal is to establish long-term patency either via endovascular means or by surgical bypass.
- CLI limb salvage
  - Goal is to rapidly establish arterial flow to the area of ulceration/gangrene in hopes of preventing limb amputation.
  - Improving perfusion to the lower leg is the primary factor affecting wound healing, preventing progression of ulceration, and avoiding limb loss.
  - If a patient is not suitable for revascularization secondary to comorbidities, medical management should be initiated, and amputation must be considered.

⊚ LITERATURE REVIEW

- A 2011 study of 1 million Medicare beneficiaries with critical limb ischemia (CLI) by Henry et al. showed that the act of performing an angiogram decreased the odds of amputation by 90%, but an angiogram was only performed in 27% of patients.
- A 2012 study of 20,464 CLI patients by Goodney et al. demonstrated that 54% of patients had no angiogram and 71% had no revascularization attempt prior to major amputation.
- The CLEVER (Claudication: Exercise Versus Endoluminal Revascularization) trial randomized peripheral artery disease patients to receive either supervised exercise, stenting, or optimal medical care. There was no significant difference in improvement in pain-free walking times between the groups randomized to supervised exercise or to stenting.

INDICATIONS

- For PAD, elective revascularization is an option if the disease interferes with activities of daily living despite adherence to optimal medical therapy.
- For CLI, urgent revascularization may be necessary if the patient has rest pain, ischemic ulcers, or gangrene corresponding to Rutherford class 4, 5, and 6, respectively.

CONTRAINDICATIONS

- Patients that will not necessarily benefit from limb salvage (i.e., contracted immobile nursing home patient)
- Stenosis that is not hemodynamically significant
- Any general contraindication to angiography or contrast use

ANATOMY (Figs. 20.3 and 20.4)

- Three distinct layers of the arterial wall:
  - *Intima* consisting of endothelial cells
  - *Media* made up of smooth muscle cells
  - *Adventitia* made up of collagen fibers and fibroblasts
- Common collateral pathways to the lower extremities in **aortoiliac occlusive disease**
  - Subclavian artery → internal mammary artery → superior epigastric artery → inferior epigastric artery → external iliac artery
  - Aorta → intercostal/lumbar arteries → superior gluteal artery → retrograde flow through the internal iliac artery → external iliac artery
  - Aorta → intercostal/lumbar arteries → deep circumflex iliac arteries → external iliac artery

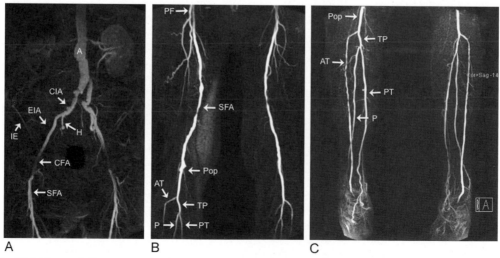

Fig. 20.3 Magnetic Resonance Angiogram of the Lower Extremity. Magnetic Resonance Angiogram of the (A) lower abdomen/pelvis, (B) thigh and popliteal, and (C) politeal and calf. *A*, Aorta; *AT*, anterior tibial artery; *CFA*, common femoral artery; *CIA*, common iliac artery; *EIA*, external iliac artery; *H*, hypogastric artery (internal iliac artery); *IE*, inferior epigastric artery; *P*, peroneal artery; *PF*, profunda femoris; *Pop*, popliteal artery; *PT*, posterior tibial artery; *SFA*, superficial femoral artery; *TP*, tibioperoneal trunk. (Courtesy Robert Beasley, MS, MD, FSIR.)

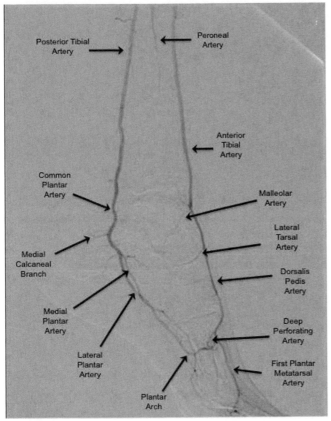

Fig. 20.4 Lateral oblique digital subtraction angiography image demonstrating the pedal arterial vasculature. (Courtesy Robert Beasley, MS, MD, FSIR.)

- Superior mesenteric artery (SMA) → marginal artery of Drummond + arc of Riolan → inferior mesenteric artery (IMA) → superior rectal artery → middle and inferior rectal arteries → retrograde flow through internal iliac artery → external iliac artery

- Revascularization strategy follows the geographic distribution of **angiosomes**.
  - An angiosome (Fig. 20.5) is a 3D anatomic unit of tissue fed by a source artery. It includes skin and the underlying subcutaneous tissue, fascia, fat, muscle, and bone.
  - *Anterior tibial artery angiosome* involves the anterior lower leg.
    - Dorsalis pedis branch feeds the dorsum of the foot.
  - *Posterior tibial artery angiosome* involves the posterior lower leg.
    - Calcaneal branch feeds the medial ankle.
    - Medial plantar artery branch feeds the medial plantar instep.
    - Lateral plantar artery branch feeds the lateral plantar forefoot.
  - *Peroneal artery angiosome* involves the anterior upper ankle.
    - Calcaneal branch feeds the lateral artery.
  - Direct revascularization of the artery supplying the angiosome has been shown to lead to better wound healing than indirect revascularization. That is, if a patient has a wound on the dorsal aspect of the forefoot, it would likely heal faster and more completely if the patient's occluded anterior tibial artery were to be revascularized rather than if the occluded peroneal artery were to be revascularized.

EQUIPMENT

Refer to *Basics* chapter for a thorough discussion on the wires, catheters, angioplasty balloons, stents, atherectomy devices, and thrombectomy devices commonly used in PAD/CLI.

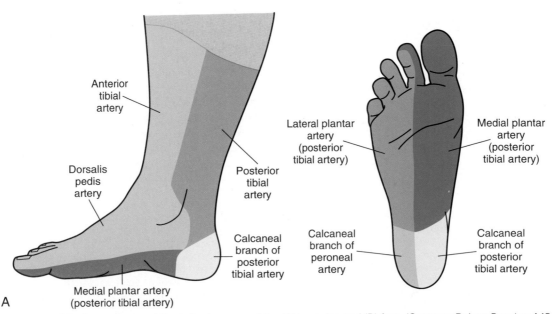

Fig. 20.5 Angiosomes of the Lower Leg and Foot. Angiosomes of the (A) lower leg and (B) foot. (Courtesy Robert Beasley, MS, MD, FSIR.)

PROCEDURAL STEPS

Diagnostic Aortoperipheral Angiogram

While the number of solely diagnostic angiographies has decreased due to the excellent anatomic preprocedural imaging with **computed tomography angiography (CTA)** and **magnetic resonance angiography (MRA)**, many physicians perform a full diagnostic angiogram just prior to undergoing intervention.

1. Standard retrograde access is obtained with the contralateral common femoral artery. Obtaining contralateral access facilitates treatment of the affected leg during the same session.
2. A diagnostic 4-Fr catheter (pigtail or Omni flush) is advanced over the wire into the abdominal aorta and formed just above the renal artery ostia (approximately at the level of the L1–L2 vertebral body).
3. Diagnostic catheter is spun to ensure no visceral arteries have been inadvertently selectively catheterized prior to power injection.
4. Images are taken of the abdominal aorta with power injector settings of 15 mL/s for 30 mL of total contrast.
5. Diagnostic catheter is retracted to approximately 2 cm above the aortic bifurcation.
6. Oblique runs of the iliac and common femoral arteries are performed with power injector settings of 7 mL/s for 14 mL of total contrast volume.
   a. 30-degree left anterior oblique (LAO) enhances visualization of the right common iliac and left common femoral bifurcations.
   b. 30-degree right anterior oblique (RAO) enhances visualization of the left common iliac and right common femoral bifurcations.
7. Lower extremity run-off images are performed in posterior-anterior (PA) projection using the bolus-chase method or serial descending overlapping runs to the level of the toes.
   a. Both PA and lateral views of the foot are necessary to completely depict the complex vascular anatomy of the foot.
8. Proceed to intervention (Fig. 20.6) or complete the diagnostic procedure.
   a. To complete the procedure, equipment is removed, pressure is applied for 15 minutes, and a sterile dressing is applied. Patient is monitored with bedrest for 4 hours.

Procedural Considerations

- **Angiography** obtained with selective catheterization of more distal vessels (catheter tip in popliteal artery) may demonstrate flow channels through stenoses or collateral pathways that are not seen on more proximal, non-selective injections.
- Patients with knee arthroplasties will need lateral views at the level of the knee to fully image the popliteal artery.
- To ensure complete visualization of the pedal vessels, Manzi et al. established the following criteria for correct foot positioning during pedal angiography:
  - The base of the first metatarsal should project outward from the base of the foot in lateral oblique view.
  - The first proximal metatarsal interspace should be seen on PA view.

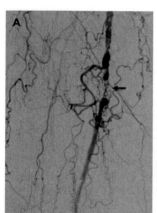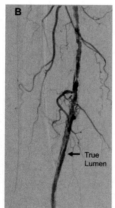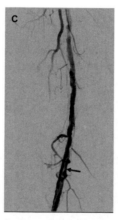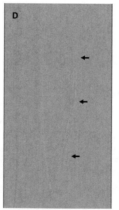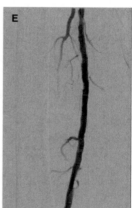

Fig. 20.6 (A) Digital subtraction angiography images of the distal superficial femoral artery revealed extensive calcified plaque with a short-segment complete occlusion with reconstitution distally by collateral vessels. The aortoiliac, common femoral (inflow), popliteal, and infrapopliteal arteries were patent (not shown). (B) Despite attempts to stay intraluminal, the guidewire tracked along a sub-intimal course around the occlusion before again re-entering the true lumen of the vessel. (C) After preparing the vessel lumen with balloon angioplasty with a 6 × 150-mm Ultraverse percutaneous balloon (Bard PV, Tempe, AZ) with excellent luminal gain, drug-coated balloon angioplasty was performed with a 6 × 100-mm Lutonix drug-coated balloon PTA catheter (Bard PV, Tempe, AZ) because of the strong patency results afforded by drug-coated technology. Unfortunately, post-angioplasty films revealed a flow-limiting dissection (black arrow = dissection flap). (D, E) To tack down the flow-limiting dissection flap and restore flow, stenting was performed with 6 × 150-mm LifeStents (Bard PV, Tempe, AZ) *(black arrows)* with excellent postprocedural results. The patient resumed his daily activities with no further claudicant symptoms. (Courtesy Robert Beasley, MS, MD, FSIR.)

- To correct for patient motion and thinning of the contrast bolus, digital postprocessing is usually necessary for adequate vessel visualization in pedal angiography.

TREATMENT ALTERNATIVES

- Although surgical bypass is a viable alternative to endovascular treatment strategies, an endovascular-first strategy is increasingly being adopted by interventionalists.
- The TransAtlantic Inter-Society Consensus for the Management of Peripheral Arterial Disease (TASC) sought to provide guidance on optimal revascularization strategies (endovascular versus surgical) through the creation of a classification system that ranges from least complex (TASC A—focal stenosis) to most complex (TASC D—diffuse and/or occlusive disease). TASC A lesions can be treated endovascularly and TASC D lesions usually with surgery.
- An endovascular approach is generally considered less morbid and has gained popularity as the primary management choice of even the most complex lesions (TASC C and D lesions).
- The BASIL (Bypass versus Angioplasty in Severe Ischemia of the Leg) trial compared endovascular to surgical revascularization.
  - Patients were randomized to either surgical infrainguinal saphenous vein bypass or balloon angioplasty.
    - Equivalent rates of amputation-free survival at 1 year (71% vs. 68%) and 3 years (52% vs. 57%)
    - Balloon angioplasty was associated with significantly lower morbidity and was less costly at 1-year follow-up when compared to the surgical bypass contingent.
    - Beyond 3 years, a trend emerged for better overall and amputation-free survival in the surgical bypass group.
  - A major limitation of the BASIL trial is that the angioplasty group was only treated with plain balloon angioplasty. Additional benefits that may have been conveyed with stenting and drug-eluting technology were thereby not seen.

COMPLICATIONS

Minor Complications

- Allergic reaction to injected contrast
- Leg swelling
- Lymphocele

Access Site Complications

- Hematoma occurs in 1% to 3% of causes. Causes include:
  - Inadequate compression of an arterial puncture site below the femoral head (inadequate compression)
  - Closure device failure (secondary to calcified vessels, maldeployment)

- May need surgery fixation if there is continued enlargement or signs of femoral nerve compression.
- Pseudoaneurysms occur in less than 1% of cases.
  - Small pseudoaneurysms can be followed up with ultrasound in 1 to 2 weeks to assess for resolution; 89% of those less than 3 cm in size resolve within 21 days. If it persists on follow-up ultrasound or is greater than 3 cm in size, it should be treated with thrombin injection, ultrasound compression, or surgery.
- Arteriovenous fistulas occur in less than 1% of cases.
  - Puncture of the profunda femoris is the most common cause.
    - 80% resolve spontaneously by 1 month. If the patient develops arterial steal or other hemodynamic changes, it should be treated surgically.
- Retroperitoneal hemorrhage occurs in less than 0.5% of cases.
  - Caused by high puncture, usually of the external iliac artery.
  - The potential for delayed diagnosis, due to the large amount of retroperitoneal space in which to bleed into, results in the high morbidity and mortality associated with this complication. If it is suspected, a non-contrast CT should be ordered urgently.
  - It is treated endovascularly by obtaining contralateral access, inflating tamponade balloon, and placing a covered stent.

Major Complications

- Contrast-induced nephropathy
- Anaphylaxis
- Embolism
  - Air
  - Atheroembolism
    - Wires and arterial manipulation embolizes plaque distally. Interventionalist should look for blue toe syndrome and livedo reticularis.
- Arterial perforation/rupture
  - Caused by use of hydrophilic wires, which have less tactile feedback, and oversized balloons.
  - Most small perforations resolve on their own. Large perforations and ruptures require balloon tamponade, covered stent placement, and potentially open surgery.
- Limb loss and major amputation
  - Can be caused by dissection, distal atheroembolism, or thrombosis secondary to an occlusive sheath in the small artery or a vascular closure device complication.
- Death
  - Often secondary to access site complications (retroperitoneal hematoma), aortic dissection/rupture, or severe cardiovascular disease.

🏠 TAKE-HOME POINTS

- Most patients with peripheral artery disease (PAD) will die from cardiovascular disease; therefore, cardiovascular risk reduction is of paramount importance.
- In patients with claudication (Rutherford-Baker Classification 1, 2, and 3), endovascular options should be entertained only after the failure of maximum medical therapy.
- Guidewire selection is dependent on the situation, as different aspects of guidewire design confer specific advantages and disadvantages when treating PAD.

- Stents provide a scaffold to increase luminal diameter but have shortcomings that affect their long-term patency including foreign body reaction, fracture risk, and decreased potential surgical options for the stented segment.
- Drug-eluting balloon technology demonstrates promise for good long-term patency without leaving behind a foreign body.
- Various atherectomy technologies have been developed to remove plaque from the vessel.

REVIEW QUESTIONS

1. A 76-year-old male with history of smoking, diabetes, and hypertension arrives to your office with lifestyle-limiting right calf claudication. He is found to have a physiologically significant high-grade right SFA stenosis. What is your first step in treatment?
   a. Consult vascular surgery for potential bypass
   b. Maximize the patient's medical therapy
   c. Schedule the patient for urgent diagnostic angiography and intervention
   d. Schedule the patient for elective endovascular revascularization
   e. Since the patient likely has neurogenic claudication, no further treatment for vascular disease is necessary

2. Which choice best describes atherectomy?
   a. Debulking plaque by either removing it from the vessel or vaporizing it.

   b. Opening an obstruction by compressing the plaque against the arterial wall.
   c. Injecting anti-thrombolytic medication at the site of obstruction to open the vessel.
   d. Deploying a stent that applies outward radial pressure on the obstruction to open the vessel.

3. Revascularization of which artery would likely most contribute to wound healing in a patient with an ulcer over the medial plantar aspect of the instep of the foot?
   a. Dorsalis pedis artery
   b. Anterior tibial artery
   c. Posterior tibial artery
   d. Peroneal artery

SUGGESTED READINGS

Conde ID, Erwin PA. Evaluation of the patient who presents with critical limb ischemia: diagnosis, prognosis, and medical management. *Tech Vasc Inter Radiol.* 2014;17(3):140–146.

Dippel EJ, Makam P, Kovach R, et al. Randomized controlled study of excimer laser atherectomy for treatment of femoropopliteal in-stent restenosis: initial results from the EXCITE ISR Trial (EXCImer Laser Randomized Controlled Study for Treatment of FemoropopliTEal In-Stent Restenosis). *J Am Coll Cardiol Interv.* 2015;8(1 Pt A):92–101.

Duda SH, Bosiers M, Lammer J, et al. Drug-eluting and bare nitinol stents for the treatment of atherosclerotic lesions in the superficial femoral artery: long-term results from the SIROCCO Trial. *J Endovas Ther.* 2006;13(6):701–710.

Duda SH, Bosiers M, Lammer J, et al. Sirolimus-eluting versus bare metal nitiniol stent for obstructive superficial femoral artery disease: the SIROCCO II trial. *J Vasc Interv Radiol.* 2005;16(3):331–338.

Fanelli F, Cannavale A, Corona M, et al. The "DEBELLUM"—lower limb multilevel treatment with drug eluting balloon—randomized trial: 1-year results. *J Cardiovasc Surg (Torino).* 2014;55(2):207–216.

Goodney PP, Travis LL, Nallamothu BK, et al. Variation in the use of lower extremity vascular procedures for critical limb ischemia. *Cardiovasc Qual Outcomes.* 2012;5:94–102.

Henry AJ, Hevelone ND, Belkin M, et al. Socioeconomic and hospital-related predictors of amputation for critical limb ischemia. *J Vasc Surg.* 2011;53:330–339. e1.

Hirsch AT, Criqui MH, Treat-Jacobson D, et al. Peripheral arterial disease detection, awareness, and treatment in primary care. *JAMA.* 2001;286(11):1317–1324.

Hirsch AT, Hiatt WR. PARTNERS Steering Committee. PAD awareness, risk, and treatment: new resources for survival—the USA PARTNERS program. *Vasc Med.* 2001;6(3 suppl):9–12.

Manzi M, Cester G, Palena LM, et al. Vascular imaging of the foot: the first step toward endovascular recanalization. *Radiographics.* 2011;31:1623–1636.

Murphy TP, Cutlip DE, Regensteiner JG, et al. Supervised exercise, stent revascularization, or medical therapy for claudication due to aortoiliac peripheral artery disease: the CLEVER study. *J Am Coll Cardiol.* 2015;65:999–1009.

Olivieri B, Beasley R. SFA and BTK Interventions with the Chocolate® PTA Balloon Catheter. *Endovasc Today Suppl.* 2014;13–15.

Rastan A, McKinsey JF, Garcia LA, et al. One-year outcomes following directional atherectomy of infrapopliteal artery lesions: subgroup results of the prospective, multicenter DEFINITIVE LE trial. *J Endovasc Ther.* 2015;22(6):839–846.

Rosenfield K, Jaff MR, White CJ, et al. Trial of a paclitaxel-coated balloon for femoropopliteal artery disease. *N Engl J Med.* 2015;373:145–153.

Tepe G, Laird J, Schneider P, et al. Drug-coated balloon versus standard percutaneous transluminal angioplasty for the treatment of superficial femoral and/or popliteal peripheral artery disease: 12-month results from the IN.PACT SFA randomized trial. *Circulation.* 2015;131:495–502.

Walker C. Guidewire selection for peripheral vascular interventions. *Endovasc Today.* 2013;80–83.

Pulmonary Embolism

Christopher R. Bailey, Muhammad Umair, Clifford R. Weiss

CASE PRESENTATION

A 53-year-old male presents to the emergency department in marked respiratory distress after a recent transatlantic flight. On presentation, he is afebrile with a heart rate of 123 beats/min, respiratory rate of 32 breaths/min, and blood pressure of 108/72. Pulse oximetry demonstrates an oxygen saturation of 92%, which only improved to 94% with supplemental oxygen delivered by nasal cannula. Physical examination is significant for tachycardia, tachypnea, and a painful and swollen calf. ECG demonstrates sinus tachycardia with no signs of ischemia or right heart strain, and his chest x-ray is unremarkable. D-dimer is elevated on initial laboratory workup. Pulmonary embolism (PE)-protocol computed tomography (CT) is obtained and is positive for an acute PE in the right pulmonary artery.

The patient is started on parenteral unfractionated heparin. One hour after initiating heparin therapy, he develops worsening chest pain. He remains hypoxic on 6 L of oxygen delivered by nasal cannula. ECG reveals evidence of right heart strain. His troponins are now elevated to 0.09. The PE rapid response team is called, and the decision is made to take him to the interventional radiology suite for catheter-directed thrombolysis.

- The incidence of **pulmonary embolism** (PE) in the United States is approximately 600,000 per year. The most common cause of PE is a deep venous thrombosis (DVT) (further discussed in the *DVT* chapter). PE-related mortality in the United States amounts to roughly 60,000 to 100,000 deaths per year.
- Pulmonary emboli can be classified into three subtypes (Table 21.1).
- Signs and symptoms of an acute PE include:
  - Pleuritic chest pain
  - Dyspnea
  - Diaphoresis
  - Palpitations
  - Lightheadedness
  - Cough/hemoptysis
  - Lower extremity swelling
  - Fever
- Risk factors for the development of PE include:
  - Immobilization
  - Malignancy
  - Recent surgery
  - Inherited disorders (Factor V Leiden, Protein C and S deficiency)
  - Pregnancy
  - Smoking
  - Cirrhosis
  - Severe burns, infections, trauma
- **Wells criteria** (Tables 21.2 and 21.3) can be used to risk stratify patients when there is clinical suspicion for PE.
- **D-dimer**, a fibrin degradation product, can be used to further stratify patients with moderate or low pretest probability of having a PE per Wells criteria.
  - A D-dimer level greater than 500 µg/L generally warrants further diagnostic testing but may be falsely elevated in rheumatologic conditions, malignancy, and liver disease.
- **Computed tomography pulmonary angiography** (CTPA) is the definitive modality used to diagnosis PE (Fig. 21.1).
- If the patient cannot receive iodinated contrast (renal failure or anaphylactic contrast allergy), a **ventilation-perfusion (V/Q) scan** may be used to evaluate for PE (Fig. 21.2).
- For low-risk PEs and a proportion of submassive PEs, the mainstay of treatment is anticoagulation.
- In cases of massive PEs, submassive PEs with hemodynamic instability, or PEs with evidence of right heart strain, additional therapies are needed to improve perfusion.
- Catheter-directed therapies are rapidly becoming a standard of care for the treatment of massive and submassive PE (Table 21.4).
  - Catheter-directed therapies provide benefit to patients with submassive PE by potentially preventing conversion to massive PE, preventing heart failure, and preventing development of pulmonary hypertension.
- Catheter-directed therapies use endovascular pharmacomechanical techniques to debulk clot and/or infuse thrombolytic drug directly into the thrombus, leading to rapid clot lysis. Treatment can be initiated rapidly at properly equipped medical centers and is generally well tolerated in patients who are hemodynamically unstable with multiple comorbidities.

TABLE 21.1 Subtypes of Pulmonary Emboli

Subtype	Criteria
Massive (5%)	• Acute PE with sustained hypotension (systolic BP <90 mm Hg OR decrease in baseline SBP of 40 mm Hg or more for more than 15 min OR persistent bradycardia <40 bpm) • Mortality >50% at 90 days

Submassive (40%)	• Acute PE without hypotension
	• Signs of right ventricular (RV) dysfunction or myocardial necrosis including:
	  • Right ventricle to left ventricle ratio >0.9 on CT or echo
	  • Elevated proBNP
	  • EKG changes: RV strain, ischemic changes, SIQIIITIII pattern
	  • Elevated troponins
	• Mortality estimated at 16%–22% at 90 days

Low risk (55%)	• Acute PE without the clinical markers that define massive or submassive pulmonary embolism • Mortality estimated at 15% at 90 days

PE, pulmonary embolism; *BP*, blood pressure; *SBP*, systolic blood pressure; *EKG*, electrocardiogram; *proBNP*, pro b-type natriuretic peptide.

TABLE 21.2 Wells Criteria for Pulmonary Embolism

Criteria	Points
Clinical signs and symptoms of a DVT	3
PE is the most likely diagnosis	3
Heart rate >100 bpm	1.5
Immobilization ≥3 days or surgery in the previous 4 weeks	1.5
Prior history of DVT or pulmonary embolism	1.5
Hemoptysis	1
Malignancy	1

DVT, Deep venous thrombosis; *PE*, pulmonary embolism.

TABLE 21.3 Pulmonary Embolism Probability Based on Wells Score

High risk	Score > 6
Moderate risk	2 ≤ score ≤ 6
Low risk	Score < 2

- By directly delivering medication into the pulmonary artery, catheter-directed thrombolysis uses lower doses of thrombolytics compared to systemic thrombolysis, which confers a lower risk of adverse bleeding events.
- Current literature suggests that a combination of mechanical disruption to expose more thrombus surface area and direct thrombolytic infusion may be the most efficacious and safe approach. New endovascular technologies have

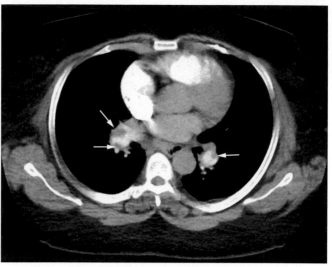

Fig. 21.1 A Chest CT with Bilateral Pulmonary Emboli. Computed tomography pulmonary angiography showing multiple filling defects *(arrows)* consistent with pulmonary emboli within the bilateral lobar and segmental branches. Central location suggests acute pulmonary emboli. This patient had enlargement of the main pulmonary artery to 3.5 cm, suggestive of pulmonary artery hypertension. There was no straightening or bowing of the interventricular septum, nor reflux of contrast into the IVC, to suggest right heart strain. (Courtesy Dr. Justin Shafa.)

led large institutions to develop multidisciplinary PE rapid response teams to evaluate and treat patients with hemodynamically significant PEs.

LITERATURE REVIEW

- The SEATTLE II study (Piazza, 2015) showed that ultrasound-assisted catheter-directed thrombolysis in both massive and submassive pulmonary embolisms (PEs) resulted in a significant reduction in right ventricular/left ventricular (RV/LV) diameter ratio, mean pulmonary artery (PA) peak systolic pressure, and PA angiographic obstruction over the subsequent 48 hours.
- The PERFECT study reported catheter-directed thrombolysis clinical success rates—measured in hemodynamic improvement, resolution of hypoxia, and survival to discharge—as high as 85.7% in massive PEs and 97.3% in submassive PEs.

INDICATIONS

- Massive PE with enough reserve to tolerate an endovascular procedure and without contraindications to thrombolysis
- Massive PE after failed systemic thrombolysis
- Submassive PE with hemodynamic instability
- Medically complex patient with a massive or submassive PE who is a poor surgical candidate

CONTRAINDICATIONS

- Absolute contraindications:
  - Active internal bleeding
  - Absolute contraindication to anticoagulation

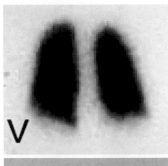

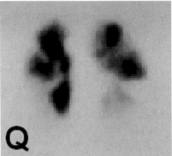

Fig. 21.2 Ventilation-Perfusion Lung Scan Demonstrating Pulmonary Emboli. The ventilation scan (V) is normal, whereas the perfusion scan (Q) shows multiple defects. (From Goldman L, Schafer A. *Goldman-Cecil Medicine*. 25th ed. Philadelphia: Elsevier, 2016, Fig. 98.3.)

- However, patients with contraindications to pharmacologic thrombolysis may undergo mechanical thrombectomy if the equipment and expertise are available.
- Neurosurgery (intracranial or spinal), stroke, or intracranial trauma within the previous 3 months

- Relative contraindications:
  - Stroke within the previous 6 months
  - Known intracranial neoplasm, arteriovenous malformation, or aneurysm
  - Gastrointestinal bleed within the previous 3 months
  - Bleeding diathesis or thrombocytopenia
  - Severe uncontrolled hypertension
  - Pregnancy
  - Severe renal or hepatic dysfunction

ANATOMY (FIG. 21.3)

- Pulmonary emboli typically originate from the deep venous system of the lower extremities; rarely, they can originate in the pelvis (May-Thurner syndrome), upper extremities, or heart.
- To reach the pulmonary system, thromboemboli travel up the inferior vena cava (IVC), through the right atrium, through the right ventricle, and into the pulmonary artery (PA).
  - A large embolus that straddles the bifurcation of the pulmonary trunk, extending into both the right and left pulmonary arteries, is referred to as a *saddle embolism*. This can commonly cause near-immediate death.
- Differentiating between an acute and chronic PE is important in determining treatment plan.
  - Imaging findings with an acute PE include:
    - The involved artery may appear enlarged in comparison to adjacent vessels.
    - Partial occlusion may appear as a *donut sign* or *tram track sign*.

TABLE 21.4	Summary of Catheter-Directed Treatments		
Modality	**Mechanism**	**Efficacy**	**Relevant Studies**
Standard catheter-directed thrombolysis (Uni*Fuse, Angiodynamics)	**Pharmacologic** Infuses thrombolytic directly at the site of thrombus	• Significant reduction in PA pressures and resolution of RV dysfunction in massive and submassive PEs • No difference between standard and ultrasound-assisted techniques	PERFECT
Ultrasound-assisted thrombolysis (EKOS, EkoSonic Endovascular)	**Pharmacomechanical** Utilizes high-frequency ultrasound to disrupt fibrin strands to allow for better penetration by the thrombolytic agent	• Significant reduction in PA pressures and resolution of RV dysfunction in massive and submassive PEs	SEATTLE II, PERFECT, ULTIMA
Thrombus fragmentation (e.g., standard pigtail catheter)	**Mechanical** Manual disruption of the thrombus by rotating the catheter to fragment it into smaller pieces	• Hemodynamic improvement seen with massive PEs when used alone • Increased efficacy when combined with catheter-directed thrombolysis	
Rheolytic embolectomy (AngioJet, Boston Scientific)	**Mechanical** Uses pressurized saline and suction (*Venturi-Bernoulli effect*) to break up and remove thrombus	• Improvement in obstruction, perfusion, and RV dysfunction • Higher complication rate compared to other modalities	
Suction embolectomy (AngioVac, Angiodynamics)	**Mechanical** Direct aspiration of the thrombus	• Reduction of clot burden and improvement of PA pressures • Increased efficacy when combined with catheter-directed thrombolysis	

PA, Pulmonary angiography; *PE*, pulmonary embolism; *RV*, right ventricular.

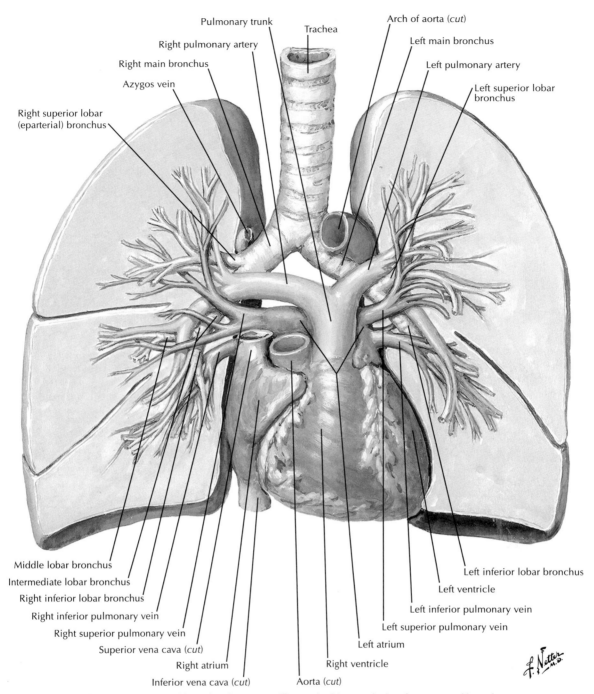

Fig. 21.3 Cardiopulmonary Vascular Anatomy. (Reused with permission from www.NetterImages.com, Elsevier; 2018.)

- A small PE may appear as a wedge-shaped infarct or discoid atelectasis.
- Imaging findings with a chronic PE include:
  - Complete occlusion of the involved vessel, which appears smaller than adjacent vessels
  - Abrupt cutoff of small arteries
  - Dilated collateral vessels

EQUIPMENT

- Ultrasound
- Micropuncture access kit
- Basic angiography set
- Iso-osmolar contrast (i.e., Visipaque)
- 7-Fr vascular sheath(s)
- Berman wedge catheter (Fig. 21.4), a compliant balloon catheter that will accept a 0.035 inch wire and allow for simultaneous pressure monitoring
- Tip-deflecting wire to cross into the right ventricle and provide guidance into the pulmonary arteries
- Exchange length Rosen and Bentson wires, both 0.035 inch
- Pressure transducer kit
- Tissue plasminogen activator (TPA) infusion system (EKOS, Unifuse, etc.)

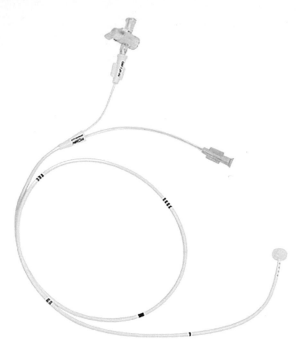

Fig. 21.4 Berman Angiographic Catheters. Berman angiography products available in two configurations: standard Berman catheter and the reverse Berman catheter. (Reused with permission from Teleflex Incorporated.)

PROCEDURE

Preprocedure Preparation

- Basic labs—Complete blood count (CBC), Basic metabolic panel (BMP), platelet count, PT/international normalized ratio (INR), and aPTT
- Review available imaging (CT or computed tomography angiography [CTA]) for a more targeted endovascular approach
- Obtain an ECG to look for left bundle branch block (LBBB), since catheter-directed thrombolysis can lead to right bundle branch block. In the presence of LBBB

(Fig. 21.5), a temporary pacemaker should be placed prior to the procedure.

Procedural Steps

1. Access site is sterilely prepped. Preferred site is the right internal jugular vein, followed by the left internal jugular, the right common femoral vein, and the left common femoral vein.
2. Access via the Seldinger technique followed by exchange with a micropuncture set to pass the guidewire. Micropuncture set is then exchanged for a vascular sheath.
3. Berman wedge catheter is then inserted and inflated with air once in the right atrium.
4. Catheter is hooked up to the pressure transducer and the right atrium and right ventricle pressures are recorded as the balloon catheter is advanced into the PA.
5. PA pressures and simultaneous systemic blood pressure are compared:
   - Normal right atrium pressure is 2 to 6 mm Hg
   - Normal systole right ventricle pressure is 15 to 25 mm Hg
   - Normal diastolic right ventricle pressure is 8 to 15 mm Hg
   - Normal PA pressure is 8 to 20 mm Hg
   - Pulmonary hypertension is a pressure $p > 25$ mm Hg
6. Performing a PA angiogram in the main PA is optional at this stage (Fig. 21.6). If PA pressures are elevated, the injection rates should be lowered.
7. Inflated Berman wedge catheter is advanced into the target PA. A tip-deflecting wire or a soft-tipped or steerable wire (Bentson or Glide) can be used.
8. Once in position, exchange length Rosen wire is advanced into the target artery, the balloon is deflated, and the Berman wedge is removed.
9. The infusion system is set up per manufacturer specifications. It must be flushed frequently so that the side holes do not become occluded with thrombus.

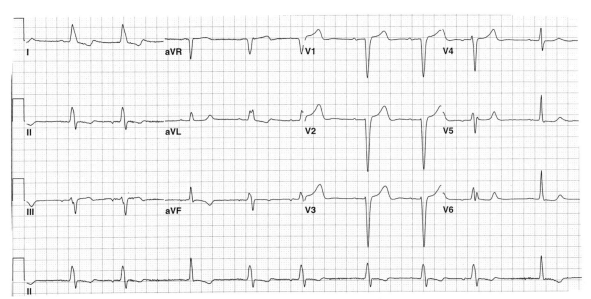

Fig. 21.5 ECG Showing Left Bundle Branch Block. (Reused with permission from Surawicz B, Knilans TK. *Chou's Electrocardiography in Clinical Practice.* Philadelphia; Elsevier; 2008:75–94, Fig. 4.11.)

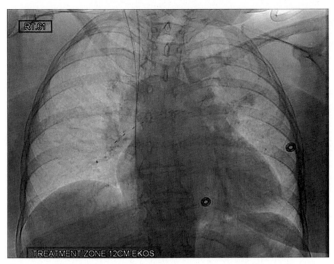

Fig. 21.6 Example of Bilateral Ultrasound-Assisted Catheter-Directed Thrombolysis. A catheter is placed into each pulmonary artery.

10. Steps 7 through 9 are repeated for the contralateral side, as needed.
11. Sheath is sutured in place and catheters secured.
12. tPA is infused overnight. The standard is to deliver a total of 24 mg, typically at a rate of at of 1 mg/h per catheter.
13. Heparinized saline is infused through the sheaths so that it does not become occluded.

Postprocedure Care

- The patient is typically transferred to an ICU level monitored bed.
- Access site monitoring, neuro checks, and a bleeding assessment are performed every 4 hours. Labs (fibrinogen, PT/PTT) are done every 8 hours.
  - If fibrinogen is between 100 and 150, the tPA dose should be cut in half.
  - If fibrinogen is <100, tPA should be stopped and replaced with full-dose heparin. Cryoprecipitate should be administered to replete fibrinogen with the goal to restart tPA if possible.
- After the full dose of tPA is delivered, the catheter can be transduced to determine PA pressures at bedside to assess the effect of the therapy.
- After completion of therapy, the catheters and sheaths are removed at bedside, and pressure is held over the access site. Standard goal heparin protocol is then started.

COMPLICATIONS

- Minor procedure-related complication rate of 7.9%. Such complications include:
  - Bradycardia
  - Minor access site hematoma not requiring transfusion
  - Minor hemoptysis not requiring transfusion
- Major procedural complications of 2.4%. Such complications include:

- Access site hematomas requiring transfusion
- Non-cerebral hemorrhages requiring transfusion
- Massive hemoptysis requiring transfusion
- Cardiac tamponade requiring surgical repair
- Renal failure requiring hemodialysis (rare)
- Death (rare)
  - Secondary to bradyarrhythmia, widespread distal embolization or cerebrovascular hemorrhage
- PA perforation (rare)

ALTERNATIVE TREATMENTS

Medical Therapy

- Mainstay of treatment for low-risk and some submassive PEs is anticoagulation.
- Anticoagulation usually begins with short-term parenteral therapy, usually unfractionated or low-molecular-weight heparin. The parenteral choice is eventually converted to an oral medication with long-term options including warfarin, a vitamin K antagonist, or novel oral anticoagulants (NOACs) such as rivaroxaban, apixaban, or dabigatran.
  - The choice of oral anticoagulant depends on characteristics such as renal function (NOACs are contraindicated in severe renal dysfunction) and patient preference.
  - Warfarin therapy requires regular INR monitoring to make sure that the drug is at a therapeutic level.
  - NOACs have the advantage of not requiring therapeutic monitoring.

Systemic Thrombolysis

- Systemic thrombolysis should be started as soon as possible for hemodynamically unstable massive PEs. Doing so does not preclude subsequent catheter-directed therapies.
- This technique involves an injection of tPA, streptokinase, or urokinase through a peripheral IV, delivering a systemic dose of thrombolytic.
- Systemic thrombolysis carries a higher risk of bleeding complications compared to catheter-directed therapies. Some studies have demonstrated a 22% rate of significant hemorrhage and a 3% to 5% rate of intracranial bleeds with systemic thrombolysis.

Surgical Thrombectomy

- Surgical thrombectomy is usually performed as a last resort in patients who:
  - Have contraindications to both systemic and catheter-directed (both mechanical and pharmacomechanical) therapies
  - Are unstable and require immediate therapy and/or extracorporeal membrane oxygenation (ECMO).
- This approach has high mortality, estimated at between 6% and 46%, depending on age and comorbidities.

🏠 TAKE-HOME POINTS

- Pulmonary emboli can be classified into three subtypes—massive, submassive, and low risk. This generally correlates to emboli located in the main pulmonary artery, segmental artery, or subsegmental arteries, respectively.
- Both the Wells criteria and D-dimer level can be used to risk stratify patients with suspected pulmonary embolism (PE).
- Computed tomography pulmonary angiography is the typical first choice for diagnosing PEs, but in patients with severe renal insufficiency or anaphylactic contrast allergy, ventilation/perfusion scanning can be performed.
- Systemic anticoagulation is the mainstay of treatment for and prevention of low-risk and a subset of submassive PEs. Advanced endovascular therapies may be required for the management of submassive and massive PEs to prevent progression, worsening heart strain/failure, and the development of pulmonary hypertension.

- Catheter-directed modalities for thrombolysis include pharmacologic, mechanical, or a combination of the two. There is no consensus approach, but current evidence suggests that the combined pharmacomechanical approach is rapid, efficacious, and safe.
- New endovascular technologies have led to the creation of multidisciplinary PE rapid response teams, which, depending on the institution, can include representatives from interventional radiology, pulmonology, critical care, hematology, vascular surgery, anesthesiology, and cardiothoracic surgery.
- In cases where the use of thrombolytic medication is contraindicated, the patient needs immediate therapy, or extracorporeal membrane oxygenation is required, surgical thrombectomy can be performed.

REVIEW QUESTIONS

1. A 76-year-old female presents with acute-onset chest pain and shortness of breath. She recently underwent intramedullary nail placement for a femur fracture. Her vitals on admission were significant for a blood pressure of 120/76, a heart rate of 130, and an oxygen saturation of 90% on room air. ECG reveals right heart strain, and her troponins are elevated to 0.09. CTPA reveals acute PE with an RV:LV ratio of 1.8. What subtype of PE does she likely have?
   a. Massive PE
   b. Saddle PE
   c. Submassive PE
   d. Low-risk PE
   e. Subsegmental PE

2. The majority of patients with PE have which subtype?
   a. Massive
   b. Submassive
   c. Low risk

3. Which of the following criteria is NOT included in the Wells score for PE?
   a. Respiratory rate >22
   b. Heart rate >100
   c. Clinical signs and symptoms of DVT
   d. Hemoptysis
   e. Immobilization ≥3 days or surgery in the previous 4 weeks

SUGGESTED READINGS

Agnelli G, Becattini C. Acute pulmonary embolism. *New Engl J Med.* 2010;363(3):266–274.

Kucher N, Boekstegers P, Müller OJ, et al. Randomized, controlled trial of ultrasound-assisted catheter-directed thrombolysis for acute intermediate risk pulmonary embolism. *Circulation.* 2014;129(4):479–486.

Kuo WT. Endovascular therapy for acute pulmonary embolism. *J Vasc Interv Radiol.* 2012;23(2):167–179.

Kuo WT, Banerjee A, Kim PS, et al. Pulmonary Embolism Response to Fragmentation, Embolectomy, and Catheter Thrombolysis (PERFECT): initial results from a prospective multicenter registry. *Chest.* 2015;148(3):667–673.

Kuo WT, Gould MK, Louie JD, et al. Catheter directed therapy for the treatment of massive pulmonary embolism: systematic review and meta-analysis of modern techniques. *J Vasc Interv Radiol.* 2009;20(11):1431–1440.

Piazza G, Hohlfelder B, Jaff MR, et al. A prospective, single-arm, multicenter trial of ultrasound-facilitated, catheter-directed, low-dose fibrinolysis for acute massive and submassive pulmonary embolism: the SEATTLE II study. *JACC Cardiovasc Interv.* 2015;8(10):1382–1392.

Sacks D, McClenny TE, Cardella JF, et al. Society of Interventional Radiology clinical practice guidelines. *J Vasc Interv Radiol.* 2003;14(9):S199–S202.

Sobieszczyk P. Catheter-assisted pulmonary embolectomy. *Circulation.* 2012;126(15):1917–1922.

Weiss CR, Scatarige JC, Diette GB, et al. CT pulmonary angiography is the first-line imaging test for acute pulmonary embolism: a survey of US clinicians. *Acad Radiol.* 2006; 13(4):434–446.

Renal Artery Stenosis

Myles Nightingale, Priyanka Ramesh, Anthony Febles

CASE PRESENTATION

A 55-year-old male presents with uncontrollable blood pressure despite being on multiple antihypertensive drugs. On examination, his mean arterial pressure is 140 mm Hg. Serum creatinine is 3.1 mg/dL, and magnetic resonance angiography (MRA) shows renal artery stenosis. Interventional radiology is consulted for possible **percutaneous transluminal renal angioplasty.**

- In 1964, Charles Dotter developed the technique of **percutaneous transluminal angioplasty** for the treatment of peripheral vascular stenosis. In 1974, Andreas Gruntzig modified percutaneous transluminal angioplasty (PTA) by developing soft, flexible, double-lumen balloon catheters for use in coronary arteries. And in 1978, **percutaneous transluminal renal angioplasty (PTRA)** was introduced as a highly effective modality for the correction of renal artery stenosis (Fig. 22.1).
- **Renal artery stenosis** is a common cause of secondary hypertension. Disease process pathophysiology involves:
  - Decreased blood flow to the juxtaglomerular apparatus secondary to stenosis leading to secretion of renin → renin converts angiotensinogen to angiotensin I, which is then converted to angiotensin II → angiotensin II causes a rise in blood pressure.
- In the setting of decreasing renal function (ischemic nephropathy) or renal hypertension, a non-invasive imaging study is performed prior to intervention to diagnose and quantify the degree of renal artery stenosis:
  - Doppler ultrasound
  - Contrast-enhanced CTA
  - Contrast-enhanced (or phase contrast) MRA
- Percutaneous angiography yields high diagnostic specificity but is an invasive procedure and risks contrast nephropathy. Benefit includes concurrent treatment, which can be performed if the angiogram is positive.
- Choice of the endovascular treatment depends on the type of lesion:
  - Non-atherosclerotic, non-ostial stenosis (e.g., **fibromuscular dysplasia**) → PTRA with balloon angioplasty
  - Atherosclerotic ostial stenosis (Fig. 22.2): PTRA with primary stent placement

- Percutaneous transluminal renal intervention is the first-line treatment of symptomatic renal artery stenosis refractory to medical treatment. Surgical intervention is an alternative for patients with difficult anatomy.
- Studies of selected patients with ischemic nephropathy after revascularization show that 25% to 30% will recover some kidney function with others avoiding progression to end-stage renal disease.

INDICATIONS

- Indications for PTRA with angioplasty:
  - Progressive, unexplained renal function decline. This entity is termed **ischemic nephropathy**. A decline in glomerular filtration rate (GFR) after administering an angiotensin-converting enzyme (ACE) inhibitor or angiotensin receptor blocker (ARB) raises suspicion for this entity.
  - Patients undergoing infrarenal abdominal aortic aneurysm repair with high-grade renal artery stenosis.
  - Greater than 75% stenosis seen in the bilateral renal arteries or trans-stenotic gradients of 10 mm Hg (mean) or 20 mm Hg (systolic) AND any of following factors:
    - Hypertension that is controlled by three or more medications
    - Labile hypertension
    - A short duration of high blood pressure prior to the diagnosis of ischemic nephropathy (best predictor of procedural success)
    - Concurrent chronic renal insufficiency with creatinine less than 3.0 mg/dL
    - Inability to tolerate optimum medical therapy
    - Difficult-to-control congestive heart failure, particularly with episodes of flash pulmonary edema
- Indications for renal artery stenting:
  - Ostial atherosclerotic renal artery stenosis
  - Re-stenosis after a previous PTRA
  - Stenosis in a renal artery bypass or a transplanted renal artery
  - Highly eccentric calcified plaque as the cause of renal artery stenosis
  - Iatrogenic or spontaneous renal artery dissection

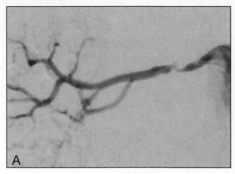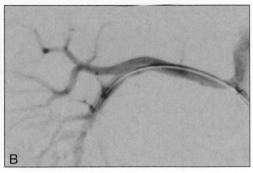

Fig. 22.1 **Treatment of Renal Artery Stenosis.** Atheromatous stenosis in the mid-renal artery (A) before angioplasty and (B) after angioplasty. (From Kessel D. *Interventional Radiology.* 3rd ed. Philadelphia, PA: Elsevier, 2011. Fig. 15.21.)

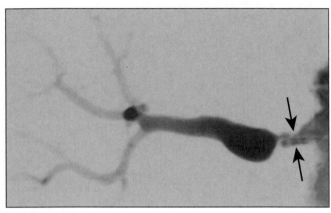

Fig. 22.2 Atheromatous ostial renal artery stenosis *(arrows)* with poststenotic dilation. (From Kessel D. *Interventional Radiology.* 3rd ed. Philadelphia, PA: Elsevier, 2011. Fig. 15.20A.)

CONTRAINDICATIONS

- Contraindications to PTRA:
  - Creatinine greater than 3 to 4 mg/dL or kidney length less than 7 cm. In either case, canalization of the arteries is unlikely to provide benefit.
  - Comorbidities or a poor operative candidate (bleeding diathesis, recent myocardial infarction, pregnancy, limited life expectancy, etc.)
- Contraindications to renal artery stenting:
  - Lesion in a branch artery (to avoid the possibility of the stent excluding the branch)
  - Diffuse intrarenal vascular disease such as a vasculitis (e.g., polyarteritis nodosa)
  - Non-compliant lesion

EQUIPMENT

- Guidewire
  - TAD-II, 0.035-inch or a thinner 0.014-inch wire may be necessary to cross tight lesions
- Angiographic 4-Fr catheter
- Guiding 5- to 8-Fr catheter
- 20- to 30-cm Ansel arterial sheath
- 4- to 6-mm balloon catheter system

- Balloon-expandable metallic stents
  - Preferred over self-expanding stents as (1) ostial lesions have high radial force and (2) the interventionalist can more accurately deploy the stent
- Contrast
  - CO_2 angiography should be considered as most patients will have chronic renal insufficiency, which increases the risk of contrast nephropathy
- Pressure monitoring equipment for measuring transstenotic gradients

ANATOMY (FIG. 22.3)

- Each kidney is usually supplied by a single renal artery that originates from the aorta below the superior mesenteric artery (SMA) at roughly the L1/L2 disk space (Fig. 22.4).
- The renal arteries are typically posterior to the renal veins and anterior to the renal pelvis.
- Right renal artery:
  - Originates slightly anteriorly on the aorta
  - Longer than the left
  - Passes posteriorly to the IVC with a downward course to the right kidney
- Left renal artery:
  - Arises at a higher level than the right and takes an upward course
  - Originates in a more lateral location on the aorta
- Congenital abnormalities in renal position and configuration are often associated with aberrant locations of renal artery origins.
- Accessory renal arteries should be sought. These may have stenosis as well.

PROCEDURAL STEPS

1. The preferred approach to the renal artery is right common femoral artery (CFA) access, which is accessed with standard Seldinger techniques.
2. The curve of the sheath or guide catheter is selected to match the angle of the renal artery as it arises from the aorta.

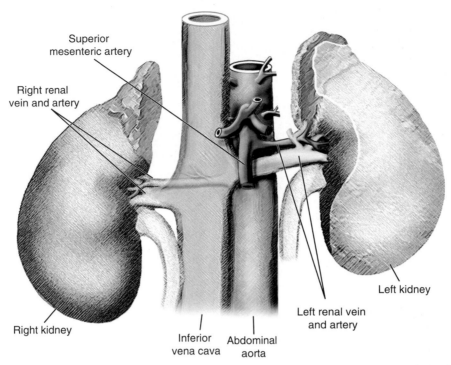

Superior
mesenteric artery

Right renal
vein and artery

Left kidney

Right kidney

Inferior
vena cava

Abdominal
aorta

Left renal vein
and artery

Fig. 22.3 Renal Vasculature. (From Mauro MA. *Image-Guided Interventions: Expert Radiology Series.* Philadelphia, PA: Elsevier; 2014, Fig. 57.1.)

3. Heparin (5,000–10,000 units) is administered prior to selecting the renal artery.
4. A long curved 6- or 7-Fr sheath or a 7- or 8-Fr guiding catheter is inserted into the CFA.
5. A guidewire, followed by the catheter, is advanced across the lesion.
6. The guidewire is removed, blood is aspirated, and contrast is injected followed by 100 to 200 µg of nitroglycerin.

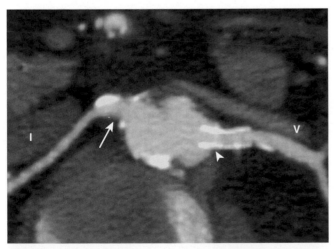

Fig. 22.4 Axial Computed Tomography Angiogram Displaying Renal Artery Origins. The origin of the right renal artery *(arrow)* is slightly anterior on the aorta. The origin of the left renal artery *(arrowhead)* is lateral on the aorta. A patent stent is located within the left renal artery and protrudes into the aortic lumen. *I,* Inferior vena cava; *V,* left renal vein. (From Kaufman JA. *Vascular and Interventional Radiology: The Requisites.* 2nd ed. Philadelphia, PA: Elsevier; 2014, Fig. 12.1.)

7. Trans-stenotic gradients are obtained between the aorta and the renal artery distal to the stenosis.
   a. Additional heparin can be administered if there is complete stasis of the intrarenal branches due to blockage of the lesion by the catheter.
8. The catheter is advanced through the lesion, and contrast is injected to confirm intraluminal position (Fig. 22.5).
9. A stiff 0.035-inch guidewire with a short straight floppy tip or 0.014- to 0.018-inch stiff guidewire with short soft platinum tips is inserted.
   a. J-tipped guidewires are more likely to induce spasm or cause dissection of intrarenal branches. A stiff guidewire can change the angle of the renal artery, facilitating the procedure.
10. Balloon-expandable stent is deployed over the guidewire. Stent should be deployed so that it protrudes into the aorta a few millimeters to ensure adequate displacement of the aortic plaque.
    a. Ostial lesions will almost always require stent placement. Proximal renal artery atherosclerotic lesions, located more than 1 cm from the aortic lumen, may respond well to angioplasty alone, but stents are still routinely used in practice.
11. After stent placement and balloon deflation, the balloon is removed while the guidewire is maintained in position across the treated site. The guidewire is always left in place in case of vessel dissection or rupture, should a bailout procedure be necessary.
12. If there is satisfactory post-stenting angiographic appearance and no residual trans-stenotic gradient, the procedure is complete.

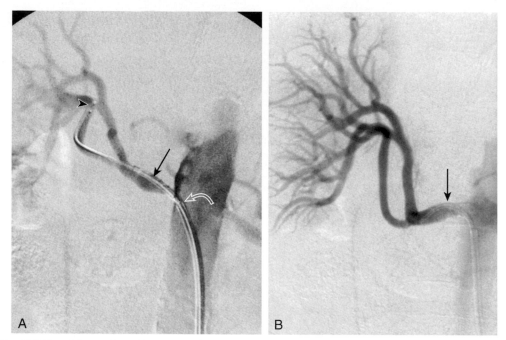

Fig. 22.5 Renal Artery Stent Placement. (A) Digital subtraction angiogram (DSA) obtained through the sheath (curved arrow) while positioning a balloon-mounted stent (arrow) across the ostial renal artery stenosis. A Rosen guidewire is in the posterior division (arrowhead). (B) DSA after stent deployment and removal of the guidewire. Note the change in angle of the main renal artery (arrow) after stent deployment. (From Kaufman JA. *Vascular and Interventional Radiology: The Requisites.* 2nd ed. Philadelphia, PA: Elsevier; 2014, Fig. 12.16.)

13. All catheters and wires are removed, pressure is applied to the arterial access site (if an arterial closure device is not used), and a sterile dressing is applied.
14. Patient should be monitored for post-op complications for 4 to 6 hours afterward.

TREATMENT ALTERNATIVES

Medical Therapy

- First-line pharmacologic agents used in the treatment of renal artery stenosis include ACE inhibitors and angiotensin II receptor blockers (ARBs).
- Studies in patients with unilateral renal artery stenosis have shown that, although the angiotensin II–mediated compensatory response (efferent arteriole vasoconstriction) is eliminated with the use of an ACE inhibitor/ARB, the total GFR is usually well maintained due to a roughly equal rise in filtration in the contralateral kidney. Even in patients with bilateral renal stenosis, a decline in renal function can be seen, but the decrease is typically small and usually reversible by discontinuation of medications.
- ACE inhibitors and ARBs are efficacious in blood pressure control, but thiazide diuretics and calcium channel blockers can be started as well if needed.

Surgical Revascularization

- This approach has significantly declined in popularity due to efficacy of antihypertensive drug therapy and developments in endovascular techniques.

- Surgical intervention is still preferred for patients with complex anatomic lesions such as:
  - Multiple small renal arteries
  - Early primary branching of the main renal artery
  - Requirement for concurrent aortic reconstruction for other pathologies such as aneurysm repair

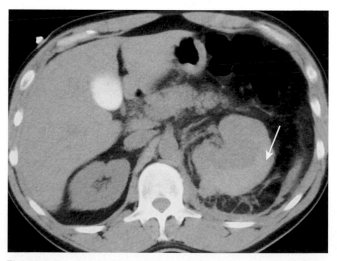

Fig. 22.6 Renal capsular hematoma, (A) which likely occurred due to guidewire perforation of kidney during angioplasty. The patient presented with flank pain several hours after the procedure. (From Kaufman JA. *Vascular and Interventional Radiology: The Requisites.* 2nd ed. Philadelphia, PA: Elsevier; 2014, Fig. 12.20.)

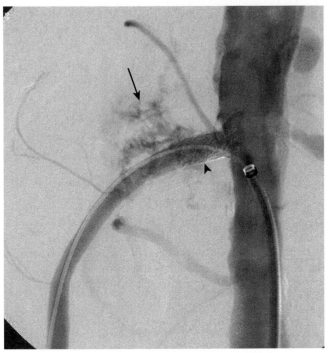

Fig. 22.7 Rupture of renal artery (arrow) during placement of 6-mm-diameter stent (arrowhead) in an elderly woman with hypertension, a very rare complication that likely occurred due to placement of an oversized stent for this particular patient. Following deployment, the patient remained hemodynamically stable and was pain free. However, rupture was discovered on completion angiogram. (From Kaufman JA. *Vascular and Interventional Radiology: The Requisites.* 2nd ed. Philadelphia, PA: Elsevier; 2014, Figs. 12–19.)

COMPLICATIONS

- Renal angioplasty and stenting is an inherently challenging procedure given the varying types and locations of lesions, the size of the renal vessels, the sharp angles between renal arteries and the aorta, movement of the renal arteries with respiration, and poor collateral supply to the kidneys.

- Generally, complications occur more frequently with stent placement (15% of cases) than with angioplasty alone (5%–10% of cases).
- Commonly seen complications are summarized in Table 22.1.

TABLE 22.1 Complications Seen With Renal Angiogram and Stenting

Complication	Incidence (%)
Death (within 30 days of the procedure)	0.5
Renal artery perforation (Fig. 22.6) and rupture (Fig. 22.7)	<1
Renal artery thrombosis	<1
Cholesterol embolization	1
Branch artery occlusion	3
Flow-limiting dissection	5
Renal failure	5
Access site issue (hematoma, pseudoaneurysm)	5
Stent infection	Anecdotal

🏠 TAKE-HOME POINTS

- Atherosclerosis primarily affects patients over 45 and typically involves the aortic orifice or proximal main renal artery.
- The primary technical success rate for renal artery angioplasty cases exceeds 90% in most reported series.
- Compared to percutaneous transluminal renal angioplasty (PTRA) alone, PTRA with stenting decreases the rate of restenosis and is more effective in improving blood pressure.
- Patients with bilateral or solitary kidney renal artery stenosis with ischemic nephropathy, renal hypertension, or difficult-to-control congestive heart failure (CHF) are most likely to benefit from renal artery revascularization.

REVIEW QUESTIONS

1. All the following are clinical findings suggestive of secondary hypertension due to renovascular disease except:
   a. Acute elevation in serum creatinine of at least 30% after administration of ACE inhibitor or ARB
   b. Paroxysmal elevations in blood pressure (pheochromocytoma)
   c. Moderate to severe hypertension in patients with recurrent episodes of flash pulmonary edema
   d. Systolic or diastolic abdominal bruit

2. Which of these is an absolute contraindication of renal artery revascularization with stent?
   a. Branch artery lesion
   b. Diffuse intrarenal vascular disease such as polyarteritis nodosa
   c. Non-compliant lesion
   d. None of the above

SUGGESTED READINGS

Kandarpa K and Machan L. *Handbook of Interventional Radiologic Procedures: Renal Artery Angioplasty and Stents.* 4th ed. Philadelphia, PA: Lippincott, Williams, and Wilkins; 2011.

Trude C, Elma J, Johanna L, et al. Stent placement for renal artery stenosis: where do we stand? A meta-analysis. *Radiology.*

2000;216(1)(2000). http://pubs.rsna.org/doi/abs/10.1148/radiology.216.1.r00jl0778.

Wheatley K, Ives N, Gray R, et al. Revascularization versus medical therapy for renal-artery stenosis. *N Engl J Med.* 2009;361:1953–1962. https://doi.org/10.1056/NEJMoa0905368.

23

Thrombolysis and Thrombectomy

Viky Y. Loescher, Brandon Olivieri, Timothy Yates

CASE PRESENTATION

A 29-year-old male recreational tennis player presents to the emergency department with acute-onset right upper extremity swelling, pain, and redness. The patient has no significant past medical or family history. He denies smoking, alcohol consumption, and drug use. Upper extremity duplex ultrasound reveals complete occlusion of right axillary-subclavian vein as well as the peripheral deep and superficial veins to the elbow. Workup for coagulopathies is negative. Further investigation reveals strenuous exercise, including rigorous tennis serve training the day before presentation. Interventional radiology (IR) is consulted for workup and potential treatment of Paget-Schroetter syndrome.

- **Paget-Schroetter syndrome (PSS)** (also referred to as "effort thrombosis" and "venous variant of thoracic outlet syndrome") is defined as subclavian-to-axillary or upper extremity deep vein thrombosis (DVT) associated with repetitive trauma to the venous endothelium after strenuous and repetitive activity.
- There are three types of **thoracic outlet syndrome (TOS)**:
  - Neurogenic (most common, seen in 90% to 95% of cases)
  - Arterial
  - Venous
- This endothelial trauma activates the coagulation cascade and leads to intimal hyperplasia and inflammation, which results in venous webs, formation of extensive collateral vessels, and perivenular fibrosis.
- While anticoagulation is necessary to prevent thrombus propagation, this treatment alone without any adjuncts is not recommended because of poor overall outcomes.
  - Residual obstruction in seen in up to 78% of patients, persistent symptoms in 41% to 91%, and 39% to 68% of cases are associated with permanent disability.
- In patients with PSS, **catheter-directed thrombolysis (CDT)** or **mechanical thrombectomy** are appropriate endovascular options.
  - CDT has a 62% to 100% success rate depending on the age of the thrombus, with a 30% re-thrombosis rate within 30 days.

- For these reasons, thrombolysis is recommended to improve short-term and long-term venous patency as well as prevent the development of subsequent **post thrombotic syndrome (PTS)**.

INDICATIONS

- Patients who meet the following criteria, as described by the 2016 Chest Guidelines, are most likely to benefit from thrombolysis:
  - Symptoms that have preferably lasted, but not limited to, less than 14 days
  - Anatomic cause for PSS
  - Thrombus involving most of the subclavian and axillary veins
  - Acute limb compromise
  - Maintained functional status or physiologic reserve (~20–70 years old)
  - Life expectancy of greater than 1 year
  - Low bleeding risk

> ## CLINICAL POINT
>
> - In patients with acute upper extremity deep vein thrombosis (DVTs) involving the axillary or peripheral deep veins, the Chest Guidelines recommend anticoagulation without thrombolysis (Grade 2C).
> - In patients with upper extremity DVTs who undergo thrombolysis, the same dosing and duration of anticoagulation are recommended as in patients with upper extremity DVTs who do not undergo thrombolysis (Grade 1B).

CONTRAINDICATIONS

- Bleeding diathesis/thrombocytopenia
- Organ-specific bleeding risk (recent cardiac ischemia, cerebrovascular event, gastrointestinal bleeding, surgery, or trauma)
- Renal or hepatic failure
- Malignancy

EQUIPMENT

- Trellis-8 rotating sinusoidal dispersion wires
- AngioJet or EKOS system
- Multi-sidehole infusion catheter (Fig. 23.1)

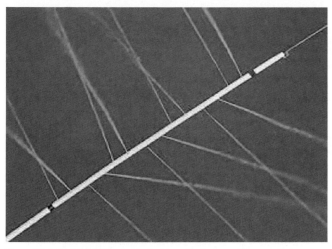

Fig. 23.1 Multi-Sideport Infusion Catheter. The catheter has two black (radiopaque) markers delineating the "infusion length," spray of fluid through multiple infusion side holes, and a distal tip-occluding wire. (Courtesy E. Tamussino http://www.tamussino.com.br/en/produto-det.php?rp=428.)

ANATOMY

- Familiarity with the anatomy of the thoracic outlet plays an important role in understanding disease pathogenesis. Anatomic variants play an important role in deciding therapeutic approach, whether endovascular or surgical.
- The three spaces of the **thoracic outlet** are the (1) interscalene triangle, (2) costoclavicular space, and (3) pectoralis minor space, as depicted in Fig. 23.2.
- A thorough evaluation of the skeletal and soft tissue structures outlining the thoracic outlet must be performed in order to avoid disease recurrence. Variations include:

- Bony abnormalities: abnormal first cervical rib, elongated C7 transverse process, exostosis or tumor of the first rib or clavicle, or excess callus of the first rib or clavicle
- Soft tissue abnormalities: fibrous band, congenital muscle abnormalities, variations in muscle insertion, or supernumerary muscles
- Other abnormalities: posttraumatic fibrous scarring, postsurgical scarring, postural variations, or weak muscular support in thin women
- Different maneuvers are used to dynamically induce compression of the structures in the thoracic outlet in order to reproduce symptoms and identify the components causing compression.
  - The Wright test is performed with the shoulder hyperabducted and externally rotated, as elevation of the upper limb has been reported to elicit symptoms.
  - In a patient without PSS, elevation of the arm does not produce a change in the size of the interscalene triangle but does cause narrowing of both the costoclavicular and pectoralis minor spaces.
    - The subclavian vein does not cross the interscalene triangle. It runs beneath the anterior scalene muscle before joining the internal jugular vein to form the brachiocephalic vein.

PROCEDURAL STEPS

- Two important principles must be observed to ensure successful CDT.
  - The thrombolysis catheter must be directly embedded within the thrombosed venous segment.
  - Constant flow across the treated segment is necessary to wash out lysed by-products and to promote further thrombolysis.

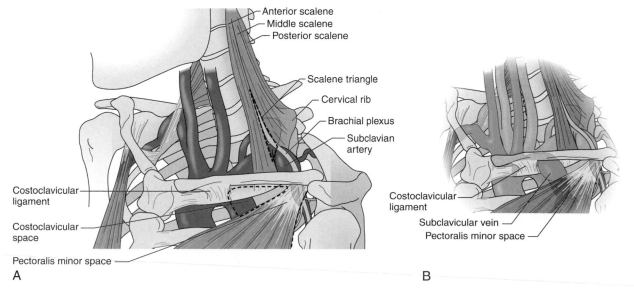

Fig. 23.2 Illustration of the thoracic outlet showing the scalene triangle, costoclavicular space, and pectoralis minor space. (A) The subclavian vein is most commonly compressed in the costoclavicular space between the costoclavicular ligament, first rib, and subclavius tendon. The subclavian artery is most commonly compressed in the scalene triangle by a variably present accessory cervical rib. (B) Inlet of the costoclavicular space (Reused with permission from Hussain MA, Aljabri B, Al-Omran M. Vascular thoracic outlet syndrome. *Semin Thorac Cardiovasc Surg.* 2016;28[1]:151–157, Fig. 1.)

Steps

1. After sterile preparation, ultrasound-guided venous access is achieved, typically in the affected arm in a superficial vein such as the basilic or cephalic. Alternate access sites include the common femoral vein and, less commonly, either the internal jugular vein or contralateral upper extremity.

2. A 5- or 6-Fr vascular sheath is then placed within the vein to maintain access, acting as a port for venography and saline infusion.

3. Upper extremity venography is performed with contrast followed from the peripheral to the central veins in multiple fluoroscopic stations. Absolute impeccable venography is paramount for success with crossing devices, and two access points may be necessary to adequately define the target for the crossing device.

4. Once the entire thrombus burden is delineated venographically, a 0.035-, 0.018-, or 0.014-inch wire and appropriately sized catheter are used coaxially to traverse the occlusion, typically at the subclavian/brachiocephalic confluence.

   a. Occasionally with chronic thrombosis/stenosis, an auxiliary crossing device, such as a radiofrequency wire or chronic total occlusion wire, may be needed to cross the lesion.

5. Once the site of stenosis is traversed, the wire can be secured in the superior or inferior vena cava.

6. The multi-sidehole thrombolysis catheter is then advanced across the lesion, ensuring that its entire length is embedded within the thrombus.

7. **Tissue plasminogen activator (TPA)** infusion is then started through the lysis catheter using institution-specific guidelines. A continuous heparinized saline solution is infused through the sheath (if no history of heparin-induced thrombocytopenia) to ensure constant forward flow.

8. Adjunctive therapy at this stage includes:
   - **Pharmacomechanical thrombolysis/thrombectomy** for more rapid thrombolysis (i.e., AngioJet)
   - **Suction thrombectomy** for direct thrombus removal (i.e., Indigo System)
   - **Balloon venoplasty**
     - This is almost always necessary after thrombolysis to open chronic stenoses and webs at the thoracic inlet that were responsible for the initial flow blockage (Fig. 23.3).
   - **Stenting**
     - Stenting can be performed in patients who are not potential surgical candidates; however, long-term patency rates with stenting are lower than that with multiple angioplasty sessions. Stenting is strictly contraindicated in patients who may require surgery (e.g., PSS caused by a cervical rib).
     - It has been suggested that the overall decreased patency in the stent group is likely related to stent fatigue and fracture at the previously identified anatomic compression point. Stenting of the vein running through the non-decompressed costoclavicular junction has been shown to be complicated by fracture in some, deformation in nearly all, and rethrombosis rates as high as 40%.

ALTERNATIVE TREATMENTS

Surgical Decompression

- Transaxillary first rib resection (most common)
  - First rib resection via a supraclavicular approach has traditionally been the leading treatment strategy.
  - Some have recently adopted a highly selective approach in which supraclavicular scalenectomy is the principal treatment for PSS, reserving first rib resection solely for arterial forms of TOS.

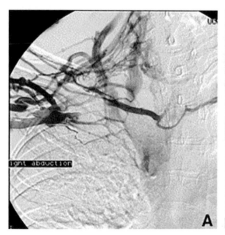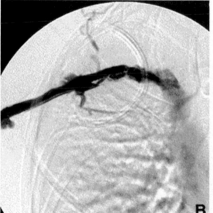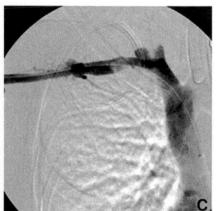

Fig. 23.3 Right Upper Extremity Venograms in a 19-Year-Old Woman. (A) Preoperative venogram during arm abduction demonstrates positional occlusion of the right subclavian vein with multiple venous collateral vessels. (B) Intraoperative venogram after surgical decompression still shows subclavian vein stenosis with residual chronic thrombus. (C) Completion venogram after balloon angioplasty demonstrates a patent subclavian vein. (Reused with permission from Schneider DB, Dimuzio PJ, Martin ND, et al. Combination treatment of venous thoracic outlet syndrome: open surgical decompression and intraoperative angioplasty. *J Vasc Surg.* 2004;40 [4]:599–603, Fig. 1.)

- First rib resection and subclavian vessel reconstruction is required when any arterial aneurysm is present, particularly if the patient has had prior symptoms of digital thromboembolism.
- Thoracic outlet decompression
  - Includes scalenectomy, brachial plexus neurolysis, resection of the first rib, and circumferential venolysis
- Debulking of subclavius muscle/tendon
- Resection of fibrotic tissue
- Circumferential release of the vein from the clavicle

COMPLICATIONS

Complications of Untreated Venous Thoracic Outlet Syndrome

- *Phlegmasia cerulea dolens* is characterized by limb cyanosis and swelling as a result of thrombosis at a capillary level. This can potentially lead to limb-threatening venous gangrene and severe morbidity secondary to chronic venous hypertension.
- *Postthrombotic syndrome* is caused by chronic venous hypertension secondary to venous reflux, venous obstruction, and valvular dysfunction. Clinical sequelae include leg pain, edema, venous trophic changes, and chronic ulceration. It is estimated that up to 80% of patients with a lower extremity DVT may go on to develop symptoms of PTS, while 15% progress to leg ulceration.

Procedural Complications

- Bleeding
  - Most CDT-associated bleeding complications are local.
  - Reported to occur with prolonged infusion time and high dosing of thrombolytic agent.
  - Routine use of ultrasound-guided venous access can reduce puncture site complications by avoiding multiple punctures.

- Limiting thrombolytic agent infusion time and/or dose in addition to strict enforcement of patient exclusion criteria further limited bleeding complications.
- Pulmonary emboli (PE)
  - There is debate as to whether CDT increases the risk of PE in the process of clot lysis. PEs occur in up to 30% of general patients with acute DVTs, most of these being in the lower extremities, and many having subclinical presentations. In PSS treated with CDT, PEs had been reported in as many as 1% to 4.5% of cases.

🏠 TAKE-HOME POINTS

- Paget-Schroetter syndrome (PSS) describes an upper extremity deep vein thrombosis typically related to repetitive venous trauma.
- PSS occurs secondary to venous endothelial injury from strenuous and repetitive activity of the upper extremities. The typical patient may be a young athletic male or female tennis player, pitcher, or swimmer.
- Anticoagulation alone is not an effective therapy to reduce rates of PTS. Catheter-directed thrombolysis is recommended to improve short-term and long-term venous patency as well as prevent the development of subsequent postthrombotic syndrome.
- Balloon venoplasty is almost always necessary after thrombolysis to open chronic stenoses and webs at the thoracic inlet that were responsible for the initial blockage.
- Stenting is not a standard of care and is rarely used when symptoms are persistent despite multiple sessions of venoplasty. Stenting is contraindicated in patients who may require surgery in the future but can be performed in those who have already undergone surgical decompression and present with recurrent obstruction.

REVIEW QUESTIONS

1. CDT therapy is effective in treating PSS but is prone to an approximate _____ rate of procedural-related PE.
   a. 1%
   b. 5%
   c. 10%
   d. 25%
2. Which anatomic factor does not play a role in TOS?
   a. Bony abnormalities such as an abnormal first cervical rib, elongated C7 transverse process, exostosis or tumor of the first rib or clavicle, or excess callus of the first rib or clavicle.
   b. Soft tissue abnormalities such as fibrous band, congenital muscle abnormalities, insertion muscle variations, or supernumerary muscles.
   c. Soft tissue abnormalities including posttraumatic fibrous scarring, postsurgical scarring, postural variation, and weak muscular support in thin women.
   d. Vascular abnormalities such as May-Thurner syndrome
3. How should the dose of anticoagulation in PSS patients undergoing CDT be titrated?
   a. Decreased, as they are already receiving fibrinolytic therapy.
   b. Unchanged
   c. Increased, secondary to expected hypercoagulability post operatively.

SUGGESTED READINGS

Alla VM, Natarajan N, Kaushik M, et al. Paget-Schroetter syndrome: review of pathogenesis and treatment of effort thrombosis. *West J Emerg Med.* 2010;11(4):358–362.

Demondion X, Herbinet P, Van Sint Jan S, et al. Imaging assessment of thoracic outlet syndrome. *Radiographics.* 2006;26(6): 1735–1750.

Grunwald MR, Hofmann LV. Comparison of urokinase, alteplase, and reteplase for catheter-directed thrombolysis of deep venous thrombosis. *J Vasc Interv Radiol.* 2004;15(4): 347–352.

Illig KA, Doyle AJ. A comprehensive review of Paget-Schroetter syndrome. *J Vasc Surg.* 2010;51(6):1538–1547.

Kearon C, Akl EA, Ornelas J, et al. Antithrombotic therapy for VTE disease: CHEST guideline and expert panel report. *Chest.* 2016;149(2):315–352.

Lee JT, Karwowski JK, Harris EJ, et al. Long-term thrombotic recurrence after nonoperative management of Paget-Schroetter syndrome. *J Vasc Surg.* 2006;43(6):1236–1243.

Sabeti S, Schillinger M, Mlekusch W, et al. Treatment of subclavian-axillary vein thrombosis: long-term outcome of anticoagulation versus systemic thrombolysis. *Thromb Res.* 2002;108(5–6):279–285.

Urschel Jr. HC. Anatomy of the thoracic outlet. *Thorac Surg Clin.* 2007;17(4):511–520.

Transjugular Intrahepatic Portosystemic Shunts

Paul B. Lewis, Sara E. Smolinski, Jacob W. Fleming, Ron C. Gaba

CASE PRESENTATION

A 57-year-old male has recurrent ascites that is poorly controlled with medications and requires large-volume paracentesis two to three times a month. He has had one episode of hepatic encephalopathy since being diagnosed with alcoholic cirrhosis 8 years prior. As a candidate for liver transplant, he undergoes regular surveillance imaging and laboratory evaluation. A recent triple-phase liver computed tomography scan demonstrates no masses, and a cardiac echo showed normal chamber pressures and ejection fraction. Labs include an INR of 2; total bilirubin, 1.2 mg/dL; creatinine, 1.3 mg/dL; and serum sodium, 140 mEq/L (Model for End-stage Liver Disease [MELD] = 14). His hepatologist recommends **transjugular intrahepatic portosystemic shunt** creation.

- In the normal physiologic state, blood from the abdominal viscera drains into the portal vein, passes through the hepatic parenchyma (via microscopic vascular spaces termed *hepatic sinusoids*), and ultimately exits by the hepatic veins. The hepatic vein then joins the inferior vena cava to drain into the right atrium. This normal blood flow pattern is called hepatopetal.
  - This arrangement allows for (1) the metabolism of a number of molecules by hepatocytes before entering the systemic circulation and (2) the simultaneous nourishment of the liver parenchyma by nutrient-rich blood.
- In portal hypertension, elevated pressures develop in the portal vein secondary to increased vascular resistance. This change in vascular tone ultimately leads to a reversal in the direction of blood flow through the portal vein, which is described as hepatofugal.
  - The underlying etiology of increased vascular resistance can be classified as presinusoidal, sinusoidal, and postsinusoidal in relation to the hepatic sinusoids.
- The most common etiology is cirrhosis (i.e. scarring of the liver), which is a sinusoidal process.
  - Worldwide, the most common cause of cirrhosis is chronic viral hepatitis (frequently by the hepatitis C virus). In the United States, non-alcoholic steatohepatitis (NASH) and alcoholic liver disease (ALD) are the second and third most prevalent causes, respectively.
- Through a different mechanism, presinusoidal "masses" such as cancers or portal vein thromboses can physically block blood flow through the liver and, as a result, reverse the direction of blood flow.

- The gold standard to objectively appraise portal hypertension is measuring the hepatic venous pressure gradient (HVPG).
  - HVPG = wedged hepatic vein pressure − free hepatic vein pressure
  - Portal hypertension is diagnosed with a gradient >5 mm Hg and is considered clinically significant when >10 to 12 mm Hg.
  - HVPG is in contrast to portosystemic pressure gradient (PSPG).
    - PSPG = portal vein pressure − right atrial pressure
- The two principal consequences of portal hypertension are varices and recurrent ascites.
  - Blood flowing "backward" into the tributaries of the portal vein from the liver cause collateral veins in the gastrointestinal tract to become engorged. These varices are thin-walled and are at increased risk of rupture (principle of Laplace's Law), ultimately resulting in massive bleeds, especially in the esophagus.
  - The other consequence of portal hypertension is ascites, the pathologic collection of fluid in the peritoneal space.
  - The development of ascites in portal hypertension is ultimately the result of (1) increased hydrostatic pressure, (2) increased vascular wall permeability, and (3) decreased oncotic fluid retention/resorption.
  - Ascites refractory to typical medical treatment requires frequent drainage by paracentesis. Refractory ascites has major negative effects on quality of life and predisposes the patient to spontaneous bacterial peritonitis, a major infection.
- Measures of clinical status in liver failure:
  - Model for End-stage Liver Disease (MELD) Score
    - Scoring system to assess the severity of chronic liver disease
    - Developed for prognosticating the survival of patients undergoing elective transjugular intrahepatic portosystemic shunt (TIPS) but was also found useful in organ allocation for liver transplant
      - A MELD score of 14 or less is a good predictor of survival post TIPS in elective cases and emergent settings.

- In elective TIPS, the risk of early mortality is higher in patients with a MELD score of 18 or greater.
- In emergent TIPS, poorer outcomes are more likely in patients with a MELD score of 14 or greater.
- The 30-day mortality for a patient with a MELD score of >24 is 60%.
- **Child-Pugh Score** (Table 24.1)

TABLE 24.1   Child-Turcotte-Pugh Classification for Severity of Cirrhosis

Clinical and Lab Criteria	POINTS[a]		
	1	2	3
Encephalopathy	None	Mild to moderate (grade 1 or 2)	Severe (grade 3 or 4)
Ascites	None	Mild to moderate (diuretic responsive)	Severe (diuretic refractory)
Bilirubin (mg/dL)	<2	2–3	>3
Albumin (g/dL)	>3.5	2.8–3.5	<2.8
Prothrombin time			
Seconds prolonged	<4	4–6	>6
International normalized ratio	<1.7	1.7–2.3	>2.3

[a]Child-Turcotte-Pugh Class obtained by adding score for each parameter (total points).
Class A = 5 to 6 points (least severe liver disease).
Class B = 7 to 9 points (moderately severe liver disease).
Class C = 10 to 15 points (most severe liver disease).
Reused with permission from Pugh RN, Murray-Lyon IM, Dawson JL, et al. Transection of the oesophagus for bleeding oesophageal varices. *Br J Surg.* 1973;60:646–649.

- Similar to the MELD score, the Child-Pugh score provides a succinct evaluation of the patient's liver function.
- The Child-Pugh score is calculated using serum bilirubin, albumin, and INR with assessment of the presence and degree of ascites and encephalopathy.
- Due to difficulties with the inclusion of subjective metrics, some clinicians prefer the use of the MELD score over the Child-Pugh score.

>> **CLINICAL POINT**

Model for End-stage Liver Disease-Na is a modified scoring system that takes into account a patient's serum sodium value. Hyponatremia results from solute-free water retention in patients with cirrhosis, and hyponatremia is considered an indirect marker of portal hypertension in these cases. Several studies have shown that hyponatremia is a strong predictor of early mortality in patients with severe liver disease.

- The goal of TIPS is **decompression of the portal vein** by creating an intrahepatic shunt directly from the portal vein (portal system) to a hepatic vein (systemic vasculature system).
  - This shunt **reduces the HVPG**, which decreases the risk of variceal rupture and hemorrhage.
  - TIPS serves to alleviate portal hypertension, which ultimately improves the effective circulating blood volume.
  - TIPS does not increase the oncotic pressure of the portal venous system.
    - TIPS creation may cause liver damage that can lead to a further decrease in protein production and commensurate decrease in oncotic pressure. For this reason, liver function needs to be appraised prior to TIPS creation.

INDICATIONS

- TIPS is a treatment for portal hypertension, but not all patients with portal hypertension should have the procedure; appropriate patient selection with consideration of the patient's MELD and/or Child-Pugh score is crucial.
- The American College of Radiology (ACR), Society of Interventional Radiology (SIR), and Society for Pediatric Radiology (SPR) currently consider the following to be indications for TIPS creation:
  - Emergent uncontrollable variceal hemorrhage
  - Current or prior variceal hemorrhage not amenable to endoscopic therapy
  - Prophylaxis against recurrent variceal hemorrhage in high-risk patients
  - Portal hypertensive gastropathy or intestinopathy
  - Refractory ascites
  - Hepatic hydrothorax
  - Budd-Chiari syndrome (thrombosis or compression of the hepatic vein)
  - Hepatopulmonary syndrome
  - Hepatorenal syndrome
  - Decompression of portal collateral circulation prior to abdominal surgery

>> **CLINICAL POINT**

What is the first-line treatment for esophageal varices in patients with cirrhosis? For small or medium varices found on endoscopy, nonselective β-blockers such as nadolol are preferred. For large varices prone to rupture, esophageal variceal ligation (EVL) is recommended.

CONTRAINDICATIONS

- The creation of a TIPS is not without risks, and these must be considered in patient selection.
- There are no absolute contraindications, but the ACR, SIR, and SPR list the following as relative contraindications:
  - Elevated right or left heart pressures
    - Decompression of the portal circulation increases cardiac preload and can put additional strain on the heart.

- Heart failure or valvular insufficiency
- Marked pulmonary hypertension
- Rapidly progressive liver failure
  - The liver parenchyma receives most of its blood flow by way of the portal vein. Diverting this flow in a patient with underlying liver failure could compromise liver function.
- Severe, uncorrectable coagulopathy
  - One of the chief functions of the liver is synthesis of clotting enzymes, and so diverting portal flow could theoretically compromise the liver's reserve synthetic function.
- Clinically significant hepatic encephalopathy
  - TIPS often leads to worsening of hepatic encephalopathy, so this must be taken into account in a patient with an underlying history.
- Uncontrolled systemic infection or sepsis
- Unrelieved biliary obstruction
- Extensive primary or metastatic hepatic malignancy

EQUIPMENT

- Ultrasound for internal jugular access
- Guidewires:
  - 3-mm J-wire
  - Regular and stiff curved hydrophilic wire
  - Regular and stiff Amplatz or Newton wire
- Cobra or MPA catheter
- Angioplasty balloons: 8 mm × 4 cm, 10 mm × 4 cm, 12 mm × 4 cm
- Vascular pressure transducer
- Contrast medium and/or CO_2
- TIPS set:
  - 40-cm 10-Fr introducer sheath with end marker
  - 51-cm curved guide catheter with stiffener
  - 60-cm sheathed needle ("TIPS needle")
- TIPS stents:
  - Standard practice calls for covered stents, as uncovered stents have a propensity for failure but still have success in certain clinical settings.
    - Viatorr (Gore Medical; Flagstaff, AZ) (Fig. 24.1) and Wallstent (Boston Scientific; Marlborough, MA) are popular options.
- Several kits (Figs. 24.2) are available that provide the instruments needed for TIPS creation. A few examples include (but are not limited to):
  - Fine-needle TIPS set (AngioDynamics; Glens Falls, NY)
  - Haskal set (Cook Medical; Bloomington, IN)
  - Ring set (Cook Medical; Bloomington, IN)
  - Rösch-Uchida transjugular liver access set (Cook Medical; Bloomington, IN)

ANATOMY

Why Use the Right Hepatic Vein?

- The right hepatic vein is preferred, given its typically large caliber and posterior and cephalad position relative to the

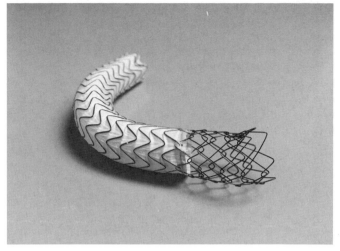

Fig. 24.1 Viatorr Transjugular Intrahepatic Portosystemic Shunt Stent. The Viatorr has a portion coated with polytetrafluoroethylene (PTFE), a polymer that reduces neointimal hyperplasia as well as transmural leakage of mucin and bile, leading to better long-term rates of patency. (Courtesy Paul Lewis, MD.)

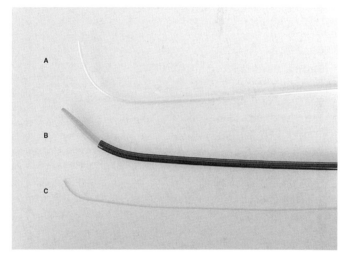

Fig. 24.2 TIPS Kit. (A) 5-Fr multipurpose catheter. (B) 10-Fr introducer sheath with end marker and stiffening cannula. (C) 0.035-inch-diameter Roadrunner wire guide (hydrophilic wire). (Courtesy Sara Smolinski, MD.)

right portal vein. Puncturing the right hepatic vein lessens the probability of injuring the liver capsule.
- The middle or left hepatic vein may be used if the right hepatic vein is absent, too small, or at a suboptimal angle arising from the IVC.

Why Use the Right Portal Vein?

- Assuming the right hepatic vein is used, the right portal vein is in a satisfactory position for access via a transparenchymal tract.
- The right portal vein is also large and profiles well on anteroposterior (AP) fluoroscopy projection.

Why Measure Right Atrial Pressure?

- TIPS increases cardiac preload by diverting the high-pressure portal circulation to the right atrium.

- If right atrial (RA) pressure exceeds 20 mm Hg, the patient has a predisposition for acute right heart failure after TIPS creation.

Why Measure the Portosystemic Pressure Gradient?

- It is important to measure the gradient prior to the procedure to ensure that the TIPS will be effective in treating symptoms and in order to limit the risk of complications such as hepatic encephalopathy. In some cases, a competitive shunt, such as a splenorenal shunt, may be present, and the gradient between the RA and portal vein may already be low, in which case the TIPS should not be placed.
- The gradient measurement itself is used to gauge the degree of shunting post TIPS and to reassess TIPS function should symptoms recur.
  - For treatment of esophageal varices, a post-TIPS gradient of less than 12 mm Hg is preferred.
  - In the setting of refractory ascites, the ideal gradient is less defined, but a final PSPG less than 12 mm Hg is recommended.

PROCEDURAL STEPS

Preprocedural Steps

- Labs: Complete blood count (CBC), platelets, hemoglobin/hematocrit (H/H), PT/INR, PTT, LFTs, serum creatinine, and type and cross if transfusion is a possibility
- Level of anesthesia: moderate conscious sedation
- Antibiotics: yes (ciprofloxacin)
- Patient position: supine with right neck prepped
- The patient is preferably euvolemic to mitigate the risk of overloading the heart.
  - A successful TIPS leads to increased preload due to diverting higher pressure portal blood to the right atrium.

Steps

1. Local anesthesia is administered, and standard Seldinger technique is used to access the right internal jugular vein.
2. 5-Fr micropuncture sheath is placed over the 0.018-inch microwire.
3. The 3-Fr inner dilator and 0.018-inch microwire are removed in tandem, leaving the 5-Fr micropuncture sheath in place.
4. A hydrophilic guidewire is inserted through the sheath, and the micropuncture sheath is then exchanged for a 9- or 10-Fr introducer sheath with an end marker (Fig. 24.3).
5. The introducer sheath is guided into the right atrium. Atrial and inferior vena cava (IVC) pressures are measured.
6. A 5-Fr multipurpose curved catheter (e.g., MPA catheter) is guided into the right hepatic vein.
7. After advancing the introducer sheath into the right hepatic vein, a hepatic venogram with iodinated contrast or CO_2 is done to confirm positioning. As CO_2 can cause capsular rupture, its use is limited.
8. The curved catheter is then exchanged for an occlusion balloon (Fig. 24.4) to measure free and wedged hepatic venous pressures.

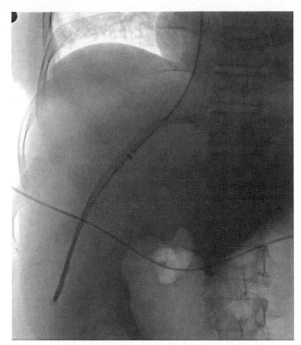

Fig. 24.3 Advancement into the Right Hepatic Vein. Fluoroscopic image demonstrates advancement of the 9-Fr vascular sheath into the right hepatic vein and contrast infused through the 5-Fr curved catheter to opacify the right hepatic vein. The free hepatic venous pressure is then measured. (Courtesy Ron Gaba, MD, and Paul Lewis, MD, at University of Illinois, Chicago.)

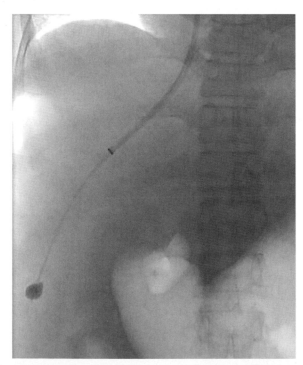

Fig. 24.4 Measuring Free and Wedged Hepatic Pressure. An occlusive balloon is inflated in a distal branch of the right hepatic vein to measure the wedged hepatic pressure. The free hepatic venous pressure is then measured with the occlusion balloon deflated. (Courtesy Ron Gaba, MD, and Paul Lewis, MD, at University of Illinois, Chicago.)

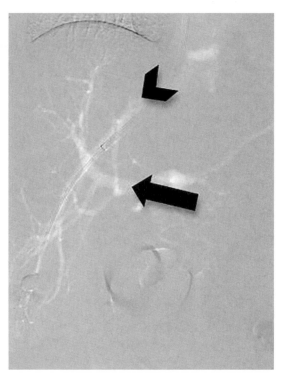

Fig. 24.5 Hepatic Venography. Hepatic venography is performed with CO_2 as a digitally subtracted angiography. The CO_2 gas perfused back into the portal system. This step maps out the target for transhepatic needle advancement from the right hepatic vein *(chevron = arrowhead)* to the portal vein *(arrow)*. (Courtesy Ron Gaba, MD, and Paul Lewis, MD, at University of Illinois, Chicago.)

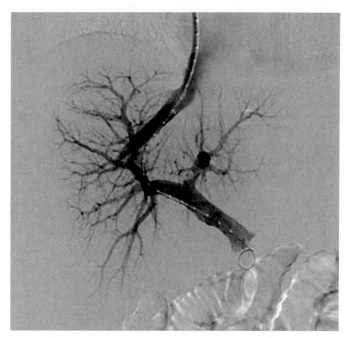

Fig. 24.6 Transhepatic Bridge. Digitally subtracted angiogram demonstrates simultaneous contrast infusion through the pigtail catheter in the portal vein and the vascular sheath in the right hepatic vein. The new transhepatic bridge is identified by the segment of the catheter not immediately surrounded by contrast medium. The pre-TIPS portal venous pressure would be acquired at this step. (Courtesy Ron Gaba, MD, and Paul Lewis, MD, at University of Illinois, Chicago.)

9. With the occlusion balloon inflated, contrast is infused into the right hepatic vein (Fig. 24.5). Due to the occlusion balloon, the contrast or CO_2 transmits into the portal system.
10. The puncture needle is pierced through hepatic parenchyma from the hepatic vein to the right portal vein.
11. Aspiration while withdrawing the puncture needle is performed until blood is obtained. If no blood is aspirated, step 10 is repeated.
12. After blood is aspirated, contrast is infused under fluoroscopy to confirm that the blood is coming from the portal system and not a hepatic artery.
13. After confirming the needle is within the portal system, a 0.038-inch stiff guidewire is advanced through the needle into the portal or splenic vein.
14. A pigtail catheter is then advanced over the guidewire to measure the portal venous pressure and calculate the pre-TIPS PSPG.
15. Contrast is then infused through this pigtail catheter to measure the transhepatic bridge (Fig. 24.6) and allow for appropriate sizing of the shunt.
16. The parenchymal tract is then dilated with an 8-mm or 10-mm angioplasty balloon.
17. A self-expandable stent graft (Fig. 24.7) is deployed across the portosystemic tract with the uncovered portion (2 cm in length) positioned within the portal vein. The covered portion of the stent should extend into the hepatic vein but not into the IVC.
18. The stent is dilated until the appropriate PSPG is reached (12 mm Hg) (Figs. 24.8–24.10).

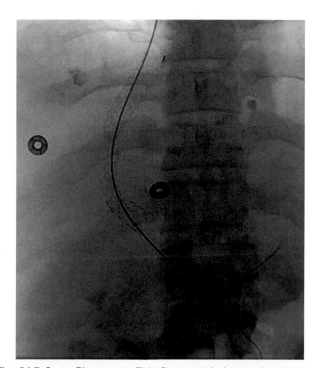

Fig. 24.7 Stent Placement. This fluoroscopic image demonstrates that the self-expanding Viatorr stent (Gore Medical, Flagstaff, AZ) has been deployed but not yet fully expanded by intrastent balloon angioplasty. (Courtesy Ron Gaba, MD, and Paul Lewis, MD, at University of Illinois, Chicago.)

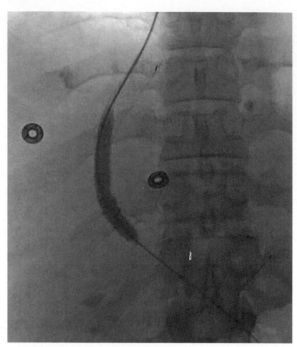

Fig. 24.8 Stent Expansion. In this fluoroscopic image, the angioplasty balloon is further expanding the Viatorr stent (Gore Medical, Flagstaff, AZ). (Courtesy Ron Gaba, MD, and Paul Lewis, MD, at University of Illinois, Chicago.)

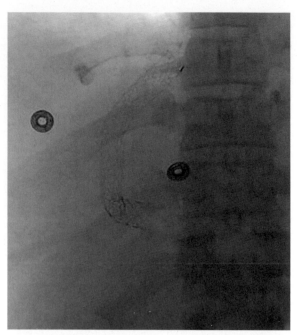

Fig. 24.10 Final Image. Final fluoroscopic image demonstrates the newly placed transjugular intrahepatic portosystemic shunt. (Courtesy Ron Gaba, MD, and Paul Lewis, MD, at University of Illinois, Chicago.)

> ## ▶ CLINICAL POINT
>
> - Take care not to extend TIPS into the IVC or extrahepatic PV, which could compromise future candidacy for liver transplantation.
> - The optimal post-TIPS PSPG is less than 12 mm Hg for variceal hemorrhage. It is a subject of debate for ascites, but optimal gradient is probably less than 12 mm Hg as well.

19. Embolization of varices can be performed, if necessary.
20. Equipment is removed, pressure is applied, and a sterile dressing is applied.
21. Patients should be monitored for postprocedural complications, typically for one to two nights. Liver function tests (LFTs) should be monitored, patient should be observed for development/worsening of hepatic encephalopathy, and Doppler ultrasound for baseline shunt function should be performed (at discharge, 3-month intervals for the first year, and 6- to 12-month intervals indefinitely).

> ## ▶ CLINICAL POINT
>
> Can a 24-hour baseline ultrasound be performed on a covered stent graft?
> No, gas within the ePTFE covering creates "dirty" shadow artifact that obscures the stent lumen. These air bubbles resolve within 2 to 4 days.

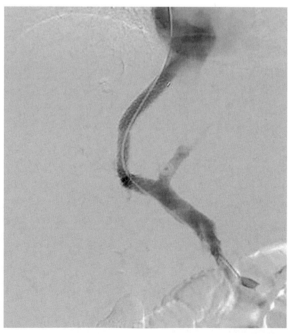

Fig. 24.9 Completion Angiogram. Final portography digitally subtracted angiogram image demonstrates opacification of the newly created TIPS as well as the main and left portal vein. (Courtesy Ron Gaba, MD, and Paul Lewis, MD, at University of Illinois, Chicago.)

ALTERNATE TREATMENTS

- Management guidelines for portal hypertension have undergone rigorous discussion and revision since the first Baveno consensus workshop in 1990.
- Guidelines focus on management of the most common sequelae of portal hypertension and those that cause the most morbidity—namely, variceal hemorrhage and ascites.
- TIPS is reserved as a treatment for advanced portal hypertension refractory to medical management (usually Child-Pugh class B or C).
- Prior to referral of a patient for TIPS placement, patients are managed medically or with serial paracentesis (in cases of recurrent ascites).
- Prior to the advent of the TIPS procedure, surgical shunts were used.
- Liver transplantation is the definitive treatment for portal hypertension.

Gastroesophageal Varices (Fig. 24.11)

- No prior hemorrhage
  - Small bleeds (*red wale sign*; Child B or C) are treated with nonselective β-blockers (propranolol, nadolol).
  - Medium/large bleeds are treated with nonselective β-blockers or endoscopic variceal ligation.
- Acute hemorrhage
  - Resuscitate with IV fluids, blood transfusion to hemoglobin of 8 g/dL, vasoactive drugs as needed, and prophylactic antibiotics (norfloxacin, ciprofloxacin)

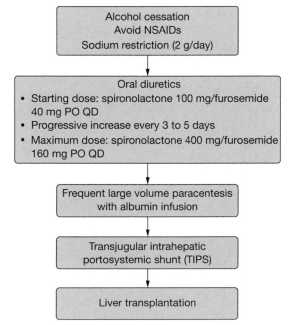

Fig. 24.11 Treatment algorithm for cirrhotic patients with refractory ascites.

- Procedure of choice is **endovascular variceal ligation** (survival benefit over TIPS)
- "Early" TIPS within 72 h in those likely to fail ligation (Child B or C) is controversial, but a survival benefit has been demonstrated.
- Prevention of rebleeding
  - Therapy of choice is a combination of **nonselective β-blockers** and **endoscopic variceal ligation**. TIPS can be performed in patients with Child A or B cirrhosis and recurrent bleeding.
  - Endoscopic sclerotherapy has been largely replaced by endoscopic variceal ligation, given the risk of rebleed and the greater number of treatments required for complete ligation. Sclerotherapy also carries risks of ulceration and stricture.

Ascites

- Medical management includes abstinence from alcohol, low = sodium diet (2000 mg/day), and diuretics (spironolactone and furosemide).
- Large = volume paracentesis
  - <5 L drained has no hemodynamic consequences.
  - If >5 L drained, give albumin 6 to 8 g/L of fluid removed.

Surgical Shunting

- Surgical options, as described below, have largely been replaced with medical management, endoscopic options, and endovascular therapy. Medical management has been shown to have a survival benefit over surgical treatment in patients with gastroesophageal varices.
- Surgical shunt creation carries a high risk of encephalopathy, and the technical skill required limits number of surgeons who can consistently achieve satisfactory outcomes.
- Surgical options include:
  - **Total portal systemic shunt**: end-to-side or side-to-side shunt created by anastomosing the main portal vein to the IVC
  - **Partial portal systemic shunt**: graft placed between the portal vein and the IVC
    - This procedure maintains some flow to the liver but carries a higher risk of shunt occlusion.
  - **Selective variceal decompression**: creation of a distal splenorenal shunt
    - Requires maintenance of portal hypertension by interrupting the gastroepiploic arcade and ligating the right and left gastric veins.
  - **Devascularization**: splenectomy, ligation of all vessels of the distal esophagus and proximal stomach, and possible esophageal transection

Orthotopic Liver Transplant

- Depends on clinical status of the patient (cirrhosis with Child-Pugh score of 7 or a MELD score of 15), etiology of cirrhosis, promise of abstinence from alcohol and drugs, social support system, and availability of a donor organ, among other factors.

COMPLICATIONS

- Complications during or as a result of TIPS are population based.
- Based on the clinical setting, individual cases may have significantly greater or less probability of complications or adverse events occurring.
- Major complications, as defined by the Society of Interventional Radiology, overall occur in about 5% of cases and further decrease with increased operator experience.

Intraprocedural

- TIPS creation has the same access site–related complications as seen with transjugular liver biopsy (TJLB).
- Tract formation (i.e., piercing for the portal vein) can cause similar complications as tissue sampling during a TJLB.
- **Biliary complications**
  - While traversing the liver parenchyma, the needle can transect a bile duct. This can later lead to TIPS-associated infection, biloma formation, or biliary occlusion by mass effect.
  - With the use of covered stents, a biliary-venous fistula is remarkably rare.
- Transcapsular puncture
  - Occurs in about one-third of cases with <3% of those cases developing intraperitoneal hemorrhage.
  - The gallbladder is the most common non-target organ punctured, and inadvertent puncture leads to hemobilia, cholangitis, and intrabiliary thrombus.
  - There are only a few sequelae from non-target puncture of the right kidney, colon, and duodenum.
- Shunt maldeployment
  - Due to operator error. Most commonly, the shunt is inadvertently deployed on the back table or when inserting it into the sheath.
- Shunt malpositioning
  - The TIPS device can be too short, too long, or have appropriate length but be "off center" within the parenchymal tract.
- Right heart failure
  - TIPS increases cardiac preload by diverting high-pressure portal circulation to the right atrium.
  - Right atrial pressure >20 mm Hg increases the propensity for acute right heart failure.
- **Major hemorrhage and death**
  - Estimated to be 1% in the ACR-SIR-SPR Practice Parameter for the Creation of a TIPS (Amended 2014 [Resolution 39]).
- **Radiation dermatitis and ulceration**
  - Dermatitis and ulceration present weeks after intraprocedural radiation exposure.
  - This complication is reduced by remaining attentive to reducing radiation exposure and procedural time.

Intravenous ultrasound, ultrasound-assisted hepatic vein puncture, and MRI techniques have been researched as means of decreased radiation exposure for both the patient and interventionalist.

Postprocedural

- **New or worsening hepatic encephalopathy**
  - Occurs in about 30% of patients and as early as one day post TIPS.
  - Related to the increased shunting of non-metabolized blood away from the liver and into systemic circulation after a technically successful TIPS placement
  - Almost all cases can be managed medically. If medical management fails, it may be necessary to reduce the inner diameter of the TIPS ("**TIPS reduction**") or occlude it all together.
- **Hepatic failure**
  - A rare but momentous complication secondary to insult to an already compromised liver. Possible causes include:
    - TIPS diverting too much of the portal perfusion from the liver to the systemic venous system. In the normal liver, around 70% of the organ's perfusion is from the portal system. So, if too much is diverted—or shunted—the liver is markedly compromised.
    - Mass effect from the TIPS compressing vital hepatic arteries or portal veins.
    - Covered stent traversing the orifice of an important branch of the hepatic or portal veins and ultimately occluding that branch.
- **Flow-limiting stenosis or occlusion**
  - Incidence of 20% to 50%
  - Development and use of covered stent grafts has significantly decreased problems related to stent stenosis and thrombosis.
  - Stenosis occurs most commonly at the hepatic vein end of the TIPS. The second most common place is within the TIPS.
  - Workup includes TIPS venography with portosystemic gradient measurements.
  - Stenosis in the locations mentioned above responds well to balloon angioplasty.
    - TIPS occlusion or hemodynamically significant stenosis recalcitrant to balloon angioplasty can be addressed with placing a second, parallel TIPS.
- **Shunt migration**
  - May occur during or after the procedure
  - Hepatoatrial migration (centrally into the right atrium) is much more difficult to address than hepatoportal migration.
- **Persistent ascites**
  - No response or partial response to TIPS occurs in 10% to 50% of patients.
  - Workup includes TIPS venography with portosystemic gradient measurements.
  - Can be addressed with placing a second, parallel TIPS.

CASE PRESENTATION

A patient who underwent transjugular intrahepatic portosystemic shunt creation 6 months ago experiences persistent, recurrent symptomatic ascites that fails medical management, and so he presents for **TIPS revision**. The TIPS extends from the right portal vein to the right hepatic vein. The initial portogram demonstrates a patent 8-mm Viatorr TIPS shunt. The PSPG is 17-mm Hg (Fig. 24.12).

Final portogram demonstrates the original 8-mm Viatorr covered stent graft and the new 10-mm Viatorr stent graft (containing the pigtail catheter). The new parallel TIPS extends from the left portal vein to the right hepatic vein. The new PSPG is 7 mm Hg, representing a reduction of 10 mm Hg (Fig. 24.13).

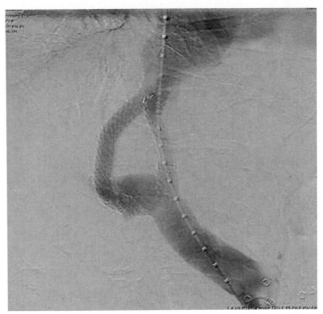

Fig. 24.13 Post-TIPS Reduction. Final portogram demonstrating the original 8-mm Viatorr covered-stent graft and the new 10-mm Viatorr stent graft (containing the pigtail catheter). The new parallel transjugular intrahepatic portosystemic shunt extends from the left portal vein to the right hepatic vein. The portosystemic pressure gradient was 7 mm Hg, representing a reduction of 10 mm Hg. (Courtesy Ron Gaba, MD, and Paul Lewis, MD, at University of Illinois, Chicago.)

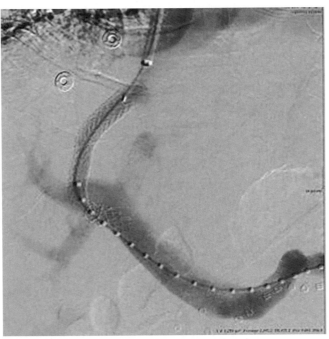

Fig. 24.12 Recurrent Ascites Following TIPS. A patient 6 months post transjugular intrahepatic portosystemic shunt (TIPS) creation experienced persistent, recurrent symptomatic ascites that failed medical management and presented to undergo TIPS revision. The TIPS extends from the right portal vein to the right hepatic vein. The initial portogram demonstrating a patent 8-mm Viatorr TIPS shunt. The portosystemic pressure gradient was 17 mm Hg. (Courtesy Ron Gaba, MD, and Paul Lewis, MD, at University of Illinois, Chicago.)

- **Recurrent variceal bleeding**
  - TIPS placement alone has 20% incidence of recurrent variceal bleeding at 6 months.
  - When TIPS is done with concurrent variceal embolization, the incidence of recurrent bleeding is only about 6% at 6-month follow-up.
  - Ectopic varices (e.g., colonic, ileal, jejunal, duodenal, and parastomal varices) are at increased risk for rebleeding.
- **Infection**
  - Called *tipsitis* or *endotipsitis*, this complication rarely occurs.

TAKE-HOME POINTS

- Transjugular intrahepatic portosystemic shunt (TIPS) creation is a safe and effective procedure to decompress the portal venous system as a means of treating and preventing variceal bleeding and ascites in an elective or emergent clinical setting.
- TIPS is a technically difficult procedure that creates a transhepatic shunt from the portal venous system (portal vein) to the systemic venous shunt (hepatic vein). This shunt reduces the hepatic venous pressure gradient and portal venous hydrostatic pressure but does not increase the portal venous oncotic pressure.

- Common indications for TIPS creation include emergent uncontrollable variceal hemorrhage, variceal hemorrhage not (or incompletely) controlled by endoscopic therapy, refractory ascites, or hepatic hydrothorax. These indications and associated morbidity need to be balanced with the relative contraindications and risks of TIPS creation.
- The gold standard to objectively appraise TIPS creation is measuring the hepatic venous pressure gradient; a gradient less than 12 mm Hg is technically successful.

Continued

TAKE-HOME POINTS—cont'd

- The routine follow-up after TIPS creation includes, but is not limited to, TIPS Doppler ultrasound and liver function tests 2 to 3 weeks post procedure, in 3-month intervals for the first year and then 6- to 12-month intervals thereafter. Patient should be closely monitored for signs of hepatic encephalopathy from the first post procedure day and thereafter.

- The 2-year survival rate after TIPS with a covered stent is approximately 75%. Patients undergoing elective TIPS creation with a Model for End-stage Liver Disease (MELD) score of 18 tend to have poorer outcomes. In the emergent setting, patients with a MELD score of 14 have increased risk of mortality.

REVIEW QUESTIONS

1. An intrahepatic shunt typically shunts between which two blood vessels?
   a. Right hepatic vein, right portal vein
   b. Right hepatic vein, left portal vein
   c. Middle hepatic vein, right portal vein
   d. Middle hepatic vein, left portal vein
2. In which patient scenario is TIPS placement most indicated?
   a. In a patient with a small amount of ascites
   b. In a patient with Child's A cirrhosis and small varices
   c. In a patient with Child's B cirrhosis and recurrent variceal hemorrhage
   d. In a patient with hepatic hydrothorax and uncontrolled hepatic encephalopathy
3. The pathophysiologic consequences of concomitant portal hypertension and liver failure include which of the following within the portal circulation?
   a. Increased hydrostatic pressure, increased oncotic pressure
   b. Increased hydrostatic pressure, decreased oncotic pressure
   c. Decreased hydrostatic pressure, increased oncotic pressure
   d. Decreased hydrostatic pressure, decreased oncotic pressure

SUGGESTED READINGS

Fidelman N, Kwan SW, LaBerge JM, et al. The transjugular intrahepatic portosystemic shunt: an update. *AJR Am J Roentgenol.* 2012;199:746–755.

Haskal ZJ, Duszak R, Furth EE. Transjugular intrahepatic transcaval porto-systemic shunt: the gun-sight approach. *J Vasc Interv Radiol.* 1996;7:139–142.

Rösch J, Hanafee WN, Snow H. Transjugular portal venography and radiologic portacaval shunt: an experimental study. *Radiology.* 1969;92(5):1112–1114.

Stephen T, Kee AG. MR-guided transjugular intrahepatic portosystemic shunt creation with use of a hybrid radiography/MR system. *J Vasc Interv Radiol.* 2005;16:227–234.

Uflacker R, Reichert P, D'Albuquerque LC, et al. Liver anatomy applied to the placement of transjugular intrahepatic portosystemic shunts. *Radiology.* 1994;191:705–712.

Transjugular Liver Biopsy

Justin Shafa, Justin P. McWilliams

CASE PRESENTATION

A 57-year-old female with a history of cirrhosis secondary to non-alcoholic steatohepatitis status post orthotopic liver transplantation in 2010 subsequently complicated by chronic rejection is postoperative day 15 from a second transplantation. She presents to the emergency department in a confused state with a moderate amount of new-onset ascites. Her INR is found to be elevated at 2.1. Her primary team requests a **transjugular liver biopsy** to assess for acute transplant rejection.

- In 1883, German immunologist Paul Ehrlich performed the first **percutaneous liver biopsy (PLB)**.
- In 1964, Dr. Charles Dotter performed the first series of **transjugular liver biopsies (TJLBs)** in dogs.
- In 1973, Dr. Josef Rosch performed TJLBs in 44 patients. He obtained quality diagnostic samples in 39 of these cases.
- PLB is considered the **gold standard** for obtaining liver specimens.
  - Tissue analysis obtained via biopsy is used to determine diagnosis and assess prognosis in patients with acute liver failure (ALF) due to unknown causes and chronic viral hepatitis.
  - This technique, by definition, penetrates the liver capsule and can cause hematoma, blood loss, and hemorrhage. Therefore, PLB should not be performed in patients with bleeding diathesis or those on anticoagulation.
- The transjugular approach is the first-line backup to the percutaneous approach.
  - Many patients with liver disease suffer from coagulopathy and/or ascites, which are both contraindications to the percutaneous approach. Therefore, in this patient subclass, the transjugular approach is widely utilized.
  - Historical concern that smaller specimens provided by the transjugular approach were inadequate for diagnosis has largely been negated by the development of newer biopsy needle systems.
- Type and gauge of needle are important factors in obtaining adequate samples. In terms of efficacy:

- Tru-cut needle = quick-core needle > Menghini needle > aspiration needle

◎ LITERATURE REVIEW

Kalambokis et al. (2007) reviewed 64 series reporting on 7,649 TJLBs, concluding that the transjugular approach was as safe as the percutaneous approach and provided comparable samples.

- Tissue samples (Table 25.1) are graded based on:
  - Size
  - Minimization of fragmentation
  - Number of *complete portal tracts* (CPTs), the most important factor

◎ KEY DEFINITION

A **complete portal track** (Fig. 25.1) contains a portal vein, hepatic artery, and bile duct, and its total circumference must be at least 75% visible for the sample to be considered adequate by the pathologist.

TABLE 25.1 Desired Tissue Sample Quality

	Noncirrhotic Livers	Cirrhotic Livers
Size (mm)	15	20–25
# of Complete portal tracts (CPTs)	6–8	11

- Failed attempts at TJLBs are uncommon and are usually due to:
  - Inability to catheterize a suitable hepatic vein
  - Failure to cannulate the jugular vein
  - Failure to obtain a liver sample
- **Hepatic venous pressure gradient (HVPG)** is the gold standard for evaluating the presence and severity of portal hypertension.
  - HVPG = wedged hepatic venous pressure (WHVP) − free hepatic venous pressure (FHVP)

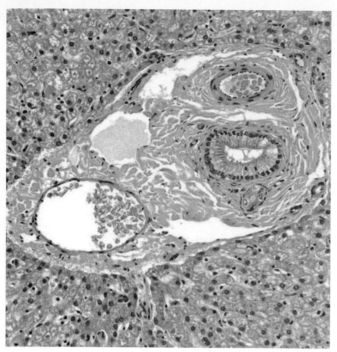

Fig. 25.1 Representative portal triad consisting of a portal vein, hepatic artery, and bile duct. (Courtesy of Fred Hutchinson Cancer Research Center.)

- HVPG = HVPG can concurrently be obtained during TJLB; it cannot be obtained during PLB.
- HVPG is used to assess:
  - Risk of variceal bleeding
  - Efficacy of drug treatment in patients with portal hypertension
- Patients who experience a reduction in HVPG of $\geq$20% or to <12 mm Hg are defined as responders to drug therapy.
  - HVPG $\leq$5 mm Hg: normal
  - 5 mm Hg < HVPG <10 mm Hg: subclinical portal hypertension
  - 10 mm Hg $\leq$HVPG: clinically significant portal hypertension
  - 12 mm Hg $\leq$HVPG: risk for variceal bleeding
  - 16 mm Hg $\leq$HVPG: increased mortality risk

▶▶ CLINICAL POINT

Hepatic resection for hepatocellular carcinoma is contraindicated in patients with HVPG >10 mm Hg due to risk of irreversible decompensation within 3 months of surgery.

INDICATIONS

- TJLB is performed when hepatic tissue is needed for pathologic analysis and PLB is contraindicated.
- Advantages over the percutaneous approach include:
  - Reduced risk of bleeding complications
  - Opportunity to perform concurrent hepatic venography
  - Opportunity to measure hepatic pressures to assess for portal hypertension

- General indications for all liver biopsies include:
  - Diagnosis, grading, and staging of infectious (chronic hepatitis B and C) and non-infectious liver diseases (non-alcoholic steatohepatitis, alcoholic liver disease, and autoimmune hepatitis)
  - Diagnosis of hemochromatosis with measurement of iron levels
  - Diagnosis of Wilson's disease with measurement of copper levels
  - Diagnosis of primary biliary cirrhosis and primary sclerosing cholangitis
  - Detecting adverse effects of drug treatment
  - Further evaluating abnormal biochemical tests and inconclusive serology reports
  - Evaluating liver status after transplantation
    - Gold standard for evaluating acute rejection. Histopathologic analysis of samples obtained by biopsy is key in evaluating posttransplant complications.
    - General 1-, 3-, and 5-year survival rates after liver transplantation are 87%, 78%, and 72%, respectively.
  - Evaluating donor liver before transplantation
  - Evaluating patients who presents with **acute liver failure (ALF)**
    - ALF is the combination of symptoms (jaundice, coagulopathy, and encephalopathy) and severe liver dysfunction presenting with acute onset, typically within 8 weeks, in a patient without a known history of liver disease.
    - Mortality rate of 65% to 85%. Liver necrosis and cirrhosis are predictors of poor long-term prognosis for patients with ALF.
    - Early and accurate diagnosis is key in determining a patient's eligibility for liver transplantation.
  - Evaluating patients with fever of unknown origin

Indications for Transjugular Liver Biopsy

BOX 25.1 Specific Indications for Transjugular Liver Biopsy

Major
- Coagulopathy (platelets <60,000, INR $\geq$2, or PT <60% normal)
- Moderate or severe ascites

Minor
- Massive obesity
- Concurrent procedures (TIPS)
- Need for additional concurrent diagnostics (venography, HVPG)
- Post–liver transplant patients with complications
- Patients with liver failure (fulminant and alcoholic types)
- Cirrhotic liver

HVPG, Hepatic venous pressure gradient; *TIPS*, transjugular intrahepatic portosystemic shunt.

Unique Indications for a Left Internal Jugular Approach

- History of difficult catheterization via the right IJ vein
- Partial or total occlusion of the right IJ vein
- Skin infection overlying the right IJ
- Existing right IJ tunneled dialysis catheter
- Anatomic variations and distortions that make right-sided approach impossible

Unique Indications for a Right Common Femoral Vein Approach

- Hyper-acute angle of the origin of the hepatic vein with the inferior vena cava (IVC) necessitating an approach from below.

Unique Indications for a Transcaval Approach

- Cannulation of the hepatic vein not being possible due to conditions including Budd-Chiari syndrome.

CONTRAINDICATIONS

- No absolute contraindications.
- Relative contraindications include:
  - Severe renal impairment
  - Contrast allergy
  - The TJLB approach should not be used to biopsy focal liver lesions as localization under fluoroscopy is not possible (unless mass is large and adjacent to a hepatic vein).
  - The TJLB patient often has an abnormal coagulation profile. Attempts should be made to correct this preprocedurally, if possible. However, this is not a contraindication to proceeding.

EQUIPMENT

- Key equipment (Fig. 25.2)
  - **Biopsy set** typically containing a 7-Fr sheath with curved metal stiffening cannula, a 5-Fr straight catheter, a 5-Fr curved catheter, and an 18G or 19G biopsy needle
  - Basic angiography set

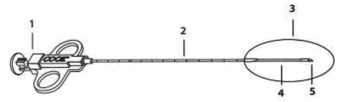

Fig. 25.3 Tru-Cut Needle. *(1)* Plunger, *(2)* cutting cannula, *(3)* approximate length of cut specimen, *(4)* specimen notch, *(5)* inner stylet. Tissue prolapses into the specimen notch when plunger is pressed in until resistance is met, and tissue is cut by advancement of the outer cutting cannula when plunger is clicked in. (Courtesy of Cook Group Incorporated.)

- 9-Fr sheath
- 5-Fr occlusion balloon (if obtaining pressures)
- Hydrophilic guidewire, Bentson wire, and Amplatz wire
- Biopsy needle options:
  - **Tru-cut** needle (Fig. 25.3)
  - **Quick-Core** needle

ANATOMY

Why the Right Internal Jugular?

- This approach offers a straighter route for the 7-Fr sheath and metal guide to reach the IVC and right hepatic vein.
- In certain circumstances, alternate sites such as the left internal jugular vein, right common femoral vein, and inferior vena cava can be used.
- The internal jugular vein lies anterior and lateral to the carotid artery just above the clavicle.
  - A mid-internal jugular puncture is ideal.
  - A low puncture increases the risk of pneumothorax, and a high puncture increases the risk of inadvertent arterial puncture, as the artery lies more posterior to the vein in the neck.

Why the Right Hepatic Vein?

- The right and middle hepatic veins (Fig. 25.4) are the preferred routes of biopsy because of the larger volumes of

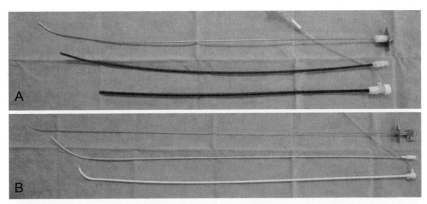

Fig. 25.2 Rosch-Uchida Transjugular Liver Access Set (A) From top to bottom: 14-G stiffening metallic cannula, modified 10-Fr outer catheter, and a 10-Fr introducer sheath. (B) From top to bottom: Brockenbrough needle, dilator, and 8-Fr introducer sheath. (Reused with permission from Okuno T, Yamaguchi M, Okada T, et al. Endovascular creation of aortic dissection in a swine model with technical considerations. *J Vascular Surg.* 2012;55(5):1410–1418, Fig. 1.)

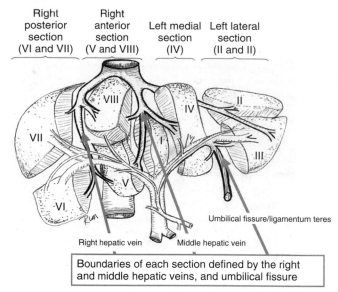

Right posterior section (VI and VII)   Right anterior section (V and VIII)   Left medial section (IV)   Left lateral section (II and II)

Right hepatic vein   Middle hepatic vein

Umbilical fissure/ligamentum teres

Boundaries of each section defined by the right and middle hepatic veins, and umbilical fissure

Fig. 25.4 Couinaud Classification. Division of the liver into eight functionally independent segments, each with its own vascular inflow, outflow, and biliary drainage. (Reused with permission from Coran AG. *Pediatric Surgery.* 7th ed. Philadelphia, PA: Elsevier; 2012, F33-34.)

adjacent liver, which decreases the risk of inadvertent liver capsule perforation. Adequate liver tissue is available anteriorly, and the metal guide can easily be directed anteriorly by turning the metallic guide counter-clockwise.

PROCEDURAL STEPS

Preprocedure

- Labs: Complete blood count (CBC), platelets, coagulation profile, Basic metabolic panel (BMP), Prothrombin time (PT)/International normalized ratio (INR), Partial thromboplastin time (PTT), Liver function tests (LFTs), and serum creatinine
- Anesthesia level: moderate sedation
- Antibiotics: none
- Patient position: supine with head turned slightly to the left

Steps

1. Local anesthesia is administered, and standard Seldinger technique is used to access the right internal jugular vein (Fig. 25.5). Access site is immediately anterior to the sternocleidomastoid muscle about an inch above the clavicle.
2. A 5-Fr micropuncture sheath is placed over the microwire, and the microwire is exchanged for a longer 0.035-inch Amplatz or Bentson guidewire, which is then advanced into the IVC.
3. Micropuncture sheath is exchanged for a long 9-Fr introducer sheath, which is placed over the wire.
4. Under fluoroscopy, the right hepatic vein is selectively catheterized with a 5-Fr curved catheter and guidewire. In difficult cases, a multipurpose catheter or Cobra II catheter may prove useful.
5. Venography is performed to confirm positioning and vessel patency (Fig. 25.6).

> ## CLINICAL POINT
>
> If obtaining pressures, they may be obtained in the right atrium and IVC following *Step 3*. Following initial venography in *Step 5*, the catheter would then be exchanged for a 5-Fr occlusion balloon, which is placed in the mid-portion of the right hepatic vein. Free hepatic pressure is obtained, and then, with the balloon inflated, wedge hepatic venous pressure is obtained.

6. Guidewire is exchanged for a stiffer Amplatz (if not initially used) or Rosen for increased structural support.
7. Over the catheter and stiff guidewire, the introducer sheath is advanced into the right hepatic vein. Venography can be repeated through the catheter to assess the position of the sheath tip, ideally 3 to 4 cm from the IVC.
8. The catheter is removed, and the curved metal cannula is advanced into the right hepatic vein.
9. On the table, the biopsy needle is prepared by pulling back on the plunger until there is a click.
10. The needle is introduced into the cannula to the exact point where the black mark on the needle shaft is at the entry point of the cannula (Fig. 25.8).

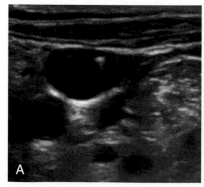
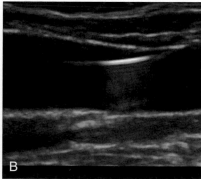

Fig. 25.5 Accessing the Right Internal Jugular Vein. Ultrasound of a guidewire in the internal jugular vein in short (A) and long (B) axis views. (Reused with permission from Duke J. *Duke's Anesthesia Secrets.* 5th ed. Philadelphia, PA: Elsevier; 2016, Fig. 23.2.)

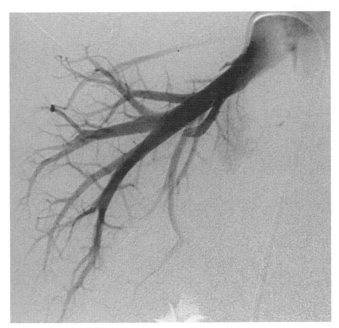

Fig. 25.6 Hepatic Vein Catheterization. Venogram demonstrating a patent right hepatic vein. (Reused with permission from Valji K. *The Practice of Interventional Radiology.* 1st ed. Philadelphia, PA: Elsevier; 2012, Fig. 12.4.)

11. The cannula is rotated accordingly, anteriorly (counterclockwise) if in the right hepatic vein or posteriorly (clockwise) if in the middle hepatic vein.
12. Needle is fired, and specimen is transferred to biopsy cup (three passes minimum) (Fig. 25.7 and Fig. 25.9).
13. The cannula is removed from the sheath and a completion venogram is performed through the side arm of the introducer sheath to evaluate for capsular perforation.
14. Remainder of the equipment is removed, pressure is held, and a sterile dressing is applied.
15. Patients should be monitored for postprocedure complications for 6 hours afterward.

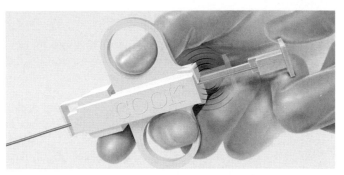

Fig. 25.8 Positioning the Needle at the Tip of the Cannula. (© 2014 Lisa Clark courtesy of Cook Medical. Used with permission from Cook Medical, Bloomington, IN, USA.)

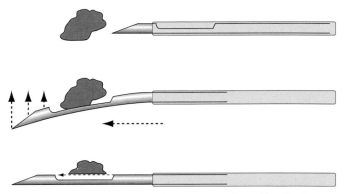

Fig. 25.9 Graphic Depiction of Automated Core Needle Biopsy Throw Mechanism. The needle deploys as a multistage process. The portion of the needle containing the sampling notch has a beveled leading tip, causing it to arc as it deploys. Upon reaching full throw, it restraightens, impressing the tissue firmly into the notch. A cutting cannula extends over the notch, shearing off a cylinder of tissue, the specimen. (From Newell MS, Mahoney MC. Image-guided percutaneous biopsy. In: Bassett LW, Mahoney MC, et al. *Breast Imaging.* Philadelphia, PA: Elsevier; 2011:563–596, Fig. 29.2.)

> ## ⟫ CLINICAL POINT
>
> One pass with a 14-gauge needle yields the same sample size as three passes with an 18-gauge needle and six passes with a 20-gauge needle.

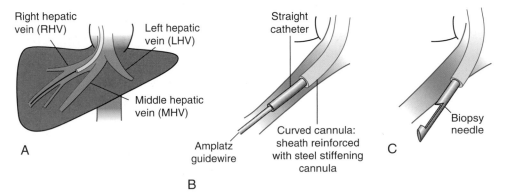

Fig. 25.7 Transjugular Liver Biopsy Technique. (A) Catheterization of the right hepatic vein *(RHV)* and exchange for an Amplatz wire. (B) Advancing the curved cannula into the right hepatic vein using a straight catheter and the Amplatz. (C) Introduction of the biopsy needle. (Reused with permission from Kessel D, Robertson I. *Interventional Radiology: A Survival Guide.* Philadelphia, PA: Elsevier; 2017, 191–198, Fig. 38.3.)

TREATMENT ALTERNATIVES

- As previously discussed, there are several methods for procuring liver tissue: percutaneous core biopsy, transjugular core biopsy, laparoscopic biopsy, and ultrasound/CT-guided fine-needle aspiration.
  - Each method has its particular advantages and disadvantages; the decision to select one over another is based upon available expertise and the clinical situation.
- **PLB** is the simplest, quickest, and the most commonly performed technique.
- **Fine-needle aspiration** provides cells for cytological examination but is not a true tissue biopsy. It is used most often when a specific identifiable lesion needs to be sampled.
- **Laparoscopic liver biopsy** provides a higher diagnostic yield in patients with cirrhosis compared to PLB and is used for staging in patients with intraabdominal malignancies. Requires that the patient be placed under general anesthesia, which is associated with increased risk and cost and is therefore often used when a patient is being taken to the operating room for another planned procedure.
- **Transjugular biopsy** approach is more invasive than the percutaneous technique but is useful in patients with a bleeding diathesis or in whom the percutaneous technique is otherwise contraindicated.

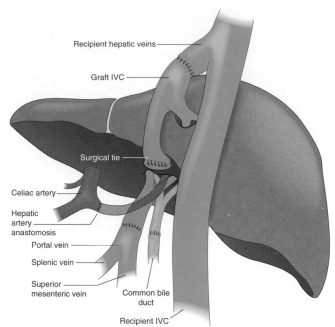

Fig. 25.10 Piggyback Technique. Venous outflow reconstruction is performed between the suprahepatic donor inferior vena cava *(IVC)* and a common orifice created by opening the native right, middle, and left hepatic veins or only the middle and left veins. (Modified from Office of Visual Media, Indiana University School of Medicine used in Cameron JL. *Current Surgical Therapy.* 12th ed. Elsevier; 2016, Liver Transplantation, Fig. 4.)

▶ CLINICAL POINT

The Post-transplant Patient
- As the vignette that began this chapter alluded to, the post-transplant patient presents a unique case in determining what method and anatomic approach to biopsy is best. These patients will likely have indications—coagulopathy and/or ascites—that indicate transjugular liver biopsies over percutaneous liver biopsy. However, depending on what type of hepatic venous anastomosis the transplant surgeon used, transjugular cannulation might be more technically challenging in the posttransplant patient depending on the angle between the inferior vena cava (IVC) and the hepatic vein.
- The two main surgical techniques include:
  - Traditional **in-line venous anastomosis** in which the donor IVC is anastomosed to the recipient's IVC, leaving the anatomic relationship intact.
  - **Piggyback technique** (Fig. 25.10) in which the end of the donor IVC is anastomosed to the side of the recipient's IVC. This acute angle makes cannulation with a transjugular approach difficult. Cannulation is still possible—using stiffer guidewires, reshaping the cannula, and timing catheterization with patient respiration helps.
    - Advantages to the piggyback technique include maintenance of caval flow, improved maintenance of core body temperature, and improved cardiac hemodynamic stability.

COMPLICATIONS

- Accesst site related:
  - Neck hematoma
  - Accidental carotid puncture
  - Transient Horner syndrome
  - Transient dysphonia
- Sample site related:
  - Abdominal and shoulder pain (13%)
  - Postprocedural fever
  - Pneumothorax
  - Capsular perforation
    - Among the most commonly seen complications
    - Can be avoided in most cases by confirmed entry into the right or middle hepatic veins with appropriate rotation of the cannula anteriorly (if in the right hepatic vein) or posterolaterally (if in the middle hepatic vein).
    - Can be treated by immediate embolization of the needle track with Gelfoam pledgets.
  - Hemoperitoneum
    - Most common cause of procedure-related death.
    - Most commonly seen in percutaneous liver biopsies but seen in transjugular biopsies as well secondary to capsular perforation.
    - Incidence increases as the biopsy site becomes more peripheral.

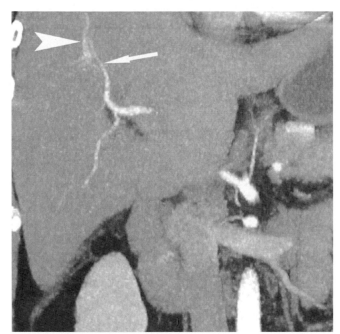

Fig. 25.11 AV Fistula Creation following TJLB. CT (computed tomography) scan of a 36-year-old man with hepatic cirrhosis who had TJLB because of suspected acute alcoholic hepatitis shows an arteriorvenous fistula between a segmental arterial branch of the right hepatic artery (arrow) and right hepatic vein (arrowhead). (From Dohan A, Guerrache Y, Dautry R, et al. Major complications due to transjugular liver biopsy: incidence, management and outcome. *Diagn Interv Imaging.* 2015;96[6]:571–577.)

- It has been shown that up to three passes with the TJLB approach does not increase complication rate, but any more than one pass with PLB does increase the complication rate.
- Fistula formation (Fig. 25.11)

LITERATURE REVIEW

Complications were noted in 7.1% of the 7,649 cases reviewed by Kalambokis et al. (2007):
- 6.5% of these were deemed minor per Society of Interventional Radiology (SIR) classification.
- 3.2% of these were due to puncture of the liver capsule.

- Catheterization related complications:
  - Cardiac arrhythmias (10%)
  - Due to passing of equipment through the right atrium and into the IVC.
  - Transient supraventricular tachycardia commonly resolves with removal of guidewires and catheters from the right atrium

LITERATURE REVIEW

Kalambokis et al. (2007) reported a 0.3% rate of Supraventricular tachycardia (SVT) and a 0.03% death rate from arrhythmias in their review of 7,469 transjugular liver biopsies.

TAKE-HOME POINTS

- Transjugular liver biopsy is a safe and highly effective alternative for obtaining diagnostic liver tissue specimens in patients with diffuse liver disease when the gold standard percutaneous approach is either suboptimal or contraindicated.
- Common indications for the transjugular approach include severe coagulopathy, ascites, evaluating posttransplant complications, need for hepatic venous pressure gradient readings, and need to do a concurrent transjugular intrahepatic portosystemic shunt (TIPS) procedure. Attempts should still be made to correct any coagulopathy preprocedurally.
- By accessing the liver parenchyma through the hepatic vein, this approach avoids puncturing the hepatic capsule as is done in the percutaneous approach.
- Complications include cardiac arrhythmias, capsular perforation, fistula formation, hemoperitoneum, and hemobilia.
- Multiple passes with the percutaneous approach results in added capsular damage that increases the risk of complication; up to three passes with the transjugular approach do not increase complication rate.
- The transjugular approach successfully obtains liver specimens in 80% to 100% of cases, and these samples are diagnostic in 85% to 100% of cases.

REVIEW QUESTIONS

1. Which of the following is not an advantage of the transjugular approach versus the percutaneous approach?
   a. Higher quality of obtained tissue sample
   b. Reduced risk of bleeding and its associated complications
   c. Opportunity for concurrent performance of hepatic venography
   d. Opportunity for concurrent measurement of hepatic pressures
2. TJLB is routinely performed to diagnose all the following except:

   a. Nonalcoholic steatohepatitis (NASH)
   b. Acute hepatitis
   c. Chronic hepatitis
   d. Hemochromatosis
   e. Wilson disease
3. Which is the preferred access site?
   a. Left internal jugular vein
   b. Right internal jugular vein
   c. Right femoral artery
   d. Right femoral vein

SUGGESTED READINGS

Behrens G, Ferral H. Transjugular liver biopsy. *Semin Intervent Radiol.* 2012;29(2):111–117. https://doi.org/10.1055/s-0032-1312572.

Kalambokis G, Manousou P, Vibhakorn S, et al. Transjugular liver biopsy—indications, adequacy, quality of specimens, and complications—a systematic review. *J Hepatol.* 2007;47:284–294.

Kaufman J, Lee M. *Vascular and Interventional Radiology: The Requisites.* Philadelphia, PA: Saunders; 2013.

Kessel D, Robertson I, Sabharwal T. *Interventional Radiology: A Survival Guide.* Edinburgh; New York: Churchill Livingstone/Elsevier; 2011.

Krohmer S, Bhagat N. Transjugular liver biopsy. In: Geschwind J, Dake M, eds. *Abrams' Angiography: Interventional Radiology.* Philadelphia, PA: Wolters Kluwer/Lippincott Williams & Wilkins Health; 2013.

Mauro M, Murphy K, Thomson K, et al. *Image-Guided Interventions.* Philadelphia, PA: Saunders/Elsevier; 2014.

Varicose Veins

Daniel E. Fuguet, Nadia V. Silva, Tameem M. Souman

CASE PRESENTATION

A 64-year-old Caucasian female with a history of venous insufficiency presents with worsening pain and swelling in her right calf that is alleviated by elevating her legs and lying in bed. She contributes the pain to her varicose veins. She wears compression stockings and states that they "barely make a difference." Recently, she has noticed that the skin surrounding the affected area has started to ulcerate. Her primary doctor refers her to an interventional radiologist for evaluation.

- In the 4th century BC, Hippocrates described treating varicose veins using a metal apparatus to induce thrombosis.
- In the 1680s, the first reports of sclerotherapy arose.
- In 1939, McCausland introduced sclerotherapy in the United States in a series with 10,000 patients.
- In 1999, the Food and Drug Administration (FDA) approved percutaneous endovenous radiofrequency (RF) thermal ablation, and in 2002, the FDA approved laser ablation therapy.
- **Chronic venous insufficiency (CVI)** and **varicose veins** arise from **chronic venous hypertension** secondary to reflux or venous obstruction. Elevated pressure can cause the venous tissue to dilate, resulting in damage to the venous wall, pain (due to stretching of receptor fibers), and skin manifestations (ulcers).
  - The most common cause is **venous reflux** due to insufficient venous valves.
    - Venous blood normally flows toward the heart. Retrograde gravitational flow is limited by valves. Failure of these valves will cause retrograde flow defined as reflux. Significant reflux lasts longer than 0.5 or 1.0 seconds.
  - The second most common cause is **venous obstruction**, most likely due to thrombosis in a venous segment from a **prior deep-vein thrombosis (DVT)**.
  - Less common causes include muscular pump dysfunction and congenital abnormalities.
- **CEAP** (clinical status, etiology, anatomy, and pathophysiology) is a system that helps establish the clinical status of the patient with CVI (Table 26.1).
- **Duplex ultrasound** (DUS) is the primary imaging modality used to evaluate CVI. DUS should be performed in patients with CEAP class C2 or higher. The patient must be standing during the exam.
  - Venous reflux is diagnosed on DUS if there is retrograde flow for **more than 0.5 second**, following dorsiflexion or mechanical compression of the calf or foot by the examiner.
- Conservative management includes leg elevation, exercise, and compression stockings, and these measures should be tried before any endovascular intervention.
- Interventional therapies used in the treatment of CVI and varicose veins include **endovascular thermal ablation (EVTA)** and **sclerotherapy**. In practice, a combination of these is likely to be used.
  - The goal of **EVTA** is to convey enough energy to the walls of an incompetent vein to cause collapse and fibrosis of the target venous segment. EVTA uses a catheter with **laser or RF emissions** to deliver high thermal doses that achieve resolution of clinical symptoms.
  - **Sclerotherapy** involves the ultrasound-guided injection of a sclerosing agent into the target vein that causes sufficient endothelial damage to dissolve the vessel wall.
- Catheter access is obtained either **percutaneously** or by **open venotomy**.
- Generally, this procedure does not require sedation or admission. Local anesthesia in the ambulatory setting is appropriate.

◎ LITERATURE REVIEWS

Min et al. (2003) reviewed 499 limbs treated with **endovenous laser ablation** and found a recurrence rate of less than 7% at 2-year follow-up. These results were superior or comparable to other treatment options available including RF ablation, US-guided sclerotherapy, and surgery.

The **EVOLVeS study** (Endovenous Radiofrequency Obliteration [Closure] versus Ligation and Stripping) by Lurie et al. (2003) reviewed 86 limbs and showed many advantages of radiofrequency ablation over surgery including faster recovery times, fewer adverse effects, and better quality of life outcomes.

INDICATIONS

- Symptoms affecting quality of life including:
  - Aching
  - Throbbing

TABLE 26.1   CEAP Classification of Chronic Venous Disease

Classification	Description/Definition
C (Clinical)—can be subdivided into A for asymptomatic and S for symptomatic	
0	No venous disease
1	Telangiectases, small varicose veins
2	Large varicose veins
3	Edema
4	Skin changes without ulceration
5	Skin changes with a healed ulcer
6	Skin changes with an active ulcer
E (Etiology)	
Congenital	Present since birth
Primary	Undetermined etiology
Secondary	Associated with prior DVT or trauma
A (Anatomic)	
Superficial	Great and short saphenous veins
Deep	Cava, iliac, gonadal, femoral, popliteal, tibial, and muscular veins
Perforator	Thigh and leg perforating veins
P (Pathophysiologic)	
Reflux	Axial and perforating veins
Obstruction	Acute and chronic
Combination of both	Valvular dysfunction and thrombus

CEAP, Clinical status, etiology, anatomy, and pathophysiology; *DVT*, deep-vein thrombosis.

- Heaviness
- Fatigue
- Pruritus
- Night cramps
- Restlessness
- Pain/discomfort
- Lower extremity swelling
- DUS showing reflux for more than 0.5 second with skin changes associated with CVI (Fig. 26.1) including:
  - Ulcers (healed or active)
  - Edema
  - Atrophie blanche pigmentation
  - Corona phlebectasia
  - Lipodermatosclerosis
  - Superficial thrombophlebitis
- For EVTA, the venous segment must be straight and large enough to allow for the catheter to be introduced. Segments that do not allow for passage of the device may be treated with sclerotherapy.
- Somewhat unique in the realm of interventional radiology, varicose veins may also be treated for purely cosmetic reasons, per patient's request.

CONTRAINDICATIONS

- No absolute contraindications
- Relative contraindications for EVTA and sclerotherapy include:
  - Currently pregnant or nursing
  - Liver dysfunction

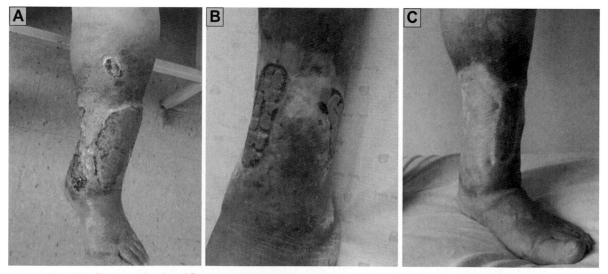

Fig. 26.1 Preprocedural and Postprocedural Pictures. (A) Preprocedural large ulcers with a 32-year chronic history. (B) Ulcers healing at 28 days after popliteal vein external banding and synchronous skin grafting. (C) At 1 year, the ulcers remained cured, and they did not recur within the 52-month follow-up. The patient wears no compression stockings. (Reused with permission from Ma T, Fu W, Ma J. Popliteal vein external banding at the valve-free segment to treat severe chronic venous insufficiency. *J Vasc Surg.* 2016;64:2:438-445.e1, Fig. 3. Copyright © 2016 Society for Vascular Surgery.)

- Allergy to local anesthetic agent (cold saline is an alternative) or sclerosing agent
- Severe uncorrectable coagulopathy
- Active DVT
- Inability to ambulate after the procedure or inability to wear compression stockings
- Active systemic infection
- Severe arterial disease
- Relative contraindications for EVTA only include:
  - Target segment within the great saphenous vein (GSV) with an aneurysm >2.5 cm
  - Target veins <1 cm deep to skin dermis after tumescent anesthesia administration (to avoid possible skin burns)
  - Chronic or recurrent phlebitis in the target vein causing sheath access difficulty secondary to synechiae formation
  - Tortuous veins that would not allow for passage of the ablation device

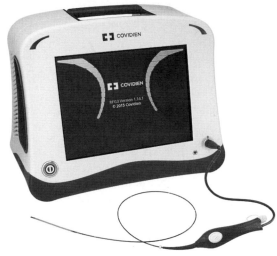

Fig. 26.2 The ClosureFast™ system utilizes segmental radiofrequency ablation to deliver uniform heat to close the vein *(Courtesy of Medtronic, Minneapolis, Minnesota)*

EQUIPMENT

- Duplex ultrasound for vein mapping and procedural guidance
- Skin marker
- Local anesthetic
- Tumescent anesthesia
  - 0.05% to 0.1% lidocaine
  - Saline
  - Bicarbonate
  - 30-mL syringe
  - 16- to 20-gauge needle used to draw anesthetic; 25- to 30-gauge needle to inject

> ◎ **KEY DEFINITION**
>
> **Tumescent** means swollen. Tumescent anesthesia refers to the injection of a large volume of dilute lidocaine into the subcutaneous space to cause the tissue to become firm and swollen. This is beneficial as it decreases the incidence and severity of postprocedural paresthesia and thermal injury and contributes to faster recovery time.

- No. 11 scalpel
- Heparinized saline
- Laser safety goggles
- 0.9% saline
- Cotton-roll wrap or elastic adhesive bandage
- Compression stockings
- Wound dressing with adhesive or Steri-Strips
- For **EVTA or Radiofrequency Ablation (RFA)** cases:
  - Micropuncture kit containing:
    - 18- to 21-G echogenic micropuncture needle
    - 0.018-inch micropuncture guidewire
    - 5-Fr or 6-Fr vascular introducer sheath
  - Catheter sheath kit containing:
    - 0.035-inch J-tipped guidewire
    - 6-Fr or 8-Fr dilator/sheath

- Ablation device; options include:
  - 400- or 600-μm endovascular diode laser fiber
    - Wavelengths: 810 nm (most common), 940 nm, 980 nm, 1064 nm, 1320 nm, 1470 nm
  - RF catheter
    - RF generator (Fig. 26.2)
    - 7-Fr vascular introducer sheath
- For sclerotherapy:
  - 18- to 25- gauge needle
  - Sclerosant
    - Polidocanol, purified sodium tetradecyl sulfate, or sodium morrhuate
  - For a foaming system, the following is needed:
    - Two 10-mL syringes
    - 10-cm infusion set tubing
    - Three-way stopcock

ANATOMY

- The **superficial venous system** (Fig. 26.3) is superficial to the deep muscular fascia and drains into the deep venous system. This includes the GSV and short saphenous vein (SSV).
  - GSV
    - Its course begins in the dorsal foot, and it ascends along the medial leg adjacent to the saphenous nerve before eventually draining into the femoral vein near the groin at the **saphenofemoral junction (SFJ)**.
    - Procedural considerations: catheter should be inserted 2.5 cm below the SFJ, and the sheath should be above the knee in order to avoid injuring the saphenous nerve.

> ▷ **CLINICAL POINT**
>
> The most common cause of symptomatic chronic venous insufficiency is great saphenous vein reflux. Discomfort originates from the pressure applied to nearby nerves from dilated veins.

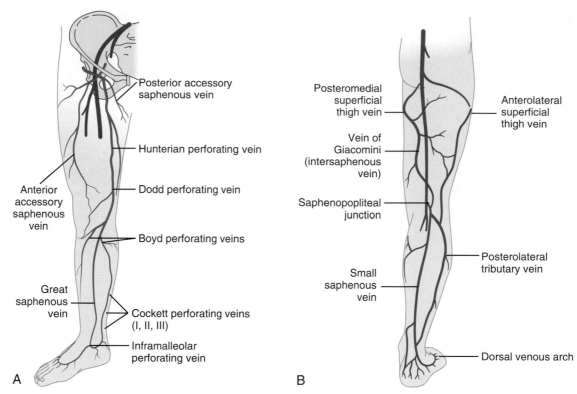

Fig. 26.3 Drawings of the Superficial Veins of the Leg. (A) The great saphenous vein with tributary and perforating veins. (B) Posterior superficial veins. (Modified from Bergan JJ. Varicose veins: treatment by surgery and sclerotherapy. In: Rutherford RB, ed. *Vascular Surgery*. 5th ed. Philadelphia, PA: WB Saunders; 2000, Fig. 16.2.)

- **Short (or small) saphenous vein**
  - Begins in the lateral foot and ascends in the midline of the lower leg alongside the sural nerve before draining into the popliteal vein (in two-thirds of patients) or further superior in the posterior thigh (one-third of patients).
  - Procedural consideration: catheter tip is introduced at the "fascial curve" before joining the popliteal vein, with the sheath at the inferior edge of the gastrocnemius muscle, to avoid injuring medial cutaneous sural nerve.
  - The **Giacomini vein** is a communication between the GSV and SSV.
- The **deep venous system** lies beneath the deep muscular fascia and can be either intramuscular or intermuscular. This includes, but is not limited to, the femoral, peroneal, popliteal, sinusoidal, and tibial veins.
- The **perforating veins** traverse the muscle fascia as a communication between the superficial and deep veins. This includes Boyd, Cockett, Dodd, and Hunterian perforators.
  - Procedural considerations: catheter tip should be 5 to 10 mm above the deep muscular fascia to prevent thermal injury to deep veins.

PROCEDURAL STEPS

Preprocedural Steps

- Sclerotherapy is used primarily in the management of spider veins, telangiectasias, and reticular veins—in other words, vessels that is not easily accessible by EVTA.

- The amount and strength of sclerosant are directly proportional to the diameter of the target vessel:
  - **Small spider veins** (1-mm diameter) can be treated with glycerin/lidocaine/epinephrine combination (glycerin 72% mixed 2:1 with 1% lidocaine with epinephrine 1:100,000) or 0.1% sodium tetradecyl sulfate (Fibrovein).
  - **Telangiectasias** (1–3-mm diameter) can be treated with hypertonic saline or microfoams prepared from sodium tetradecyl 0.1% to 0.3% depending on the diameter.
  - **Reticular veins** and tributary varicosities can be treated with hypertonic saline or microfoams prepared from 0.3% or 1% sodium tetradecyl sulfate.
  - **Saphenous vein** and large tributaries can be treated with 3% sodium tetradecyl sulfate.
  - Veins >4 mm normally do not respond to hypertonic saline. Hypertonic saline can be used in patients with liver dysfunction or an allergy to sclerosant.

Sclerotherapy Steps

1. Draw the necessary amount of sclerosant into a 3- or 5-mL syringe with a 30-gauge needle (can be bent at an angle if preferred).
2. Prepare the skin with alcohol.
3. Enter the target vein as parallel to skin as possible. Proper position in the vessel can be confirmed by drawing back a small amount of blood into the syringe. Use ultrasound guidance when dealing with large-diameter or deep veins such as the saphenous veins (Fig. 26.4).
4. Proceed to administer the sclerosant until there is blanching around the injection site or resistance is felt. When treating

saphenous veins, the ultrasound probe can be used to occlude junction points between the target vessels and the non-target deep venous system (such as the saphenofemoral or saphenopopliteal junction or a perforating vein).

▶ CLINICAL POINTS

- A wheal formation is evidence of sclerosant extravasation. Stop injecting sclerosant immediately.
- Do NOT use more than 10 mL of glycerine/lidocaine/ epinephrine in one session as it may cause transient hematuria. For sodium tetradecyl sulfate, a maximum of 10 mL of 3% is recommended.

Endovascular Thermal Ablation

1. Begin by using the ultrasound to map the target vessels and segments, marking their course on the skin.
2. The treatment area must be sterilely prepped and draped.
3. Utilizing ultrasound guidance (either transverse or sagittal), access the vein using the standard Seldinger technique. The best point of access is caudal to the most inferior segment of reflux.

▶ CLINICAL POINT

Avoid accessing the saphenous vein between 10 and 15 cm inferior to the knee to prevent saphenous nerve injury since both travel in close proximity at this level.

4. Insert the guidewire and vascular introducer sheath into the vein.
5. Position the device in the most central location of the target vein. A 0.025-inch guidewire may be used to assist the catheter in accessing tortuous segments. If treating reflux in the GSV at the SFJ, placing the device inferior to the junction of a competent epigastric vein decreases the risk of DVT formation and neovascularization.
6. Place the patient in the Trendelenburg position to allow for venous emptying. A heparin infusion may be required when performing RF ablation to completely empty the vessel (Fig. 26.5).
7. Perivenous tumescent anesthesia is delivered along the entire target segment under ultrasound guidance. This serves as a vasoconstrictor to improve the delivery of energy to the vein. It also serves as a barrier to prevent skin burns.

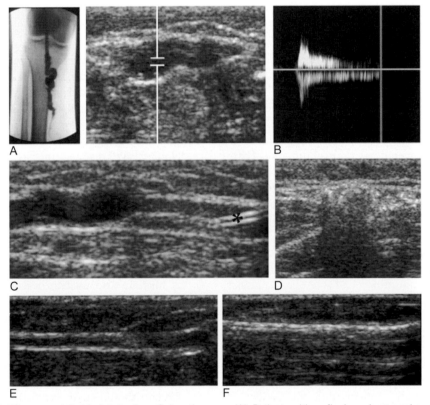

Fig. 26.4 Ultrasound-Guided Injection Sclerotherapy. (A) Patient with refluxing short saphenous vein. Attempted radiofrequency ablation of the vein was unsuccessful because the vessel was too tortuous for catheterization. (B) Transverse ultrasound image of the SSV caudal to the saphenopopliteal junction before injection sclerotherapy. (C) Doppler tracing shows prolonged reflux after augmentation. (D) Longitudinal ultrasound image of the SSV shows a 20G Angiocath (*) inserted under real-time ultrasound guidance. Approximately 3 mL of microfoam created from 3% sodium tetradecyl sulfate 1:5 with room air was injected under real-time sonographic monitoring. When the column of microfoam approached the saphenopopliteal junction, this point of potential communication was compressed for 5 minutes to prevent the spilling of microfoam into the popliteal vein. (E) Transverse image of the SSV at about the same level as (B) showing echogenic microfoam filling the vessel lumen. (F) In a different patient, longitudinal image of residual great saphenous vein lumen after attempted endovenous ablation. (From Worthington-Kirsch RL. Injection sclerotherapy. *Semin Intervent Radiol.* 2005;22[3]:209–217. https://www.ncbi.nlm.nih.gov/pmc/articles/PMC3036677/figure/f22209-3/.)

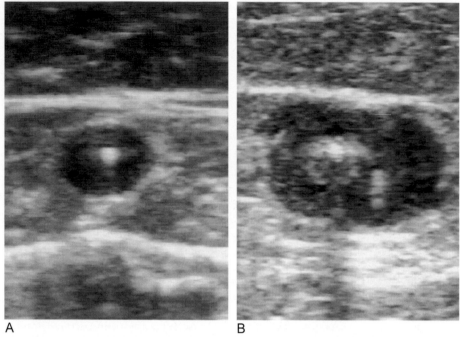

A   B

Fig. 26.5 Duplex US (transverse view) demonstrating appearance of the great saphenous vein (GSV) before and after proper delivery of tumescent anesthesia. (A) Intraluminal position of laser fiber and catheter within an enlarged GSV. (B) Tumescent anesthesia delivered by echogenic needle tip adjacent to laser fiber and catheter with fluid surrounding the compressed GSV. (Reused with permission from Min RJ, Khilnani N, Zimmet SE. Endovenous laser treatment of saphenous vein reflux: long-term results. *J Vasc Interv Radiol.* 2003;14 [8]:991–996, Fig. 1.)

▶▶ CLINICAL POINT

Make sure that the most superficial part of the target vein is **at least 1 cm** from the skin surface to prevent skin burns.

---

8. Thermal energy is delivered per the technique's specifications:
   a. For laser ablation, the device is pulled back to maintain energy delivery at a rate of 80 to 100 joules/cm at 12 to 14 watts.
   b. For RF ablation, the probe is heated to 85°C. For the first 5 cm, the device is pulled back at a rate of 1 cm/min. Over the remainder of the vein's course, it is retracted at 2 to 3 cm/min.
9. Catheter is removed.
10. Venous entry site is manually compressed.
11. The treated vein is reimaged with ultrasound. Absence of flow, concentric narrowing, and wall thickening signal successful treatment.
12. Compression stockings (thigh-high class II) or ACE bandages are placed on the patient, and the patient is observed for at least 30 minutes prior to discharge.
13. Follow-up should include a repeat ultrasound to verify success and evaluate for a potential DVT (Fig. 26.6).

ALTERNATE TREATMENTS

- Treatment of CVI should begin conservatively with behavior modification and noninvasive techniques (compression stockings) in an attempt to prevent further disease progression.
- CEAP classification and Venous Severity Score (VSS) have been used to characterize CVI and can help the physician in planning appropriate treatment approaches.
- Noninvasive treatment options include:
  - **Behavioral modification:** including leg elevation, exercising, and reducing intraabdominal pressure (i.e., weight loss).
  - **Compression stockings:** use of graded external compression helps to improve oxygen transport and opposes hydrostatic forces, thereby decreasing lower extremity edema, inflammation, and discomfort. Stockings are also used to heal venous ulcers and prevent their recurrence.
    - Elasticity is graded between 20 and 50 mm Hg.
    - Better patient compliance is seen with knee-length compression stockings rather than thigh-high stockings.
- **Skin care** including moisturizers and emollients to help prevent skin breakdown and subsequent complications. Patients should be advised to use a mild non-soap cleanser in order to prevent drying out the skin. Topical steroids are used for stasis dermatitis while silver-impregnated dressings are used for infected ulcers.
- **Pharmacologic management** may include aspirin, antibiotics, diuretics, vasoconstrictors, and anti-inflammatory agents.
- **Microphlebectomy,** also known as ambulatory or stab phlebectomy, is best performed on varicose tributaries.

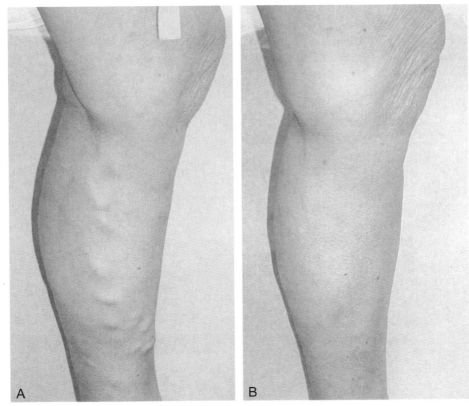

Fig. 26.6 Significant improvement in appearance of varicose tributaries after endovenous laser treatment of an incompetent left great saphenous vein (GSV). (A) Typical appearance of varicose veins caused by GSV reflux. (B) The same leg 1 month after endovenous laser treatment. (Reused with permission from Min RJ, Khilnani N, Zimmet SE. Endovenous laser treatment of saphenous vein reflux: long-term results. *J Vasc Interv Radiol.* 2003;14[8]:991–996, Fig. 3.)

Multiple 3- to 4-mm skin incisions are made to allow small hooks to remove target vein.

- **Stripping and ligation** involves the removal of affected vein under general or spinal anesthesia. This option is reserved for severe, refractory, or recurrent CVI as there is high perioperative morbidity. The same technique is performed to harvest veins during coronary artery bypass surgery.
- **Valve reconstruction** describes open valvuloplasty or transcommissural valvuloplasty on deep veins. There is a high incidence of postprocedural DVT.

COMPLICATIONS

◎ LITERATURE REVIEW

The Comparison of Laser Surgery and foam sclerotherapy (**CLASS**) trial by Brittenden et al. (2015) reported the following general procedural complication rates:
- EVTA—1%
- Foam sclerotherapy—7%
- Surgery—8%

Endovascular Thermal Ablation and Radiofrequency Ablation
- Anatomy treatment failure (Table 26.2)
- Venous complications:

TABLE 26.2 Anatomic Failure

Type 1	Nonocclusion	Vein not occluded initially or at follow-up.
Type 2	Recanalization	Vein occluded initially; recanalization seen at follow-up.
Type 3	Groin reflux	Vein occluded; reflux demonstrated at groin.

  - Superficial phlebitis (5%)
    - An expected complication to some extent at the target ablated vein. However, retrograde extension of a thrombus causes both inflammation and pain.
    - Symptomatic patients can be offered compression stockings and anti-inflammatory agents (nonsteroidal anti-inflammatory drugs [NSAIDs]), and are advised to walk.
    - Can be followed with serial duplex ultrasounds until resolution.
  - DVT (<1%)
  - Arteriovenous (AV) fistula
- Regional complications:
  - Delayed tightness, "pulling" (90%)
  - Bruising (24%)
  - Paresthesia (15%–22%)
    - Due to thermal or mechanical nerve irritation.

- Usually transient and symptoms can be prevented or blunted with the use of tumescent anesthesia.
- Occurs more commonly in the leg than the thigh due to the relative proximity of the saphenous nerve and sural nerve to the GSV and SSV, respectively.
- Skin burns (0.5%–3%)
- Lidocaine toxicity from tumescent anesthesia (<1%)

> ## ▶▶ CLINICAL POINT
>
> More complications are reported with laser wavelengths ≥1064 nm.

Sclerotherapy

- Acute complications
  - Visual disturbances (1.5%)
    - Typically transient, subsiding within 30 minutes, but may periodically recur.
    - Increased risk associated with migraines with aura.

- Transient confusion
- Transient paresthesia
- Delayed complications
  - Thrombophlebitis (5%)
  - DVT (1%)
  - Skin necrosis (<1%)
  - Skin hyperpigmentation
  - Gait disturbances
    - Often attributed to calf muscle fibrosis
    - This may be due to sclerosant extravasation or local complications in blood flow following the procedure.
    - Patients may subsequently develop ankle contractions.

> ## ▶▶ CLINICAL POINT
>
> Foam sclerotherapy causes less immediate postprocedure pain than EVTA.

🏠 TAKE-HOME POINTS

- Chronic venous insufficiency (CVI) and varicose veins result from chronic venous hypertension.
  - Great saphenous vein (GSV) reflux due to insufficient valves is the most common cause.
- Venous reflux is diagnosed on Doppler ultrasound if there is retrograde flow for more than 0.5 s following dorsiflexion or mechanical compression of the calf or foot by the examiner.
- Interventional therapies used in the treatment of CVI and varicose veins include endovascular thermal ablation (EVTA) and sclerotherapy. Before any interventional procedure, conservative management must be tried first.
  - Sclerotherapy is used primarily for the treatment of spider veins, telangiectasias, and reticular veins (vessels that are not easily accessible by EVTA).

- Tumescent anesthesia not only helps enhance intra- and post-procedural analgesia but also works to decrease thermal-related injuries and post procedure paresthesias.
- The saphenous nerve and sural nerve are at greatest risk of injury due to their anatomic proximity to the GSV and short saphenous vein (SSV), respectively.
- The Comparison of LAser Surgery and foam Sclerotherapy (CLASS) trial found the procedural complication rates of EVTA (1%) to be less than that documented in foam sclerotherapy (7%) or surgery (8%).
- Up to 90% of patients will experience a delayed tightness or pulling sensation following EVTA and RFA.
- Superficial phlebitis is a relatively common complication of EVTA and sclerotherapy and can often be managed conservatively with compression stockings, NSAIDs, and early ambulation.

▌ REVIEW QUESTIONS

1. Mrs. Smith, a 62-year-old Caucasian female, is referred to your clinic due to progressive discomfort in her lower extremities with accompanying edema and skin hyperpigmentation. Feelings of heaviness and fullness in her legs worsen throughout the day and are exacerbated by prolonged standing. She admits she believed this was a normal part of aging as her mother developed the same issues. Her past medical history includes obesity and hypertension. You suspect she has developed sequelae of chronic venous insufficiency. What is the most likely etiology of this patient's symptoms?
   a. May-Thurner syndrome
   b. GSV reflux

   c. Primary muscle pump dysfunction
   d. Perforator vein incompetence

2. After confirming the diagnosis of CVI, Mrs. Smith inquires about her treatment options. In addition to encouraging behavior modification, like weight loss and leg elevation, which of the following are you likely to offer first?
   a. Transcommissural valvuloplasty
   b. Sclerotherapy
   c. Compression stockings
   d. EVTA

3. A 68-year-old Hispanic male with a history of type II diabetes mellitus undergoes EVTA for symptomatic CVI. Following the procedure, the patient's skin overlying the

treatment area is erythematous and has decreased sensation to pinprick. Due to his long-standing diabetes and underlying neuropathy, the overlying skin begins to break down, and his condition worsens. What potentially could have prevented or decreased the severity of this patient's complication?

a. Postprocedural application of ice packs
b. EVTA laser wavelength >1064 nm
c. Thoroughly cleaning leg with soap and water
d. Tumescent anesthesia

SUGGESTED READINGS

Brittenden J, Cotton SC, Elders A, et al. Clinical effectiveness and cost-effectiveness of foam sclerotherapy, endovenous laser ablation and surgery for varicose veins: results from the Comparison of LAser, Surgery and foam Sclerotherapy (CLASS) randomised controlled trial. *Health Technol Assess.* 2015; 19(27):1–342. http://www.ncbi.nlm.nih.gov/pubmed/25858333. Accessed March 3, 2016.

Gloviczki P, Comerota AJ, Dalsing MC, et al. The care of patients with varicose veins and associated chronic venous diseases: clinical practice guidelines of the Society for Vascular Surgery and the American Venous Forum. *J Vasc Surg.* 2011;53(5): 2S–48S.

Khilnani N, Grassi C, Kundu S, et al. Multi-society consensus quality improvement guidelines for the treatment of lower-extremity superficial venous insufficiency with endovenous thermal ablation from the Society of Interventional Radiology, Cardiovascular Interventional Radiological Society of Europe, American College of Phlebology, and Canadian Interventional Radiology Association. *J Vasc Interv Radiol.* 2010;21(1):14–31. https://doi.org/10.1016/j.jvir.2009.01.034.

Lurie F, Creton D, Eklof B, et al. Prospective randomized study of endovenous radiofrequency obliteration (closure procedure) versus ligation and stripping in a selected patient population (EVOLVeS Study). *J Vasc Surg.* 2003;38(2):207–214. https://doi.org/10.1016/s0741-5214(03)00228-3.

Min RJ, Khilnani N, Zimmet SE. Endovenous laser treatment of saphenous vein reflux: long-term results. *J Vasc Interv Radiol.* 2003;14(8):991–996.

O'Donnell TF, Passman MA, Marston WA, et al. Management of venous leg ulcers: clinical practice guidelines of the Society for Vascular Surgery and the American Venous Forum. *J Vasc Surg.* 2014;60(2):1S–2S.

Zhan HT, Bush RL. A review of the current management and treatment options for superficial venous insufficiency. *World J Surg.* 2014;38(10):2580–2588.

Zygmunt J, Dauplaise T. Pre-, intra-, and post-treatment use of duplex ultrasound. In: Pichot O, ed. *Practical Phlebology: Venous Ultrasound.* New York: CRC Press; 2013:111–130.

Useful Videos

Injection Sclerotherapy at https://www.youtube.com/watch?v=nZ82mxgDcUo&feature=youtube. Accessed September 2018.

Treatment of Great Saphenous Vein with Radial EndoVenous Laser Ablation (EVLA) at https://www.youtube.com/watch?v=1nukdMXpMUc&feature=youtube. Accessed September 2018.

Venous Access

Mohammed F. Loya, Salman S. Shah

CASE PRESENTATION

A 48-year-old female with type II diabetes presents with worsening back pain for 2 weeks. She was found to be febrile and has an elevated white blood cell count. MRI was obtained, and the patient was diagnosed with osteomyelitis. Her primary team would like to discharge the patient on 4 weeks of IV antibiotics and have requested that a peripherally inserted central catheter (PICC) be placed.

- In 1929, Werner Forssmann, a German surgical resident, gained access to his own antecubital vein and advanced a ureteric catheter 35 cm centrally. He then obtained an X-ray of himself to confirm its location (Fig. 27.1). His goal was to show he could gain access into the right atrium as a means of administering medication for cardiac resuscitation.
  - Subsequently, he administered radiopaque contrast and demonstrated that this technique allowed him to image not only the heart but the pulmonary arteries as well.
- In 1953, Sven Ivar Seldinger introduced the **Seldinger technique**, which became instrumental in arterial and venous access.
- **Central venous access** is one of the most commonly performed interventional procedures. It is likely the first encounter many patients will have with the interventional radiology service.
- This technique involves placing a catheter, allowing for long-term, yet temporary, venous access. The catheter may be tunneled, a more elaborate procedure that reduces the risk of line infection, or non-tunneled, a simpler procedure in which the line more often gets infected.
- Prior to placement, one should consider the type of catheter, reason for venous access, and site of access.
- Access may be obtained peripherally (i.e., arms), as Forssmann did, or centrally (jugular, femoral, or subclavian veins). The selected approach is contingent on several factors (which can be remembered with the mnemonic *RADS*):
  - **R**eason for the consult
    - Follow up with the consulting service to understand the patient's condition and goals of care
  - **A**ssessment of the patient
    - Check labs, including complete blood count (CBC), creatinine, coagulation panel, prior imaging, and vital signs over the past 48 hours
    - Evaluate for contraindications
    - Interview the patient
    - Explain why the interventional radiology team was consulted
    - Describe the procedure including benefits and risks
  - **D**etermine the approach
    - Determine laterality based off of patient's history and prior imaging
    - Perform a physical exam
      - Assess the patient's body habitus (i.e., obese vs. thin, contracted vs. full range of motion) and any sites of skin infection or scarring as this will help determine which approach will be best for the patient
  - **S**can and See
    - Evaluate the venous anatomy with ultrasound
    - Evaluate contralateral side as a potential alternative site of access
    - Choose most appropriate venous access site

INDICATIONS (TABLE 27.1)

- Acute causes
  - Large-volume resuscitation
  - Emergency hemodialysis
- Long-term course of IV antibiotics
- Chemotherapy
- Hemodialysis (may or may not be waiting for an arteriovenous [AV] fistula to mature)
- Parenteral nutrition
- Repeated blood sampling
- Plasmapheresis
- Blood product transfusion

CONTRAINDICATIONS

- Absolute contraindications:
  - Placement of a tunneled catheter or port in a patient who is septic or has been febrile in the past 48 hours
  - Local skin infection at the access site (an alternative access site should be chosen)

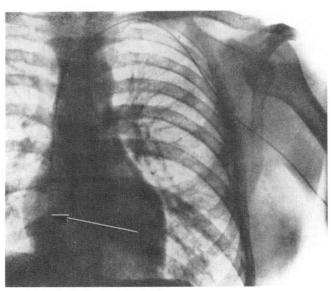

Fig. 27.1 Werner Forssmann's 1929 Radiograph of His Self-Catheterization. (Reused with permission from Meyer JA. Werner Forssmann and catheterization of the heart, 1929. 1990;49[3]:497–499, Elsevier, Fig. 2.)

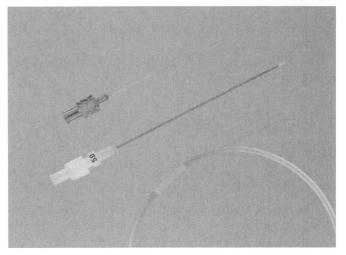

Fig. 27.2 **Micropuncture access set** from Cook, which contains a 21-gauge access needle *(top)*, a coaxial catheter *(middle)*, and a microwire *(bottom)*. (Courtesy COOK MEDICAL LLC, https://www.cookmedical.com/products/e4790704-1c72-48bc-95f7-6c5bd6ea3b53/.)

- Relative contraindications:
  - Coagulopathy
    - Should be corrected prior to the procedure. If not, intraoperative measures can be taken (i.e., fresh frozen plasma).
  - Use of the ipsilateral extremity in patients with prior mastectomy or lymph node resection
    - The contralateral extremity should be strongly considered for access.
  - Patients who are anticipated to require dialysis in the future
    - PICC lines are associated with a 23%-57% percent incidence of thrombosis of the vein in which they are inserted. The use of PICCs in CKD patients is guarded.

EQUIPMENT

- Micropuncture access set (Fig. 27.2), which includes:
  - An access needle to enter the vein and pass a microwire through
  - A microwire to secure access as the needle is removed

- A 5-Fr coaxial catheter that is advanced over the microwire and allows for larger wires to be inserted
- Guidewire(s) (Figs. 27.3 and 27.4)
  - Many types of guidewires are available, differing on their size, stiffness, shape, and flexibility.
  - Dilator, catheter, and sheath exchanges are made over the secured guidewire so that access is not lost.
- Peel-away sheath
  - Allows for intraluminal introduction of the catheter
- Access device
  - Note that most devices come in pre-packaged kits that include a majority of the needed supplies (needles, catheters, dilators, wires, scalpel, etc.).
  - Long-term central venous access devices (Fig. 27.5)
  - Short-term central venous access device

ANATOMY (FIG. 27.6)

- The site of access is best determined by the patient's venous anatomy and preference.
- Portions of the vein proximal and distal to the site of access should be scanned and evaluated to ensure the vein is appropriate for insertion of a central venous catheter.

TABLE 27.1	Types of Central Venous Access Devices and Uses		
Device	**Duration**	**Uses**	**Suggested Coagulation Parameters**
Nontunneled central catheter	7–14 days	Acute resuscitation, dialysis, blood transfusion, short course of antibiotics, vasopressors, and inotropes	INR < 2, PTT < 50, Platelets ≥ 15,500
Non-tunneled PICC	1–12 weeks	Long-term antibiotics, TPN	As above.
Tunneled catheter	>1 month	Chemotherapy, dialysis, TPN, plasmapheresis	INR < 1.5, PPT < 50, Platelets ≥ 30,000
Implantable port	>3 months	Chemotherapy, chronic blood transfusions, repetitive blood sampling	INR-Normal, PPT-Normal, Platelets ≥ 30,000

PICC, Peripherally inserted central catheter; *TPN,* total parenteral nutrition; *PTT,* partial thromboplastin time.

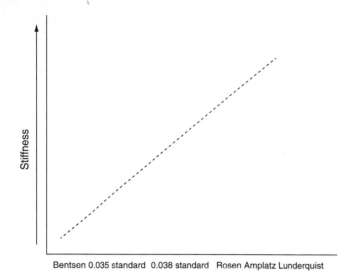

Fig. 27.3 Guidewire Stiffness.

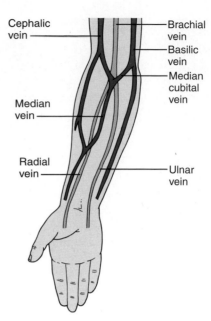

Fig. 27.6 Normal Venous Anatomy of the Arm and Forearm. (From Soni N, Arntfield R, Kory P. *Point-of-Care Ultrasound*. Philadelphia, PA: Elsevier; 2015, Fig. 29.1.)

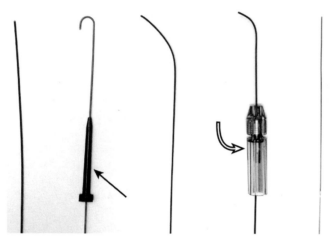

Fig. 27.4 Common Guidewires. From left: Straight 0.038-inch; J-tipped 0.038-inch with introducer device *(arrow)* to straighten guidewire during insertion into needle hub; angled high-torque 0.035-inch; angled hydrophilic-coated 0.038-inch nitinol wire with pin vise *(curved arrow)* for increased control; 0.018-inch platinum-tipped microwire. (From Kaufman JA. *Vascular and Interventional Radiology: The Requisites*. 2nd ed. Philadelphia, PA: Elsevier; 2014, Fig. 2.3.)

Areas of active infection or venous thrombosis/stenosis should be avoided.

- Basilic (medial arm), brachial, and cephalic (lateral arm) veins are the common sites for midline/peripherally inserted central catheter (PICC) placement.
- The venous structures in the arm can be categorized into two sections, superficial and deep.

Superficial Veins

- **Basilic vein**
  - Ascends medially along the upper limb
  - Courses deep into the arm at the border of the teres major muscle, where it drains into the brachial vein to form the axillary vein

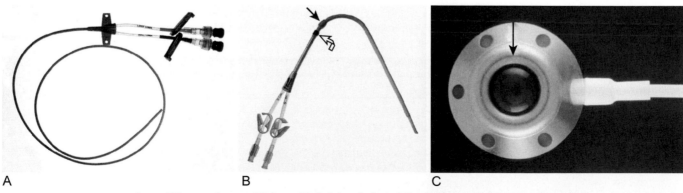

Fig. 27.5 Central Venous Access Devices. (A) Peripherally inserted central catheter, double lumen. (B) Tunneled catheter; characterized by the presence of a cuff for tissue ingrowth *(straight arrow)* that stabilizes the catheter after 3 to 4 weeks. Also seen is a silver-impregnated cuff *(curved arrow)* to reduce infections. (C) Port for subcutaneous implantation. A silicone membrane *(arrow)* for access with a needle is characteristic. (From Kaufman JA. *Vascular and Interventional Radiology: The Requisites*. 2nd ed. Philadelphia, PA: Elsevier; 2014, Fig. 7.19.)

- Considerations
  - Generally safe to access given its superficial location
  - Not accompanied by a neurovascular bundle or artery, which lessens potential complications
- **Cephalic vein**
  - Originates from the dorsal veins of the hand
  - Courses laterally between the deltoid and pectoralis major muscles and drains into the axillary vein
  - Considerations
    - Prone to vasospasm
    - Angle of the access needle to the skin may need to be less than 30 degrees, given its superficial location
    - Access is generally contraindicated if the patient has acute or chronic kidney disease. The cephalic serves as possible salvage for a future AV fistula.

Deep Veins

- **Brachial vein** (Fig. 27.7)
  - Ulnar and radial veins combine to form the brachial vein, which courses alongside the brachial artery and nerve
  - Ends at the border of the teres major muscle, joining the basilic vein to form the axillary vein
  - Considerations
    - Given close juxtaposition, the brachial artery and neurovascular bundle are both at risk of inadvertent injury with brachial vein access.
    - Again, access is generally contraindicated if the patient has acute or chronic kidney disease. The brachial serves as possible salvage for a future AV fistula.
- **Internal jugular vein**
  - Formed by the inferior petrosal and sigmoid venous sinus
  - Receives venous drainage from the face and neck

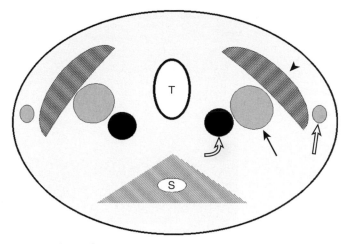

Fig. 27.8 Cross-Sectional Vascular Anatomy of the Neck. *Arrowhead*, Sternocleidomastoid muscle; *curved arrow*, common carotid artery; *open straight arrow*, external jugular vein; *S*, spine; *straight arrow*, internal jugular vein; *T*, trachea. (From Kaufman JA. *Vascular and Interventional Radiology: The Requisites*. 2nd ed. Philadelphia, PA: Elsevier; 2014, Fig. 2.41.)

- Courses between the heads of the sternocleidomastoid muscle alongside the internal carotid artery and CN X (Fig. 27.8) before joining the subclavian vein to form the brachiocephalic vein
- Considerations
  - Widely used given ease of access to the superior vena cava and hepatic vein
  - Preserves venous structures in the arm for future hemodialysis
  - Ultrasound guidance can provide accurate puncture at the optimal location
    - Access that is too cephalad increases risk of carotid artery injury
    - Access that is too caudal increases risk of pneumothorax
- **Subclavian vein**
  - Courses posterior to the clavicle and is fed by the external jugular branch before draining into the superior vena cava (SVC)
  - Considerations
    - Difficult to sonographically visualize
    - High associated risk of subclavian vein thrombosis
    - Lowest risk of infection among the aforementioned access sites
    - Long-term access in this region is not recommended due to a complication known as "pinch-off syndrome," which involves physical compression of the catheter by the first rib

PROCEDURAL STEPS

Non-tunneled Central Venous Catheter

1. Prior to sterilely prepping the site of insertion, perform a preliminary ultrasound evaluation to determine the window for insertion. Look for clot, stenosis, spasm, tortuosity, and a valve at the insertion site.

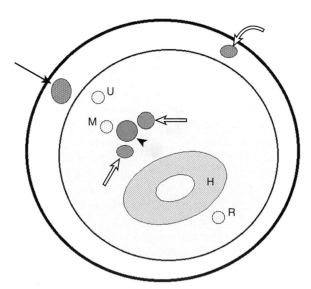

Fig. 27.7 Cross-Sectional Anatomy of the Upper Arm Proximal to the Antecubital Fossa. *Arrowhead*, Brachial artery; *curved arrow*, cephalic vein; *H*, humerus; *M*, median nerve; *open straight arrows*, brachial veins; *R*, radial nerve; *straight arrow*, basilic vein; *U*, ulnar nerve. (From Kaufman JA. *Vascular and Interventional Radiology: The Requisites*. 2nd ed. Philadelphia, PA: Elsevier, 2014, Fig. 2.44.)

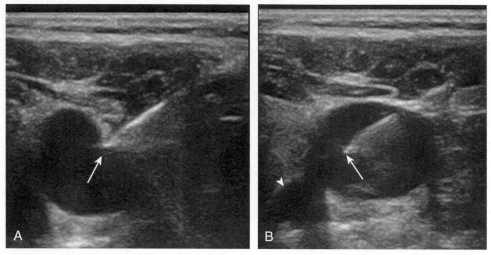

Fig. 27.9 Ultrasound of the Internal Jugular Vein. (A) Using a linear ultrasound probe, the needle tip *(arrow)* is seen tenting the internal jugular vein just before entering it. (B) The needle tip *(arrow)* is confirmed to be in the vein. Note the proximity to the common carotid artery *(arrowhead)*. (From Kaufman JA. *Vascular and Interventional Radiology: The Requisites.* 2nd ed. Philadelphia, PA: Elsevier; 2014, Fig. 2.42BC.)

2. After local anesthesia is administered, the standard Seldinger technique is used to gain access into the desired vein under ultrasound guidance (Fig. 27.9).
3. Advance the guidewire into the superior vena cava to secure access.
4. Remove the micropuncture needle.
5. Use a scalpel to create a nick at the needle site to ease passage of the sheath and catheter.
6. Insert a peel-away sheath.
7. Under fluoroscopy, advance the wire to the cavoatrial junction.
8. To determine the length of the catheter, clamp the wire at this point, and then subtract an amount, usually about 2 cm, to account for the peel-away sheath's hub.
9. Remove the wire, cut the catheter to the desired length, and flush it with normal saline.
10. Insert the catheter through the sheath, and peel to advance the catheter.
11. An X-ray should be performed to ensure the catheter is in the proper position. Keep in mind as the patient stands up or sits up the catheter will retract 1 to 3 cm.
12. Apply biopatch, flush the catheter, and secure to the skin.

Tunneled Central Venous Catheter

Steps 1 through 5 as above.
6. Advance a coaxial catheter over the wire.
7. Under fluoroscopy, advance the wire to the cavoatrial junction, which will allow for appropriate catheter length measurement. Clamp the wire at this point as this will represent, taking into account the catheter hub, the appropriate catheter length.
8. A site on the chest wall is chosen, local anesthesia is administered, and a superficial dermatotomy is created (Fig. 27.10). The size of the dermatotomy depends on the type of catheter being used.

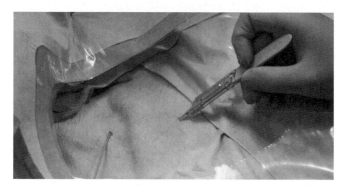

Fig. 27.10 Dermatotomy. Scalpel is used to create a dermatotomy at appropriate exit site for subcutaneous tunnel. (Reused with permission from Yu H, Kim KR, Burke CT. Hemodialysis access: catheters and ports. In: Mauor MA, Murphy KPJ, Thomson KR, et al. Image-Guided Interventions, Second Edition, e121-5, pgs 891-898.e3, 2014, Elsevier.)

9. Local anesthesia is administered along a path from the site of the dermatotomy to the internal jugular (IJ) access site, staying in the subcutaneous plane.
10. Using the provided tunneling apparatus, catheter is pushed from the dermatotomy site through the subcutaneous tissue through the nick at the IJ access site (Fig. 27.11). The tunneling apparatus can then be separated off of the catheter.
11. Thread the catheter through the peel-away sheath, and peel to advance the catheter. Confirm with fluoroscopy to ensure positioning and lack of kinking in the catheter.
12. Aspirate and flush the catheter with saline. Catheter may be locked with heparin solution to prevent thrombosis.
13. Secure the catheter with skin sutures, and apply Steri-Strips (or Dermabond) and a sterile dressing to the venous access and venotomy site.

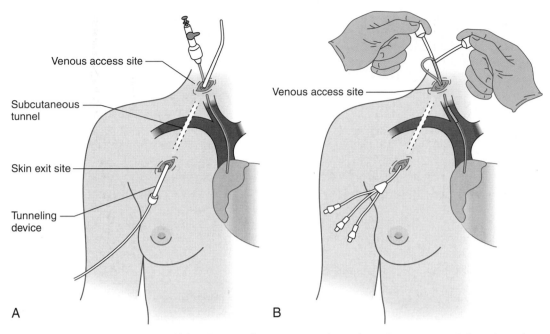

A   B

Fig. 27.11 Tunneling Process. Using the tunneling apparatus, the catheter is maneuvered through to the venous access site. (From Abrams HL, Baum S, Pentecost MJ. *Abrams' Angiography: Interventional Radiology.* 3rd ed. Philadelphia, PA: Lippincott Williams & Wilkins; 2013.)

Port Placement

 CLINICAL POINT

In patients with breast cancer, place the device on the side contralateral to the cancer in case the patient requires radiation therapy in the future, which may erode the skin and cause complications with an ipsilateral port.

Steps 1 through 7 as above.

8. A site on the chest wall is chosen, local anesthesia is administered, and a superficial dermatotomy is created. Blunt and sharp dissection may be used to create a pocket to accommodate the port reservoir.
9. Local anesthesia is administered along a path from the site of the dermatotomy to the IJ access site, staying in the subcutaneous plane.
10. Using the provided tunneling apparatus, the catheter is pushed from the dermatotomy site through the subcutaneous tissue through the nick at the IJ access site (see Fig. 27.11). The tunneling apparatus can then be separated off of the catheter.
11. Secure the proximal end of the catheter to the port with the provided lock.
12. Cut the catheter to the calculated length.
13. Thread the distal end of the catheter through the peelaway sheath, and peel to advance the catheter. Confirm with fluoroscopy to ensure positioning and lack of kinking in the catheter.
14. Using the provided angled Huber needle (which will not core the port), aspirate blood and then flush with saline.

Port may be locked with heparin solution to prevent thrombosis.
15. The dermatotomy site can be closed using 3-0 absorbable sutures for the deep fascial layers. A subcutaneous absorbable running stitch or Dermabond can be used as needed.
16. Steri-Strips and sterile dressings should be applied to the dermatotomy and venous access sites.

ALTERNATIVE TREATMENTS

• **Non-tunneled central venous catheters** may be placed emergently, if the clinical situation necessitates, not under imaging guidance. It is typically placed in the internal jugular, subclavian, or femoral vein.
• **Peripherally inserted central catheters** are typically placed in the basilic, brachial, or cephalic veins and terminate at the cavoatrial junction. These are placed with ultrasound and fluoroscopic guidance. Most common indications include TPN and long-term antibiotic administration in patients preparing for discharge
• Traditional **peripheral intravenous lines (pIV)** provide short-term access (up to 3 days) but have a high rate of malfunction.
• **Midline catheters** are similar to PICCs except they do not reach the central circulation. These provide longer access than peripheral IVs (average of 7–10 days) and are typically placed in patients with poor veins (e.g., volume depleted, injection drug user with depleted veins, sickle cell patients, etc).

COMPLICATIONS

With the use of ultrasound and fluoroscopic guidance, many of the following complications have been minimized. Ninety-eight percent of central lines are placed successfully without any immediate complications.

Early Complications

- Hematoma (1%) occurs secondary to accidental arterial puncture.
  - Can usually be treated by compression; however, pro-thrombotic agents may be used if severe.
- Pneumothorax (<2%) occurs when visualization of the needle tip is lost.
  - Small pneumothoraces can be monitored with serial X-rays and vitals checks.
  - Moderate to large pneumothoraces may require a chest tube placement.
- Air embolism (<2%) is usually caused by the patient inspiring during catheter placement into the venous system.
  - Can be avoided by asking the patient to hold his/her breath at strategic points during the procedure.
  - A small amount of air is of no clinical significance as it can be auto-reabsorbed.
  - If the amount is large (20–30 mL), a density can be seen outlining the pulmonary valve under fluoroscopy. If the patient is unstable, place him/her in a left lateral decubitus position to trap the air in the right atrium and aspirate the air with a catheter placed in the right atrium.

Late Complications

- Catheter malfunction (10%–20%)

- Due to inadequate flushing of the catheter
- A fibrin sheath deposits in or around the tip of the catheter.
- Infection (5%–10%)
  - If the patient is febrile, the recently placed catheter is usually the culprit without definite evidence otherwise.
  - If not responsive to antibiotics, the catheter may need to be removed.
  - If the patient is septic or neutropenic, the catheter must be removed urgently, and the patient must be afebrile for 48 hours before a new access line is placed.
- Symptomatic venous thrombosis
  - If the patient still requires the venous access, start anti-coagulation if there are no contraindications.

🏠 TAKE-HOME POINTS

- Patent venous access assists in patient care for long-term medical and pharmacologic treatment goals.
- Different options for central venous access exist depending on the patient's clinical history and the length of expected treatment. Central lines may be tunneled or non-tunneled, or may be implanted under the skin in the form of a port.
- Alternatives to central lines include rotating peripheral IVs, midlines, and peripherally inserted central catheters (which is a central line placed in the upper arm terminated at the cavoatrial junction).
- With the use of image guidance, catheter placement is a safe procedure with a low rate of early and late complications. These potential complications include pneumothorax, cardiac arrhythmia, catheter malfunction, venous thrombosis, and infection.

REVIEW QUESTIONS

1. Which of the following statements are FALSE?
   a. The cephalic vein is prone to vasospasm.
   b. Sonographic evaluation of a vein includes compressibility and color Doppler.
   c. The basilic vein is a deep structure.
   d. The subclavian vein can be easily visualized with ultrasound.
2. The distal tip of a tunneled dialysis catheter should be at what expected location?
   a. High right atrium
   b. Proximal superior vena cava
   c. Axillary vein
   d. Subclavian vein
3. Which of the following is NOT a primary indication for a peripherally inserted central catheter?
   a. Long-term IV antibiotics
   b. Emergent fluid resuscitation
   c. Chemotherapy
   d. Total parenteral nutrition

SUGGESTED READING

Banerjee S. Dialysis catheters and their common complications: an update. *Scientific World Journal.* 2009;9:1294–1299.

Biffi R, de Braud F, Orsi F, et al. Totally implantable central venous access ports for long-term chemotherapy. A prospective study analyzing complications and costs of 333 devices with a minimum follow-up of 180 days. *Ann Oncol.* 1988;9(7):767–773.

Butler PJ, Sood S, Mojibian H, et al. Previous PICC placement may be associated with catheter-related infections in hemodialysis patients. *Cardiovasc Intervent Radiol.* 2011;34(1):120–123.

Crowley JJ. Vascular access. *Tech Vasc Interv Radiol.* 2003;6(4):176–181.

Pirotte T. Ultrasound-guided vascular access in adults and children: beyond the internal jugular vein puncture. *Acta Anaesthesiol Belg.* 2008;59(3):157–166.

Siegel JB. Tunneled dialysis catheters: pearls and pitfalls. *Tech Vasc Interv Radiol.* 2008;11(3):181–185.

Simpson KR, Hovsepian DM, Picus D. Interventional radiologic placement of chest wall ports: results and complications in 161 consecutive placements. *J Vasc Interv Radiol.* 1997;8(2):189–195.

Y-90 Embolization

Hunaid Nasir Rana, Shivang Patel, Poyan Rafiei

CASE PRESENTATION

A 57-year-old male with a history of metastatic colon cancer (KRAS +) to the lungs, liver, and abdominal lymph nodes is status post left colectomy and chemotherapy (FOLFOX + Avastin, FOLFIRI + Avastin, and Stivarga). Most recent chemotherapy with Stivarga was completed in September 2017. CT abdomen/pelvis demonstrates interval progression of metastatic disease burden in the lower chest with multiple new pulmonary nodules and an increase in the size and number of bilobar hepatic masses. He currently reports mild abdominal pain relieved by Prilosec, and he denies recent fever, nausea, and vomiting. He presents today for evaluation for hepatic locoregional therapy.

- The first successful **transarterial chemoembolization (TACE)** for treatment of **hepatocellular carcinoma (HCC)** was reported by Doyon et al. in 1974.
- In 1983, Yamada et al. reported transcatheter hepatic artery embolization in 120 patients with unresectable HCC. The cumulative 1-year survival rate was 44%. Follow-up angiography showed that in most cases there was disappearance of tumor vessels, and CT demonstrated a significant decrease in tumor density without changes to normal liver parenchyma.
- Recently, **yttrium-90 (Y-90)** has emerged as a radiotherapeutic agent with encouraging results in the treatment of liver malignancies. The first reports of human Y-90 application were released in the late 1980s and early 1990s.

◎ KEY DEFINITION

The process of clogging tumor vessels as a means of blocking their nutrient arterial supply is known as *embolization*.

- Injection of radiotherapeutic material through the hepatic artery allows for targeted treatment of a hepatic tumor with significantly reduced damage to surrounding tissue. Tumor angiogenesis creates preferential arterial flow to the tumor bed, increasing delivery of particles to the tumor tissue rather than normal liver parenchyma (which mainly receives flow from the portal venous system).

- Y-90 emits β radiation and is the principle agent of two FDA-approved, commercially available radioembolization therapies: **TheraSphere**, in the form of glass Y-90 microspheres, and **SIR-Spheres**, in the form of resin microspheres.
  - Principal differences between the two forms are in the amount of activity per microsphere, the number of microspheres injected per treatment, and their indications.
    - Less than 5 million microspheres per TheraSphere (glass) treatment versus 10 to 30 million microspheres per SIR-Spheres (resin) treatment.
    - The glass form has a higher activity per sphere than resin.
    - Glass form is FDA approved under a humanitarian device exemption for HCC and needs IRB approval to be used. Resin is FDA approved for colorectal metastases in conjunction with intrahepatic floxuridine (no longer performed), and IRB approval is not required.
- Y-90 is a form of localized radiotherapy. The radiation dose absorbed is dependent on microsphere distribution within the tumor vascularization. Equal distribution is necessary to ensure tumor cells are not spared due to a 2.5-mm mean tissue penetration, with maximum penetration up to 11 mm.
- Y-90 radioembolization is indicated in primary intermediate and metastatic liver-dominant cancers where surgical resection is not possible.
- Transarterial radioembolization is a two-stage process. The first stage, *pretreatment evaluation*, encompasses screenings, imaging, and tests that assess a patient's viability for Y-90 treatment, guide treatment planning, and prepare the liver for radiation. This includes:
  - **Imaging work-up** includes computed tomography and/or magnetic resonance imaging of the liver for the 3D volumetric assessment of tumor and nontumor volume, portal vein patency, and the extent of extrahepatic disease.
  - **Pretreatment angiography** allows for tailoring of Y-90 microsphere delivery based on individual arterial variation of hepatic tumors. This helps to avoid non-target embolization.
  - **99mTc-macroaggregated albumin scintigraphy** determines the presence of possible shunts to the lungs that

are characteristic of HCC. When administered, 99mTc-MAA particles mimic the distribution of Y-90 microspheres, and this information is then used in the planning process to avert Y-90 deposition into the lungs.

- A successful radioembolization practice is dependent on the development and establishment of an interdisciplinary team represented by members from interventional radiology, hepatology, oncology, liver transplant surgery/surgical oncology, radiation oncology, and nuclear medicine. Patient referral, screening, and treatment will involve cooperation of all these members.

INDICATIONS

 CLINICAL POINT

Ideal candidates are those with ECOG performance status of 0, 1, or 2. Generally, life expectancy should be greater than 3 months.

- Unresectable HCC
- Patients with preserved liver function
- HCC patients ineligible for liver transplantation
  - Y-90 can be used to decrease tumor size to potentially make these patients eligible for transplantation.
- HCC patients with partial or branch portal vein thrombosis
- Metastatic colorectal cancer
- Metastatic neuroendocrine tumor
- Patients with liver-dominant disease where primary and secondary therapies have failed

CONTRAINDICATIONS

- Absolute
  - Exaggerated hepatopulmonary shunting
  - Demonstrable gastrointestinal deposition
  - Pregnancy/breastfeeding
  - Use of capecitabine, a chemotherapeutic agent, is contraindicated starting 4 weeks prior to radioembolization session and cannot be resumed after treatment
- Relative
  - Compromised liver function
  - Renal failure
  - Biliary blockage
  - Prior hepatic radiotherapy
  - Right-to-left cardiopulmonary shunting

CLINICAL POINT

The calculated pulmonary ionizing radiation dose in Y-90 is >30 Gy per treatment and >50 Gy cumulative. If a patient has compromised pulmonary function (from COPD or prior lung resection), dosing is limited to 15 Gy per treatment and 30 Gy cumulative.

EQUIPMENT

- For arterial mapping and prophylactic coiling:
  - Femoral puncture set
  - 1% lidocaine
  - 5-Fr or 6-Fr sheath connected to pressure bag with heparinized saline
  - Multiple guidewires (stiff, glide, etc.)
  - Curved selective catheter for celiac and SMA angiography (Table 28.1)
  - Microcatheter and microwire for selective hepatic artery angiogram
  - Coils for potential embolization of the GDA and other collateral vessels
- For treatment, same equipment as above and additionally (Figs. 28.1–28.4):
  - Y-90 embospheres
  - Geiger counter

TABLE 28.1 Catheter Options

Artery	Typical Catheters	Injection (mL/s/total volume)	Filming
Celiac	Cobra-2, Rosch celiac, Sos Omni	5–7/30–60	2–4/s × 10 s, then 1s
Splenic	Cobra-2, Simmons-2	5–6/30–50	Same
Hepatic	Cobra-2, Rosch hepatic, Simmons-2	4–5/15–30	Same
Left gastric	Cobra-2	3–4/6–16	Same
Gastroduodenal	Cobra-2, Rosch celiac	3–4/6–16	Same
Superior mesenteric artery	Cobra-2, Rosch celiac, Sos Omni	5–7/30–60	Same; may require two injections with overlapping upper and lower fields to include all of bowel
Inferior mesenteric artery	Sos Omni, Rosch IMA Simmons-1	3–5/9–20	Same; for gastrointestinal bleed, use left posterior oblique projection and include anal verge on image

Reused with permission from Kaufman JA. *Vascular and Interventional Radiology: The Requisites.* 2nd ed. Philadelphia: Elsevier; 2014: Table 11.3.

- 10 + 20-mL syringes
- Acrylic box and labeled tubing
- Container for radioactive waste disposal

ANATOMY

- The liver is divided into eight anatomic segments in the Couinaud system, each with independent vascular supply, outflow, and biliary drainage.
  - The middle hepatic vein divides the left and right hepatic lobes.
  - The falciform ligament divides the left lobe into a medial segment (IV) and lateral segments (II and III).
  - The right hepatic vein divides the right hepatic lobe into anterior and posterior segments.
  - The portal vein divides the liver into superior and anterior segments.

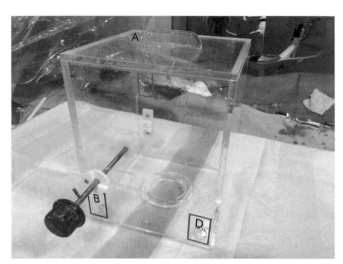

Fig. 28.1 **Acrylic Administration Box.** Note the openings labeled *A*, *B*, and *D*. The black control knob is used to control a three-way stopcock inside the box.

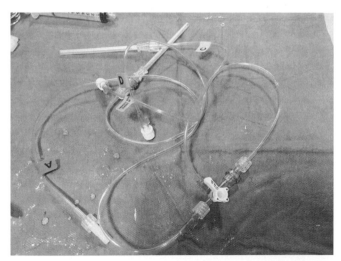

Fig. 28.2 Tubing Labeled *A*, *C*, and *D*. Line *A* will be connected to the microcatheter in the patient.

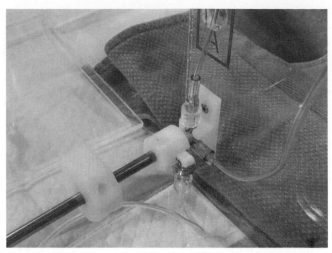

Fig. 28.3 View From the Inside of the Acrylic Box at the Three-Way Stopcock.

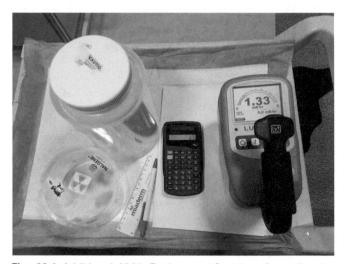

Fig. 28.4 **Additional Y-90 Equipment.** Container for radioactive waste disposal *(left)*. Radiation survey meter *(right)*.

- The common hepatic artery, a branch of the celiac trunk, gives off the proper hepatic artery, right gastric artery, and gastroduodenal artery.
  - The proper hepatic artery in turn branches into the left hepatic artery and right hepatic artery (which gives off the cystic artery feeding the gallbladder).
- Common variations of this basic branching pattern include an aberrant (or replaced) right hepatic artery that arises from the superior mesenteric artery and an aberrant (or replaced) left hepatic artery that arises from the left gastric artery. Accessory hepatic arteries, which exist in addition to the normal anatomic pattern, also exist.
- Hepatic tumors may parasitize extrahepatic arteries (commonly the right inferior phrenic artery), so pre-Y-90 angiography is crucial for planning purposes.

PROCEDURAL STEPS

Preprocedure

- Pretreatment with prophylaxis antacid, steroid, and/or antiemetic.
- Informed consent should include a discussion about post-procedure leg immobility (2–6 hours), post-radioembolization syndrome, treatment failure, potential need for additional treatment, potential liver failure, risk of non-target embolization, etc...

Steps

1. Use fluoroscopy and a metal instrument to locate the femoral head; entry site will be 1 to 2 cm distal to this point.
2. Place second and third digits along length of pulsating artery, with a 1- to 2-cm gap between fingers.
3. Advance vascular access needle between fingers at a 45-degree angle until pulsatile blood return is visualized.
4. Insert a microwire under fluoroscopic guidance.
5. Make a small dermatotomy over the needle, perpendicular to the artery.
6. Remove the needle and advance an arterial sheath over the wire. The wire can be removed once the sheath is in place.
7. Connect the sheath to a pressurized heparinized saline flush bag.
8. Insert the Glidewire into the aorta up to the level of the diaphragm.
9. Place a selective catheter over the wire, and remove the Glidewire.
10. Use the selective catheter to catheterize the superior mesenteric artery. Perform an angiogram, and continue to visualize until the venous phase to identify portal vein patency.
11. Catheterize the celiac trunk, and perform a celiac angiogram.
12a. If this is a mapping case, coil embolization of the gastroduodenal and other collateral arteries can be performed as necessary to avoid non-target embolization.
12b. If this is a treatment session, place the selective catheter at the proximal area of delivery. An anti-reflux catheter (ex. Surefire) can be used here. Ideally, a high-flow microcatheter (greater than or equal to 2.7 Fr) should be used to avoid catheter clogging and to tolerate the higher pressures during particle delivery.
13. **Y-90 radioembosphere delivery** (Fig. 28.5): preparation of the Y-90 delivery system is beyond the scope of this text. Please refer to the specific package insert for TheraSphere or SIR-Spheres, whichever is used at your facility. Useful links:
    - Dose Administration Procedure for SIR-Spheres Y-90 resin microspheres (https://www.youtube.com/watch?v=1mWhQtD2cyc, accessed October 2018)
    - TheraSphere Yttrium-90 Glass Microspheres Instructions for Use (https://www.btg-im.com/BTG/media/

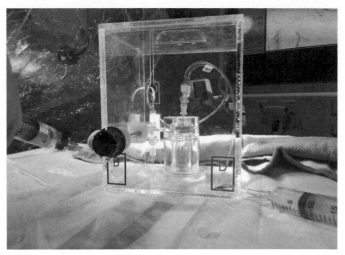

Fig. 28.5 Embolization in Action. With the control knob in the 12 o'clock position, contrast/saline or contrast/D5W injected into the *B* line will flow through the *A* line, testing the tubing connection. A hand contrast run can be performed to confirm the microcatheter's position within the patient. With the control knob in the 3 o'clock position, D5W/water/contrast injected into the *D* line will cause the microspheres contained in the vial in the center of the acrylic box to agitate into suspension, passing through the *C* needle into the *A* line. Once the *A* line is preloaded with microsphere, 2 to 3 cm outside the box, the control knob should be turned back to the 12 o'clock position. Contrast injected at this time through the *B* line will push the microspheres into the patient. The process is then repeated.

TheraSphere-Documents/PDF/10093509-Rev8_English-searchable.pdf; accessed October 2018)
- SIR-Spheres Y-90 resin microspheres instruction manual (https://www.sirtex.com/media/155126/ssl-us-13.pdf; accessed October 2018)

14. Continue drug delivery until either the entire dose of yttrium is delivered or arterial stasis is achieved (as seen by contrast stasis for 4–5 heartbeats).
15. Dispose of the microcatheter, vial holder, delivery set assembly, and gloves into the waste container (Fig. 28.6).
16. Hold direct pressure at puncture site for a minimum of 15 minutes, or place a vascular closure device (prior to removing the wire).
17. Everyone in contact with Y-90 needs to have his/her hands and feet scanned to check for radioactivity.

Postprocedure

- Send to recovery unit for pain control and groin monitoring.
- Limb immobility for 2 to 6 hours given femoral puncture
- Continue PPI. Add a 5-day steroid taper, which can help counter postradioembolization syndrome fatigue. Prescribe, as needed, an antiemetic and pain control medications upon discharge.
- Set up a follow-up appointment in about 14 days (>4 half-lives of Y-90).

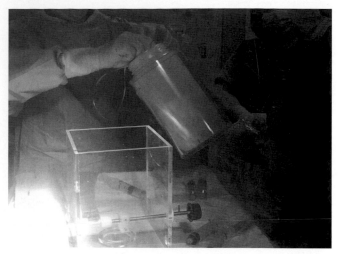

Fig. 28.6 Conclusion of the Procedure. At the end of the procedure, equipment is carefully disposed of into the radioactive waste container.

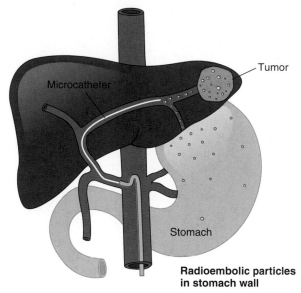

Fig. 28.7 Schematic representation of aberrant microsphere deposition in the stomach/intestine, which can occur due to hepaticogastric communicating arteries. (Reused from Riaz A, Awais R, Salem R. Side effects of yttrium-90 radioembolization. *Front Oncol.* 2014;4:198. doi:10.3389/fonc.2014.00198.)

ALTERNATE TREATMENTS

- Depending on a patient's functional status, hepatic reserve, and level of pulmonary shunting, Y-90 may not be appropriate.
  - A large tumor burden with little hepatic reserve could leave the patient with hepatic failure if he/she undergoes radioembolization. A discussion with the patient's medical oncologist should occur to determine safe alternatives.
- **Surgical resection** is a possible alternative, but the inherent invasiveness of the open procedure carries a higher morbidity than Y-90.
  - Comorbidities may exclude Y-90 candidates from major surgery.
- **External beam radiation** has less risk of non-target embolization but delivers a lower overall dose to the tumor, potentially resulting in incomplete therapy.
- If a patient has a life expectancy of less than 3 to 6 months, a goals-of-care discussion with consideration of **palliation / hospice care** should be had among the patient, the treatment team, and the patient's family.

COMPLICATIONS

- Postradioembolization syndrome
  - Symptoms include fatigue, nausea, vomiting, fever, abdominal pain, and cachexia.
  - Administration of prophylaxis antacid, steroid, and/or antiemetics prior to and after treatment will help.
- Non-target embolization
  - Gastroduodenal ulcers (Fig. 28.7), pneumonitis (Fig. 28.8), and cholecystitis (Fig. 28.9) are the most common sequela.
  - Preventable with pretreatment angiogram and coil embolization of collateral arteries as necessary.
- Gastritis

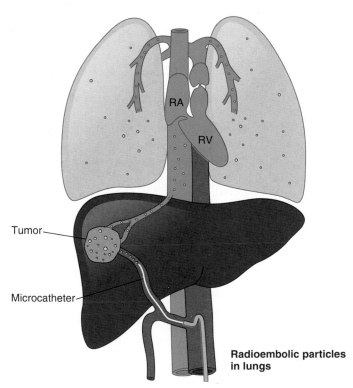

Fig. 28.8 Schematic Representation of Aberrant Microsphere Deposition in the Lungs. (RA = Right Atrium; RV = Right Ventricle) (Reused from Riaz A, Awais R, Salem R. Side effects of yttrium-90 radioembolization. *Front Oncol.* 2014;4:198. doi:10.3389/fonc.2014.00198.)

- Pancreatitis
- Transient elevated liver enzymes
- Radiation-induced liver disease (RILD)
- Hepatic fibrosis, which can lead to portal hypertension
- Fulminant liver failure

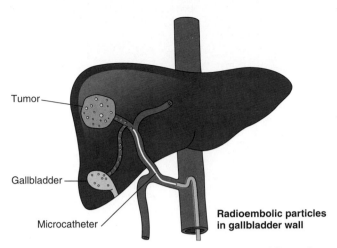

Tumor

Gallbladder

Microcatheter

Radioembolic particles in gallbladder wall

Fig. 28.9 Schematic Representation of Aberrant Microsphere Deposition in the Gallbladder Wall. (Reused from Riaz A, Awais R, Salem R. Side effects of yttrium-90 radioembolization. *Front Oncol.* 2014;4:198. doi:10.3389/fonc.2014.00198.)

TAKE HOME POINTS

- Y-90 radioembolization can be performed for primary and secondary liver malignancies for cure, palliation, or as a bridge to orthotopic liver transplant.
- General indications include unresectable tumors, those with sufficient reserve hepatic function, and those with lung shunt fractions less than 20%.
- Pretreatment arterial mapping and coiling of collaterals is necessary to prevent non-target embolization and damage to other tissues.
- Most common complications will be related to post-radioembolization syndrome and include fatigue, nausea, vomiting, fever, and abdominal pain.

REVIEW QUESTIONS

1. What type of radiation is delivered from Y-90?
   a. Alpha
   b. Beta
   c. Gamma

2. What artery most commonly needs prophylactic embolization before treatment?
   a. Splenic
   b. Left gastric
   c. Gastroduodenal
   d. Pancreaticoduodenal

SUGGESTED READINGS

Doyon D, Mouzon A, Jourde AM, Regensberg C, Frileux C. Hepatic, arterial embolization in patients with malignant liver tumours. *Annales de Radiologie.* 1974;17(6):593–603.

Guha C, Kavanagh BD. Hepatic radiation toxicity: avoidance and amelioration. *Semin Radiat Oncol.* 2011;21(4):256–263.

Madoff DC, Murthy R, Kee ST. Clinical Interventional Oncology. *Elsevier Health Sciences*; 2014.

Kennedy A, Nag S, Salem R, et al. Recommendations for radioembolization of hepatic malignancies using yttrium-90 microsphere brachytherapy: a consensus panel report from the radioembolization brachytherapy oncology consortium. *Int J Radiation Oncol Biol Phys.* 2007;68(1):13–23.

Riaz A, Awais R, Salem R. Side effects of yttrium-90 radioembolization. *Front Oncol.* 2014;4:198.

Edeline J, Gilabert M, Garin E, et al. Yttrium-90 microsphere radioembolization for hepatocellular carcinoma. *Liver Cancer.* 2015;4(1):16–25.

Kennedy A, Nag S, Salem R, et al. Recommendations for radioembolization of hepatic malignancies using yttrium-90 microsphere brachytherapy: a consensus panel report from the radioembolization brachytherapy oncology consortium. *Int J Radiat Oncol Biol Phys.* 2007;68(1):13–23.

Lewandowski RJ, Salem R. Yttrium-90 radioembolization of hepatocellular carcinoma and metastatic disease to the liver. *Semin Intervent Radiol.* 2006;23(1):64–72.

Mosconi C, Cappelli A, Pettinato C, Golfieri R. Radioembolization with yttrium-90 microspheres in hepatocellular carcinoma: role and perspectives. *World J Hepatol.* 2015;7(5):738–752.

Murthy R, Kamat P, Nuñez R, et al. Radioembolization of yttrium-90 microspheres for hepatic malignancy. *Semin Intervent Radiol.* 2008;25(1):48–57.

Salem R, Thurston KG. Radioembolization with 90yttrium microspheres: a state-of-the-art brachytherapy treatment for primary and secondary liver malignancies. Parts 1–3, *J Vasc Interv Radiol.* 2006;17(8):1251–1278; 17(9):1425–1439; and 17(10):1571–1593.

Singh P, Anil G. Yttrium-90 radioembolization of liver tumors: what do the images tell us? *Cancer Imaging.* 2013;13 (4):645–657.

Yamada R, Sato M, Kawabata M, Nakatsuka H, Nakamura K, Takashima S. Hepatic artery embolization in 120 patients with unresectable hepatoma. *Radiology.* 1983;148(2):397–401.

29

Abscess Drainage

David H. Ballard, Sarah T. Flanagan, Horacio B. D'Agostino

CASE PRESENTATION

A 64-year-old female who is 5 days status post laparoscopic right hemicolectomy for a sessile cecal polyp develops a fever of 102°F, abdominal distention, pain, nausea, and leukocytosis. Cessation of oral intake, nasogastric tube insertion, initiation of broad-spectrum intravenous antibiotics, and resuscitative efforts are initiated; however, these measures fail to improve her clinical status. A CT scan of the abdomen and pelvis reveals a 10.5 × 6.2 cm multiloculated complex fluid collection in the right lower quadrant. The general surgery service has consulted interventional radiology for percutaneous abscess drainage.

- An adage in medicine states *ubi pus, ibi evacua*, meaning "where [there is] pus, there evacuate [it]."
- Image-guided percutaneous drainage is the insertion of a catheter or needle through the skin (percutaneous) or body orifices (transorificeal) for evacuation of an abnormal fluid collection in an anatomic cavity.
- Imaging modality of choice is most commonly ultrasound, combined ultrasound and flouroscopy, or CT, depending on the depth and location of the abscess.
- Percutaneous drainage is the treatment of choice rather than open surgical drainage due to reduced morbidity, reduced mortality, and shorter overall hospital stays with the former.

◉ LITERATURE REVIEWS

- vanSonnenberg et al. (2001) reviewed 45 series on percutaneous abscess drainage, totaling 2048 cases, and concluded that it has become the procedure of choice for treatment of most intraabdominal abscesses. It is the prototypical interventional radiology procedure, providing localization by imaging, diagnosis by needling, and therapy by catheterization.

◉ LITERATURE REVIEWS

- Levin et al. (2015) reviewed Medicare part B procedural billing records from 2001 to 2013 and found that a greater proportion of intraabdominal abscesses are drained percutaneously versus surgically (63% percutaneous vs. 37% surgical in 2001, and 82% percutaneous vs. 18% surgical in 2013).

- This chapter focuses predominantly on intraabdominal fluid collections as this is the most common anatomic site an interventional radiologist drains. Drainage of intrathoracic collections is described briefly. It follows many of the same principles as intraabdominal drainage, but there are important differences and nuances in technique and principles.
- Curative abscess drainage is defined as complete resolution of an infection that does not require subsequent operative intervention, and this occurs in more than 80% of patients following percutaneous drainage.
  - Partial success is adequate abscess drainage followed by surgery to correct the causative problem. This occurs in 5% to 10% of patients.
  - Failure to drain and abscess recurrence each occur in 5% to 10% of patients.

INDICATIONS

- **Percutaneous needle aspiration** can be used for both diagnostic and therapeutic indications with infected or sterile fluid collections.
  - **Diagnostic aspiration** is a single-stage procedure aimed at obtaining fluid samples for cytology, microbiology, chemistry, and other diagnostic tests.
  - **Therapeutic aspiration** is a single-stage procedure that completely evacuates symptomatic fluid collections to alleviate pain and discomfort.
  - Diagnostic and therapeutic aspiration includes thoracenteses, paracenteses, and aspiration of fluid collections in the chest, abdomen, pelvis, and soft tissues.

- Sterile collections (cysts, pseudocysts, and ascites) are drained when they become symptomatic, causing pain, discomfort, and/or gastrointestinal/biliary obstruction.
  - Small collections (<4 cm in diameter) of clear or bloody fluid are drained by therapeutic aspiration with a needle or needle cannula.
  - Larger collections (>4 cm in diameter) are drained by single-step catheter drainage (a small catheter is inserted and removed at the end of the therapeutic aspiration).
- **Percutaneous catheter drainage** and antibiotic therapy are the first-line treatments for most infected intraabdominal fluid collections.
  - Therapeutic aspiration is performed when the collection is too small (2–3 cm in diameter) to hold a drainage catheter.
  - Larger collections (>4 cm in diameter) require that a drainage catheter be placed in the patient until the **CLIC criteria** are accomplished.

CONTRAINDICATIONS

- No safe pathway for transabdominal, transrectal, or transvaginal catheter insertion
  - Usually due to overlying bowel or blood vessels
  - Single-step needle aspiration may be more appropriate in these cases
- Uncorrectable coagulopathy
- Suspected gangrene or other necrotic tissue process that will require surgical debridement, although percutaneous drainage may still be attempted in certain situations
  - Percutaneous drainage may still be a reasonable first step in selected cases (e.g., necrotizing pancreatitis or necrotic tumors causing abscesses).

EQUIPMENT

- Choice of imaging modality
  - Sonography, alone or combined with fluoroscopy or CT
  - CT
  - MRI (need special non-paramagnetic materials)
- Localizing needles (Table 29.1)
- Single-lumen catheter, typically between 8 and 28 Fr in size

> ⊚ **KEY DEFINITION**
>
> The French scale is used to measure the size of a catheter. 1 Fr = 1/3 mm. For example, if the French size is 12, the outer diameter of the catheter is 4 mm.

TABLE 29.1   Localizing Needles

Type	Size	Length
Micropuncture sets	21–22 gauge	7–10 cm
Seldinger needle	18–19 gauge	7–10 cm
Chiba	18–20–22 gauge	10–20 cm
Angiocath	16 gauge	7–15 cm

- Three-way stopcock
- Wires
  - For intraabdominal drainages, 0.035-inch J-tip wire
  - For transvaginal and transrectal placement, 0.035-inch Amplatz
- Retention mechanism
  - Internal fixation to prevent dislodgment:
    - Locking pigtail (e.g., Cope loop)
    - Balloon (e.g., Foley)
    - Mushroom tip (e.g., Malecot, Pezzer)
  - External fixation:
    - Nonabsorbable suture
    - Adhesive tape (e.g., Elastikon)
    - Adhesive dressings (e.g., Tegaderm)
- Collection device
  - Drainage bag
  - Jackson-Pratt closed-suction drain
  - Water-sealable device for thoracic drainages (e.g., Atrium)

ANATOMY

Intrathoracic Collections

- Accessed by intercostal chest tube insertion
- Tube is inserted superior to the subjacent rib to avoid intercostal vessel injury, which is exposed at the lower margin of the ribs near the costovertebral joint.
- Typically placed along the posterior axillary line and above the diaphragm so that the patient can lie down in bed without occluding the drainage tube
- Use caution when inserting a tube on the left side to avoid injury to the heart, aorta, and spleen.

Intraabdominal Collections

- Most abdominal and pelvic collections can be accessed transabdominally, with the exception of deep (true) pelvic collections (Fig. 29.1A).
- Imaging determines the safest pathway to the collection.
- Most important anatomic consideration is the avoidance of blood vessels and bowel loops, which can be identified on pre- and intraprocedure CT abdomen/pelvis.
  - Rectus sheath vessels are prone to injury. The internal mammary vessels run caudally from the thorax and anastomose with the epigastric vessels, which run cephalad from the pelvis. These vessels are located in the posterior aspect of the rectus muscles fascia at the junction of the lateral and medial third of the rectus muscles.
  - Distended bowel loops with thickened walls can be difficult to distinguish from abscess cavities on noncontrast imaging.

Deep (True) Pelvic Collections

- Defined as collections below the innominate line of the pelvis
- Often cannot be safely accessed transabdominally and require special insertion sites/techniques such as transgluteal, transrectal, or transvaginal catheter placement (see Fig. 29.1B)

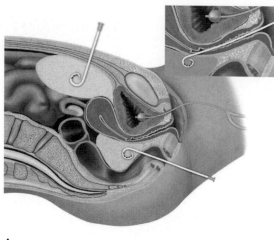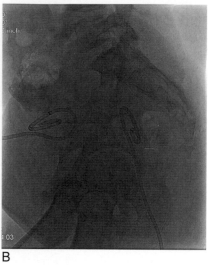

A   B

Fig. 29.1 Tranabdominal, Transrectal, and Transvaginal Drainage. Case showing concurrent transabdominal and transrectal drainage catheter insertion for true (lesser) and false (greater) pelvis collections. The true pelvis is below the innominate line (not pictured), and the false pelvis is above it. (A) Illustration depicting transabdominal catheter drainage of an infected false pelvis collection and transrectal catheter drainage of an infected true pelvis collection. The upper right-hand corner depicts transvaginal drainage of a sterile true pelvis collection. A Foley catheter is seen inserted into the bladder; visualization of the Foley balloon serves as a key landmark on ultrasound imaging. (B) Fluoroscopic image depicting two drainage catheters—one draining an abscess in the upper (false) pelvis inserted transabdominally and a transrectal catheter evacuating a lower (true) pelvic abscess. (A, Courtesy Ms. Lory Tubbs. B, Courtesy Dr. Horacio D'Agotino.)

PROCEDURAL STEPS

Preoperative Preparation

- Review the patient's chart, laboratory tests, and imaging studies. Image-guided drainage is part of the general management of the patient. Therefore, discussion among all teams involved in the patient's management is essential. Coagulation studies (PT/INR, PTT, and platelet count) are requested for most patients who will undergo percutaneous drainage of an intraabdominal fluid collection.
- NPO status for 6 to 8 hours, tailored to the urgency of the situation
- If the patient is allergic to iodinated contrast agents and CT-guided drainage is being considered, premedication with the institution's steroid/antihistamine protocol is appropriate.
- Local anesthetic (lidocaine 1% with or without epinephrine) ± conscious sedation (intravenous midazolam/fentanyl) is appropriate.

> **CLINICAL POINT**
>
> Coagulopathies must be corrected before drainage. This is facilitated by stopping heparin infusion 2–4 h before the planned procedure and administering blood products (red blood cells, fresh frozen plasma, and platelets) as needed.

Steps

- Patient positioning is dependent on the location of the fluid collection.
  - Prone, supine, or lateral decubitus for transcutaneous drainage

  - Prone, supine, lateral decubitus, jackknife, or lithotomy for transrectal and transvaginal drainage
  - Prone, supine, lateral decubitus, or upright for thoracic drainage
- Operator is positioned on the same side as the fluid collection with rare exceptions.

Seldinger Technique

1. Perform a preliminary imaging scan:
   a. Select the shortest, safest pathway from the skin to the collection, usually where it is largest, avoiding intervening viscus and vessels
   b. Mark with indelible ink the appropriate skin entry site with help from a CT biopsy grid
   c. Measure the distance between the entry site and the collection
2. Prep and drape the overlying skin in a sterile fashion.
3. Inject subcutaneous local anesthetic at the skin entry site.
4. Insert the access needle, penetrating the skin and underlying tissue until the needle is within the target collection (Fig. 29.2A).
5. Insert the guidewire and coil it within the collection (Fig. 29.2B).
6. Use a No. 11 scalpel to enlarge the skin entry site. Make a stab incision at the skin and separate the soft tissues widely with a curved or straight hemostatic clamp.

> **CLINICAL POINT**
>
> Enlarge the entry site so that it is larger than the size of the catheter to be inserted. When you insert a catheter you should not have to "fight the soft tissues."

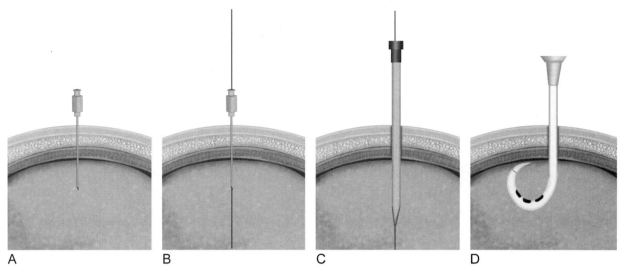

Fig. 29.2 Seldinger Technique. (A) A needle is used to access the collection. (B) A guidewire is passed through the needle. (C) Following nicking the skin with a No. 11 blade (not pictured), a dilator is advanced over the guidewire. (D) The dilator is then removed and the drainage catheter is inserted over the wire to take its characteristic pigtail form. (Courtesy Ms. Lory Tubbs.)

7. While holding the proximal end of the guidewire, remove the access needle slowly, grabbing the proximal end of the guidewire once the needle is out of the skin. Always make sure you have control of the wire.

8. Insert dilators over the guidewire from the skin to the collection cavity, performing serial dilatations up to the size of the drainage catheter (Fig. 29.2C).

9. Insert the drainage catheter with its stiffening cannula (plastic or metallic) over the guidewire and into the collection cavity, making sure all side holes are inside the cavity and there is enough catheter length within the cavity to form the pigtail.

10. Remove the plastic stiffener together with the guidewire, and activate the catheter's internal locking mechanism (e.g., pigtail) (Fig. 29.2D).

11. Aspirate fluid using a Luer-Lok or catheter tip 60-mL syringe, aiming for complete cavity evacuation.

12. Use imaging to assess for residual collections. This may necessitate catheter repositioning or insertion of additional drainage catheters.

13. Catheter irrigation is performed with saline solution aliquots one-third to one-fourth of the total drainage volume. Do not irrigate with larger volumes as it may cause pain, septic reaction, or rupture of the collection wall. If feasible and practical, irrigate the collection cavity until the irrigant returns clear.

14. Secure the catheter to the skin using a suture (e.g., 2-0 silk) and an adhesive dressing (e.g., Tegaderm).

15. The catheter may be connected to a drainage bag, a water-seal device (Atrium), or JP drain depending on the collection type.

Tandem-Trocar Technique

1. The beginning of this procedure follows steps 1 through 4 as listed in "Seldinger Technique" above.

2. Enlarge the skin entry site with a No. 11 blade or larger. Make a stab incision at the skin, and separate widely the soft tissues with a curved or straight hemostatic clamp.

3. A drainage catheter is loaded with the metal stiffening cannula and inner stylet. The measured distance from the skin to the collection is marked on the drainage catheter shaft with a Steri-Strip or tape.

4. The stiffener/stylet/catheter is inserted into the enlarged skin entry site. The catheter is placed parallel to the access needle, confirmed by imaging, and is safely inserted within the collection cavity. The access needle and the catheter are held together with one hand as the other hand advances the catheter the measured depth into the collection cavity.

> ### ⟫ CLINICAL POINT
>
> When performing CT-guided drainage, this is a blind catheter insertion. Otherwise, if using fluoroscopy or ultrasound, catheter advancement may be monitored in real time.

5. When the catheter has been inserted to the measured depth, the stylet is removed and the cannula is aspirated to confirm correct location within the collection. If no fluid is obtained, the catheter may need to be repositioned to a new depth (either advanced or retracted). In this case, a CT scan should be performed to determine the catheter's position in relation to the collection.

6. Once the catheter is confirmed to be in the collection, a guidewire is inserted and coiled within the cavity.

7. The catheter is deployed within the collection cavity over the guidewire.

8. The remainder of this procedure follows steps 10 through 15 as listed in "Seldinger Technique" above.

Direct Trocar Placement

1. The beginning of this procedure follows steps 1 through 3 as listed in "Seldinger Technique" above.
2. The skin incision is enlarged by blunt dissection to the diameter of the catheter to be inserted.
3. The drainage catheter is loaded with the metal stiffening cannula and inner stylet. The measured distance from the skin to the collection is marked on the drainage catheter shaft with a Steri-Strip or tape.
4. The stiffener/stylet/catheter is inserted slowly, repeating CT as needed to confirm positioning until the catheter is within the collection cavity.
5. The stylet is removed and the cannula aspirated. Aspiration of fluid confirms catheter position.
6. The catheter is deployed directly in the collection and the inner retention mechanism is activated.
7. The remainder of this procedure follows steps 11 through 15 as listed in "Seldinger Technique" above.

WHICH PROCEDURE IS RIGHT FOR MY PATIENT?

Tandem-Trocar Advantages
* The rigidity of the stiffener and catheter combination allows more directional control of the catheter.
* Simpler, single-step technique that does not require serial dilation and is quicker than the Seldinger technique.

Seldinger Technique Advantages
* Allows for better drainage of large, multiloculated fluid collections than the tandem-trocar technique due to a greater number of side holes and easier ability to reposition.
* Better control allows access to deeper, more difficult-to-access fluid collections.

Direct Trocar Placement Advantages
* Safe and quick in large and very superficial collections.

Postprocedure

* Specimen should be sent for:
  * **Microbiology**
    * Gram stain, culture, and antibiotic sensitivities for aerobic and anaerobic bacteria and fungi
    * If indicated by clinical suspicion, tuberculous bacillus culture and sensitivities may be requested
  * **Chemistries** in certain collection locations and clinical situations (e.g., lipase for pancreatic collections, cell count for lymphoceles).
  * **Cytology** if malignancy is suspected.
* Daily rounds on inpatients to follow catheter output and perform irrigation aspirations (if not being performed by the primary team or nursing team).
* In patients with persistent high catheter output, a catheter sinogram can be performed to evaluate the collection size. Drain revision versus surgical exploration should be considered.

* If the patient is discharged home with a drain, he/she should be set up with a home health aide for drain care, if help is needed, and a clinic appointment should be scheduled when drainage has subsided to less than 10 mL/day.
* CLIC criteria for catheter removal:
  * **Clinical improvement:** improvement of fever and pain, return of appetite, and subjectively feeling better
  * **Laboratory improvement:** WBC normalizing
  * **Imaging improvement:** resolution of the abscess cavity by CT/ultrasound or sinogram/abscessogram
    * Not always necessary to perform imaging if the other three criteria are present
  * **Catheter evaluation:** daily output volume is <10 mL/day (with the catheter having previously been confirmed to be in good position within the abscess cavity)

Catheter Flow Principles

* Bodily fluids are non-Newtonian and flow through drainage catheters follows Poiseuille's Law.
* Poiseuille's Law states that the laminar flow rate of the fluid through the drainage catheter is influenced by the difference in pressure inside (P_1) and outside (P_2) the fluid cavity, the radius of the catheter (r), the length of the catheter (l), and the viscosity (μ) of the fluid to be evacuated. The equation is visually depicted in Fig. 29.3.
* Drainage can be optimized by creating negative external pressure (P_2) or increasing intraabdominal pressure (P_1).
  * Negative external pressure is achieved mechanically by using low intermittent or continuous wall suction, a closed-suction JP drain, or manual aspiration.

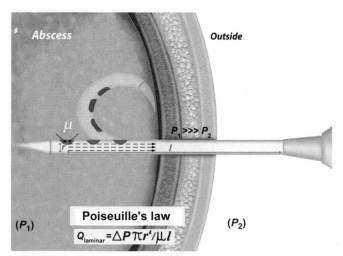

Fig. 29.3 Poiseuille's Law. Illustration of catheter drainage of an intraabdominal abscess highlighting the principles of Poiseuille's law. $Q_{laminar}$ = laminar flow rate; $\triangle P$ = change in pressures (P_1 = inside pressure; P_2 = outside pressure); π = 3.14; r = radius; μ = viscosity; l = length. Solid black arrows represent the flow of fluid into the side hole of the catheter; dashed black arrows represent laminar flow within the lumen of the catheter; solid red arrows depict the radius (r) and length (l) of the catheter. (Courtesy Ms. Lory Tubbs.)

- Increased intraabdominal pressure is achieved physiologically by asking the patient to Valsalva or use incentive spirometry.
- Drainage can be optimized by using larger diameter catheters.
  - Radius is the most influential factor in Poiseuille's law as it is amplified to the fourth power.
  - A large catheter can be downsized as drainage volume decrease and clinical status improves to facilitate eventual cavity closure.

> **CLINICAL POINT**
>
> Keep in mind that the limiting factor here is the connection devices (e.g., stopcocks) that have a fixed diameter. The effects of larger catheters (e.g., 20 + Fr) may be negated when connected to a connection device of a smaller diameter.

- Drainage can be optimized by using the shortest safe anatomic pathway to the fluid collection.
  - Length is measured to the most proximal side hole, not the distal end of the catheter, so the position of this side hole is key. It should be positioned as close to the body surface as possible while still being in the fluid collection to shorten this distance.
  - If the most proximal side hole is occluded, the catheter will malfunction. It may be occluded by malposition (not positioned within the collection) or by intraluminal thrombus/debris. Drains can be flushed daily or twice daily with 10 mL of normal saline to prevent this.
  - If all distal holes are occluded but the most proximal hole is still patent, the catheter will continue to drain.
- Drainage can be optimized by decreasing the viscosity of the collection contents either by irrigating the catheter or injecting antithrombotic agents.
  - Irrigation is done with saline or antiseptic solutions (e.g., Dakin solution 0.125%).
  - Antithrombotic agents (e.g., alteplase [tPA], urokinase) are injected directly into the cavity. These may also break septations in a multiloculated abscess cavity.

> **CLINICAL POINT**
>
> In summary, drainage is enhanced by increasing catheter radius, decreasing catheter length, decreasing drainage fluid viscosity, or increasing intraabdominal pressure.

SPECIAL CONSIDERATIONS

Paired Catheter Drainage (Fig. 29.4)

- Insertion of two drainage catheters into a single collection cavity
- Reasons for paired drainage include:
  - Primary insertion: initial insertion of multiple catheters into a single collection, usually a complex fluid collection, that would not otherwise completely drain
  - Salvage therapy: insertion of an additional drainage catheter to improve evacuation of a single collection that a single catheter failed to effectively drain

> ◎ **KEY DEFINITION**
>
> Complex fluid collections include collection with high-viscosity fluid, collections with particulate/necrotic debris, abscesses associated with fistulas, or collections larger than 6 cm.

Abscess-Fistula Complexes (Fig. 29.5)

- Defined as an intraabdominal abscess caused or fed by an internal enteric fistula
- Etiology:
  - ~75% are postprocedural, resulting from abdominal surgery, endoscopic procedures, or percutaneous interventions
  - ~25% occur spontaneously in patients with inflammatory conditions (e.g., Crohn's, perforated diverticulitis, perforated appendicitis, or necrotic tumors)
- Goal of catheter insertion is to effectively evacuate the abscess cavity, which facilitates healing of the fistula.
- High-output fistulae (output >200 mL/day) or recurrent low-output fistulae may benefit from catheter cannulation of the tract.

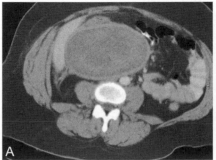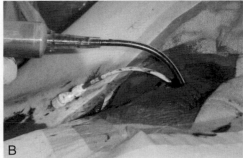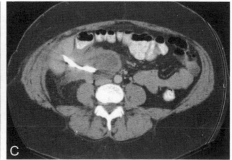

Fig. 29.4 Case Showing Paired Catheter Insertion. A 39-year-old morbidly obese female with a postoperative hematoma following laparoscopic cholecystectomy for symptomatic cholelithiasis. (A) Preprocedural CT showing the massive hematoma. (B) Paired drainage with two drainage catheters. (C) Status post initial percutaneous evacuation, the hematoma resolved with serial post-drainage irrigation-aspirations. (Courtesy Dr. Horacio D'Agotino.)

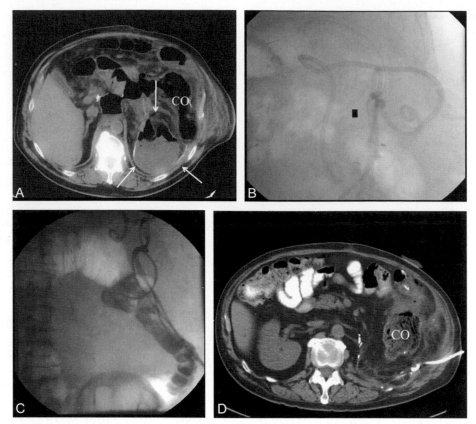

Fig. 29.5 Case Using Paired Catheter Insertion and Fistula Cannulation. A 69-year-old male with postoperative abscess and colonic fistula after an extensive debulking operation for recurrent retroperitoneal liposarcoma that included partial pancreatectomy, splenectomy, left nephrectomy, and partial left colectomy with colo-colonic anastomosis. (A) Postoperative retroperitoneal abscess post-resection *(arrows)* (CO = colon). (B) Paired drainages with 24-Fr and 10-Fr drainage catheters. (C) Catheter cannulating the fistulous tract in the colon. (D) CT prior to catheter removal (CO = colon) showing resolution of the abscess savity. (Courtesy Dr. Horacio D'Agotino.)

- Effective abscess cavity drainage precludes tract cannulation.
- In cases appropriate for cannulation, a drainage catheter is left in the abscess cavity, and another catheter, either a drainage catheter or feeding tube, is used to cannulate the fistulous tract.

Lower (True) Pelvis Collections

- Describes fluid collections in the pelvis below the innominate line
- Collections in the true pelvis often cannot be accessed transabdominally, requiring the following special insertion sites:
  - Transgluteal drainage
    - A painful procedure that involves insertion of a drainage catheter through the buttock
    - CT is typically needed to plan trajectory; some have reported success with ultrasound guidance
    - Difficult in morbidly obese patients
  - Transrectal drainage (Fig. 29.6)
    - Insertion of a drainage catheter through the rectum
    - Used for infected lower pelvis collections as this is not a sterile insertion site
    - Can be performed with only ultrasound guidance
    - Does not require an anoscope

- Requires that a Foley catheter be inserted into the bladder to empty it, thereby dropping the collection caudally to facilitate its safe access
- Transvaginal drainage
  - Insertion of a drainage catheter through the vagina
  - Can be performed with only ultrasound guidance
  - Used for both sterile or infected lower pelvis collections as the vaginal flora is typically not colonized with pathogenic bacteria and can be prepped with iodine
  - Does not require a speculum
  - Requires that a Foley catheter be inserted into the bladder to empty it, thereby dropping the collection caudally to facilitate its safe access

Thoracic Drainage

- Placement of a chest tube in the lung or pleural space for drainage of an infected or uninfected fluid collection
- Inserted under sonographic or CT guidance
  - Ultrasound is preferred for free-flowing pleural effusions
  - CT is preferred for multiloculated pleural collections, lung abscesses, and mediastinal abscesses
- Chest tubes or catheter drains are connected to a collection atrium (e.g., Pleur-evac) that is placed on continuous low-wall suction at −20 cm.

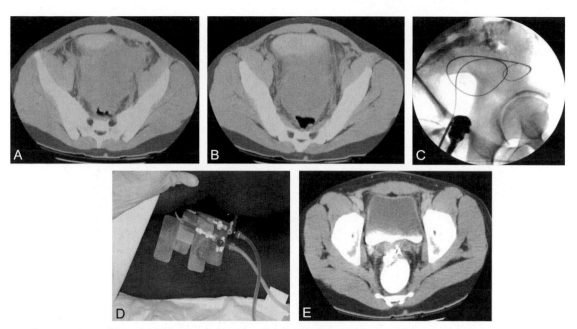

Fig. 29.6 Case of Transrectal Drainage for a True Pelvis Collection. A 23-year-old male with a gunshot wound to the abdomen underwent two exploratory laparotomies for trauma for damage control and resection of perforated bowel and developed postoperative leukocytosis. (A and B) CT demonstrating large, ill-defined pelvic collection. (C and D) The patient underwent transrectal insertion of two drainage catheters using fluoroscopy and ultrasound. (E) Postdrainage CT showing improvement and near resolution of the collection (Courtesy Dr. Horacio D'Agotino.)

- Empyema drainage
  - Often, a diagnostic thoracentesis immediately precedes any attempts at drainage
  - Drainage fluid with the following characteristics is concerning for empyema:
    - Purulent fluid
    - pH <7.2
    - Bacteria on Gram stain
    - Glucose <40 mg/dL
  - Empyema stages include:
    - Acute (exudative)
    - Subacute (fibrinopurulent)
    - Chronic (organizing)
    - Percutaneous drainage only has a role during the first two stages; surgical decortication is necessary with a chronic empyema.
- Lung abscess drainage (Fig. 29.7)
  - Percutaneous drainage is successful in resolving ~90% of lung abscesses.
  - Percutaneous drainage of a lung abscess establishes a controlled bronchocutaneous fistula.
  - CT guidance is often required to plan insertion tract and map out affected and healthy lung tissue.
    - Catheter insertion through abnormal lung tissue en route to the abscess is preferred.

ALTERNATE TREATMENTS

- Open surgical drainage
  - Requires the patient be placed under general anesthesia and is a more invasive option, leading to longer hospital stays.

- Antibiotic therapy
  - Antibiotics alone can be curative if the abscess is simple and less than 3 cm in diameter. With larger abscesses or those with thick walls, antibiotics are unlikely to penetrate into the cavity without adjunctive drainage.

◎ LITERATURE REVIEWS

Ballard et al. (2016) deemed surgical drainage appropriate in certain scenarios:
- An abscess less than 3 cm in diameter that fails to improve with antibiotic therapy, especially when the cause of the abscess has not been elucidated
- There is no safe window for percutaneous drainage
- Generalized peritoneal debridement would be appropriate
- Both source control and abscess drainage are required
- Interventional radiology drainage is not available, and transfer to a higher level of care is not an option

In a survey study of the practice patterns of radiologists who performed image-guided drainage of intraabdominal abscesses, 61% (89 of 147) answered that they would not drain an abscess less than 3 cm in diameter.

In a 2011 study, Politano et al. reported the largest comparison of open surgical versus percutaneous drainage in a retrospective review of 686 drainage cases in 500 patients (240 percutaneous vs. 260 surgical). Open surgical drainage was associated with significantly high mortality and longer hospital stay. Even after adjusting severity of illness and other mortality-associated factors, percutaneous drainage was still associated with better survival compared to surgical drainage.

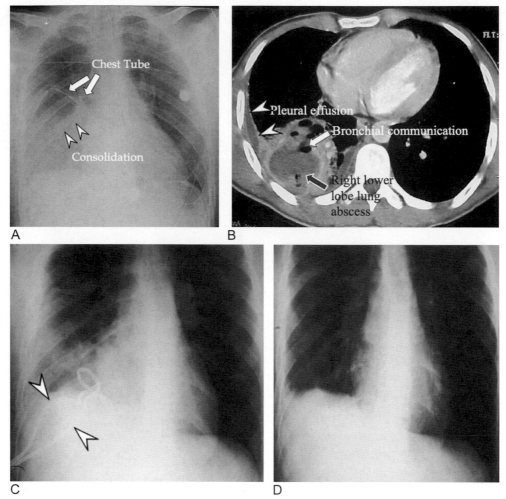

Fig. 29.7 Case of Lung Abscess Drainage. A 16-year-old male was initially triaged in the trauma bay following a motor vehicle collision. Assessment at that time showed a large pneumohemothorax which was alleviated by chest tube insertion in the trauma bay. (A) Six days following chest tube insertion *(arrows)*, the patient was febrile and had an elevated WBC, with a consolidative process seen on chest x-ray *(arrowheads)*. (B) CT showed a right-sided small pleural effusion and a bronchial communication *(white arrow)* with an irregular rim-enhancing fluid collection consistent with an abscess *(dark arrow)*. (C) Patient underwent image-guided placement of two catheters within the collection *(arrowheads)*. (D) The patient clinically improved, catheter output had decreased prompting removal of the catheters, and his post catheter removal chest x-ray showed no evidence of residual abscess. (Courtesy Dr. Horacio D'Agotino.) (Courtesy Dr. Horacio D'Agotino.)

COMPLICATIONS

- The complication rate for percutaneous drainage is approximately 10% (see Table 29.1)
- Major complications of abscess drainage include:
  - Septic shock (1%–2%)
  - Bacteremia requiring significant new intervention (2–5%)
  - Hemorrhage requiring transfusion (1%)
  - Superinfection, including infection of a sterile fluid collection (1%)
  - Pleural transgression requiring subsequent intraabdominal intervention (1%)
  - Bowel perforation requiring intervention (1%)

- If a bowel loop is penetrated by the catheter only with an entry wound, it is important to leave the catheter in and re-assess the site 7 to 10 days later. This essentially creates a percutaneous enterostomy.
- If a bowel loop is penetrated through and through, with entry and exit wounds, failure to withdraw the catheter may cause a bowel obstruction. If the bowel "kebab" is identified and the catheter is pulled out, intestinal content may spill and cause an additional intraabdominal infection. The situation can best be handled by withdrawing the catheter until the tip or the pigtail is within the bowel lumen and leaving it there, thus creating a percutaneous enterostomy.

TAKE-HOME POINTS

- Know who you are draining
  - Obtain history and perform physical exam. The patient's age group, performance status, and body complexion (i.e., pediatric population, elderly, critically ill, morbidly obese, comorbidities, coagulopathy) are essential for drainage strategy planning and material selection.
- Know what you are draining
  - Knowing if the collection is sterile or infected is key for patient preparation with or without preprocedure antibiotics.
  - Knowing if it is a simple or complex collection guides drainage catheter selection.

- Drain it well
  - Aim for complete evacuation at initial drainage.
  - Large collections with viscous fluid and particulate matter benefit from multiple or large diameter drainage catheters (18–24 Fr) for effective evacuation.
- Follow up
  - The catheter should be flushed once or twice daily to maintain its effectiveness and irrigated to remove any residual collection content.
  - The patient should be seen daily on inpatient IR rounds, and outpatient follow-up should be set up for catheter management and removal, as determined by the CLIC criteria.

REVIEW QUESTIONS

1. A 54-year-old female with Crohn disease and severe COPD is admitted to the intensive care unit under the medical intensivist team for fever, abdominal pain, and leukocytosis. The patient has generalized abdominal pain without signs of guarding or rebound tenderness. A CT of the abdomen reveals multiple intraabdominal complex fluid collections consistent with abscesses, three of which are 6 cm or larger. Broad-spectrum intravenous antibiotics, cessation of oral intake, and resuscitative efforts are initiated. Interventional radiology is consulted and deems that percutaneous drainage is the most appropriate course of action. Multiple drains at multiple sites will be required for effective drainage, including a transrectal drain for a deep pelvic collection.

   The patient's primary team is concerned about the anesthesia requirements for the procedure. The patient was previously deemed an inappropriate candidate for general anesthesia for an elective inguinal hernia repair due to her pulmonary impairment. The team also states that she "screamed her head off" when a right internal jugular central venous catheter was placed under local anesthesia this admission. What is the most appropriate response concerning the patient's anesthesia requirements for image-guided percutaneous catheter placement?
   a. Delay the procedure and ask the team to optimize the patient for general anesthesia with endotracheal intubation
   b. Proceed with the procedure using general anesthesia with endotracheal intubation
   c. Proceed with the procedure using both intravenous sedation and local anesthesia
   d. Proceed with the procedure using local anesthesia only
   e. Abort considerations for the procedure at this time and recommend intravenous antibiotics and supportive care with a repeat CT in 2 days

2. A 63-year-old male with a history of a low anterior resection with ileostomy creation for rectal adenocarcinoma also treated with adjuvant chemoradiation therapy presents to the hospital for elective ileostomy takedown. The procedure is technically successful, and the patient is admitted for postoperative recovery. On postoperative day 5, he develops abdominal distention, fever, and leukocytosis. Abdominal CT reveals a left lower quadrant intraabdominal fluid collection. Interventional radiology is consulted and successfully places a transabdominal drainage catheter, which evacuates 400 mL of purulent fluid. Four days following the drainage procedure, the patient is doing clinically well, and his primary team decides to discharge him to a short-term skilled nursing facility. The daily drainage catheter output the past 2 days has been 60 mL and 50 mL, respectively. After providing instructions for the facility's nursing staff to record daily catheter drainage, what is the most appropriate course of action with regard to follow-up?
   a. Give instructions to the surgery team to follow up with the patient in 1 to 2 weeks and remove the drainage catheter if the output is less than 10 mL/day
   b. Give instructions to the skilled nursing facility to remove the drainage catheter if the output is less than 10 mL/day
   c. Schedule follow-up in interventional radiology clinic in 6 weeks, and remove the drainage catheter if the output is less than 10 mL/day
   d. Schedule an outpatient sinogram with catheter manipulation procedure within 1 to 2 weeks following discharge
   e. Refer the patient to a physical therapy wound specialist to monitor the catheter output and remove when indicated

3. A 34-year-old male comes to the trauma bay following an abdominal gunshot wound. The patient is awake and alert with no respiratory compromise or hemodynamic instability. There is a single gunshot wound to the left upper quadrant with no exit wound. The abdomen is distended and tender to palpation in the upper quadrants with elements of involuntary guarding and rebound tenderness. Focused assessment with sonography for trauma is positive for intraperitoneal fluid. The patient is brought

emergently to the operating room where laparotomy reveals the bullet tract through the splenic flexure of the colon and the ballistic fragment lodged in the violated spleen. Splenectomy and partial colectomy with end colostomy are performed, and no other injuries are observed. On postoperative day 7, the patient develops abdominal pain and leukocytosis. Abdominal CT reveals a left upper quadrant intraabdominal fluid collection suspicious for an abscess. Interventional radiology performs transabdominal catheter drainage and evacuates the collection, leaving the catheter indwelling. In the interim, the patient clinically improves and is discharged with the drainage catheter in place. Ten days following the initial abscess drainage (17 days following the laparotomy), the patient is brought back for catheter revision. A sinogram reveals a residual abscess cavity and also a fistulous tract that appear to communicate with the small bowel. Which of the following is the most effective strategy to treat this patient's abscess-fistula complex?

a. Position one catheter to effectively drain the abscess and use another catheter to cannulate the fistulous tract

b. Position one catheter to effectively drain the abscess and position a second catheter at the dependent effluent portion of the fistulous tract without cannulating it

c. Use the current catheter to effectively drain the abscess irrespective of the fistula, and once the abscess cavity is resolved, attempt fistula closure using a percutaneous fistula plug

d. All of the above strategies are effective, and none has been shown to be superior to the other

e. None of the above; recommend general surgery consultation for open surgical repair

SUGGESTED READINGS

vanSonnenberg E, Wittich GR, Goodacre BW, et al. Percutaneous abscess drainage: update. *World J Surg.* 2001;25(3):362–369. Discussion 370–372, https://doi.org/10.1007/s002680020386.

Ballard DH, Flanagan ST, Griffen FD. Percutaneous versus open surgical drainage: surgeon's perspective. *J Am Coll Radiol.* 2016;13(4):364. https://doi.org/10.1016/j.jacr.2016.01.012.

Politano AD, Hranjec T, Rosenberger LH, et al. Differences in morbidity and mortality with percutaneous versus open surgical drainage of postoperative intra-abdominal infections: a review of 686 cases. *Am Surg.* 2011;77(7):862–867.

vanSonnenberg E, D'Agostino HB, Casola G, et al. Lung abscess: CT-guided drainage. *Radiology.* 1991;178(2):347–351. https://doi.org/10.1148/radiology.178.2.1987590.

van Sonnenberg E, Casola G, D'Agostino HB, et al. Interventional radiology in the chest. *Chest.* 1992;102(2):608–612.

Levin DC, Eschelman D, Parker I, et al. Trends in use of percutaneous versus open surgical drainage of abdominal abscesses. *J Am Coll Radiol.* 2015;12:1247–1250.

Chon KS, vanSonnenberg E, D'Agostino HB, et al. CT-guided catheter drainage of loculated thoracic air collections in mechanically ventilated patients with acute respiratory distress syndrome. *AJR Am J Roentgenol.* 1999;173(5):1345–1350. https://doi.org/10.2214/ajr.173.5.10541116.

Pfitzner J. Poiseuille and his law. *Anaesthesia.* 1976;31(2):273–275.

Lee SH, vanSonnenberg E, D'Agostino HB, et al. Laboratory analysis of catheters for percutaneous abscess drainage. *Minim Invasive Ther Allied Technol.* 1994;3:233–237.

Ballard DH, Alexander JS, Weisman JA, et al. Number and location of drainage catheter side holes: in vitro evaluation. *Clin Radiol.* 2015;70(9):974–980. https://doi.org/10.1016/j.crad.2015.05.004.

D'Agostino HB, Park Y, Moyers JP, et al. Influence of the stopcock on the efficiency of percutaneous drainage catheters: laboratory evaluation. *AJR Am J Roentgenol.* 1992;159(2):407–409. https://doi.org/10.2214/ajr.159.2.1632367.

Hoyt AC, D'Agostino HB, Carrillo AJ, et al. Drainage efficiency of double-lumen sump catheters and single-lumen catheters: an in vitro comparison. *J Vasc Interv Radiol.* 1997;8(2):267–270.

Ballard DH, Hamidian Jahromi A, Li AY, et al. Abscess-fistula complexes: a systematic approach for percutaneous catheter management. *J Vasc Interv Radiol.* 2015;26(9):1363–1367. https://doi.org/10.1016/j.jvir.2015.06.030.

vanSonnenberg E, D'Agostino HB, Casola G, et al. US-guided transvaginal drainage of pelvic abscesses and fluid collections. *Radiology.* 1991;181(1):53–56. https://doi.org/10.1148/radiology.181.1.1887056.

D'Agostino HB, Hamidian Jahromi A, et al. Strategy for effective percutaneous drainage of pancreatic collections: results on 121 patients. *J La State Med Soc.* 2013;165(2):74–81.

Ballard DH, Erickson A, Ahuja C, Vea R, Sangster G, D'Agostino H. Percutaneous Management of Enterocutaneous Fistulae and Abscess–Fistula Complexes. *Digestive Disease Interventions.* 2018; 02(02):131–140. https://doi.org/10.1055/s-0038-1660452.

Pope MC, Ballard DH, Sticker AL, Adams S, Ahuja C, D'Agostino HB. Fluid Flow Patterns Through Drainage Catheters: Clinical Observations in 99 Patients. *J La State Med Soc.* 2018; 170(5):146–150.

Ballard DH, Flanagan ST, Li H, D'Agostino HB. In vitro evaluation of percutaneous drainage catheters: Flow related to connections and liquid characteristics. *Diagn Interv Imaging.* 2018; 99(2):99–104. https://doi.org/10.1016/j.diii.2017.07.010.

Ballard DH, Mokkarala M, D'Agostino HB. Percutaneous drainage and management of fluid collections associated with necrotic or cystic tumors in the abdomen and pelvis. *Abdom Radiol (NY).* 2019; 44(4):1562–1566. https://doi.org/10.1007/s00261-018-1854-z.

Ballard DH, Gates MC, Hamidian Jahromi A, Harper DV, Do DV, D'Agostino HB. Transrectal and transvaginal catheter drainages and aspirations for management of pelvic fluid collections: technique, technical success rates, and outcomes in 150 patients. *Abdom Radiol (NY).* [Ahead of print]. https://doi.org/10.1007/s00261-019-01974-9.

Biliary Drains and Biliary Stenting

Daniel M. DePietro, Brittany K. Nagy, Scott O. Trerotola

CASE PRESENTATION

A 76-year-old female presents to the physician with increasing jaundice and pruritus. History reveals an unexplained 15-pound weight loss over the past 6 months. Total bilirubin is found to be 7.6 mg/dL, and a computed tomography (CT) scan of the abdomen reveals biliary ductal dilatation proximal to a stricture of the common hepatic duct by an enveloping mass. A diagnosis of cholangiocarcinoma is made. The patient is not a surgical candidate. She is seen by IR for placement of an internal/external biliary drainage tube to relieve her pruritus and hyperbilirubinemia prior to the initiation of chemotherapy.

After 6 months of chemotherapy and multiple tube exchanges, the tumor has not responded to treatment and therapy is stopped. The patient would like the drainage tube removed but does not want her prior symptoms of jaundice and pruritus to return. The patient is seen again by interventional radiology for removal of her internal/external biliary drain and placement of a permanent metal stent.

- Percutaneous biliary drainage was first described by Molnar and Stockholm in 1974. They described the first use of catheters capable of both **external** (into a drainage bag) and **internal** (into the small intestine) **drainage**, the latter of which was achieved by having side holes in the catheter distal to the site of obstruction. These initial catheters were used to relieve obstructive jaundice due to benign strictures and malignant tumors.
- Palliative drainage through the use of internal/external catheters, and later internal **plastic stents**, continued through the 1970s and 1980s, but these early devices were prone to complications including stent occlusion and cholangitis.
- In the late 1980s, multiple clinical trials using **metal stents** were published. Metal stents proved to be less prone to occlusion due to an increased internal diameter and now are the treatment of choice for palliative biliary drainage.
- Biliary stent insertions usually occur in two stages. Initial decompression is achieved by placing an internal/external drainage catheter that, in the next stage, is replaced by a permanent metal stent.

> ## CLINICAL POINT
>
> Many chemotherapy regimens for gastrointestinal (GI) malignancy require bilirubin levels below 2 mg/dL, although some only require levels below 5 mg/dL.

BENIGN BILIARY STRICTURE

- **Internal/external drainage** is performed for the treatment of benign biliary strictures.
- The majority of **benign biliary strictures** are iatrogenic, occurring after surgery or endoscopic retrograde cholangiopancreatography (ERCP), or due to inflammation secondary to choledocholithiasis, pancreatitis, primary sclerosing cholangitis, or autoimmune disease.
- Treatment generally includes temporary (approximately 3–12 months) placement of a plastic stent along with internal/external drainage catheter placement. In addition to stenting, the stricture is often treated with balloon dilation.
- Permanent metal stents are not used in the treatment of benign biliary strictures as they cannot be removed.
- Techniques, including length of stenting and timing of balloon dilation, vary significantly among institutions.

MALIGNANT BILIARY STRICTURE

- Malignancies that cause biliary strictures can be divided into two categories—those that cause proximal bile duct obstruction and those that cause distal obstruction.
- Proximal bile duct obstructions are less amenable to endoscopic stenting techniques by the interventional GI team. Common causes include:
  - Cholangiocarcinoma (Klatskin tumor) (most common)
  - Gallbladder cancer extending into the liver
  - Advanced gastric cancer
  - Liver metastases compressing the hilum
- Distal bile duct obstructions are often amenable to endoscopic stenting. These are treated percutaneously if endoscopic intervention is contraindicated (due to altered biliary anatomy such as a bilo-enteric anastomoses) or after endoscopic techniques have failed. Causes of distal bile duct obstructions include:
  - Pancreatic adenocarcinoma (most common)
  - Distal cholangiocarcinoma
  - Periampullary tumors

- Metal stents are placed in cases involving malignant obstruction whereas plastic stents are used for benign strictures. While more expensive, metal stents have the following advantages over plastic stents:
  - Better patency, reducing reintervention rates and increasing cost-effectiveness
  - No external tube is required
  - Small-diameter delivery system (metal stents are self-expanding, plastic stents are not)
- Cholangiocarcinoma is graded using the Bismuth-Corlette classification system (Fig. 30.1). This system (Table 30.1) is helpful in planning an approach in the percutaneous management of biliary obstruction as caused by cholangiocarcinoma.

INDICATIONS

- **Hilar obstruction** presenting with:
  - Jaundice (hyperbilirubinemia)
  - Need to reduce bilirubin levels prior to the initiation of chemotherapy
  - Pruritus
  - Cholangitis (less common)
- History of failed endoscopic drainage
- Prior biliary-enteric anastomoses (e.g., choledochojejunostomy)

⟫ CLINICAL POINT

What is the **Charcot's triad** of cholangitis? Fever, jaundice, and right upper quadrant abdominal pain.

CONTRAINDICATIONS

- Relative contraindications to percutaneous biliary drainage include:
  - Platelet count <50,000/dL
  - International Normalized Ratio (INR) ≥1.5
- Contraindications to the placement of a **metal** stent:
  - Possibility of future surgical intervention
  - Desire for future removal

EQUIPMENT

- Equipment for internal/external drain placement:
  - 21- or 22-gauge needle (e.g., Chiba needle)
  - 5- to 7-Fr coaxial percutaneous access kit (e.g., Jeffrey set)
    - Includes a metal trocar, an inner plastic trocar, and an outer sheath
  - Stiff 0.018-inch or 0.035-inch guidewire (e.g., Amplatz SuperStiff)
  - Hydrophilic 0.035-inch guidewire
  - Angled 5-Fr catheter (e.g., Kumpe, Berenstein)
  - Dilators
  - Internal/external biliary drainage catheter
  - Skin fixation device
- If placing a metal stent:
  - Self-expanding metal stent
    - Commonly used stents include the Wallstent and a variety of bare-metal nitinol stents. Stent grafts such as the ViaBil can also be used.

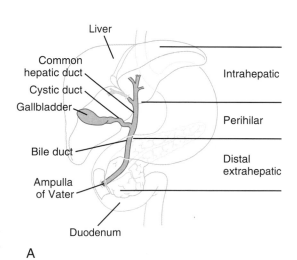

A

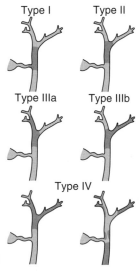

B

Fig. 30.1 Illustration of the Bismuth-Corlette Classification for Cholangiocarcinoma. A. Intrahepatic cholangiocarcinoma (CCA) denotes malignancy affecting the intrahepatic bile ducts. Extrahepatic CCAs are divided into hilar, middle, and distal tumors. B. There are 4 types of hilar CCA. Type I affects the common hepatic duct; type II involves the common hepatic duct and the confluence of the right and left hepatic ducts; types IIIa and IIIb occlude the common hepatic duct and either the right or left hepatic duct, respectively; and type IV involves the biliary confluence and extends to both the right and left hepatic ducts or refers to multifocal bile duct tumors. (From Lazaridis KN, Gores GJ. Cholangiocarcinoma. *Gastroenterology.* 2005;128:1655–1667, Fig. 4.)

TABLE 30.1   Bismuth-Corlette Classification for Cholangiocarcinoma

Type	Location
I	Common hepatic duct without involvement of the biliary confluence
II	Involves the biliary confluence, no involvement of segmental ducts
IIIa	Involves the biliary confluence and right hepatic duct
IIIb	Involves the biliary confluence and left hepatic duct
IV	Extends beyond the biliary confluence into both the right and left hepatic ducts or is multifocal

- PTA balloon
  - Used for post-stent dilation or post-stent graft placement

ANATOMY

Liver Anatomy

- The liver is functionally divided into two lobes, left and right, based on biliary drainage (Fig. 30.2). This is not to be confused with the anatomic right and left lobes of the liver, whose division is based on the anatomic location of the falciform ligament.
- It is the functional division of the liver that is of interest to interventional radiologists.
  - The functional left lobe contains segments II, III, and IV.
  - The functional right lobe contains segments V, VI, VII, and VIII.
  - The caudate lobe is found on the posterior surface of the liver and consists of segment I.

Biliary Anatomy (Fig. 30.3)

- Biliary ducts from segments II, III, and IV join to form the left hepatic duct.
- Biliary ducts from segments V, VI, VII, and VIII join to form the right hepatic duct.
  - The right lobe can be further divided into an anterior and posterior drainage system.
    - The right anterior hepatic duct drains segments V and VIII, whereas the right posterior hepatic duct drains segments VI and VII.
- Segment I drains into both the left hepatic and right posterior hepatic ducts.

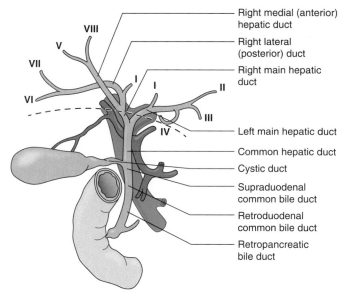

Fig. 30.3 Biliary Anatomy. The anatomy of the bile duct system demonstrating the segmental drainage of the liver and the route of biliary drainage from the liver to the duodenum. (From Ellis H. Anatomy of the gallbladder and bile ducts. *Surgery (Oxford).* 2011;29(12):593–596.)

- The right anterior and posterior ducts join to form the right main hepatic duct prior to the confluence of the left and right ducts, which form the common hepatic duct. The common hepatic duct joins with the cystic duct to form the common bile duct. The common bile duct descends through the head of the pancreas, where it joins the pancreatic duct prior to draining into the duodenum via the major duodenal papilla.

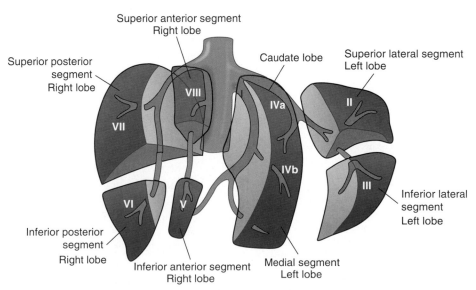

Fig. 30.2 Couinaud's Hepatic Segments Divide the Liver Into Eight Segments. The three hepatic veins are the longitudinal boundaries. The transverse plane is defined by the right and left portal pedicles. The caudate lobe (segment I) is situated posteriorly. Segment I includes the caudate lobe. Segments II and III include the left superior and inferior lateral segments. Segments IVa and IVb include the medial segment of the left lobe. Segments V and VI are caudal to the transverse plane. Segments VII and VIII are cephalad to the transverse plane. (From Hagen-Ansert SL. *Textbook of Diagnostic Sonography.* 8th ed. Philadelphia: Mosby Elsevier; 2018:chap 9, 190–247, Fig. 9-3.)

Anatomic Variations

- Knowledge of the segmental drainage of the liver and its variations is important in the planning of interventional biliary procedures. Classical biliary anatomy occurs in approximately 60% of patients, leaving 40% of patients with some type of aberrant anatomy. It is therefore common to encounter anatomic variations in biliary drainage, making preprocedural imaging a valuable resource in procedural planning.

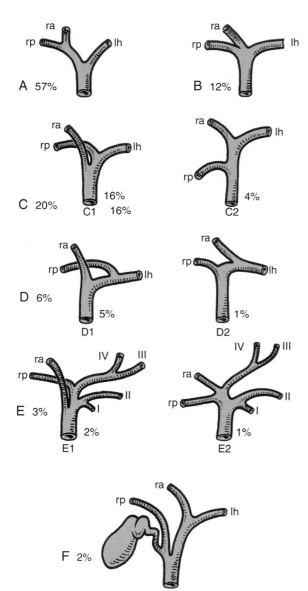

Fig. 30.4 Variations of the Hepatic Duct Confluence. A. Typical anatomy of the confluence. B. Triple confluence. C. Ectopic drainage of a right sectoral duct into the common hepatic duct (CHD) (C1, right anterior (ra) duct draining into the CHD; C2, right posterior (rp) duct draining into the CHD). D. Ectopic drainage of a right sectoral duct ino the left hepatic ductal system (D1, right posterior sectoral duct draining into the left hepatic (lh) ductal system; D2, right anterior sectoral duct draining into the left hepatic ductal system). E. Absence of the hepatic duct confluence. F. Absence of the right hepatic duct and ectopic drainage of the right posterior duct into the cystic duct. (From Jarnagin WR. *Blumgart's Surgery of the Liver, Pancreas and Biliary Tract: Expert Consult-Online.* London: Elsevier Health Sciences; 2012, Fig. 2.25.)

- One should be familiar with the most common anatomic variations in biliary anatomy, notably variations of the biliary confluence (Fig. 30.4).
- For example, if an anatomic variation results in the right posterior duct aberrantly draining into the left hepatic duct, rather than the right main hepatic duct, a strategically placed stent in the distal left hepatic duct can drain both the right posterior duct and the left hepatic duct. This would require accessing the biliary tree from patient's left side, rather than the right, directly impacting procedural planning.

> ### ▶ CLINICAL POINT
>
> Magnetic resonance cholangiopancreatography (MRCP) is particularly useful in evaluating biliary anatomy in patients with biliary obstruction and is the preferred imaging modality for preprocedural planning.

Right-Sided Biliary Access

- Most common approach for biliary drainage
- Puncture is typically made from the right flank inferior to the lowest rib (subcostally) in the mid-axillary line.
  - Puncture can be achieved under fluoroscopic or ultrasound guidance.
  - Finding a horizontal duct with a course consisting of gentle curves, rather than acute angles, toward the biliary confluence is preferred.
- Care must be taken to avoid the pleural reflection, which is directly above the liver and extends to the bottom of the rib cage.

Left-Sided Biliary Access

- More difficult approach compared to right-sided access due in part to the left lobe's relationship to the costal margins and xiphoid process, but is more patient friendly.
- Puncture is best achieved under ultrasound and fluoroscopic guidance but can be achieved with fluoroscopy alone.
  - If a bilateral approach is being performed, the biliary ducts can first be opacified using the more easily achieved right biliary access to aid in obtaining left biliary access.
- Segment II or III ducts are used for access.
  - Segment II ducts have a more horizontal course but are not always large enough to allow access.
  - Segment III ducts may have acute angles in their course to the biliary confluence, making maneuvering of equipment through these ducts difficult.

PROCEDURAL STEPS

Percutaneous Transhepatic Biliary Drainage (Biliary Tube Placement)

The right hemiliver is more often entered owing to its larger volume and ease of accessibility; therefore, a right-sided access is discussed here.

1. Right-sided drainage begins with selection of a low intercostal approach, ideally even subcostal to minimize pain

and pleural complications. Puncture is typically made along the mid-axillary line. Fluoroscopy can aid in initial needle placement by ensuring that puncture is not too cranial and potentially transpleural. Local anesthesia is administered at the skin entry site, and using ultrasound or fluoroscopic guidance, a Chiba needle is used to access a dilated peripheral bile duct percutaneously.

2. After puncture, the stylet is removed, and a syringe with connection tubing is attached to the needle.

3. The needle is slowly withdrawn while contrast is injected under fluoroscopic guidance until a duct opacifies. It will be evident that a bile duct has been opacified if the branching structure remains opacified. A hepatic artery will wash contrast vigorously to the periphery with pulsatile flow; a portal vein will demonstrate nonpulsatile flow of contrast toward the periphery; a hepatic vein will have nonpulsatile contrast flow directed centrally/toward the heart; lymphatics will appear beaded with slow contrast flow toward the hilum.

4. Following successful bile duct cannulation, a percutaneous cholangiogram is performed to assess for the best approach to biliary catheter placement and to ensure the access is peripheral enough (Fig. 30.5). Central access and long tracts through the hepatic parenchyma can increase the risks of hemorrhage and poor drainage. Additionally, an obtuse angle between the needle and duct is preferred as this makes catheter manipulation and drain/stent placement easier.

5. A guidewire is advanced centrally after an appropriate duct is accessed. A small dermatotomy is made adjacent to the needle, the needle is then removed and exchanged for a transitional dilator. A coaxial 6-Fr dilator with an inner stiffener is placed, the inner stiffener is removed, and a 0.035-inch guidewire is advanced.

> ## CLINICAL POINT
>
> In cases of emergent decompression for infection or/and cholangitis, or if the patient's clinical state is tenuous, an external biliary drain can be placed. In this instance, after step 5, the external drain is placed over the 0.035-inch wire. Attempts to internalize the drain can be made after the patient's clinical status improves.

6. The 0.035-inch wire is used to try and cross the obstruction with the goal of getting the wire into the proximal small bowel. A 5-Fr angled catheter can also be used to navigate past the obstruction. Once the wire has reached the duodenum, the catheter is advanced and the hydrophilic wire is exchanged for a stiffer working wire such as an Amplatz Super Stiff.

7. The tract is then serially dilated, if necessary, and the internal/external biliary drain (usually between 10 and 12 Fr) is placed (Fig. 30.6).

Biliary Tube Exchange

1. A 0.035-inch Amplatz wire is placed through the existing biliary tube.

2. The tube is removed over the wire.

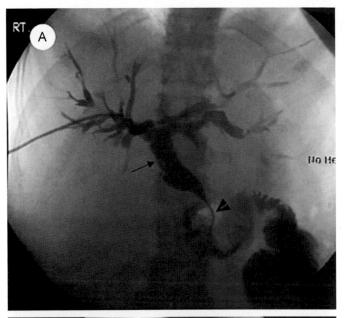

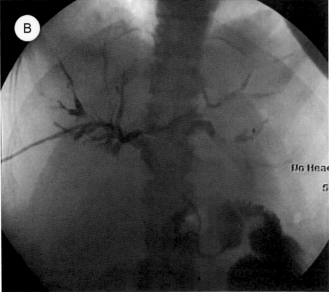

Fig. 30.5 Cholangiogram Demonstrating Bile Duct Obstruction. (A) Cholangiogram with drainage catheter in place demonstrates low bile duct obstruction. The common hepatic duct *(arrow)* is patent, and there is occlusion of the common bile duct *(arrowhead)* by a pancreatic carcinoma. (B) After catheter placement, all bile segments are adequately drained. (Reused with permission from Covey AM, Brown KT. Percutaneous transhepatic biliary drainage. *Tech Vasc Interv Radiol.* 2008;11(1):14–20, Fig. 1.)

3. The tract can be serially dilated, if needed.

4. A new internal/external biliary drain is placed over the wire. Placement can be confirmed with a cholangiogram.

Biliary Stent (Internal Metallic Stent) Placement

1. A 0.035 inch Amplatz wire is placed across the obstruction.

2. A sheath large enough to accommodate stent deployment is placed over the wire.

3. A sheath cholangiogram is performed to evaluate the length and extent of the obstruction so that an appropriately sized stent can be selected.

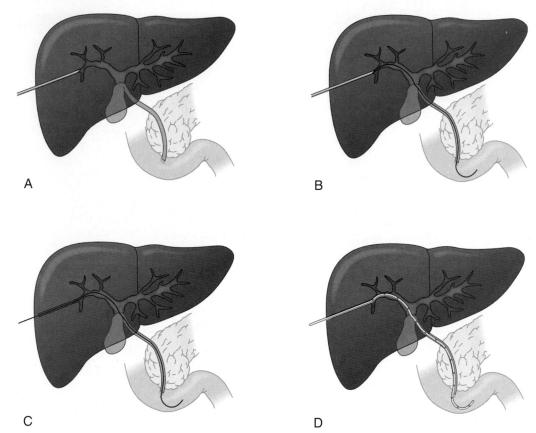

Fig. 30.6 Percutaneous Transhepatic Biliary Drainage. (A) A peripheral bile duct is identified and entered with a needle. (B) A guidewire is passed through the needle across the obstructing lesion into the duodenum. (C) The needle is withdrawn. (D) An internal-external catheter is inserted over the guidewire. (From: Stockland AH, Baron TH. *Endoscopic and Radiologic Treatment of Biliary Disease. Sleisenger and Fordtran's Gastrointestinal and Liver Disease.* Philadelphia: Elsevier Saunders; 2010, Fig 70.8.)

4. The self-expanding stent is deployed a few centimeters distal to the final desired position. After initiation of deployment, the stent, depending on its design, can be retracted to its final position.

5. A post-deployment sheath cholangiogram is performed to confirm antegrade passage of contrast through the stent and into the duodenum. If the appearance of contrast passage through the stent is suboptimal or hemobilia is present, an external biliary drain can be left to maintain access.

ALTERNATE TREATMENTS

- Endoscopic intervention: decompression with plastic stent placement
- Surgical intervention: hepaticojejunostomy, cholecystojejunostomy, or choledochoduodenostomy

COMPLICATIONS

- Bacteremia and sepsis (most common)
- Hemorrhage
  - Portal or hepatic vein injury (more common)
  - Hepatic artery injury (less common)
- Intractable pain
  - Resulting from a right-sided drain placed too close to a rib resulting in periosteal irritation and/or intercostal nerve injury
- Pleural transgression
  - Results in pneumothorax, hemothorax, and biliary pleural effusions
- Pericatheter leakage
- Stent occlusion
  - Multiple interventions over time are common to maintain stent patency

TAKE-HOME POINTS

- Biliary drainage is performed for many reasons, including as treatment for strictures due to benign as well as malignant causes.
- Metal stents are used for palliative biliary drainage in patients with malignant strictures. Consideration should be given to placing a metallic stent for palliation and to improve the quality of life in a terminally ill patient when clinically appropriate. The patient should be made aware that multiple interventions may be needed to maintain stent patency. Metallic stents should not be placed in patients who are potential surgical candidates.
- Biliary stent placement usually occurs in two stages—initial decompression is achieved with an internal/external drainage catheter, which is later replaced by a permanent metal stent.
- If an internal/external biliary drain is being placed, a 12-Fr drain can be placed if the patient is adequately sedated. In cases of

- emergent decompression for infection/cholangitis, an external biliary drain can be placed. Attempts to internalize the drain can be made in the future after the patient has clinically improved.
- Knowledge of the biliary drainage system, including the segmental anatomy of the liver, normal biliary duct anatomy, and variations in normal anatomy, is necessary to adequately plan and properly perform biliary drainage procedures.
- Preprocedural imaging is important in determining the anatomy of the biliary tree and planning a treatment approach.
- Right-sided biliary drainage is the most common approach, beginning with a low subcostal approach below the 11th subcostal space in the mid-axillary line. Needle trajectory is directed toward the left mid-clavicular line.

REVIEW QUESTIONS

1. What is the preprocedural imaging modality of choice for assessing biliary anatomy?
   a. CT scan
   b. Ultrasound
   c. Magnetic resonance cholangiopancreatography (MRCP)
   d. Endoscopic retrograde cholangiopancreatography (ERCP)

2. A 57-year-old female with a recent history of laparoscopic cholecystectomy is experiencing fever, nausea, and chills and is found to have abdominal distention on physical exam. There is a concern for bile leak due to an injury sustained during the recent cholecystectomy. The biliary system is accessed from the patient's right side, and the right anterior hepatic duct is catheterized. Contrast dye is flushed into the biliary system. No active extravasation from contrast is noted, despite filling of all apparent ducts on the right with contrast and multiple flushes. What variation in biliary anatomy is most likely present in this patient?

   a. Absence of the right posterior hepatic duct
   b. Drainage of the right anterior hepatic duct into the cystic duct
   c. Triple confluence of the right posterior, right anterior, and left hepatic ducts
   d. Drainage of the right posterior hepatic duct into the left hepatic duct

3. A 39-year-old male with a history of orthotopic liver transplant presents with jaundice and increased liver function tests. Ultrasound reveals biliary ductal dilatation and a narrowing of the bile duct at the bilo-enteric anastomosis. What is not indicated in this patient?
   a. Long-term biliary stenting
   b. Evaluation of biliary anatomy with an MRCP
   c. Metal stent placement
   d. Peri-procedural antibiotics

SUGGESTED READINGS

Molnar W, Stockum AE. Relief of obstructive jaundice through percutaneous transhepatic catheter—a new therapeutic method. *AJR Am J Roentgenol.* 1974;122(2):356–367.

DePietro DM, Shlansky-Goldberg RD, Soulen MC, et al. Long-term outcomes of a benign biliary stricture protocol. *J Vasc Interv Radiol.* 2015;26(7):1032–1039.

Sutter CM, Ryu RK. Percutaneous management of malignant biliary obstruction. *Tech Vasc Interv Radiol.* 2015;18(4):218–226.

van Delden OM, Laméris JS. Percutaneous drainage and stenting for palliation of malignant bile duct obstruction. *Eur Radiol.* 2008;18(3):448–456.

CT-Guided Lung Biopsy

Mina Makary, David Petrov, Makida Hailemariam, Laurie M. Vance

CASE PRESENTATION

A 67-year-old African American female with significant smoking history but no other comorbidities underwent routine low-dose chest CT screening. Imaging showed a 9-mm peripherally located pulmonary nodule in the lower lobe of the right lung. Per Fleischner Society recommendations, a follow-up chest CT is obtained 3 months later, which demonstrates an increase in size of the mass, now measuring 1.4 cm, with suspicious spiculated margins. The medical oncology team, in conjunction with cardiothoracic surgery and radiation oncology, consult the interventional radiology department for CT-guided biopsy of the growing pulmonary nodule.

- The first percutaneous approach in the investigation of lung pathology was described in 1883 by Leyden, who used the technique to aspirate organisms in a patient with pneumonia.
- In 1976, Haaga and Alfidi reported the first use of computed tomography in localizing target lesions and guiding percutaneous biopsy.
- Biopsy of lesions within the thoracic cavity, specifically nodules or masses arising in the lung parenchyma, is a quintessential step in the diagnosis and staging of malignancies as well as the diagnosis of other diseases requiring histologic confirmation. This is particularly true when surgical resection may not be the preferred treatment option.
- CT-guided biopsies provide a minimally invasive method to aid in tissue diagnosis. The technique has high diagnostic yield, relatively low complication risk, and lower cost and reduced morbidity compared to more invasive procedures.

◎ LITERATURE REVIEW

Schreiber and McCrory (2003) showed an overall sensitivity of 0.90 (95% CI, 0.88–0.92) for histologic yield using CT-guided lung biopsy of pulmonary lesions based on a meta-analysis of 19 studies.

- Increased spatial resolution with CT allows for biopsy of lesions <1 cm in size. Multiplanar reformatting can be used to aid in localization of subcentimeter nodules.

- CT fluoroscopy (CTF) is a tool available on many modern CT scanners that aids in percutaneous biopsying. With CTF, the radiologist, while wearing lead protection, uses a foot pedal next to the CT scanner to directly control image acquisition.
  - Advantages include:
    - Lower doses of radiation to the patient, up to a factor of 10 times less, compared to the classic technique
    - Near real-time image acquisition to localize the biopsy needle as it is advancing toward the target tissue
    - Decreased total procedure time, meaning less total anesthesia time for patient
  - Disadvantages include:
    - Interventionalist receives a small amount of radiation exposure

INDICATIONS

- Evaluation of non-benign (those that lack fat or have central, diffuse, laminated, or popcorn calcification patterns) solitary pulmonary nodules >8 mm in size
- Evaluation of suspicious nodules, including positron emission tomography (PET) positive nodules or those with documented growth
- Staging of bronchogenic carcinoma and metastatic lung lesions
- Evaluation of chronic pulmonary infections refractory to treatment
- Diagnosis of pleural thickening and chest wall masses

CONTRAINDICATIONS

- Uncorrectable bleeding diathesis (INR >1.5 or platelet count <50,000)
- Uncooperative patients (includes those with intractable cough)
- Severe bullous emphysema
- Poor lung reserve (e.g., patients with contralateral pneumonectomy)
- Intubated patients on positive pressure ventilation
- Central lesion in the setting of pulmonary arterial hypertension
- Suspected hydatid cyst (risk of anaphylaxis if biopsied)

EQUIPMENT (FIG. 31.1)

- If malignancy is highly suspected and additional molecular testing is not necessary, a fine-needle aspiration can be performed; for most lesions, however, the coaxial or core-cutting biopsy needle is most commonly used. Options include:
  - Core-cutting spring-activated 18- to 20-gauge needle (most common)
  - Coaxial needle system, consisting of a 22-gauge inner needle and a 19-gauge outer needle
  - Chiba aspiration needle, 20- to 25-gauge needle
- Pathology slides
- Formalin specimen containers
- Percutaneous pneumothorax drainage set (if needed)

ANATOMY

- The goal with thoracic and lung biopsies is to take the shortest path possible to the lesion, while avoiding vital structures, vessels, central bronchi, bullae, and fissures.
- Peripheral lesions are the safest to target as doing so avoids critical central structures and the fissures (which are pleural reflections, raising risk of pneumothorax if punctured).
- Given that emphysema is generally upper lobe predominant, careful approach planning for upper lobe and apical lesions should minimize passage through bullae.

HOW LARGE IS THE PNEUMOTHORAX?

- Size measurements of pneumothoraces on conventional radiographs correlate poorly with their actual size as determined on chest CT.
- Correlation between the size of the pneumothorax and the degree of clinical impairment is weak. Assessment of the patient's clinical status is the most important determinant in deciding whether chest tube drainage is required.
- The *2-cm rule*: if the distance between the lung margin and the chest wall at the apex is <2 cm, a chest tube is usually not needed; a distance of >2 cm usually requires chest tube placement.

Reused with permission from Herring W. *Learning Radiology: Recognizing the Basics*. 3rd ed. Philadelphia: Elsevier; 2016:Box 10.2.

PROCEDURAL STEPS

1. Patient is positioned on the table such that the skin entry site is upright.
2. Preliminary images are obtained covering the area of interest (Fig. 31.2). The skin entry site should be marked with the aid of a CT biopsy grid.
   a. Of note, all imaging should be obtained in the same phase of respiration, usually expiratory, since it represents approximately two-thirds of the respiratory phase.
3. Planned approach to the target lesion should take the shortest path possible, avoiding bullae, fissures, large vessels, central bronchi, and if possible, aerated lung. Lesions

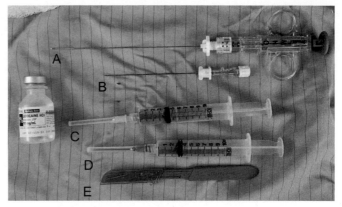

Fig. 31.1 Biopsy Equipment. (A) 20-gauge × 20-cm biopsy needle, (B) 15-cm coaxial introducer needle, (C) 10-mL 25-gauge syringe containing 1% lidocaine, (D) 10-mL syringe for tract aspiration while removing coaxial needle, and (E) scalpel for incision of coaxial needle tract.

directly below a rib can be targeted by angling the gantry or by taking an oblique approach.

4. The skin entry site is cleansed with chlorhexidine, and the area is covered with sterile drapes (Fig. 31.3).
5. The skin and subcutaneous soft tissues are anesthetized with 1% lidocaine, but the pleura should not be entered during this step (Fig. 31.4).
6. The biopsy introducer or biopsy device is advanced along the planned trajectory to the target lesion (Fig. 31.5). The goal is to have the introducer (spring-activated needle) or biopsy device (coaxial needle system) just into the lesion. Thin CT images are obtained superior and inferior to the needle tip to ensure accurate positioning.
7. If using the spring-activated needle, the biopsy needle is inserted into the introducer; if using the coaxial system, the biopsy device is advanced through the lesion (Fig. 31.6).
8. Tip position is confirmed with imaging, and the sample is obtained. Attention should be paid to the needle tip so that a vital structure is not punctured beyond the edge of the lesion.
9. One to three samples is usually sufficient volume. If there is concern for inadequate sampling, a wet prep slide can be prepared so that the on-site pathologist can ensure adequacy of the sample prior removing equipment (Fig. 31.7).
10. The biopsy device is carefully removed, an occlusive bandage is quickly placed over the skin entry site to reduce risk of pneumothorax, and the patient is turned to the side of the biopsy.
    a. Some interventionalists advocate for a **blood patch technique** to reduce the risk of pneumothorax. This involves injecting 4 mL of the patient's peripheral blood through the introducer or biopsy needle into the needle tract.
11. Postprocedural observation for at least an hour and a post-biopsy chest radiograph to evaluate for pneumothorax is common practice in many institutions.

For reference, please review the Michigan SIR RFS YouTube video recording of the procedural steps at: https://www.youtube.com/watch?time_continue=1&v=ym6lbe_UAXs (accessed October 2018).

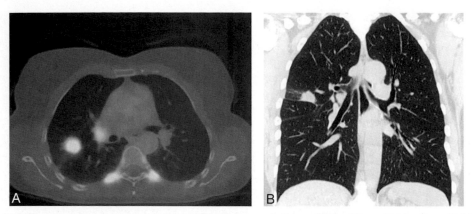

Fig. 31.2 Pre-procedure Imaging. (A) Fused PET-CT demonstrating an FDG-avid target lesion (max. SUV 6.9). (B) Preprocedure coronal reformat shows a spiculated right upper lobe lung mass abutting the minor fissure. (FDG = fluorodeoxyglucose; SUV = standardized uptake value)

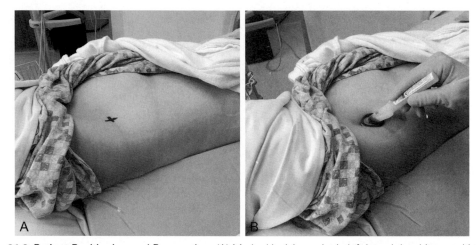

Fig. 31.3 Patient Positioning and Preparation. (A) Marked incision point in left lateral decubitus position for intercostal trajectory. (B) Chlorhexidine for antiseptic skin site cleaning. (Courtesy MSU CHM, Providence—Providence Park Hospitals, Department of Radiology.)

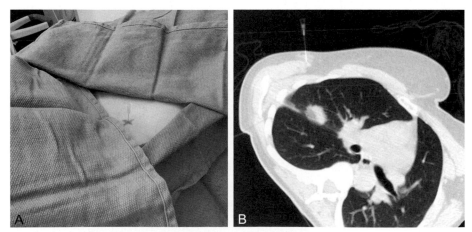

Fig. 31.4 Trajectory Planning. (A) 25-G anesthesia needle in skin to mark trajectory. (B) Redemonstration of anesthesia needle on axial views with appropriate angle trajectory toward lesion and in-plane orientation with the CT slice. (A, Courtesy MSU CHM, Providence—Providence Park Hospitals, Department of Radiology.)

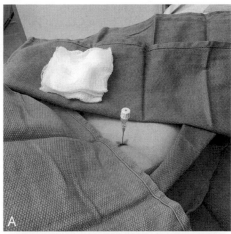

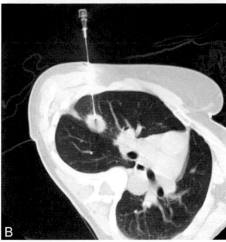

Fig. 31.5 Introducing the Coaxial Needle. (A) Coaxial needle inserted through the skin site. (B) Coaxial needle in the lesion with needle shadow demonstrating appropriate depth of tip. (A, Courtesy MSU CHM, Providence—Providence Park Hospitals, Department of Radiology.)

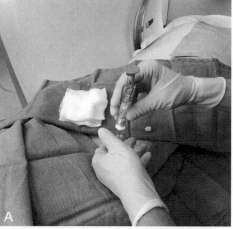

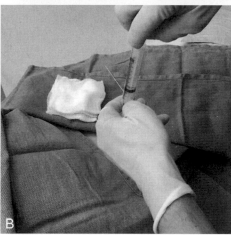

Fig. 31.6 Biopsying and Procedure Conclusion. (A) Biopsy needle is placed within the coaxial needle. (B) 10-mL syringe attached to coaxial needle for aspiration during removal. (Courtesy MSU CHM, Providence—Providence Park Hospitals, Department of Radiology.)

ALTERNATE TREATMENTS

- The combination of PET/CT staging and CT-guided percutaneous lung biopsy has nearly eliminated the need for more invasive surgical approaches and has limited the use of transbronchial biopsy. These alternative techniques include:
  - Surgical approaches, which are inherently invasive, require the patient be placed under general anesthesia and have longer recovery times
    - Open thoracotomy
    - Video-assisted thoracoscopic surgery (VATS)
  - Bronchoscopic approaches, which are less invasive compared to surgical biopsies but are largely limited to central lung lesions and lymph nodes
    - Transbronchial biopsy
    - Endobronchial ultrasound-guided transbronchial needle aspiration (EBUS-TBNA)

COMPLICATIONS

- Pneumothorax (12%–30%) (Fig. 31.8)
  - The most commonly seen complication, most post-biopsy pneumothoraces do not require intervention. Only 2% to 15% necessitate drainage or chest tube placement.
  - Risk factors for the development of a post-biopsy pneumothorax include:
    - Emphysema
    - Use of a large-gauge (18-gauge) needle
    - Crossing through the fissure during the biopsy
    - Decreased needle-to-skin angle
- Hemoptysis (5%–10%), almost always self-limited
- Parenchymal hemorrhage (5%–17%), almost always self-limited (Fig. 31.9)
- Rare but reported complications include:
  - Pericardial tamponade
  - Air embolism
  - Pulmonary infection
  - Malignant seeding of the needle tract

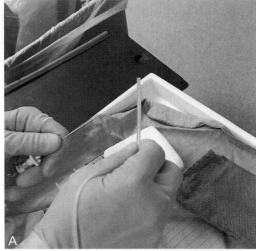

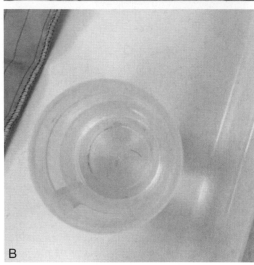

Fig. 31.7 Handling the Biopsy Sample. (A) Biopsy needle with tissue sample. (B) Sample in formalin solution. (Courtesy MSU CHM, Providence—Providence Park Hospitals, Department of Radiology.)

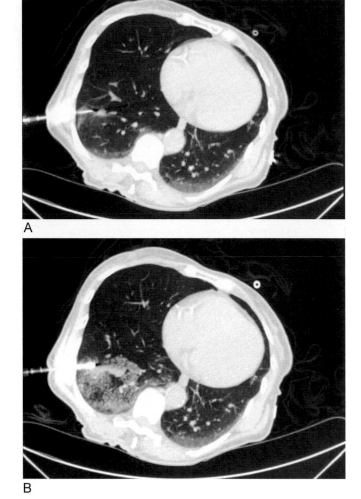

Fig. 31.9 Complications Following Biopsy. Axial CT demonstrating biopsy trajectory (A) and subsequent intraparenchymal pulmonary hemorrhage after firing of biopsy needle (B).

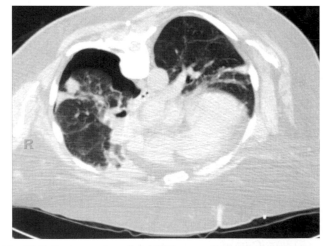

Fig. 31.8 Postprocedure Axial CT Demonstrating Left-Sided Pneumothorax Following Biopsy. (Courtesy MSU CHM, Providence—Providence Park Hospitals, Department of Radiology.)

🏠 TAKE-HOME POINTS

- Percutaneous CT-guided lung biopsy is a safe and efficacious approach for tissue sampling with an overall 93% sensitivity and 98% specificity.
- A direct vertical percutaneous approach that takes the shortest possible pathway to the lesion, evading central vessels and bronchi, is preferred.
- Precautions include avoiding bullae and fissures, and the use of large caliber needles; doing so will reduce the risk of developing a pneumothorax.
- Postprocedure care includes turning the patient onto the side where the biopsy was performed, which is also meant to reduce the risk of pneumothorax.
- The most common complication is pneumothorax, with most requiring no intervention. Other less common complications include parenchymal hemorrhage and hemoptysis, both of which are usually self-limited.

REVIEW QUESTIONS

1. Which of the following is NOT a contraindication to transthoracic lung biopsy?
   a. Bullous emphysema with FEV_1 of <50%
   b. Suspected hydatid cyst
   c. Platelet level: 30,000
   d. INR: 1.2
   e. Ventilated patient with PEEP of 8 cm H_2O
2. What is the most common complication resulting from CT-guided lung biopsy?
   a. Hemothorax
   b. Neuropathic pain
   c. Pneumothorax
   d. Chylothorax
   e. Pericardial laceration
3. Which of the following types of thoracic lesions is most amenable to CT-guided percutaneous lung biopsy?
   a. Central bronchial lesion
   b. Subcarinal lymph node
   c. Peripheral parenchymal 10-mm noncalcified nodule
   d. Peripheral parenchymal 10-mm nodule with popcorn calcifications
   e. Peripheral 15-mm serpiginous mass with early phase CT enhancement

SUGGESTED READINGS

Anderson JM, Murchison J, Patel D. CT-guided lung biopsy: factors influencing diagnostic yield and complication rate. *Clin Radiol.* 2003;58:791–797.

Heck SL, Blom P, Berstad A. Accuracy and complications in computed tomography–guided needle biopsies of lung masses. *Eur Radiol.* 2006;16:1387–1392.

House AJS. Biopsy techniques in the investigation of diseases of the lung, mediastinum and chest wall. *Radiol Clin N Am.* 1979;17:393–412.

Kandarpa K, Machan L. *Handbook of Interventional Radiologic Procedures.* Philadelphia: Wolters Kluwer/Lippincott Williams & Wilkins Health; 2010.

Lal H, Nayaz Z, Nath A, et al. CT-guided percutaneous biopsy of intrathoracic lesions. *Kor J Radiol.* 2012;13(2):210–226.

Lorenz J. Updates in percutaneous lung biopsy: new indications, techniques and controversies. *Sem Interv Radiol.* 2012;29: 319–324.

Schreiber G, McCrory DC. Performance characteristics of different modalities for diagnosis of suspected lung cancer: summary of published evidence. *Chest.* 2003;123:115S–128S.

Winokur R, Pau B, Sullivan B, et al. Percutaneous lung biopsy: technique, efficacy, and complications. *Sem Interv Radiol.* 2013;30:121–127.

Gastrostomy Tube Placement

Judy W. Gichoya, Millie Liao, John M. Moriarty

CASE PRESENTATION

A 78-year-old male with recently diagnosed esophageal squamous cell carcinoma presents to his primary care physician with generalized weakness and dysphagia secondary to obstruction from the mass. His physician requests an interventional radiology consult for percutaneous radiologic gastrostomy tube placement for long-term enteric nutrition access.

- Egeberg first proposed the concept of **surgical gastrostomy** in 1837.
- In 1846, Sedillot attempted gastrostomy placement, but his patient did not survive.
- Subsequently, in 1876, Verneuil performed the first successful surgical gastrostomy. By 1894, Stamm had standardized the technique of surgical gastrostomy tube placement.
- In 1979, Gauderer and Ponsky performed the first **percutaneous endoscopic gastrostomy (PEG)**, and in 1981, Preshaw performed the first percutaneous fluoroscopic-guided gastrostomy tube placement.
- Percutaneous gastrostomy tube placement creates direct access to the stomach through the anterior abdominal wall without exposing the stomach.
- Gastrostomy placement provides an alternative feeding route for long-term enteral nutrition in patients unable to meet caloric and nutritional requirements orally.
- Short-term access can be achieved with nasogastric and orogastric feeding tubes, but the small diameter of these tubes leads to more frequent clogging, which makes them inappropriate for long-term access.
- Gastrostomy tubes can also be used for decompressive purposes in patients with chronic small bowel or gastric outlet obstruction.
- The following specialists can place gastrostomy tubes:
  - **Surgeons** perform open, surgical gastrostomy tube placement.
  - **Gastroenterologists** perform PEG tube placement under endoscopic guidance.
  - **Interventional radiologists** perform **percutaneous radiologic gastrostomy (PRG)** tube placement under fluoroscopic guidance.

- Percutaneous gastrostomy (i.e., PRG and PEG) can be further categorized by method of gastrostomy tube (G-tube) insertion:
  - **Transoral** (or **pull-through**) technique: G-tube is inserted in the mouth, pulled through the stomach, and pulled out of the anterior abdominal wall
  - **Transabdominal** (or **push-through**) technique: G-tube is inserted through the anterior abdominal wall and pushed into the stomach

INDICATIONS

- General indications for G-tube placement include:
  - Access for long-term enteral nutrition
  - Gastric decompression
- Indications for long-term enteral nutrition access include:
  - Dysphagia:
    - Neurologic causes include cerebrovascular accidents and traumatic brain injury.
    - Neuromuscular causes include cerebral palsy and amyotrophic lateral sclerosis (ALS).
    - Physically obstructive causes include head, neck, and esophageal malignancies.
  - Chronic conditions, often seen in the pediatric population, that lead to insufficient oral caloric intake (e.g., cystic fibrosis, hydrocephalus)
- Indications for gastrointestinal decompression include:
  - Small bowel obstruction
  - Gastric outlet obstruction
  - Enteric fistula

> **CLINICAL POINTS**
>
> - A specific access method may be more appropriate than another in certain circumstances. For example:
> - PRG is favored over PEG in cases where passage of the endoscope is difficult secondary to a mass or where there is concern for spreading oral/esophageal cancer cells to the stomach.
> - PEGs are commonly placed in ALS patients for dysphagia; however, PRG is preferred in patients with greater respiratory compromise (forced vital capacity <50%), as there is less risk of respiratory complications.

CLINICAL POINTS—cont'd

- Advantages of transabdominal access:
  - Avoidance of G-tube exposure to oral flora, thus reducing the risk of infection
  - Avoidance of tumor seeding in patients with head and neck cancer
- Advantages of transoral access:
  - Increased certainty of gastric entry
  - Less risk of G-tube malpositioning
  - Reduced risk of dislodgment

CONTRAINDICATIONS

- **Absolute contraindications** include:
  - Gastrointestinal obstruction (unless the G-tube is being placed for decompression)
  - Active peritonitis
  - Uncorrectable coagulopathy - risks uncontrollable internal hemorrhage
  - Bowel ischemia
- **Relative contraindications** include:
  - Hemodynamic instability
  - Active or recent GI bleed (e.g., esophageal varices, peptic ulcer disease)
  - Gastric malignancy
  - Ascites - risks peritonitis and failure of G-tube tract maturation
  - Presence of a ventriculoperitoneal shunt - risks ascending meningitis
  - Morbid obesity - risks G-tube dislodgment from shifting panniculus prior to tract maturation
  - Anatomic abnormalities (e.g., high-lying stomach, history of partial gastrectomy)
  - Interposition of the colon between stomach and abdominal wall

LITERATURE REVIEW

In a review of 7,369 patients, Rabeneck et al. (1996) showed that despite widespread approval of the use of G-tubes, there was no evidence supporting increased patient survival rates due to the G-tube placement.

- According to the Society of Interventional Radiology (SIR), percutaneous gastrostomy procedures have a moderate risk of bleeding. SIR recommends the following:
  - INR <1.5
  - Platelet count >50,000/μL
  - Withholding clopidogrel for 5 days prior to procedure
  - Withholding 1 therapeutic dose of low-molecular-weight heparin prior to the procedure
  - No need to withhold aspirin

EQUIPMENT

- Classification of G-tubes is based on diameter, material, and retention mechanism. Anatomy of a G-tube is shown in Fig. 32.1.

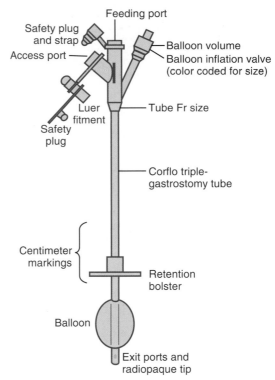

9-in (23-cm) overall length

Fig. 32.1 Parts of a G-Tube. (From Samuels LE. Nasogastric and feeding tube placement. In: Roberts JR, Hedges JR, eds. *Clinical Procedures in Emergency Medicine*. 4th ed. Philadelphia: Saunders; 2004:794–816.)

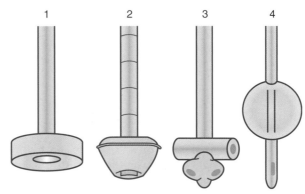

Fig. 32.2 Gastrostomy Tubes. (From Samuels LE. Nasogastric and feeding tube placement. In: Roberts JR, Hedges JR, eds. *Clinical Procedures in Emergency Medicine*. 4th ed. Philadelphia: Saunders; 2004:794–816.)

- Gastrostomy tubes are available in various French sizes and are divided into four types (Fig. 32.2), summarized as follows:
  - Silicone catheter (American Endoscopy, Bard Interventional Products; Billerica, MA)
  - Polyurethane catheter with a collapsible foam flange (CORPAK MedSystems, Wheeling, IL)
  - Latex catheter with a movable external bolster and an internal mushroom- or de Pezzer–type flange on the end (American Endoscopy)
  - Balloon (Foley) catheter (Wilson-Cooke Co., Winston-Salem, NC)

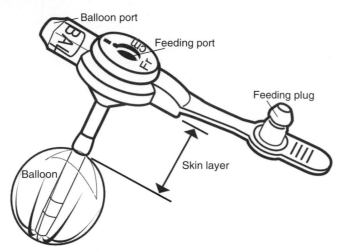

Balloon port

Feeding port

Feeding plug

Skin layer

Balloon

Fig. 32.3 Button (MIC KEY) G-Tube Parts. (Used with permission from Halyard, https://www.halyardhealth.com/.)

- T-fasteners are used to affix the stomach to the anterior abdominal wall.
- Button (MIC KEY) G-tubes are used for replacing established tracks with dedicated "stoma-lengths" for each G-tube (Fig. 32.3).

ANATOMY

- G-tubes are placed in patients with normal or near normal gastric and small bowel motility (unless being placed for decompression). The patient's anatomy should be amenable to G-tube placement. When these criteria are not met (e.g., patients with surgically altered gastric anatomy, gastric or duodenal fistulas, or patients with severe reflux), placement of a jejunal feeding tube should be considered.
- The stomach is an intraperitoneal organ that lies below the diaphragm in the left upper abdomen under a portion of the left hepatic lobe. The following anatomic correlations can be made (*portion of the stomach: organ [attachment]*):
  - Posterior: pancreas
  - Left lateral: spleen (gastrosplenic/gastrolienal ligament)
  - Superior and right lateral: liver (hepatogastric ligament/lesser omentum)
  - Superior: diaphragm (gastrophrenic ligament)
  - Inferior: transverse colon (gastrocolic ligament/greater omentum)

Stomach Anatomy (Fig. 32.4)

- **Cardia** is the portion of the stomach that is continuous with the esophagus and transitions into the **body** of the stomach.
- **Fundus** is the portion of the stomach above an imaginary horizontal line through the cardia.
- A line through the angular notch separates the body from the **antrum,** which transitions into the duodenum via the pylorus.

PROCEDURAL STEPS

Preprocedural Evaluation

- Ensure that the patient meets the moderate risk criteria by checking the INR (<1.5) and platelet count ($>50,000/\mu L$).

- Review patient history including previous surgeries and available imaging (e.g., abdominal radiographs and CT).
- Patient should be NPO for at least 6 hours prior to procedure.

New G-Tube Placement (Transabdominal Approach)

1. Place a nasogastric feeding tube, or retract the Dobhoff tube into the stomach.
2. Place the patient in a supine position and clean/drape the left hemi-abdomen. An entry location lateral to the left rectus abdominis muscle is preferred to avoid going through muscle and avoid injury to the superior epigastric branches.
3. 0.1 to 1 mg of glucagon (in nondiabetics) is given intravenously to the patient to avoid stomach decompression during inflation. An antiemetic may be administered at this point.
4. Fluoroscopic images are taken at this point to visualize the stomach. The stomach is insufflated via the NG tube until sufficient distention is visualized.
   a. The transverse colon should be identified and distinguished from the stomach. Some institutions give a patient oral contrast 12 hours before the procedure to highlight the colon.
   b. Ultrasound can be used to confirm that the inferior lobe of the liver is away from the stomach at the selected site.
   c. Color Doppler can be used to exclude the superior epigastric artery.
   d. The ideal puncture location is in the body of the stomach, facing the antrum to allow for easy conversion to a gastrojejunostomy if needed in the future.
5. To secure the stomach to the abdominal wall, the site is secured with gastropexy sutures (Fig. 32.5). Subcutaneous lidocaine is injected at all sites. The practitioner may use two to four gastropexy sutures based on the amount of subcutaneous tissue traversed to get to the stomach.
6. After administering lidocaine, an incision is made between the gastropexy sutures, and a needle is used to access the stomach directed towards the pylorus.
7. A guidewire is advanced through the needle and coiled in the stomach, and the tract is dilated with serial dilation.
8. A 10- to 20-Fr G-tube is placed through the tract. Location in the stomach is confirmed with injection of contrast into the stomach lumen.
9. The securing balloon mechanism is then inflated with up to 10 cm of sterile water.
10. The tube is retracted so as not to be too snug or too tight. The retention bolster is secured at this position using silk sutures.
11. The tube is then connected to a gravity bag to drain. The patient is made NPO with no tube feeds for 24 hours. If there are no signs of peritonitis after 24 hours, then the tube can be used for feeds and medications.
12. The patient should be seen in clinic (or the inpatient setting) in 1 to 3 weeks for gastropexy suture removal. If gastropexy sutures are left for too long, they can erode into the skin, potentially causing abscess or fistula formation.

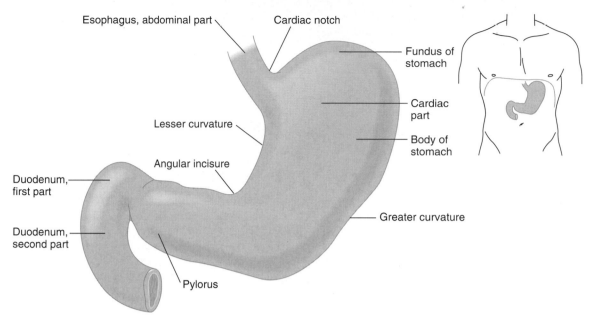

Fig. 32.4 Stomach—ventral view (From Paulsen F. *Sobotta Atlas of Human Anatomy*. 2013:69–156. Munich, Germany. © 2013, Figs. 6.5 and 6.6.)

New G-Tube Placement (Transoral Approach)

The beginning of this procedure follows steps 1 through 5 as listed in "New G-tube Placement (Transabdominal Approach)."

6. An 18-gauge needle is advanced into the stomach pointing toward the gastroesophageal junction.
7. A guidewire is inserted through the needle and advanced into the esophagus, oropharynx, and out of the mouth. The G-tube with an internal bumper is inserted in an anterograde direction over the wire until it emerges out of the abdominal wall.

Steps 9 through 12, as listed in "New G-tube Placement (Transabdominal Approach)," are repeated to secure the G-tube.

G-Tube Replacement

- Accidental tube removal occurs in 1.5% to 4.5% of cases.
- Preventative maintenance with tube exchange should occur every 3 to 6 months.
- Gastrostomy tract generally matures within the first 7 to 10 days postplacement, but this may be delayed for up to 4 weeks in immunosuppressed patients (e.g., corticosteroid users, diabetics, HIV+ patient, etc...).
- Approach to replacement of a G-tube is dependent on the interval duration since its initial placement.
  - If the tube is removed in the period where the tract is not mature, replacement should be made under fluoroscopy over a wire.
  - If the tube has been present for several months and a tract has formed, it can be changed at bedside; if the tract is not mature, exchange is made over guidewire under fluoroscopic guidance, as follows:

1. The balloon is deflated, and the existing tube is removed.
2. Lubricating jelly is added to the tract. Ensure that the patient is flat with no tense muscles. A new tube is then inserted through the preexisting tract.
3. Tube is secured using standard methods.

G-Tube Maintenance

- Gastrostomy site should be cleaned with mild soap and water.
- Excessive granulation tissue can be treated with topical silver nitrate or a high-potency topical steroid.
- Stoma adhesive powder or zinc oxide can be applied to the skin to prevent local irritation.
- Occlusive dressings should be avoided; foam dressings are preferred, as they lift drainage away from the skin.
- Persistent leakage around the tube can be treated with proton pump inhibitors, upsizing of the tube to tamponade the tract, or conversion of the gastrostomy tube into a gastrojejunostomy tube.
- Frequent flushing with sterile water prevents clogging. Pancreatic enzymes or mechanical devices to declog the tube can be used if it is already clogged. Tube replacement can be performed when the aforementioned techniques fail.

ALTERNATE TREATMENTS

- Patients who require short-term feeding needs (<6 weeks) can use a **nasogastric or nasojejunal feeding tube**.
  - Associated with an increased risk of gastroesophageal reflux and aspiration, as these keep the gastroesophageal junction open

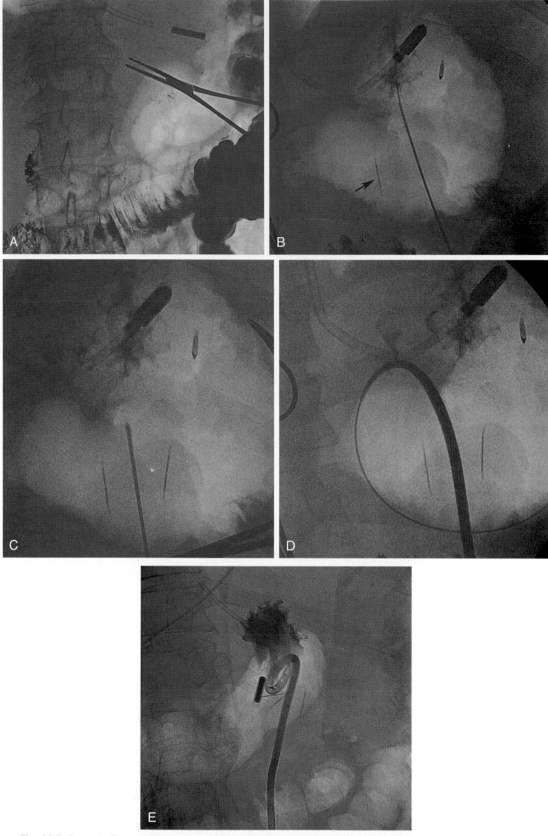

Fig. 32.5 Steps in Percutaneous Gastrostomy Tube Placement. (A) Initial localization. The hemostat marks the costal margin. Stomach is inflated with air via a preexisting nasogastric tube. The optimal access is through the greater curvature in the lower mid body of the stomach. (B) Gastropexy using T-fasteners. Image shows first T-tack already in place *(black arrow)*. A second anchor is being deployed through an 18-gauge needle. Intraluminal position is confirmed by contrast injection to outline the rugae as well as by lateral fluoroscopic imaging. (C) Needle entry for actual tube placement into the stomach. Note the two T-fasteners already in position; some operators prefer to place three fasteners. Needle puncture directed toward the pylorus would simplify future conversion to gastrojejunostomy. Care is taken to be well below the costal margin and mindful of the expected location of the superior epigastric artery. (D) Tract dilatation over an Amplatz wire. (E) Final image showing the Deutsch pigtail gastrostomy tube in the fundus of the stomach. (Reused with permission from Vaidya S, Rivera-Sanfeliz G, Lim G. *Gastrointestinal Interventions in The Practice of Interventional Radiology* edited by Karim V. 635–655, Philadelphia: Elsevier; 2012, F21.5.)

- **Intravenous total parenteral nutrition (TPN)** can be used for long-term nutrition in place of gastrostomy tube placement
  - Associated with an increased risk of sepsis and cholestatic liver disease
  - Risk of central line infection with peripherally inserted central catheter (PICC) line, which is needed for TPN infusion

COMPLICATIONS

◎ LITERATURE REVIEW

Lowe et al. (2012) conducted a multicenter study in 2012 with 684 patients and reported an overall 30-day mortality rate of 1% for PRG.

Minor Complications

- Mild pain (31%) that is relieved with oral analgesics
- Moderate pain (28%) that is relieved with IV analgesics
- Severe pain (1%) that persists 30 minutes after analgesic administration
- Peristomal leakage
  - Serial dilation for tract formation can lead to overdilation, risking gastric content and enteral formula leakage from the stoma site
  - Inserting a larger G-tube will decrease this leakage
- Peristomal wound infection (up to 5%)
- Buried bumper syndrome
  - Growth of gastric mucosa over the internal bolster of the G-tube
- Gastric ulcer formation
- Gastric bleeding

▶ CLINICAL POINT

SIR recommends leaving ~1 cm between the skin and external bolster for adequate tension and reduced pressure-related complications (pain, ulcers, peristomal infection, buried bumper syndrome, etc.).

- Tube malfunction
  - Blockage commonly occurs after the administration of crushed medications
  - Regular flushing with water prevents this

- Pneumoperitoneum (56%)
  - Generally not of clinical significance unless the volume of free air increases over time or the patient becomes symptomatic
- Tube dislodgment
  - A dislodged tube can lead to peritonitis (if it is malpositioned in the peritoneum), especially if dislodgment occurs before tract maturation, which typically takes 7 to 10 days in the nonimmunosuppressed patient.
  - Most common reason for tube replacement

Major Complications

- Tube misplacement (1%)
  - Inadvertent insertion of the G-tube into the peritoneal cavity during the procedure, which is often recognized perioperatively

▶ CLINICAL POINT

Confirm intragastric positioning of the tube **both during and after** percutaneous radiologic gastrostomy placement to reduce tube misplacement and evaluate for visceral injury.

- Peritonitis (2%)
  - Due to either malpositioning of the G-tube in the peritoneum or leakage of gastric content through the puncture site into the peritoneum
- Inadvertent perforation of the stomach, small intestine, or colon
- Tumor tract seeding
- Aspiration pneumonia
  - Often from gastroesophageal reflux secondary to underlying dysphagia
  - G-tube placement mortality rate of up to 3.2% is most often attributable to aspiration pneumonia
- Gastrocolocutaneous fistula (fistula of the stomach, colon, and skin)
  - Occurs when the procedure is inadvisably conducted with the colon lying between the stomach and anterior abdominal wall
  - Can result in acute colonic perforation, obstruction, or stool leakage around the stoma
  - Discovery of a previously created gastrocolocutaneous fistula often occurs when a replacement G-tube is placed directly into the colon rather than through the colon and into the stomach.

TAKE-HOME POINTS

- Percutaneous G-tubes are placed for nutritional support or decompression of the gastrointestinal tract.
- The Society of Interventional Radiology recommends an INR <1.5, platelets >50,000/µL, and holding Plavix for 5 days prior to the procedure.
- Absolute contraindications for G-tube placement include active peritonitis, bowel ischemia, uncorrectable coagulopathy, and gastric obstruction (unless the G-tube is being used for decompression of that obstruction).
- Placement of a G-tube requires review of prior patient history, including surgical history, and review of available imaging to ensure that there is an appropriate window to the stomach (no ascites and no overlying colon).

- Glucagon 0.1 to 1.0 mg is used to reduce peristalsis and prevent stomach decompression after air insufflation.
- The stomach is held against the anterior abdominal wall with gastropexy sutures, and access is made toward the pylorus (transabdominal approach) or the gastroesophageal junction (transoral approach). A wire is then advanced through the needle and the G-tube is placed.
- The gastrostomy tract matures in 7 to 10 days but may take up to 4 weeks in immunosuppressed patients.
- Maintenance of the G-tube includes flushing to prevent clogging, regular tube cleaning, and comfortable positioning to maintain the integrity of the skin around the tube. Preventative maintenance in the form of tube exchange should be performed every 3 to 6 months.

REVIEW QUESTIONS

1. Which of the following is a true recommendation from the Society of Interventional Radiology on laboratory and medication optimization before placement of a G-tube?
   a. INR <1.5
   b. Platelets >25,000/µL
   c. Continue Plavix
   d. Stop aspirin therapy
2. What is an absolute contraindication for placement of a percutaneous G-tube?
   a. GI obstruction in a patient with an obstructing esophageal mass

   b. Active peritonitis
   c. Uncorrectable coagulopathy
   d. Bowel ischemia
   e. All of the above
3. What is an indication for percutaneous G-tube placement?
   a. Respiratory distress
   b. Dysphagia
   c. Weight loss
   d. Increased survival rates

SUGGESTED READINGS

Black MT, Hung CA, Loh C. Subcutaneous T-fastener gastropexy: a new technique. *AJR Am J Roentgenol.* 2013;200(5):1157–1159.

Crowley JJ, Hogan MJ, Towbin RB, et al. Quality improvement guidelines for pediatric gastrostomy and gastrojejunostomy tube placement. *J Vasc Interv Radiol.* 2014;25(12):1983.

Itkin M, DeLegge MH, Fang JC, et al. Multidisciplinary Practical Guidelines for Gastrointestinal Access for Enteral Nutrition and Decompression From the Society of Interventional Radiology and American Gastroenterological Association (AGA) Institute, With Endorement by Canadian Interventional Radiological Association (CIRA) and Cardiovascular and Interventional Radiological Society of Europe (CIRSE). *J Vasc Interv Radiol.* 2011;22(8):1089–1106. https://doi.org/10.1016/j.jvir.2011.04.006.

Lang EK, Allaei A, Abbey-Mensah G, et al. Percutaneous radiologic gastrostomy: results and analysis of factors contributing to complications. *J La State Med Soc.* 2012;165(5):254–259.

Lowe A, Laasch H, Stephenson S, et al. Multicentre survey of radiologically inserted gastrostomy feeding tube (RIG) in the UK. *Clin Radiol.* 2012;67(9):843–854. https://doi.org/10.1016/j.crad.2012.01.014.

Lyon S, Pascoe D. Percutaneous gastrostomy and gastrojejunostomy. *Sem Interv Radiol.* 2004;21(3):181–185.

Ozmen M, Akhan O. Percutaneous radiologic gastrostomy. *Eur J Radiol.* 2002;43:186–195.

Rabeneck L, Wray N, Petersen N. Long-term outcomes of patients receiving percutaneous endoscopic gastrostomy tubes. *J Gen Int Med.* 1996;11(5):287–293.

Russ KB, Phillips MC, Wilcox CM, et al. Percutaneous endoscopic gastrostomy in amyotrophic lateral sclerosis. *Am J Med Sci.* 2015;350(2):95–97.

Lymphangiography and Thoracic Duct Embolization

Samuel K. Toland, Edward W. Lee

CASE PRESENTATION

A 69-year-old male with esophageal adenocarcinoma develops chylothorax on postoperative day 7 following esophagogastrectomy. High-output chylous fluid is being drained via bilateral chest tubes. His chest X-ray shows bilateral effusions (Fig. 33.1). This does not resolve following conservative management. He is referred to IR for lymphangiography with possible thoracic duct embolization.

- **Lymphangiography** was first performed in 1952 by Kinmonth et al., and the first satisfactory radiologic technique was described in 1955.
- The use of oil-based contrast agents such as **Lipiodol/Ethiodol** was first described in 1956 by Bruuns and Engstet. They showed that these agents do not diffuse from the lymphatic system, allowing for a satisfactory view of the lymph nodes.
- Historically, lymphangiography has been the **gold standard** for imaging pathologic conditions of the lymphatic system. However, with the advent of cross-sectional CT imaging, expertise in performing and interpreting lymphangiography has significantly declined.
  - Given its ability to demonstrate internal architectural derangements within the lymphatic system, lymphangiography remains the gold standard for the diagnosis and localization of lymphatic vessel damage.
- Lymphangiography involves the opacification of the lymphatic vessels with an oil-based contrast agent, typically via pedal or inguinal access sites.
- **Thoracic duct embolization (TDE)** involves transabdominal cannulation of the cisterna chyli followed by embolization of the injured thoracic duct.
  - The technique was developed by Dr. Constantine Cope. Initially working on porcine models, Dr. Cope, in 1998, published the results of thoracic duct embolization on his first five human patients.

LITERATURE REVIEW

In 1998, Dr. Cope and his team assessed the feasibility of catheterizing the cisterna chyli and embolizing the chylous fistula in patients with postoperative chyloperitoneum and/or chylothorax. They determined it to be feasible, safe, and clinically beneficial. This paper brought lymphangiography and thoracic duct embolization (TDE) to the forefront.

In a 2002 follow-up paper, Cope et al. cured lymph leak with TDE in 31 of 42 patients with no morbidity.

- Causes of lymphatic leakage include:
  - Surgical complications (e.g., following thoracic surgery, radical neck dissections, retroperitoneal lymph node dissections, coronary artery revascularization, and vascular surgery bypass)
  - Trauma
  - Radiation therapy in cancer patients
  - Any process that causes lymphatic occlusion such as:
    - Diseases of the lymph vessels
      - Gorham disease
      - Lymphangioleiomyomatosis
    - Systemic diseases
      - Sarcoidosis
    - Congenital malformations

CLINICAL POINT

Even within interventional radiology, lymph leaks have been described as a rare complication following central venous catheter insertion.

- Leaks can occur anywhere along the lymphatic system; however, the most clinically important pathway is that which goes from the intestines to the cisterna chyli to the thoracic duct.
  - Symptoms include dyspnea, tachycardia, cough, fever, and chest pain
    - The average period between injury and symptoms is 7 to 10 days

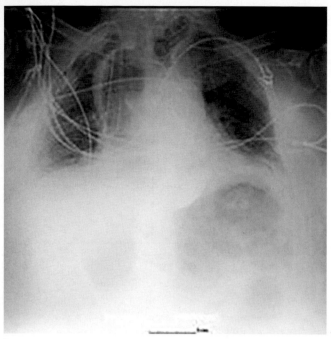

Fig. 33.1 Portable anterior-posterior (AP) chest X-ray of this patient prior to being seen by IR. (Courtesy image collected pre- and intra-procedurally during a lymphangiogram and TDE performed by Dr. E. Lee).

- Diagnosed by the presence of lymphatic fluid in the pleural space
- Most commonly seen following thoracic or esophageal surgery, although incidence is only 0.42%
- In a normal adult, the thoracic duct can transport up to 4 L of chyle a day. Injury can therefore lead to a rapid accumulation of fluid in the chest.

INDICATIONS

- Diagnosis and characterization of lymphatic abnormalities
- Detection and localization of lymphatic leaks
- Presence of lymphatic leak leading to high-output chylothorax in which conservative management has failed
- Presence of chylous ascites
- Presence of a lymphatic fistula
- Patients with filariasis, a parasitic disease, leading to filarial chyluria
  - Endemic in tropical areas such as Japan, Hong Kong, Taiwan, Philippines, and Brazil

> ### » CLINICAL POINT
>
> Chylothorax occurs when damage to the thoracic duct (or its branches) causes a chyle fistula with leakage into the pleural space.

CONTRAINDICATIONS

- Uncorrectable coagulopathy
- Patients with an active right-to-left intracardiac shunt

- Risk of cerebral embolism given the use of oil-based contrast agents
- Patients with pulmonary insufficiency or decreased respiratory reserve
  - Oil-based contrast agents may cause pulmonary embolism and/or pneumonitis

EQUIPMENT

- For pedal access:
  - Methylene blue
  - Local anesthetic
  - Scalpel and surgical dissection equipment
  - 30-gauge lymphangiography needle
- For intranodal access:
  - 25-gauge spinal needle (Fig. 33.2)
  - Short connecting tube
  - 5-mL syringe
- For embolization:
  - 22-gauge long Chiba needle (a slightly bent tip allows for easier maneuverability)
  - Floppy 0.018-inch guidewire
  - High-flow 2.3-Fr short-length microcatheter
  - Embolization material, such as:
    - Interlock coils
    - Concerto coils
    - Cyanoacrylate glue
    - Onyx glue
- Contrast material
  - Gadolinium, diluted 1:1 or 1:2 with normal saline
  - Lipiodol, an oil-based contrast agent

ANATOMY

- The **cisterna chyli** is a sac located at the L1/L2 level.
  - It is fed by the left and right lumbar trunks, the intestinal trunk (of most importance for chylothorax), the

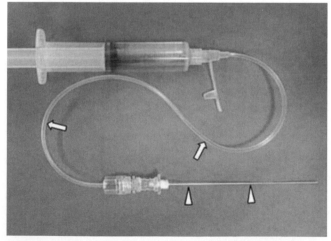

Fig. 33.2 25-G spinal needle *(arrowheads)* is assembled to connecting tube *(arrows)* and is flushed with Lipiodol contained in syringe tube. (From Lee EW, Shin JH, Ko HK, et al. Lymphangiography to treat postoperative lymphatic leakage: a technical review. *Kor J Radiol.* 2014;15 (6):724.)

lower intercostal trunks, and the hepatic lymphatic trunks.
- The **thoracic duct** is the largest lymphatic duct in the body.
  - It drains all but the right hemithorax, arm, head, and neck.
  - It originates just above the cisterna chyli in the abdomen and runs anterior to the vertebrae (for up to 45 cm) before emptying into the junction of the left internal jugular and left subclavian veins (jugulovenous angle).
- Variations of the lymphatic system and thoracic duct are seen in 40% to 60% of patients.
  - These variations are attributable to different patterns of anastomosis and diversion in embryonic development.
  - Common variants include:
    - Unilateral thoracic duct with termination at the left jugulovenous angle (90%–95%)
    - Unilateral thoracic duct with termination at the right jugulovenous angle (2%–3%)
    - Unilateral thoracic duct with termination at the bilateral jugulovenous angles (1%–1.5%)
    - Duplicated thoracic duct
    - Plexiform thoracic duct
    - Absent cisterna chyli
    - Termination of the thoracic duct into the azygos vein

PROCEDURE

- No specific preprocedure labs are indicated.
- Typically performed under general anesthesia
- There are two prevailing methods of lymphangiography:
  - The **conventional "pedal" method** isolates and cannulates lymphatic vessels on the dorsum of the foot using dye.
  - The **"intranodal" method** directly accesses lymph nodes in the inguinal region under ultrasound guidance.
    - This method was initially developed as a means of evaluating tumor involvement in inguinal, pelvic, and lumbar lymph nodes.

Pedal Lymphangiography

1. The patient is positioned in the supine position with the feet exposed.
   a. In patients with abdominal or thoracic lymphatic leakage, either foot can be used.
   b. In patients with inguinal or pelvic leakage, the foot ipsilateral to the leakage is used.
2. 0.5 mL of methylene blue is injected into the interspaces between the first and second and second and third toes in the cutaneous, subcutaneous, and intradermal layers.
3. After waiting 30 minutes to 1 hour, the lymphatics can be identified on the dorsum of the foot.
4. Local anesthesia is injected and a 2-cm incision is made on the dorsum of the foot where lymphatics are identifiable, usually at the base of the 1st metatarsal.
5. Careful dissection is performed to free the lymphatic vessel from surrounding tissue. A silk thread is looped around the vessel and pulled tight so as to distend it in order to make cannulation easier.
6. A 30-gauge lymphangiogram needle is controlled by artery forceps and held flat against the skin in alignment with the lymphatic vessel, which is then cannulated. The silk tie is relaxed, and the needle and vessel are secured together with adhesive strips, wet swabs, or 3-0 silk ties (Fig. 33.3).
7. 6 to 12 mL of Lipiodol are injected at a rate of 0.2 to 0.4 mL/min by an automatic pump.
8. Fluoroscopic images are obtained to measure the progression of the Lipiodol cranially.
9. At the conclusion of imaging, the needle is removed and the wound is sutured.

Intranodal Lymphangiography

1. A 25-gauge spinal needle is used to directly access the largest and most distal inguinal lymph using ultrasound guidance (Fig. 33.4). The needle tip is positioned in the transition zone between the cortex and the hilum of the node.
2. Lipiodol is injected and observed under fluoroscopy so as to confirm correct positioning in the node (Fig. 33.5).
3. 10 to 12 mL of Lipiodol are injected via automatic pump at a rate of 0.2 to 0.4 mL/min.
4. Serial fluoroscopic images are taken every 5 to 10 minutes to evaluate progression of the Lipiodol (Figs. 33.6 and 33.7).
5. Follow-up noncontrast CTs are obtained to delineate the lymphatic vessels, assess for sites of leakage, and identify appropriate puncture sites for potential thoracic duct embolization. These are performed immediately after the procedure and again 4 to 5 hours after.

Thoracic Duct Embolization

1. The retroperitoneal lymphatics, lumbar truck, and cisterna chyli are opacified with Lipiodol, using either of the aforementioned lymphangiography methods.

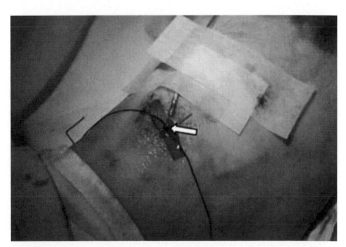

Fig. 33.3 Isolated Lymphatic of Dorsum of the Right Foot. It was cannulated using 30-G LG needle and both needle and lymphatic were firmly tied *(arrow)*. (From Lee EW, Shin JH, Ko HK, et al. Lymphangiography to treat postoperative lymphatic leakage: a technical review. *Kor J Radiol.* 2014;15(6):724.)

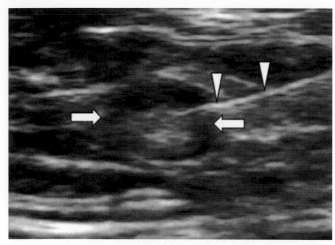

Fig. 33.4 Ultrasound-guided inguinal lymph node *(arrows)* access for initiation of intranodal LG using 25-G spinal needle *(arrowheads)*. (From Lee EW, Shin JH, Ko HK, et al. Lymphangiography to treat post-operative lymphatic leakage: a technical review. *Kor J Radiol*. 2014;15 (6):724.)

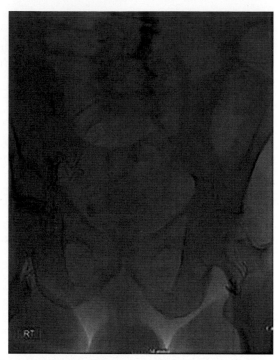

Fig. 33.6 Lipiodol Tracking up Toward the Thoracic Duct. (Courtesy Dr. E. Lee).

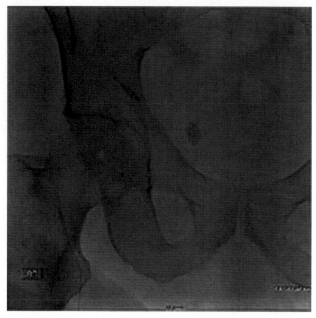

Fig. 33.5 Inguinal Lymph Nodes Accessed Directly. (Courtesy Dr. E. Lee).

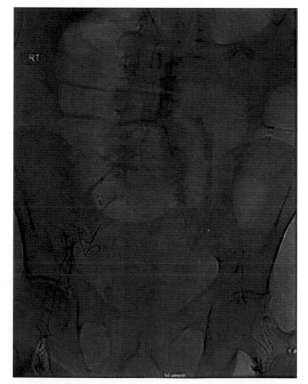

Fig. 33.7 Lipiodol Tracking Farther up the Thoracic Duct. (Courtesy Dr. E. Lee).

2. Percutaneous cannulation of the cisterna chyli is performed using a 22-gauge Chiba needle under fluoroscopic guidance. The needle should be angled slightly cranially so as to create a less acute angle for the wire to be inserted.

3. After accessing the cisterna chyli, the thoracic duct is threaded with a 0.014- to 0.018-inch microwire.

4. After the microwire is secured, a microcatheter is advanced over it and into the thoracic duct.

5. A small amount of contrast is injected to confirm correct catheter tip location and to identify any contrast extravasation/leakage.

6. The microwire and catheter are advanced past the leak, and microcoils and/or glue are used to embolize the thoracic duct both proximal and distal to the leak (Fig. 33.8).

7. After embolization, contrast is injected into the proximal duct to confirm lack of extravasation.

8. Equipment is removed.

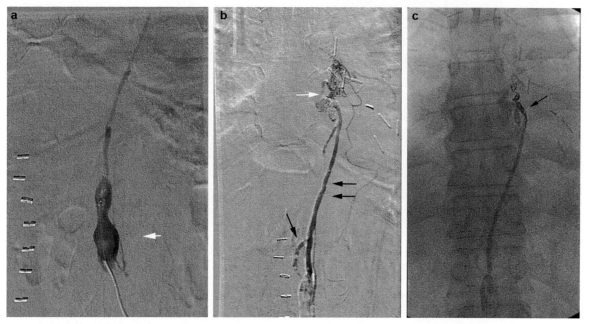

Fig. 33.8 (A) White arrow points to the cisterna chyli, opacified by Lipiodol. (B) Black arrows point to the left thoracic duct. White arrows point toward aberrant extravasation. (C) Occlusion of the leak following coiling and embolization. (From Atie M, Dunn G, Falk G. Chlyous leak after radical oesophagectomy: thoracic duct lymphangiography and embolisation (TDE)—A case report. *Int J Surg Case Rep.* 2016;23:12–16.)

COMPLICATIONS

- Overall low complication rate when less than 10 mL of Lipiodol is used
- With lymphangiography, complications include:
  - Infection
  - Pain
  - Intraalveolar hemorrhage
  - Pulmonary embolism
  - Allergic reaction to Lipiodol
  - Extravasation of Lipiodol into soft tissue
- With thoracic duct embolization, complications include:
  - Injury to solid organs and critical structures
    - Inadvertent puncture of the bowel, liver, pancreas, IVC, and aorta
- Pulmonary embolism—due to excess embolization glue escaping into the subclavian vein
- Peripheral edema—due to disruption of peripheral lymphatics

TREATMENT ALTERNATIVES

- Low-output lymphatic leaks (<500 mL) are likely to resolve with conservative management.
  - Medical management with octreotide, somatostatin, and etilefrine
  - Parenteral nutrition, a chylous diet (low-fat, high-protein), or bowel rest
- Symptomatic management with therapeutic drainage and potential chest tube placement
- Surgical ligation of the duct

🏠 TAKE-HOME POINTS

- Lymphangiography is a safe and effective method for diagnosing and localizing lymphatic leaks. It is unique in its ability to demonstrate the internal architecture of the lymphatic system.
- Lipiodol, the oil-based contrast used in lymphangiography, has been shown to have sclerosant properties. 50% to 75% of lymphatic leaks resolve after lymphangiography.
- The most common causes of a chylothorax is thoracic/esophageal surgery.

- TDE is a safe and efficacious procedure to embolize damaged lymphatic vessels causing chylous leak.
- Lymphangiogram can be performed via access through either the lymphatic vessels of the foot (pedal access) or the inguinal lymph nodes (intranodal access).
- Use of Lipiodol is absolutely contraindicated in patients with active right-to-left intracardiac shunts due to the risk of cerebral embolism. Poor respiratory reserve is also a contraindication to the use of Lipiodol due to the risk of pulmonary embolism.

REVIEW QUESTIONS

1. The most common indication for thoracic duct embolization is which?
   a. Pneumothorax
   b. Chylothorax
   c. Tracheoesophageal fistula
   d. Filariasis
2. Contraindications to TDE include which of the following?
   a. Correctable coagulopathy
   b. Chylous ascites
   c. Decreased respiratory reserve
   d. Intrahepatic shunt
3. Complications that may arise from the use of an oil-based contrast agent include which of the following?
   a. Cerebral and pulmonary emboli
   b. Lymphatic disruption
   c. Lymphocele
   d. Filariasis

SUGGESTED READINGS

Chen E, Itkin M. Thoracic duct embolization for chylous leaks. *Semin Intervent Radiol.* 2011;28(1):63–74. https://doi.org/10.1055/s-0031-1273941.

Cope C. Diagnosis and treatment of postoperative chyle leakage via percutaneous transabdominal catheterization of the cisterna chyli: a preliminary study. *J Vasc Interv Radiol.* 1998;9:727–734.

Guermazi A, Brice P, Hennequin C, et al. Lymphography: an old technique retains its usefulness1. *Radiographics.* 2003;23(6):1541–1558. https://doi.org/10.1148/rg.236035704.

Jackson D, Whittle R, Rothnie N. An introduction to lymphangiography. *Clin Radiol.* 15(4):341–346. https://doi.org/10.1016/s0009-9260(64)80011-8.

Kawasaki R, Sugimoto K, Fuji M. Therapeutic effectiveness of diagnostic lymphangiography for refractory postoperative chylothorax and chylous ascites: correlation with radiologic findings and preceding medical treatment. *AJR Am J Roentgenol.* 201(3):659–666. https://doi.org/10.2214/ajr.12.10008.

Lee E, Shin J, Ko H, et al. Lymphangiography to treat postoperative lymphatic leakage: a technical review. *Korean J Radiol.* 2014;15(6):724. https://doi.org/10.3348/kjr.2014.15.6.724.

Plotnik AN, Foley PT, Koukounaras J, et al. How I do it: lymphangiography. *J Med Imaging Radiation Oncol.* 2010; 54(1).

Syed L, Georgiades C, Hart V. Lymphangiography: a case study. *Semin Intervent Radiol.* 24(1):106–110. https://doi.org/10.1055/s-2007-971180.

Paracentesis

Andrew Sideris, Bipin Rajendran, Uma R. Prasad

CASE PRESENTATION

A 63-year-old male with a past medical history of cirrhosis and recurrent ascites presents to the emergency department with abdominal pain, fever, and chills. On exam, he is diffusely tender to palpation with severe ascites. The patient was found to have a total bilirubin of 3.1 g/mL and serum albumin of 1.5 g/dL. Interventional radiology is asked to perform a **paracentesis** to evaluate for **spontaneous bacterial peritonitis (SBP)**.

- Performed as early as 1100 BC, the first detailed description of therapeutic paracentesis has been attributed to Aulus Cornelius Celsus (30 BC–50 AD).
- In 1626, Sanctorius Sanctorius of Padua, Italy designed the first trocar that was then routinely used for paracenteses.
- Copious amounts of ascites were removed from patients (including Ludwig van Beethoven) as recently as the 1950s before the deleterious effects of large volume paracentesis (>5 L) were first described.
- In 1990, Titó et al. described the safety and efficacy of performing large volume paracentesis with subsequent infusion of albumin.
- **Paracentesis** describes the removal of fluid from the peritoneal cavity.
  - It is performed in patients with new-onset or worsening ascites of unknown etiology for diagnostic and/or therapeutic purposes.
  - In patients with recurrent symptomatic ascites of known etiology, paracentesis can be performed for therapeutic purposes.
  - Traditionally, the procedure involved insertion of a 5-Fr centesis needle and catheter combination into the peritoneum for drainage. Today, pre-packaged paracentesis kits are available, which typically include a 6- or 8-Fr drainage catheter. They are introduced into the peritoneum by an obturator which becomes blunt upon entering the abdominal cavity, preventing damage to the viscera.
  - Performing under ultrasound (Fig. 34.1) guidance allows the operator to evaluate for anatomic landmarks such as vasculature, solid organs, and viscera. Patients with ascites secondary to cirrhosis are coagulopathic and are at increased risk for subcutaneous and/or intra-peritoneal hemorrhage.
- Diagnostic paracentesis does not require a large volume for testing (30–50 mL should be adequate). Samples are sent for a variety of tests, including:
  - Cell count and differential, Gram stain, culture, total protein, albumin, carcinoembryonic antigen (CEA), amylase, lipase, and triglycerides
- Large-volume therapeutic paracentesis may be performed for symptomatic relief.
  - **Albumin replacement** should be performed in patients with ascites secondary to portal hypertension if more than 5 L is removed. However, current guidelines do not support albumin infusion if ascites is secondary to malignancy.

INDICATIONS

Diagnosis of New-Onset Ascites

- Evaluation of the ascitic fluid will help determine whether the ascites is due to portal hypertension or another process (such as cancer, infection, or pancreatitis).
  - **Cirrhosis** is the most common cause of ascites in the United States.
    - Ascites is the most common of the three major complications seen with cirrhosis. The other complications are hepatic encephalopathy and variceal hemorrhage.

Diagnosis in Preexisting Ascites

- Rule out suspected SBP. SBP is common in patients with ascites and may be life-threatening. Clinical indicators include:
  - Fever
  - Abdominal pain
  - Worsening encephalopathy
  - Worsening renal function
  - Leukocytosis
  - Acidosis
  - Gastrointestinal bleeding
  - Sepsis/shock
- Occult SBP is not uncommon in patients with cirrhosis and ascites requiring hospitalization.
- Some experts recommend a surveillance paracentesis.

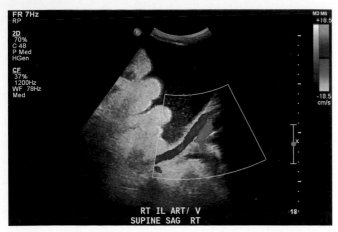

Fig. 34.1 Preprocedure ultrasound evaluation of the right lower quadrant of the abdomen demonstrates the relationship of an ascites collection to the right iliac artery and vein.

Therapeutic Drainage of Preexisting Ascites

- Performed in hemodynamically stable patients with tense ascites to alleviate discomfort and prevent respiratory compromise
- Serial large-volume paracentesis may be required in patients with refractory ascites or ascites that does not respond to diuretics.

CONTRAINDICATIONS

- The only absolute contraindication is the presence of **disseminated intravascular coagulation (DIC)**.
  - DIC is a consumptive coagulopathy that results in loss of clotting factors and platelets, and patients with DIC are at a higher risk of bleeding postparacentesis.
- With ultrasound guidance, traditional relative contraindications such as pregnancy, organomegaly, bowel obstruction, intraabdominal adhesions, and urinary bladder distention are negated.
- A relative point of contention is the need to correct anticoagulation prior to paracentesis.
  - Per the SIR consensus guidelines published in 2012, paracentesis is classified as a "Category 1" procedure that has a low risk of bleeding. The procedure should be performed when the INR and platelets have been corrected to <2.0 and >50,000/μL, respectively.
  - However, per the update to the AASLD Practice Guideline for Management of Adult Patients with Ascites due to Cirrhosis, also published in 2012, the routine prophylactic use of FFP and platelet transfusion is not recommended prior to paracentesis (a Class III, Level C recommendation).

> ◎ **LITERATURE REVIEW**
>
> In a 2004 prospective study by Grabau et al., nearly 1,100 large-volume paracenteses were performed by trained operators, and none resulted in significant bleeding complications or required pre/post-procedure transfusion. In this subset of patients, the highest INR was 8.7, and the lowest platelet count was 19,000/μL.

ANATOMY

- The abdomen houses most of the organs of the alimentary system and part of the urogenital system.
- Nine regions are used to describe the location of abdominal organs, pains, or pathologies. These regions are delineated by four planes—two sagittal (vertical) and two transverse (horizontal) planes.
- Containment of the abdominal contents is provided by:
  - Musculoaponeurotic abdominal wall anterolaterally
  - Diaphragm superiorly
  - Pelvic muscles inferiorly
- The abdominal wall dynamically contracts or distends to accommodate expansions caused by ingestion, pregnancy, fat deposition, or pathology.
- The anterolateral wall consists of skin and subcutaneous tissue (superficial fascia) composed of fat, muscles and their aponeuroses, extraperitoneal fat, and the parietal peritoneum.
  - The skin attaches loosely to the subcutaneous tissue, except at the umbilicus, where it adheres firmly.
  - The innermost component of the anterolateral abdominal wall, as well as several organs lying against the posterior wall, is covered with a serous membrane referred to as the *parietal peritoneum*. The parietal peritoneum reflects to cover the abdominal organs, which is then referred to as the *visceral peritoneum*.
- The parietal and visceral peritoneum create a potential space, the peritoneal cavity, that is formed between the abdominal walls and the viscera. This space normally contains only enough extracellular fluid (about 50 mL) to lubricate the membranes occupying the abdominal cavity. **Ascites** is the clinical condition in which one has excess fluid in the peritoneal cavity.
  - Like overlying skin, the parietal peritoneum is sensitive to pressure, pain, and temperature. Pain from puncture is generally well localized.
  - The visceral peritoneum is insensitive to touch, temperature, and pain.
  - In males, the peritoneal cavity is completely closed. In females, there is a communication pathway to the pelvis via the uterine tubes, which constitutes a potential pathway of infection.

Etiologies of Ascites

- Portal hypertension
  - Causes include:
    - Cirrhosis
    - Alcoholic hepatitis
    - Acute liver failure
    - Hepatic veno-occlusive disease
    - Heart failure
    - Constrictive pericarditis
    - Hemodialysis-associated ascites
- Hypoalbuminemia
  - Causes include:
    - Nephrotic syndrome
    - Protein-losing enteropathy

- Severe malnutrition
- Peritoneal disease
  - Causes include:
    - Malignant ascites (e.g., ovarian cancer, mesothelioma)
    - Infection peritonitis (e.g., tuberculosis, fungal infection)
    - Eosinophilic gastroenteritis
    - Starch granulomatous peritonitis
    - Peritoneal dialysis
    - Multicystic mesothelioma
  - Other etiologies include:
    - Chylous ascites
    - Pancreatic ascites (e.g., disrupted pancreatic duct)
    - Myxedema
    - Hemoperitoneum
    - Budd-Chiari syndrome

Pathophysiology of Cirrhotic Ascites

- Ascites is the most common complication of cirrhosis. Within 10 years of having compensated cirrhosis, 50% of patients will have developed ascites.
- 85% of ascites in the United States is secondary to cirrhosis
- Development of **portal hypertension (PHT)** is the first step toward fluid retention.
  - Patients with cirrhosis, but without PHT, do not develop ascites.
  - Elevated portal pressure of approximately 12 mm Hg or greater is typically seen in patients with fluid retention.
- PHT causes splanchnic arterial vasodilation that increases portal venous inflow in the setting of mechanical obstruction to portal flow.
  - Patients with cirrhosis and ascites usually have a marked reduction in systemic vascular resistance (SVR).
    - The vascular territory where the reduced SVR is most apparent is the arterial splanchnic circulation.
  - The exact mechanism through which this vasodilation occurs is an area of considerable research.
    - Current observations suggest that nitrous oxide is the primary mediator of vasodilation in cirrhosis.
- Progressive vasodilation leads to release of endogenous vasoconstrictors, sodium and water retention, and increasing renal vasoconstriction.
  - Vasoconstrictors attempt to restore perfusion pressure to normal.
  - Net effect is avid sodium and water retention because of effective volume depletion.
  - In actuality, extracellular sodium stores, plasma volume, and cardiac output are all increased.
- Retention of sodium and water increases the plasma volume.
  - Sodium retention is a sensitive marker of the overall status of a patient with cirrhosis.
  - Degree of sodium retention inversely relates to survival.
  - Urinary sodium excretion <10 mEq/day suggests a mean survival of 5 to 6 months.

- PHT is a cause of **transudative ascites**, determined by measuring the **serum-ascitic albumin gradient (SAAG)**.
  - SAAG correlates directly with portal pressure.
  - SAAG ≥1.1 g/dL is transudative.
    - Ascitic fluid total protein (AFTP) is helpful in determining etiology of ascites if the SAAG is >1.1 g/dL.
    - Cirrhotic ascites would typically have values <2.5 g/dL.
    - Cardiac ascites would be >2.5 g/dL.

CLINICAL POINT

- The differential diagnosis for ascites is based on SAAG.
- SAAG ≥1.1 suggests a transudative process. Causes include:
  - Cirrhosis (most common)
  - Hepatic malignancy (hepatocellular carcinoma or metastasis)
  - Fulminant liver failure
  - Right-sided systolic dysfunction/heart failure ("cardiac ascites")
  - Constrictive pericarditis
  - Budd-Chiari syndrome
  - Sinusoidal obstruction syndrome (SOS)
  - Portal and/or splenic vein thrombosis
  - Schistosomiasis
- SAAG <1.1 suggests an exudative process. Causes include:
  - Peritonitis (particularly tuberculosis [TB])
  - Peritoneal carcinomatosis
  - Pancreatitis
  - Myxedema
  - Pseudomyxoma peritonei
  - Struma ovarii
  - Sarcoidosis
  - Amyloidosis
  - Meigs syndrome
  - Vasculitis
  - Hypoalbuminemia
  - Bowel obstruction/infarction
  - Lymphatic obstruction/leak

EQUIPMENT

- A prepackaged catheter drainage tray (Fig. 34.2) typically contains:
  - Centesis needle
    - Alternatively, a 6- or 8-Fr catheter can be used.
  - Catheter
  - Lidocaine and a 10-mL syringe
  - 60-mL syringe for drainage
  - Specimen tubes
  - 22- and 25-gauge needles
  - Scalpel
  - Tubing for large-volume removal
  - Vacuum collection bottle or wall suction unit for large-volume drainage

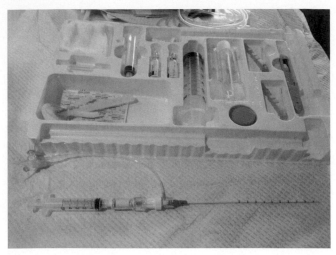

Fig. 34.2 Contents of a Prepackaged Paracentesis Kit. The catheter drainage system has been assembled below the tray.

PROCEDURAL STEPS

1. The patient is placed in a supine position with his/her head slightly elevated.
2. Drainage location is selected:
   a. Use ultrasound to locate a region containing ascitic fluid but devoid of loops of bowel or solid organs. Shifting "dullness" suggests the presence of ascites at the chosen site.
   b. Lateral approach—2 to 4 cm medial and superior to the anterior iliac spine
      i. In obese patients, the lateral approach may be preferred because the abdominal wall is thinner and the depth of ascitic fluid is deeper in comparison to the midline approach.
   c. Midline approach—2 cm below the umbilicus
      i. Relative to the lateral approach, this region is advantageously devoid of blood vessels.

> ▶▶ **CLINICAL POINT**
>
> The paracentesis catheter should not pass through sites of cutaneous infection, visibly engorged cutaneous vessels, surgical scars, or abdominal-wall hematomas.

3. Chosen entry site is marked with a skin-marking pen.
4. The site is sterilized, and a drape is applied.
5. The anticipated trajectory of the paracentesis needle is anesthetized with 1% or 2% lidocaine. A total of 5 to 10 mL of lidocaine is generally injected with a 22- or 25-gauge needle, 1.5-inch (or longer) needle.
   a. In the epidermis, a wheal is placed at the entry site with a 1-mL injection.
   b. In the deeper tissues, the needle is slowly advanced along the anticipated trajectory, alternating between injecting anesthetic and pulling back on the plunger to ensure that the needle has not penetrated a vascular structure. Sudden loss of resistance signals entry to the peritoneal cavity.

   c. Once peritoneal fluid begins to fill the syringe, an additional 3 to 5 mL of anesthetic is injected into the parietal peritoneum. This space is important to anesthetize, as it is highly sensitive.
6. A small puncture at the insertion site is made with a No. 11 blade to facilitate advancement of the paracentesis catheter through the epidermis.
7. A 5- or 10-mL syringe is attached to the catheter assembly.
8. The needle is advanced in small 2- to 3-mm increments through skin, subcutaneous tissues, and parietal peritoneum (see Fig. 34.2). The needle is held in the operator's dominant hand while the nondominant hand holds the ultrasound transducer. The syringe should be pulled back intermittently to ensure no penetration of vascular structures. Either of the following advancement techniques may be used. These methods prevent direct overlap of the cutaneous insertion site and the peritoneal insertion site, theoretically minimizing the risk of ascitic fluid leakage after the procedure.
   a. Angular insertion technique:
      i. Needle is held at 45 degrees relative to insertion site as it pierces the epidermis. This trajectory is continued through the subcutaneous tissue and into the peritoneal cavity.
   b. Z-track technique (Fig. 34.3):
      i. The cutaneous tissue is pulled 2 cm in the caudad or cranial direction. Needle is held at 90 degrees relative to the insertion site as it pierces the epidermis.
      ii. When the needle is withdrawn at the end of the procedure, the cutaneous tissue will revert to its original position, creating an offset entry/exit trajectory.
9. Sudden loss of resistance, or ascitic fluid filling the syringe, signals entry into peritoneum. At this point, the catheter is advanced over the needle, and then the needle is withdrawn.
10. Depending on indication, perform the following procedures:
    a. Diagnostic paracentesis
       i. A large syringe is attached to the catheter, and 30 to 60 mL of fluid is withdrawn to send for analysis.

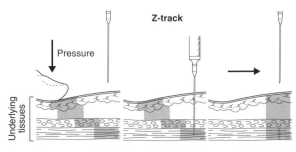

Fig. 34.3 Z-Track Injections. (Reused with permission from Hawley R, King J. *Australian Nurses' Dictionary*. 6th ed. Chatswood, NSW: Elsevier Australia [a division of Reed International Books Australia Pty Ltd]; 2016.)

b. Therapeutic (large volume) paracentesis
   i. High-pressure connection tubing is attached to the catheter hub.
   ii. Connection tubing is then attached to a large evacuated container. Additional containers can be filled as necessary.
11. Once desired quantity of fluid has been removed, the catheter is removed.
12. A sterile occlusive dressing is applied.

TREATMENT ALTERNATIVES

- Paracentesis is the gold standard for diagnosing the etiology of abdominal ascites.
- In patients with recurrent and/or symptomatic malignant ascites requiring frequent large-volume paracentesis, consideration should be given to placement of a tunneled peritoneal drainage catheter for palliation.

COMPLICATIONS

- General complications (estimated incidence of <0.2%) include:
  - Persistent leakage of ascitic fluid
  - Localized infection
  - Abdominal wall hematoma (Fig. 34.4)
- Emergent, but rare, complications include:
  - Hemorrhage
  - Injury to intraabdominal organs
  - Puncture of the inferior epigastric artery
- Late complications of paracentesis include:
  - **Paracentesis-induced circulatory dysfunction (PICD)**, first described by Ginés et al. in 1988, is a complication of large volume paracentesis that results in hypotension, hyponatremia, reaccumulation of ascites, hepatorenal syndrome, and decreased survival.

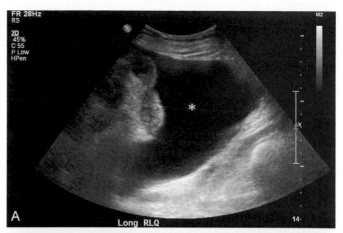

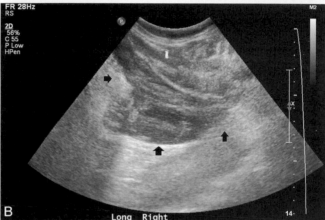

Fig. 34.4 (A) Grayscale longitudinal image of the right lower quadrant of the abdomen pre-paracentesis demonstrates hypoechoic fluid collection *(asterisk)* consistent with ascites. (B) Post paracentesis, the patient had significant abdominal wall swelling. Grayscale longitudinal image of the right lower quadrant demonstrated the ascites pocket had markedly diminished, with a mixed echogenicity collection in the subcutaneous tissues of the right abdomen *(black arrows)* consistent with abdominal wall hematoma.

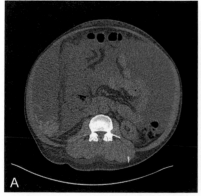
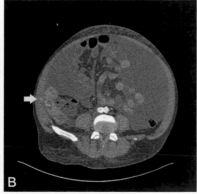
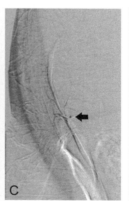
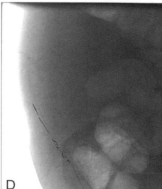

Fig. 34.5 (A) Noncontrast axial image of the abdomen after paracentesis demonstrates high-density material layering dependently in the right paracolic gutter. (B) Arterial phase image demonstrates foci of contrast extravasation with increasing density of fluid in the material *(arrow)*, consist with acute arterial bleeding. (C) Selective microcatheterization of the right deep circumflex iliac artery demonstrates focus of contrast blush *(arrow)* corresponding to known bleeding. (D) No evidence of extravasation post embolization with 300 to 500 μm embospheres and coil embolization.

- Pathophysiology of PICD is not well understood but is believed to be triggered by hypovolemia and subsequent activation of the renin-angiotensin-aldosterone (RAA) cascade.
- PICD occurs in 80% of large-volume paracenteses in which volume expanders are not used; this drops to 15% to 35% when volume expanders, such as albumin, are used.
  - This can be prevented by limiting the paracentesis to 5 to 6 L per session or by administering 6 to 8 g of intravenous albumin for every liter of ascites removed at the end of the procedure.

- Some studies have shown that 3 mg of IV terlipressin, a vasopressin analogue, is nearly as effective as albumin in reducing the incidence of PICD. Terlipressin is less costly than albumin. Terlipressin may also act synergistically with albumin.
  - Patients will have a greater than 50% increase in their baseline plasma renin activity to >4 ng/mL per hour, occurring 5 to 6 days after the paracentesis.
- **Hemoperitoneum** (Fig. 34.5) is a potentially life-threatening complication that can be caused by inadvertent puncture of the inferior epigastric artery, a branch vessel, or an abdominal wall varix.

🏠 TAKE-HOME POINTS

- Paracentesis is a relatively safe procedure recommended for determining the etiology of new-onset or worsening ascites. It is also used therapeutically for symptomatic relief of recurrent ascites of known etiology.
- SAAG and AFTP can be useful in determining the etiology of ascites.
- Ultrasound guidance in paracentesis is extremely valuable in determining the location of bowel loops, organs, and vasculature. Notably, the operator should surveil the abdominal wall for the course of the ipsilateral inferior epigastric vasculature as well as for any subcutaneous abdominal wall varices.

- The only absolute contraindication to performing a paracentesis is DIC.
- Preprocedure correction of INR and platelets has been widely debated and should be tailored to individual circumstances.
- Immediate complications include hypotension, abdominal wall hematoma, hemoperitoneum, persistent ascitic leak, perforated bowel, and traumatic organ injury. A notable late complication is PICD, which can be avoided by limiting volume of fluid drained to 5 to 6 L per session and/or administering volume expanders such as albumin or terlipressin.

REVIEW QUESTIONS

1. You are about to perform a paracentesis using ultrasound guidance. Among the following choices, which is the only absolute contraindication to performing this procedure?
   a. Intraabdominal adhesion
   b. Disseminated intravascular coagulation (DIC)
   c. Pregnancy
   d. Organomegaly
   e. Urinary bladder distension

2. A 63-year-old female with a past medical history of cirrhosis, PHT, and ascites presents to the hospital with 3 days of abdominal pain, fever, and confusion. Concerned for spontaneous bacterial peritonitis, you perform a paracentesis and send 50 mL of fluid for analysis. Which of the following ultrasound findings and laboratory results is most diagnostic of SBP?
   a. Deepest fluid pocket = 15 mm; total ascites fluid = 2500 mL; WBC = 1000; neutrophil % = 20

   b. Deepest fluid pocket = 70 mm; total ascites fluid = 6730 mL; WBC = 1200; neutrophil % = 30
   c. Deepest fluid pocket = 75 mm; total ascites fluid = 8400 mL; WBC = 1300; neutrophil % = 1
   d. Deepest fluid pocket = 70 mm; total ascites fluid = 7000 mL; WBC = 400; neutrophil % = 10

3. In cirrhotic ascites, portal hypertension is generally considered the first step toward fluid retention. Among which of the following portal pressure values would you expect ascites to be found, and what serum-albumin ascites gradient (SAAG) would be consistent with this transudative etiology?
   a. Portal pressure = 7 mm Hg; SAAG = 1.0 g/dL
   b. Portal pressure = 13 mm Hg; SAAG = 0.9 g/dL
   c. Portal pressure = 8 mm Hg; SAAG = 1.1 g/dL
   d. Portal pressure = 15 mm Hg; SAAG = 1.4 g/dL

SUGGESTED READINGS

Ginès P, Cárdenas A, Arroyo V, et al. Management of cirrhosis and ascites. *N Engl J Med.* 2004;350(16):1646–1654.

Ginès P, Titó L, Arroyo V, et al. Randomized comparative study of therapeutic paracentesis with and without intravenous albumin in cirrhosis. *Gastroenterology.* 1988;94:1493–1502.

Grabau CM, Crago SF, Hoff LK, et al. Performance standards for therapeutic abdominal paracentesis. *Hepatology.* 2004;40(2):484–488.

Lindsay AJ, Burton J, Ray CE. Paracentesis-induced circulatory dysfunction: a primer for the interventional radiologist. *Semin Intervent Radiol.* 2014;31(3):276–278.

Patel IJ, Davidson JC, Nikolic B, et al. Consensus guidelines for periprocedural management of coagulation status and hemostasis risk in percutaneous image-guided interventions. *J Vasc Interv Radiol.* 2012;23(6):727–736.

Runyon BA. Introduction to the revised American Association for the Study of Liver Diseases Practice Guideline management of adult patients with ascites due to cirrhosis 2012. *Hepatology.* 2013;57(4):1651–1653.

Titó L, Ginès P, Arroyo V, Planas R, Panés J, Rimola A, et al. Total paracentesis associated with intravenous albumin management of patients with cirrhosis and ascites. *Gastroenterology.* 1990;98:146–151.

35

Percutaneous Nephrostomy

Joanna Kee-Sampson, Thomas Powierza, Thaddeus M. Yablonsky

CASE PRESENTATION

A 41-year-old female with a recent diagnosis of stage 4 cervical cancer is admitted from an outside hospital where her serum creatinine was found to be elevated at 11. She was found to have obstructive hydronephrosis secondary to tumor burden on CT scan. Her primary team requests a **percutaneous nephrostomy** be performed for relief of her renal obstruction.

- **Percutaneous nephrostomy (PCN)** was first performed in 1955 at UCLA when urologist Dr. William Goodwin inadvertently entered the renal collecting system while performing a renal arteriogram on a patient with hydronephrosis. He left the tube in place to drain the kidney, thus placing the first tube.
- In 1976, Fernström and Johansson devised a technique for extracting kidney stones through PCN tubes.
- In 1978, Arthur Smith performed the first antegrade stent placement when he introduced a Gibbons stent through a PCN in a patient with a reimplanted ureter.
- A PCN tube is considered the **gold standard** in treating obstructive uropathy.
- PCN has a high technical success rate of close to 100% with an overall low complication rate ranging from 0.1% to 10%.

INDICATIONS

- **Obstructive uropathy** is the main indication in 85% to 90% of PCN tube placements.
  - Urinary obstruction may be due to a variety of causes, including:
    - Nephrolithiasis
    - Blood clots
    - Neoplasm
    - Scar formation following pelvic surgery
    - Retroperitoneal fibrosis
- **Gram-negative urosepsis** is an emergent indication for PCN. Mortality from gram-negative septicemia can be lowered from 40% to 8% by emergency PCN.
- **Urinary diversion** in the treatment of:
  - Urinary leaks
  - Urinary fistulas

- Decompression of a urinoma
- **Access** for percutaneous intervention, such as:
  - Extracorporeal shock wave lithotripsy (ESWL)
  - Tumor biopsy
  - Foreign body removal (e.g., catheter fragments)
  - Delivery of chemotherapy to the collecting system
- **Percutaneous nephrolithotomy (PCNL)** (Fig. 35.1)
  - Staghorn calculi or renal calculi refractory to extracorporeal shockwave lithotripsy can be managed by obtaining percutaneous access into the renal collecting system and fragmenting the stones with a nephroscope. The procedure is done in conjunction with the urology team.
  - Technique:
    - The renal collecting system is accessed in the same manner as in PCN placement. The calyx containing the stone is accessed and is punctured just peripheral to the stone. This ensures a direct path to the stone for the nephroscope.
    - The tract is dilated to 30 Fr using either a balloon catheter or serial dilators, followed by placement of a 30-Fr sheath.
    - The urologist then inserts the nephroscope through the sheath, and the stone is fragmented using either ultrasound or laser.
- **Antegrade ureteral stenting (AUS)** (Fig. 35.2)
  - Ureteral stents can be placed in an antegrade fashion through PCN access to relieve ureteric obstructions caused by malignancies, strictures, or stones or in cases of ureteric injuries.
  - Stenting are a more convenient and comfortable option compared to PCN catheters and are preferred for long-term drainage.
  - Technique considerations:
    - Midpole access is preferred over lower pole access because of a more direct angle of entry into the ureter.
    - A peel-away sheath can facilitate passage of the ureteral stent down the ureter.

Contraindications

- No absolute contraindications
- Relative contraindications include:
  - Uncorrectable coagulopathy

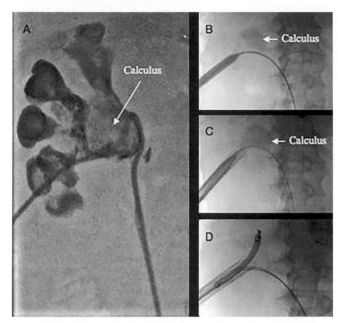

Fig. 35.1 Percutaneous Nephrolithotomy (PCNL). (A) Percutaneous access into the kidney was obtained in preparation for PCNL of the large renal calculus. (B) Balloon dilatation of the nephrostomy tract was then performed, followed by (C) placement of a sheath. (D) A flexible nephroscope was inserted through the sheath for nephrolithotomy.

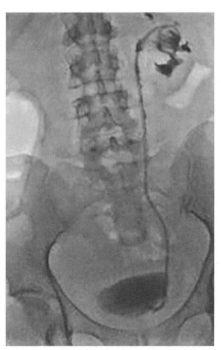

Fig. 35.2 Ureteral Stent. Antegrade ureteral stent placed through a nephrostomy access in a patient with urinary obstruction secondary to cervical cancer. The distal pigtail is formed in the urinary bladder, and the proximal pigtail is formed in the renal pelvis.

- Terminal illness with imminent death
- Antegrade ureteral stent placement is generally reserved for patients with a native functioning bladder. Relative contraindications to the placement of an antegrade ureter stent include:

- Bladder fistula
- Neurogenic bladder
- Patients with incontinence

EQUIPMENT

- Single-stick needle access system (Fig. 35.3):
  - 18-gauge to 22-gauge needles
  - Introducer sheaths
- Guidewires:
  - 0.018-inch platinum-tip wire
  - 0.035-inch J-wire or 0.035-inch Amplatz Super Stiff guidewire
- Dilators:
  - 6- to 14-Fr
- Catheters:
  - 8- to 14-Fr pigtail catheters, between 30 and 45 cm in length
  - Locking or nonlocking (Fig. 35.4)
- Double-J stent in the setting of antegrade ureteral stent placement

ANATOMY

- Why approach the kidney below the 12th rib?
  - The posterior pleural reflection is at the T12 level. To avoid entering the pleural space and potentially causing a pneumothorax or hydrothorax, the skin should be entered below the level of the 12th rib.
  - In addition, the upper poles of the kidney are often at the 11th and 12th rib levels (Fig. 35.5). For this reason, the lower poles, rather than the upper poles, are safer targets for PCN.
- Why a posterior renal calyx?
  - Puncture through a posterior calyx allows a more direct pathway for the guidewire to pass into the renal pelvis and ureter.
  - Puncture through the anterior calyx results in a suboptimal angle for guidewire passage.
- Why access the kidney dorsolaterally and peripherally, rather than centrally?
  - Accessing the kidney peripherally at a renal calyx, rather than centrally at the renal pelvis, decreases the risk of injury to the main renal artery and vein, which lie anterior to the renal pelvis.
  - There is also less risk of urine leakage and urinoma formation when the puncture traverses renal parenchyma into the calyx.
  - A dorsolateral approach to the kidney with the needle advanced along Brödels avascular line, which is a relatively avascular watershed area between the anterior and posterior renal artery divisions, reduces the risk of hemorrhage from inadvertent puncture of a large vessel.
- Approach considerations in a posttransplant patient:
  - The nephrostomy is placed with the patient supine because of the typical anterior location of a renal transplant.

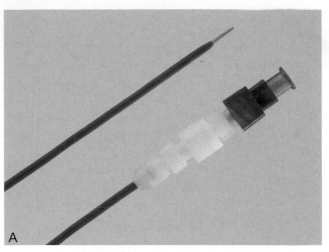

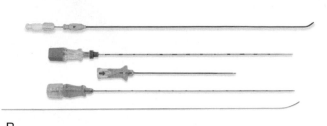

Fig. 35.3 Examples of Single-Stick Needle Access Systems. (A) Neff Percutaneous Access Set (Cook Medical, Bloomington, IN). (B) GrebSet® Micro-Introducer Kit (Teleflex) with (top) 5 Fr sheath with outer dilator, (bottom) .018-in nitinol guidewire, and (middle) multiple 21G needle options. (Courtesy of Teleflex, Inc.).

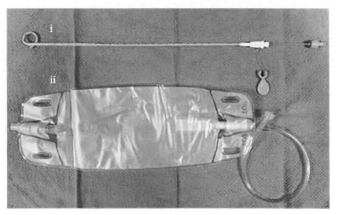

Fig. 35.4 Percutaneous nephrostomy catheter (i) with a locking pigtail and inner metal stiffener, (ii) gravity drainage bag.

- Renal transplants are easier to visualize and access under ultrasound, since they are more superficial than the native kidneys.
- Serial dilation of the tract may be necessary prior to placement of the catheter if there is extensive fibrotic tissue.

PROCEDURAL STEPS

Preprocedure

- Labs should include complete blood count (CBC), platelets, prothrombin time/international normalized ratio (PT/INR), and activated partial thromboplastin time (aPTT).
  - INR should be corrected to <1.5.
  - Transfusion is recommended for platelets ≤50,000/μL.
  - aPTT should be corrected to ≤1.5 times control.
- Level of anesthesia: conscious sedation with local
- Antibiotics—yes
  - Options include cefazolin 1 g IV, ceftriaxone 1 g IV, ampicillin/sulbactam 1.5–3 g IV, 2 g ampicillin IV and 1.5 mg/kg gentamicin IV

- If the patient is allergic to penicillin, vancomycin or clindamycin with an aminoglycoside can be used.
- Patient position: prone

Steps

1. The posterolateral flank is scanned with a 3.5- to 5-MHz ultrasound probe to identify a posterior mid- or lower pole calyx to puncture, making sure the puncture site will be below the 12th rib (Fig. 35.6).
2. Local anesthesia is administered in the direction of the target calyx.
3. A small dermatotomy is made at the skin entry site.
4. Under ultrasound guidance and using a single-stick needle access system (such as the Neff Percutaneous Access Set), the access needle is advanced into the target calyx (Fig. 35.7). The inner trocar is removed from the needle, and the needle is aspirated; it is slowly withdrawn until urine is aspirated.
5. Once urine is aspirated, a small amount of contrast is injected under fluoroscopy to confirm entry into the renal collecting system.
6. After positioning in the renal collecting system is confirmed, approximately 15 mL of air can be injected through the needle to confirm location in a posterior calyx (Fig. 35.8). Air will rise into the posterior calyces with the patient prone.

> ### ⟫ CLINICAL POINT
>
> Be sure to confirm that the access needle has entered the renal collecting system, rather than an artery or vein, before injecting air.

7. The access needle is exchanged over a 0.018-inch microwire for an introducer sheath. The size of the sheath varies between 5 and 7 Fr, depending on the access set.
8. Once the introducer sheath enters the calyx, the inner metal stiffener is unlocked, and the sheath is advanced into the renal pelvis without the metal stiffener.

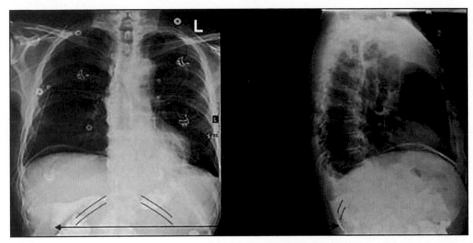

Fig. 35.5 Anatomic Location of the Posterior Pleural Reflection. Contrast extravasating and pooling in the right posterior costophrenic angle in this patient with a thoracic duct injury during a lymphangiogram shows the location of the posterior pleural reflections at the level of the 12th ribs (outlined).

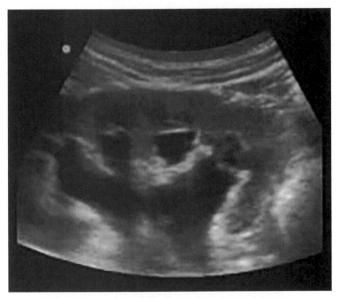

Fig. 35.6 Longitudinal Ultrasound Image of the Kidney.

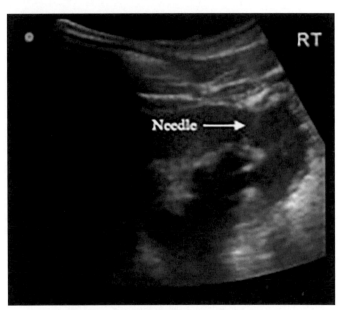

Fig. 35.7 Longitudinal Ultrasound Image of the Kidney Showing a Lower Pole Posterior Calyceal Needle Entry.

9. The microwire is exchanged for a 0.035-inch J-wire (Fig. 35.9) or Amplatz Super Stiff guidewire, either of which is coiled in the renal pelvis.
10. The introducer sheath is removed.
11. The PCN catheter is advanced over the 0.035-inch J-wire (Fig. 35.10) or Amplatz Super Stiff guidewire under fluoroscopic guidance.
12. After the catheter has entered the calyx, the inner metal stiffener is unlocked, and the remainder of the catheter is advanced over the guidewire into the renal collecting system without the metal stiffener (Fig. 35.11).
13. The guidewire is removed and the pigtail is formed in the renal pelvis by pulling on the string. The string is secured to the catheter to lock the pigtail (Fig. 35.12).

14. The PCN catheter is secured to the skin, and the catheter is connected to a gravity drainage bag.
15. Sterile dressings are applied.

> ### CLINICAL POINT
>
> Tips to removing a locking percutaneous nephrostomy catheter:
> - Be sure to release the locking mechanism before removal to avoid renal injury or catheter fracture.
> - Do not leave the catheter locking string behind, as it can lead to infection or stone formation.

TREATMENT ALTERNATIVES

- For decompression of an obstructed urinary system, a urologist may cystoscopically place a ureteral stent.

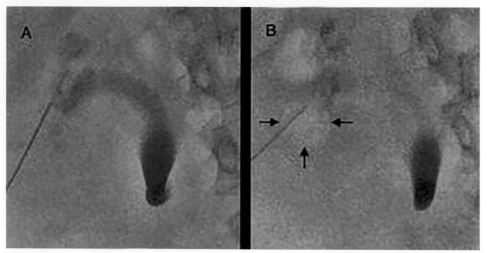

Fig. 35.8 Confirmation of Access into the Renal Collecting System and Posterior Calyx. With the patient prone, injection of a small amount of contrast under fluoroscopy (A) demonstrates opacification of the renal collecting system. This was followed by injection of a small amount of air (B) that outlines the posterior calyx *(arrows)*, confirming needle entry into a posterior calyx.

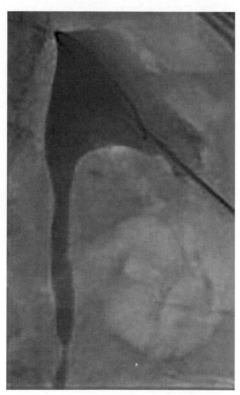

Fig. 35.9 0.035-Inch J-wire Coiled in the Renal Pelvis.

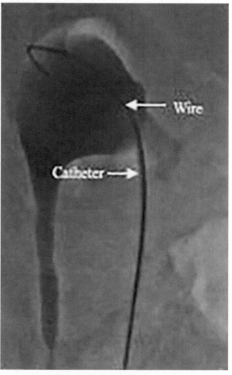

Fig. 35.10 Percutaneous Nephrostomy Catheter Advanced Into the Renal Pelvis Over a 0.035-inch J-wire.

COMPLICATIONS

◎ LITERATURE REVIEW

Farrell and Hicks (1997) noted an overall complication rate of 6.5% in a retrospective review of 454 percutaneous nephrostomy cases. Per SIR classification, 2.6% were deemed minor, and 3.9% were deemed major.

Procedure Related

- Septic shock (1%–10%)
  - Most common complication
  - Risk is increased in the presence of pyonephrosis
    - Important to minimize manipulation and distention of the collecting system in the presence of pyonephrosis
- Hemorrhage (1%–4%)

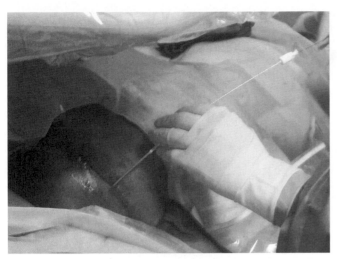

Fig. 35.11 Advancing a Percutaneous Nephrostomy Catheter Over a 0.035-inch Guidewire Without the Inner Stiffener.

- Minimized by correcting coagulopathy prior to the procedure
- Accessing the collecting system peripherally through a calyx, rather than centrally at the renal pelvis, can minimize the risk of hemorrhage
- Vascular injury (0.1%–1%)
  - Rarely, pseudoaneurysms or arteriovenous fistulas occur, which may require embolization
- Bowel transgression (0.2%–0.5%) (Fig 35.13)

- Pleural transgression (0.1%–0.6%)
  - Pneumothorax, hydrothorax, hemothorax, or empyema can be avoided by ensuring the entry site is below the 12th rib

Catheter Related

- Dislodgment
- Occlusion
- Routine PCN exchange is recommended every 3 months.

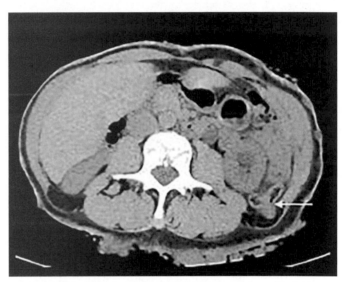

Fig. 35.13 CT of a Patient With Neurofibromatosis and Left Hydronephrosis. Note the position of the descending colon *(arrow)* behind the left kidney, which poses a risk for bowel transgression during percutaneous nephrostomy catheter placement.

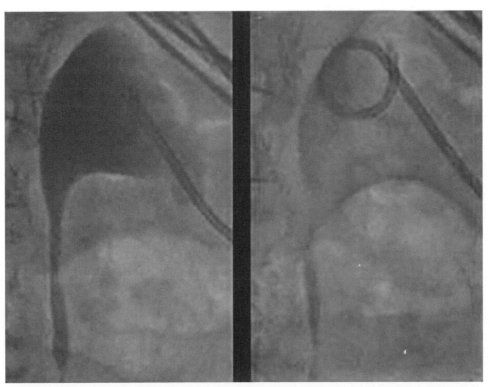

Fig. 35.12 Completion Nephrostograms Showing the Pigtail of the Catheter Formed in the Renal Pelvis.

TAKE-HOME POINTS

- Obstructive uropathy from both benign and malignant causes is the most common indication for percutaneous nephrostomy placement. Other indications include urinary diversion and access for percutaneous interventions such as antegrade ureteral stent placement and percutaneous nephrolithotomy.
- A percutaneous nephrostomy may be performed emergently in the setting of pyonephrosis and sepsis.
- There are no absolute contraindications for percutaneous nephrostomy.

- PCN is a safe and highly effective procedure when performed with good technique, which includes accessing the kidney below the 12th rib, choosing a posterior calyx for puncture, and accessing the renal collecting system peripherally.
- Preprocedural antibiotics, most commonly cefazolin, ceftriaxone, ampicillin/sulbactam, ampicillin, or gentamicin, should be given to prevent procedural-related sepsis.
- Complications include sepsis, hemorrhage, vascular injury, and bowel and pleural transgression.

REVIEW QUESTIONS

1. Which of the following is NOT an indication for percutaneous nephrostomy?
    a. Retroperitoneal mass causing obstructive hydronephrosis
    b. Septic shock secondary to pyonephrosis
    c. Urinary incontinence
    d. In preparation for percutaneous nephrolithotomy for a staghorn calculus
2. What is the optimal site for access into the renal collecting system?
    a. Renal pelvis
    b. Mid/lower pole renal calyces
    c. Upper pole renal calyces
    d. Ureteropelvic junction

3. Why is it important to exchange the initial 0.018-inch guidewire with a 0.035-inch J-wire or Amplatz Super Stiff wire for catheter advancement?
    a. To prevent any buckling of the guidewire that may result in damage of the extrarenal soft tissue or renal parenchyma
    b. For better visualization of the guidewire under fluoroscopy
    c. The 0.035-inch J-wire will dilate the tract, allowing the catheter to be advanced easily
    d. The inner diameter of the percutaneous nephrostomy catheter will not accommodate the 0.018-inch guidewire

SUGGESTED READINGS

Covey AM, Aruny JE, Kandarpa K. Percutaneous nephrostomy and antegrade ureteral stenting. In: Kandarpa K, Machan L, eds. *Handbook of Interventional Radiologic Procedures*. 4th ed. Philadelphia: Lippincott Williams & Wilkins; 2011.

Dyer RB, Regan JD, Kavanagh PV, et al. Percutaneous nephrostomy with extensions of the technique: step by step. *RadioGraphics*. 2002;22:503–525.

Farrell TA, Hicks ME. A review of radiologically guided percutaneous nephrostomies in 303 patients. *J Vasc Interv Radiol*. 1997; 8:769–774.

Fernstrom I, Johansson B. Percutaneous pyelolithotomy. A new extraction technique. *Scand J Urol Nephrol*. 1976;10(3):257–259.

Goodwin WE, Casey WC, Woolf W. Percutaneous trocar nephrostomy in hydronephrosis. *J Am Med Assoc*. 1955;891:157.

Haussegger KA, Portugaller HR. Percutaneous nephrostomy and antegrade ureteral stenting: technique, indications, and complications. *Eur Radiol*. 2006;16:2016–2030.

Pabon-Ramos WM, Dariushnia SR, Walker TG, et al. Quality improvement guidelines for percutaneous nephrostomy. *J Vasc Interv Radiol*. 2016;27(3):410–414.

Patel SR, Nakada SY. The modern history and evolution of percutaneous nephrolithotomy. *J Endourol*. 2015;29:153–157.

Smith AD, Lange PH, Miller RP, et al. Introduction of the Gibbons ureteral stent facilitated by antecedent percutaneous nephrostomy. *J Urol*. 1978;120(5):543–544.

Titton RL, Gervais DA, Hahn PF, et al. Urine leaks and urinomas: diagnosis and imaging-guided intervention. *RadioGraphics*. 2003;23:1133–1147.

Thoracentesis

Nathan Kwok, Nauman Hashmani, Ronald S. Arellano

CASE PRESENTATION

A 68-year-old female with a history of systemic lupus erythematosus (SLE) and mild kidney disease presents to the emergency room with symptoms of chest pain, shortness of breath, and cough. On physical examination, she is noted to have dullness on chest percussions, and auscultation reveals decreased breath sounds. A radiograph of the chest confirms a pleural effusion, and to help alleviate her symptoms, the physician orders an **ultrasound-guided thoracentesis**.

- A number of benign and malignant conditions can result in pleural effusions, which are the accumulation of fluid within the **pleural space.** Pleural fluid collections most frequently occur secondary to pneumonia, surgery, infection, and neoplasm. Analysis of the fluid contents can reveal the etiology of the fluid.

KEY DEFINITION

The *pleural space* is the potential space between the outer covering of the lung (parietal pleura) and the inner lining of the chest cavity (visceral pleura).

- Pleural effusions can range in size from minuscule, which are typically asymptomatic, to large collections, which can compress adjacent organs secondary to mass effect and cause chest pain and shortness of breath.
- Fluid collections in the pleural space can be treated by a variety of image-guided catheter-based procedures:
  - **Thoracentesis** is the drainage of fluid from the pleural space.
  - **Pleurodesis** is the injection of a sclerosing agent into the pleural space in order to affix the visceral and parietal pleura together and prevent fluid from accumulating.
- Fluid can be classified into four types:
  - **Transudative**—protein-poor, watery fluid that accumulates due to disturbances in Starling pressure forces (e.g., congestive heart failure)
  - **Exudative**—protein-rich, thick fluid secondary to tissue damage or increased vessel permeability due to inflammation (e.g., pneumonia)

- **Hemorrhagic**—usually occurs due to trauma, cancer, or recent surgery
- **Chylous**—lymphatic fluid that has a high lipid content, giving it a "milky" appearance, which often occurs due to a blockage or disruption of the thoracic duct (e.g., malignancy, surgery)

⟫ CLINICAL POINT: LIGHT'S CRITERIA

- Sensitivity of 98% and specificity of 83% in determining whether fluid is transudative or exudative.
- Required labs:
  - Lactate dehydrogenase (LDH) from both the serum and the effusion fluid
  - Protein from both the serum and the effusion fluid
- Fluid is **exudative** if one of the following criteria is present:
  - Effusion protein/serum protein ratio >0.5
  - Effusion LDH/serum LDH ratio >0.6
  - Effusion LDH level $>2/3$ of the upper limit of normal for serum LDH

Adapted from Lamberg J, Reghavendra M. Light's criteria. *Medscape*. Available at: http://emedicine.medscape.com/article/2172232-overview. Accessed January 30, 2016.

- Normal pleural fluid has the following characteristics:
  - Clear
  - pH range between 7.60 and 7.64
  - Protein <1 to 2 g/dL ($<2\%$)
  - WBC $<1000/mm^3$
  - Glucose approximately equal to plasma
  - LDH $<50\%$ of plasma

INDICATIONS

- Any unexplained new collection of pleural fluid should be tapped.
  - The most common reasons are to improve respiration and to obtain fluid samples for diagnostic purposes.
- Used as therapeutic treatment in patients with:
  - Large pleural effusions
  - Empyemas

CONTRAINDICATIONS

- There are no absolute contraindications.
- Relative contraindications include:
  - Variant chest wall anatomy
  - Minimal fluid volume (<1 cm in thickness on a lateral decubitus chest x-ray or on ultrasound examination)
  - Chest wall cellulitis (at the site of puncture)
  - Bleeding diathesis (uncorrectable) or coagulopathy
  - Severe pulmonary disease
  - Uncontrolled coughing
  - One functional lung

EQUIPMENT (FIGS. 36.1 AND 36.2)

- For preparation of puncture site:
  - Sterile ultrasound 3.5-MHz curvilinear transducer
  - Sterile ultrasound probe cover
  - Skin antiseptic (chlorhexidine is preferred)
  - Sterile fenestrated drape or towel

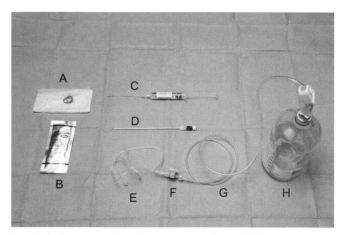

Fig. 36.1 Equipment Used for a Thoracentesis. (A) Sterile ultrasound probe cover. (B) Sterile ultrasound gel. (C) Local anesthetic. (D) 7-Fr catheter. (E) Tubing. (F) Three-way stopcock. (G) Tubing. (H) Specimen bottle.

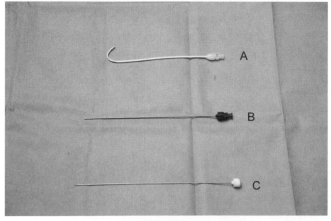

Fig. 36.2 Components of Thoracentesis Catheter. (A) 7-Fr catheter. (B) Metal stiffener. (C) Trocar needle.

- For drainage:
  - Local anesthetic
    - 1% or 2% lidocaine (5–10 mL)
    - Consider 0.5% bupivacaine for patients allergic to lidocaine
  - Three-way stopcock
  - 7-Fr catheter
  - IV connecting tube
  - Tubing
  - Specimen bottle
  - Syringes for specimens

ANATOMY

- The shortest and most direct route is often the best approach in performing a thoracentesis.

Normal Anatomy (Fig. 36.3)

- Each lung is enclosed in its own pleural space.
- Intercostal vessels vary in location but most commonly run along the inferior aspect of the rib.
- Internal mammary arteries are anterior and paramedian along the sternum.

Atypical Anatomy

- Postsurgical changes may alter the anatomy and imaging appearance.
- A single pleural space communicating bilaterally (bovine lung) can predispose to bilateral pneumothoraces.
- Avoid chest wall collaterals from venous or arterial obstruction.

PROCEDURAL STEPS

- Multiple methods exist, including the usage of large-gauge needle, IV cannula, or small catheter. The precise technique will vary slightly depending on the selected method and devices. Diagnostic aspiration is the first step and will precede any intended therapeutic fluid drainage.
- Thoracentesis can be performed more effectively by combining the traditional technique with ultrasound or CT guidance.
  - Ultrasound is preferred to CT scan as it is:
    - Less expensive
    - Offers real-time imaging
    - Does not expose the patient to ionizing radiation
    - Easier to use on a patient who cannot be moved due to a life-threatening condition or a patient requiring mechanical ventilation
- Predictors of successful drainage:
  - Anechoic collection
  - Transudative fluid
  - Lack of septations or multiple loculations
  - No pleural rind

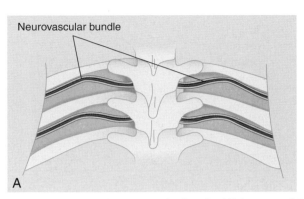

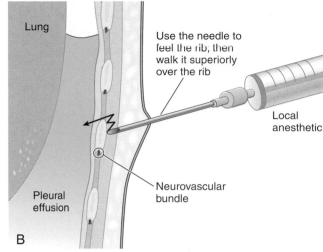

Fig. 36.3 Neurovascular Bundle. (A) Anatomy of the neurovascular bundle. The intercostal nerve, artery, and vein typically run inferior to the rib. (B) The proper approach mandates walking the needle up and over the rib to avoid these vital structures. (From Roberts JR, ed. *Roberts and Hedges' Clinical Procedures in Emergency Medicine.* Philadelphia: Elsevier; 2014:Fig. 9-15.)

⊚ LITERATURE REVIEW

There is a 16.3% reduction in risk of pneumothorax and a 38.7% reduction in risk of hemorrhage with the use of ultrasound, according to Patel et al. (2012).

⊚ KEY DEFINITION

Pleural rind refers to a clearly defined pleural border on imaging.

Diagnostic Thoracentesis

1. The patient is positioned on the stretcher or side of bed with easy access to the back or midaxillary line. The patient can be seated or supine.
2. Ultrasound is used to locate the fluid collection, and the overlying skin is marked.
3. Using sterile technique, the skin is cleansed and draped.
4. The skin is anesthetized at the desired puncture site.
5. A 21-gauge needle is advanced in the intercostal space, directly superior to the adjacent inferior rib, into the fluid collection. Advancing the needle over the top of a rib helps to avoid potential injury to the neurovascular bundle located at the inferior aspect of the rib.
6. 50 to 100 mL of fluid is aspirated for diagnostic purposes. This fluid is sent for Gram stain and culture, total protein, LDH, glucose, pH assessment, and cytology.

Therapeutic Thoracentesis

1. The patient is positioned on the stretcher similar to that for a diagnostic thoracentesis.
2. The largest area of fluid collection is located with the ultrasound.
3. The skin is sterilely prepped and anesthetized at the desired puncture site.

4. A small skin incision is made, sized appropriately for passage of a drainage catheter.
5. Under imaging guidance, the needle is advanced into the collection.
6. A small 5- to 8-Fr catheter is advanced over the needle and into the fluid collection.
7. The tubing is secured to prevent the development of kinks or positional shifts during drainage.
8. A sterile 1L vacuum bottle is connected via the tubing and three-way stopcock to the catheter. Typically 0.5 to 1 L of fluid is removed each procedure (Fig. 36.4).
9. If the drainage fluid is purulent, an attempt should be made to aspirate as completely as possible. Gentle saline irrigation of the cavity can be done to help clear pus and other semisolid debris.

ALTERNATE TREATMENTS

- **Antibiotics**—if the primary disease process is infectious, antibiotics may be preferred as an initial treatment.
- **Medical management**—treating the underlying cardiac/liver/renal condition that is causing the pleural effusion
- **Surgery**—using either an endoscope (VATS) or open (surgical decortication) approach to remove the restrictive layer of fibrous tissue overlying the lung
- **Chest tube placement**
  - Chest tubes are semistiff, clear plastic tubes placed into the chest to drain collections of fluid or air from the pleural space, allowing for restoration of intrapleural pressure and lung re-expansion.
  - Indication for placement includes the presence of pneumothorax, hemothorax, empyema, and pleural effusion.
  - In contrast to a one-time thoracentesis drainage, chest tubes are left in the patient. The patient can be discharged home with a chest tube and a PleurEvac system, if necessary.

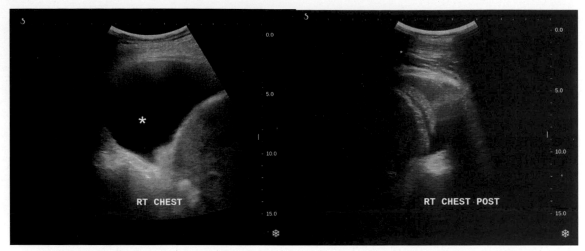

Fig. 36.4 Ultrasound Images Before and After Thoracentesis. (A) Sagittal ultrasound image of the right hemithorax demonstrating a right pleural effusion *(asterisk)*. (B) Sagittal ultrasound image of the right hemithorax immediately after removal of 500 mL of fluid. The lung has reexpanded to fill the space previously occupied by the effusion.

◎ KEY DEFINITIONS

- *PleurEvac:* a multichambered device that chest tubes are connected to in order to manage the proper outflow of fluid/air from the patient's chest. It also facilitates easy monitoring and analysis of the removed fluid.
- *Wall suction:* the PleurEvac system is connected to a wall suction unit to aid in the removal of air/fluid from the pleural space
- *Water/air seal:* both terms refer to a chamber of water that acts as a one-way valve permitting air to escape and not reenter the chest.
- *Air leak:* when the water chamber has visible bubbling, air is leaking through the system, which can be good or bad depending on the source.
- *Clamp trial:* clamping a chest tube simulates the removal of chest tube and is used to assess for an air leak.

COMPLICATIONS

- **Tube malfunction**—intraprocedural clotting, kinking, or malpositioning of the drainage catheter
- **Hemorrhage**
  - Bleeding can occur with any skilled operator, and the risk is higher in the presence of a vascular lesion/organ.
  - Risk is highest during procedures adjacent to major blood vessels or known vascular tumors, particularly when there is no surrounding normal tissue to tamponade bleeding. For high-risk patients, it is advised to type and cross-match blood prior to the procedure.
  - Injury to the lung can lead to bleeding into the bronchial tree and aspiration into the contralateral side. If bleeding appears in an endotracheal tube or the patient expectorates blood, place his/her ipsilateral side down.
- Pneumothorax
  - Rarely, a pneumothorax may occur, usually due to air being introduced during the procedure.
  - If a patient exhibits severe coughing, dyspnea, or chest pain, first titrate the rate of fluid removal. If symptoms continue, clamp the catheter, place his/her ipsilateral side down, and obtain a chest radiograph to evaluate for possible pneumothorax.
- Reexpansion pulmonary edema
  - Extremely uncommon, occurring due to the rapid evacuation of pleural fluid
  - Maintaining fluid removal slower than 500 mL/h can decrease the incidence
- **Infection**—if the operator does not adhere to proper sterile techniques
- **Death**—can occur from hemorrhage but is extremely rare following thoracentesis

🏠 TAKE-HOME POINTS

- Thoracentesis is a procedure that involves the removal of fluid or air from around the lungs by passing a needle into the pleural space.
- It is used as both diagnostic and therapeutic treatment:
  - Used diagnostically to analyze the fluid present to determine the cause of the effusion
  - Used therapeutically for patients with large amounts of fluid in their pleural space that is causing respiratory compromise or pain from mass effect
- Drainage can be made more effective by involving modern imaging, such as ultrasound or CT. Ultrasound is generally preferred to CT scan.
- The best approach is that which takes the most direct path to the fluid collection, inserting in the superior aspect of the adjacent rib.
- Thoracentesis has no absolute contraindications; some relative contraindications do exist.
- Pneumothorax is the most common complication.

REVIEW QUESTIONS

1. In which part of the body is thoracentesis performed?
   a. Lung parenchyma
   b. Pleural space
   c. Pericardial space
   d. Synovial cavity
2. In which emergency condition is a thoracentesis indicated?
   a. Increased intracranial pressure
   b. Hemorrhagic shock
   c. Pleural effusion
   d. Bacterial abscess
3. Which of these fluids, from an effusion, are characteristic of an exudate?
   a. Effusion protein/serum protein ratio >0.5
   b. Effusion protein/serum protein <0.5
   c. Effusion urea/serum urea >1.8
   d. Effusion lactate dehydrogenase/serum lactate dehydrogenase <0.6

4. Which of these is an absolute contraindication of thoracentesis?
   a. Variant chest wall anatomy
   b. Severe pulmonary disease
   c. Hemothorax
   d. None of the above
5. Which of the following reasons is NOT true regarding the advantages of ultrasound over CT for thoracentesis?
   a. Less expensive
   b. No patient exposure to ionizing radiation
   c. Detailed visualization of bony structures
   d. Convenient portability

SUGGESTED READINGS

Goljan EF. *Rapid Review Pathology.* Philadelphia: Elsevier/Saunders; 2014.

Maurelus K, Secko M, Mehta N. *Focus On: Ultrasound for Thoracentesis.* American College of Emergency Physicians; 2013. Available at: http://www.acep.org/Education/Continuing-Medical-Education-(CME)/Focus-On/Focus-On–Ultrasound-for-Thoracentesis/. Accessed 25 January 2016.

Patel P, Ernst F, Gunnarsson C. Ultrasonography guidance reduces complications and costs associated with thoracentesis procedures. *J Clin Ultrasound.* 2012. Available at: http://onlinelibrary.wiley.com/doi/10.1002/jcu.20884/abstract. Accessed 15 February 2016.

Ringel E. *The Little Black Book of Pulmonary Medicine.* Sudbury, MA: Jones and Bartlett Publishers; 2009.

Answer Key to End-of-Chapter Review Questions

CHAPTER 1: HISTORY OF INTERVENTIONAL RADIOLOGY

1. **c.** In addition to his pioneering work on transhepatic cholangiography, Seldinger is known for the eponymous technique of vascular access.
2. **c.** Palmaz invented the balloon-expandable stent that revolutionized cardiovascular medicine.
3. **d.** Gruntzig developed the technique of balloon angioplasty, which gave rise to the era of percutaneous transluminal coronary angioplasty.
4. **a.** Hawkins developed the method of carbon dioxide digital subtraction angiography.
5. **d.** Moniz pioneered cerebral angiography. He also developed Thorotrast, one of the earliest contrast agents.

CHAPTER 2: BASICS OF INTERVENTIONAL RADIOLOGY

1. **d.** 1 point for diabetes and 1 point for age greater than 65. Female, not male, would have conferred 1 more point. Therapy is recommended for scores of 2 or more.
2. **b.** This would be considered a clean-contaminated case, so preoperative antibiotics should be given. Ancef or IV vancomycin would have been appropriate choices.

CHAPTER 3: IMAGING MODALITIES

1. **c.** While acute blood appears bright on CT due to the high iron content, old hemorrhage has lower Hounsfield units because of the breakdown that occurs in pooled blood. This difference in X-ray attenuation between acute and old blood can be used to differentiate acute from old intracranial hemorrhages. The other options will all appear radiopaque, since metals (including calcium) attenuate X-rays. Arterial plaques are frequently calcified.
2. **d.** T2-weighted images highlight areas with high water content, so any kind of bleed or accumulation of fluid would be hyperintense. However, blood vessels will not be hyperintense on T2 because the flowing blood is not affected in the same way as the rest of the anatomy; as such, there is a "flow void" on noncontrast MRI, resulting in areas of hypointensity in the space of blood vessels. Note, also, that MRI contrast agents such as gadolinium are only

hyperintense on T1-weighted images, and actually appear hypointense on T2.
3. **b.** Angiogram (fluoroscopically-guided angiography) is the gold standard for vascular imaging. In this procedure, a blood vessel is catheterized and contrast agent injected to image the luminal space of a vascular network. CT angiogram and MR angiogram provide good detail of the vasculature in arterial and venous phases but do not provide the level of detail (especially in small vessels) of a true angiogram. PET does not image blood vessels, and ultrasound, while good for certain vascular studies of large vessels like the carotid arteries or abdominal aorta, is not good for imaging a large vascular network with many small vessels.

CHAPTER 4: ANATOMY

1. **b.** Answer A is incorrect because it skips the right external iliac, and an aberrant right hepatic artery, while possible, is not typical anatomy. Answer C is incorrect because the internal iliac is a separate branch from the external iliac. Answer D describes the typical pathway for TIPS or a transjugular liver biopsy, but not TACE.
2. **a.** RIPA is the most common parasitic artery, especially with tumors that are in the bare area of the liver, adjacent to the right diaphragm.
3. **a.** Coiling is relatively contraindicated in bronchial artery embolization because, should hemoptysis reoccur, it would not be possible to achieve access distal to the site of embolization.

CHAPTER 5: NEUROINTERVENTIONAL RADIOLOGY

1. **d.** All of the above are contraindications for these procedures as listed in the ACR guidelines.
2. **c.** The most common complication is transient neurological deficit.
3. **c.** PVP and KP are most often done with the use of fluoroscopy.
4. **d.** The main difference between vertebroplasty and kyphoplasty is the use of a balloon to try to restore the height of the vertebra.
5. **a.** While angiography has been the traditional gold standard, carotid ultrasonography is considered by some to

be the new gold standard. There is no consensus on which noninvasive imaging technique, ultrasound, MRA, or CTA, can replace angiography. Due to ease of access, lack of radiation exposure, efficacy, and speed, carotid ultrasound is usually the preferred first-line choice in imaging.

6. **d.** Visible thrombus is the only absolute contraindication listed due to the potential for direct embolization into the brain. The other choices listed are relative contraindications.

CHAPTER 6: INTERVENTIONAL ONCOLOGY

1. **c.** Hydrogen, helium, and neon are gases that do not cool under the Joule-Thompson effect at room temperature. The Joule-Thompson effect essentially describes the change in kinetic and potential internal energy of a gas during rapid adiabatic expansion: an adiabatic system describes one in which heat does not leave or enter so the internal energy of a gas remains stable as it expands by rapidly cooling.

2. **d.** Medical therapy with a targeted molecular agent. The imaging features of these nodules are consistent with HCC. While Mrs. S has two nodules that are each less than 3 cm in diameter, the presence of vascular invasion in multinodular HCC classifies her disease as Stage C or advanced HCC, which is best treated with targeted molecular agents such as sorafenib. Surgical resection and transplant are preferred options when possible. For patients with fewer than three lesions less than 3 cm in size without vascular invasion, ablation would be an appropriate option. TACE would be appropriate for more extensive multinodular disease without vascular invasion.

3. **d.** Hepatic abscess. The risk of hepatic abscess is increased in the setting of biliary obstruction, which was noted on Mrs. S's RUQ ultrasound.

CHAPTER 7: SURGERY

1. **c.** At a MELD score of ≥ 15, a patient becomes a candidate for liver transplantation. At a MELD score of >10, the transplant evaluation is initiated to allow sufficient time for evaluation prior to end-stage disease. Therefore at MELD scores of 5 and 10 the patient would not yet be a candidate for liver transplantation, and at 20 the patient would have already become a candidate at a MELD score of 15.

2. **a.** The first step in management in a patient showing signs of rejection/failure is to obtain an ultrasound. It is a quick, inexpensive imaging modality that does not involve radiation. CT or MRI would be the next step. A tissue biopsy is the gold standard for diagnosis but should be obtained after imaging, as it is a more invasive procedure that has potential complications.

3. **d.** A piggyback anastomosis is when the donor IVC is anastomosed to the side of the recipient IVC. This produces an acute angulation between the hepatic vein and native IVC and therefore does not maintain the anatomic relationship between the hepatic vein and IVC. Leaving the native IVC behind requires only one caval anastomosis versus two in the classic technique. This leads to a decrease in warm ischemia time and a decrease in blood loss, and it minimizes hemodynamic disturbances.

4. **d.** The Milan Criteria determine the need for transplantation in HCC. The following are components of the Milan Criteria: a single lesion ≤ 5 cm or 2 to 3 lesions none exceeding 3 cm, and no vascular invasion and/or extrahepatic spread. Choice D does not meet these criteria, as it is a single lesion that is 6 cm. A single lesion must be ≤ 5 cm. All of the other answer choices are consistent with the Milan Criteria.

5. **d.** This patient is presenting with signs of rejection/failure. Initial steps would include obtaining an ultrasound and CT scan or performing catheter angiography. However, the gold standard for diagnosis of rejection/failure is an organ biopsy.

6. **c.** Too proximal a puncture increases the risk of retroperitoneal hemorrhage, while too distal a puncture increases the risk of iatrogenic pseudoaneurysm formation. Ideal location is the common femoral artery over the femoral head.

7. **b.** A negative SMA angiogram does not rule out an active LGIB; both the SMA and IMA should be interrogated.

8. **d.** If the patient presents with signs of upper GI bleed, then the left gastric artery, celiac trunk/branches, and SMA should be interrogated.

CHAPTER 8: OBSTETRICS AND GYNECOLOGY

1. **c.** This patient would likely be best served by myomectomy.
2. **b.** Reported incidence is 0% to 3%.
3. **c.** Embolization does not preclude a patient from receiving further surgical intervention if deemed necessary.

CHAPTER 9: PEDIATRICS

1. **a.** While all of the above are possible complications, intraperitoneal bleeding is the most common and worrisome of complications after percutaneous liver biopsy. By definition, a percutaneous biopsy penetrates the liver capsule, so some degree of bleeding is expected. In patients with coagulopathy, this degree of bleeding can be life-threatening.

2. **e.** Sampling of suspected metabolic, mitochondrial, and genetic disorders requires specimens aligned along the muscle fibers. Diagnostic failure, therefore, is due to misaligned biopsy orientation. Too small a biopsy sample and degradation of samples can both result in diagnostic failure, not just of muscle biopsies but all tissue biopsies. Muscle biopsies require large specimens to allow for a variety of staining techniques, marker studies, and genetic analyses, so core biopsy is preferred to fine-needle aspiration.

3. **a.** Jejunal intussusception is more likely with a GJ tube. GJ tubes are more likely to get clogged, and they must be replaced under fluoroscopy. Because they terminate in the jejunum, patients have less risk of aspiration secondary to GERD.

CHAPTER 10: FRONTIERS OF INTERVENTIONAL RADIOLOGY

1. **d.** The prostatic artery is a branch of the anterior division of the internal iliac artery. The major branches of the posterior division are the lateral sacral, iliolumbar, and superior gluteal arteries. The remaining answer choices are all true statements.

2. **c.** Medical therapy is the first line of therapy for BPH. TURP is the most common surgical treatment for BPH for patients with significant LUTS refractory to medical therapy. The remaining answer choices are all true statements.

3. **d.** Dampening of the waveform after compression of the radial artery without recovery within 2 minutes of compression signifies an inadequate patency of the ulnopalmar arch for distal perfusion of the hand. Barbeau A, B, and C confirm patency of the ulnopalmar arch.

4. **c.** The combination of short-acting anticoagulants (heparin) and vasodilators (calcium channel blockers and nitrates) are used to prevent radial artery vasospasm and/or occlusion after radial artery access and placement of a trans-radial vascular sheath. The saline flush (choice a) prevents sheath occlusion but will not prevent radial artery vasospasm. Iodinated contrast can be used to opacify the radial artery after access and identify reasons for technical difficulties (i.e., radial artery loop).

5. **c.** Applying a compression band to the wrist over the radial artery arteriotomy site allows for adequate hemostasis without resulting in radial artery occlusion/thrombosis. Manual compression for 15 minutes may be used for groin (i.e., common femoral artery) access to achieve hemostasis. Closure devices are used for closure of larger arteries (i.e., groin access, common femoral artery after percutaneous EVAR).

6. **d.** Of all the anatomic variants related to the LGA, a replaced left hepatic artery arising from the LGA is most common. Other variants, like anomalous origin of the LGA off of the aorta or replaced CHA arising from the LGA are less common.

CHAPTER 11: ADRENAL VENOUS SAMPLING

1. **a.** Selectivity index reflects the ratio of adrenal vein cortisol to peripheral vein cortisol. Lateralization index is a comparison of aldosterone/cortisol ratio between the left and right adrenal veins. Sensitivity index is a statistic used in signal detection theory, and specificity index was made up.

2. **b.** Selectivity index reflects the ratio of adrenal vein cortisol to peripheral vein cortisol. Lateralization index is a comparison of aldosterone/cortisol ratio between the left and right adrenal veins. Sensitivity index is a statistic used in signal detection theory, and specificity index was made up.

3. **c.** In smaller veins, an appropriately placed side hole can prevent collapse of the vein walls when drawing a blood sample.

CHAPTER 12: ARTERIOVENOUS FISTULAS AND GRAFTS

1. **c.** Painful arm swelling indicates central or outflow vein stenosis. With the additional symptom of facial swelling, a central stenosis is more likely as this would not be present with outflow stenosis alone. A thrombosed fistula would not be pulsatile, and juxta-anastomotic stenosis would present as a fistula with decreased flow.

2. **d.** The potassium level is greater than 6.0 mEq/L and a fistulogram is contraindicated, since a wire will cross the myocardium and the patient would be at risk for developing an arrhythmia. A temporary dialysis catheter needs to be placed for HD. The preferred site in this patient would be the groin since the wire would not cross the myocardium during catheter placement. Once dialyzed, the fistulogram can be performed. Systemic thrombolytics would be indicated at the time of the fistulogram. An EKG would not a play a role in the management of this patient.

CHAPTER 13: ARTERIOVENOUS MALFORMATIONS

1. **b.** A sarcoma, whether of the fat, muscle, blood vessels (angiosarcoma), or other tissues, refers to a malignant tumor. The remaining choices are all benign.

2. **e.** All are potential complications. In addition to these listed, sclerosants may cause acute renal failure secondary to hemolysis.

3. **a.** This is a true statement regarding AVMs - pulsatile flow indicates the lack of a normal capillary bed between the artery and vein.

CHAPTER 14: BALLOON-ASSISTED RETROGRADE TRANSVENOUS OBLITERATION

1. **c.** This patient is a good candidate for either endoscopic therapy or BRTO because he has actively bleeding gastric varices, which may be treated by either therapy. If he were to present with isolated esophageal varices, endoscopic therapy would be the most appropriate choice. Given his history of hepatic encephalopathy, this patient is not a good candidate for a TIPS procedure as this procedure carries a relatively high risk of hepatic encephalopathy.

2. **b.** The patient's vital signs and decreased Hgb and Hct point to an acute bleeding event. Premature balloon rupture may occur in up to 15% of BRTO procedures, leading to technical failure and rebleeding of the varix. In this case, the patient would need to be emergently treated to prevent major blood loss. An anaphylactic reaction is likely to have a more rapid onset upon exposure to the contrast material and would be accompanied by symptoms such as bronchoconstriction and edema. Esophageal variceal bleeding is more likely to be a long-term complication, as redistribution of blood flow away from previously patent gastric

varices to esophageal varices typically occurs over a time frame of years rather than hours. Ethanolamine oleate is known to cause hemolysis but is unlikely to cause the systemic symptoms described in this scenario. If ethanolamine oleate is used, the patient may experience gross hematuria, but this side effect alone is not associated with an increased risk of bleeding.

CHAPTER 15: BRONCHIAL ARTERY EMBOLIZATION

1. **c.** The bronchial arteries typically arise from the aorta at the T5/6 level, with the left mainstem bronchus serving as a useful fluoroscopic landmark.
2. **c.** Massive hemoptysis is variably defined as pulmonary bleeding of between 100 to 600 mLs in a 24 hour period (we give an average of 200–300 mLs). A more relevant definition of massive hemoptysis might be the volume that is life threatening by virtue of airway obstruction or blood loss.
3. **c.** Onyx is not typically used. Gelfoam can be used, though its transient nature usually leads to recurrent episodes of hemoptysis. Embolization coils preclude future access to that bronchial artery should recurrent hemoptysis occur, which it commonly does. PVA particles are the preferred agent.

CHAPTER 16: DEEP VEIN THROMBOSIS

1. **d.** Recent surgery, active cancer, a history of DVTs, and pregnancy are all risk factors for the development of a DVT. Exercise helps to prevent DVT formation.
2. **d.** Wells criteria includes active cancer, pitting edema, immobilization, and recent surgery. Calf swelling greater than 3 cm (not 1 cm) compared to the opposite leg is an additional criteria.
3. **e.** Low molecular weight heparin is the preferred parenteral anticoagulation agent. Unfractioned heparin can be used in patients with renal failure. Warfarin and rivaroxaban are appropriate long-term oral options. Clopidogrel (Plavix) is not an appropriate choice.

CHAPTER 17: ENDOVASCULAR ANEURYSM REPAIR

1. **c.** AAAs are infrarenal in greater than 80% of cases. Repair is indicated when size is greater than 5 cm in women and 5.5 cm in men, or after having grown 5 mm in a 6-month period. Best choice is that incidence of rupture increases with aneurysm size – a 5.0 cm aneurysm has less than a 20% chance of rupturing while a 8.0 cm aneurysm has between a 30% to 50% chance of rupturing.
2. **e.** Immediate treatment is indicated in type I and III endoleaks. Type II and V endoleaks may be treated in they are shown to continue enlarging on multiple studies. Type IV endoleaks are usually self-limited.

3. **c.** Aneurysms between 6.0 cm and 6.9 cm have a 10% to 20% annual risk of rupture. Aneurysms expand at an average rate of 0.4 cm per year.

CHAPTER 18: FOREIGN BODY RETRIEVAL

1. **c.** If a patient is experiencing symptoms due to a foreign body, then removal is certainly indicated in order to ameliorate the symptoms. Regardless of the location, removal is not always indicated for a foreign body. This is especially true if a patient is terminal, a situation where removal may prove fruitless or excessive. Since there are situations where foreign bodies are not retrieved, choice e is incorrect.
2. **e.** Since a foreign body can become a nidus for infection, sepsis is a possible complication. Intravascular foreign bodies can become dislodged and embolize distally. If present in heart tissue, foreign bodies can cause an arrhythmia. Finally, depending on the geometry and material properties of an intravascular foreign body, vessel perforation is also a possible outcome. Since all options are potential complications, choice e is correct.
3. **c.** 18-gauge needles are used for venous access regardless of whether the case involves foreign body retrieval. IVC filters are not unique to foreign body retrievals. Fogarty catheters are used to remove clots from the arterial system and are not used for foreign body retrievals. C-arms used in a variety of minimally invasive image-guided procedures. Dormia baskets are a type of snare used to entrap and extract foreign bodies; therefore, c is the correct answer.

CHAPTER 19: INFERIOR VENA CAVA FILTER

1. **c.** Of the options listed, the Greenfield filter is the only permanent IVC filter. The others all may be retrieved using a variety of techniques and equipment as described in the chapter.
2. **d.** In the case of significant thrombus within the filter, retrieval is contraindicated. In many cases caval filtration is a temporary intervention, making choice *a* incorrect. Choice *b* is incorrect because ideal filter position is inferior to the renal veins. Choice *c* is incorrect because Bird's Nest filters are often selected in cases of mega cava (caval diameter >28 mm).
3. **c.** One advantage of jugular access for filter placement is the decreased risk of postinsertion thrombus. Arrhythmia, air embolus, and misplacement are all less likely with femoral access, making them the incorrect choices for this question.

CHAPTER 20: PERIPHERAL ARTERIAL DISEASE

1. **b.** Unless the patient is at immediate risk for limb loss, in which case he should be sent to the emergency department for treatment, the best course of action for this outpatient care provider is to maximize the patient's medical management and promote dietary and fitness changes.

Choices a, c, and d a, b, and d may eventually happen, but the best initial choice it to optimize noninvasive care.

2. **a.** Choice *b* describes angioplasty, choice *c* describes catheter-directed thrombolysis, and choice *d* describes vessel stenting.

3. **c.** Since this ulcer is in the angiosome of the medial plantar artery, a branch of the posterior tibial artery, the patient would most likely benefit from direct revascularization of the posterior tibial artery.

CHAPTER 21: PULMONARY EMBOLISM

1. **c.** A submassive PE is defined as an acute PE without hypotension but with signs of myocardial dysfunction or necrosis. In this case, the patient is not hypotensive but does have right heart strain on EKG (RV dysfunction), RV strain on CT (RV:LV ratio >0.9), and a positive troponin (myocardial necrosis). Answers *a* and *d* are incorrect since this patient does not meet the criteria for these subtypes based on Table 21.1. Choices *b* and *e* are incorrect because they are descriptors about a PE's configuration/location.

2. **c.** Roughly 55% of patients with PE have a low-risk PE. Answers *a* and *b* are incorrect since approximately 40% of patients with PE have a submassive PE, and 5% have a massive PE. See Table 21.1 for reference.

3. **a.** Respiratory rate is not included in the Wells criteria for PE. Choices *b*, *c*, *d*, and *e* are all included in the Wells criteria for PE. See Table 21.2. for reference.

CHAPTER 22: RENAL ARTERY STENOSIS

1. **b.** In cases of pheochromocytoma, the blood pressure is persistently high with episodes of severe hypertension (paroxysmal). ACE inhibitor/ARB use removes angiotensin II–mediated vasoconstriction to induce a decline in the GFR of the stenotic kidney. Presence of a systolic or diastolic abdominal bruit, while not very sensitive, represents turbulent flow through a stenotic vessel. Recurrent flash pulmonary edema can occur in the setting of bilateral renal artery stenosis.

2. **d.** Acute renal ischemia in which significant irreversible ischemic damage has already occurred is a major contraindication to revascularization. The patient is unlikely to benefit from renal preservation.

CHAPTER 23: THROMBOLYSIS AND THROMBECTOMY

1. **a.** In CDT-treated DVTs, PEs have been reported in as many as 4.5% of patients, although most studies suggest a rate closer to 1%.

2. **d.** May-Thurner syndrome is a condition in which the crossing right common iliac artery compresses the left common iliac vein, causing thrombosis of the left common iliac vein and leading to symptoms including discomfort, swelling, and pain. Despite both occurring in the venous system, this is an entirely different entity than PSS.

3. **b.** The same intensity and duration of anticoagulant therapy is recommended in patients undergoing CDT as in patients who do not undergo thrombolysis.

CHAPTER 24: TRANSJUGULAR INTRAHEPATIC PORTOSYSTEMIC SHUNTS

1. **a.** Right-to-right TIPS is considered optimal placement because of the relative ease of creating this shunt due to the anatomic proximity of the two vessels. The right hepatic vein is large and slopes downward, facilitating the instruments used in TIPS. In this arrangement, the needle from the hepatic vein is rotated anteriorly to access the right portal vein. The right hepatic vein and left portal vein are not in close proximity. Middle hepatic-right portal and middle hepatic-left portal are useable arrangements, depending on patient anatomy but require more complex rotational movements of the needle.

2. **c.** Recurrent variceal hemorrhage unresponsive to medical therapy in Child's B or C class is an established indication for TIPS. Refractory ascites is an established indication for TIPS, but TIPS for a small amount of ascites has been less studied. The risks of a TIPS outweigh only a small amount of ascites. While patients with Child's A cirrhosis are lower risk than patients in B or C class, small varices without hemorrhage are best managed medically. Refractory hepatic hydrothorax is an indication for TIPS, but uncontrolled hepatic encephalopathy is a relative contraindication for TIPS.

3. **b.** To answer this question, consider the consequences of portal hypertension and liver failure separately. Portal hypertension of any etiology causes increased hydrostatic pressure. Liver failure leads to decreased synthesis of a number of proteins, including albumin. As oncotic pressure is proportional to molality, the decreased protein concentration leads to decreased oncotic pressure.

CHAPTER 25: TRANSJUGULAR LIVER BIOPSY

1. **a.** TJLB and PLB have comparable technical success rates. Percutaneous biopsies tend to have higher average core lengths containing more portal tracts and therefore require slightly fewer passes on average. Percutaneous biopsies by definition penetrate the liver capsule and therefore risk bleeding. We are able to perform concurrent venography and measurement of hepatic pressures when doing transjugular biopsies but not with percutaneous biopsies.

2. **b.** Liver biopsy is not routinely done in cases of acute hepatitis unless the diagnosis is uncertain after extensive workup. It is routinely used in the diagnoses of the other mentioned conditions.

3. **b.** The right IJ vein is preferred because it gives direct access to the SVC and IVC and allows for easier catheterization of the hepatic veins. The left IJ vein or right femoral vein can be used but are not preferred. Accessing the femoral artery is not appropriate when biopsying the liver.

CHAPTER 26: VARICOSE VEINS

1. **b.** While all the answer choices may cause her lower extremity symptoms, GSV reflux is the most common cause of chronic venous insufficiency.
2. **c.** All noninvasive options should be exhausted before proceeding to intervention.
3. **d.** The symptoms being described are suggestive of post-procedure paresthesia and skin burns, both of which could have been prevented with tumescent anesthesia, which is injected into the subcutaneous space to prevent ablation-related thermal injury.

CHAPTER 27: VENOUS ACCESS

1. **d.** The subclavian vein is difficult to visualize under ultrasound to its location under the clavicle. It is the least used vessel, due to its anatomy and complications of "pinch off syndrome" and risk of developing a pneumothorax.
2. **a.** The distal tip of the tunneled dialysis catheter should be in the high right atrium ("cavoatrial junction") due to its high flow rate. This allows for appropriate use of the catheter and prevents complications such as thrombosis.
3. **b.** In the setting of emergent fluid resuscitation, a nontunneled device is used with or without image guidance. Internal jugular, subclavian, or femoral venous access is usually acquired. This form of access is usually temporary, until the patient is stabilized.

CHAPTER 28: Y-90 EMBOLIZATION

1. **b.** Y-90 is a pure beta emitter, decaying to zirconium 90. It has an average energy of 0.94 MeV, penetrating tissue up to 2.5 mm away.
2. **c.** Arteries that may require prophylactic embolization include the gastroduodenal, right gastric, and accessory left gastric. This is performed to prevent nontarget radio-embolization.

CHAPTER 29: ABSCESS DRAINAGE

1. **c.** Intravenous sedation and local anesthesia at catheter insertion sites is the most appropriate strategy in this patient. General anesthesia is typically not required for percutaneous catheter drainage of intraabdominal fluid collections, especially for a patient who is a poor candidate for the physiologic stresses of general anesthesia (choice a, b). Image-guided drainage can be achieved using only local anesthesia in appropriate, cooperative candidates; however, this vignette states the patient responded poorly to a procedure using only local anesthesia. Aborting or delaying treatment in this patient in lieu of an antibiotic-only strategy is not appropriate—she has multiple large abscesses with systemic manifestations of infection. Image-guided drainage is feasible in this patient and offers the best treatment. It should not be delayed and certainly not aborted.

2. **d.** Among the available choices, the most appropriate choice of action is to schedule a short-term outpatient sinogram with catheter manipulation procedure. This allows for assessment of the residual cavity and any associated tracts or fistulae not previously appreciated. If the daily catheter output has been acceptably low (less than 10 mL/day or whatever benchmark the interventionist chooses), this setting would be appropriate for catheter removal if the abscess cavity has completely or nearly resolved. Other maneuvers in this setting include catheter repositioning, exchange with upsizing or downsizing the diameter. Follow-up in the interventional radiology clinic within a reasonable period of time (e.g., 1–2 weeks) would be appropriate. Catheter removal does not always require a procedure—low output and clinical improvement are appropriate criteria for removal. Six weeks is too long to commence initial postprocedural follow-up. Complications requiring admissions may ensue, which may have been preventable with shorter follow-up. Delegating responsibility for catheter follow-up and removal to other physicians or health care associates loses touch with the patient and may perturb referring providers. Interventional radiology is a clinical specialty and should take responsibility for managing hardware they inserted (e.g., a drainage catheter). Surgeons are experts at abdominal drains and capable of determining appropriate removal criteria, but abandoning responsibility of this patient may hinder the surgeon-interventionist relationship.

3. **d.** Minimally invasive approaches have been shown to have similar efficacies, all in retrospective series. At the time of writing, there are no prospective trials that compare percutaneous catheter management of abscess-fistula complexes to percutaneous or endoscopic closure devices following effective abscess drainage. Although some surgeons may choose to operate in this scenario, minimally invasive techniques have been shown to be effective in fistula resolution. At this juncture, in a stable outpatient, a minimally invasive approach is a reasonable first step.

CHAPTER 30: BILIARY DRAINS AND BILIARY STENTING

1. **c.** MRCP provides detailed images of the biliary lumen in a noninvasive fashion, making it the best choice for assessing biliary anatomy pre procedure. ERCP also provides images of the biliary lumen but requires endoscopy and is thus more invasive. CT and ultrasound are useful in assessing features associated with the biliary system, such as surrounding tumor or gallstones, but does not assess the biliary lumen as well as MRCP or ERCP.

2. **d.** In this common anatomic variant, the right posterior hepatic duct converges with the left hepatic duct rather than the right anterior hepatic duct. The right posterior hepatic duct is present but is not opacified by catheterization of the right anterior hepatic duct due to its alternate drainage. Other anatomic variations may exist that would result in the same cholangiogram but are less common.

3. **c.** Metal stent placement is reserved for those with malignant biliary obstruction. Long-term stenting, an evaluation of biliary anatomy with MRCP, and periprocedural antibiotics are all indicated in this patient with a benign biliary stricture.

CHAPTER 31: CT-GUIDED LUNG BIOPSY

1. **d.** An INR >1.5 is a contraindication to biopsy. Bullous emphysema increases the risk of a pneumothorax as thin-walled bullae are easily ruptured when traversed. A hydatid cyst brings risk of anaphylactic reaction if ruptured and should not be traversed. Guidelines recommend a platelet level >50,000 for safe lung biopsy. A high PEEP level increases the likelihood of pneumothorax in ventilated patients.

2. **c.** Pneumothorax is the most common complication resulting from CT-guided lung biopsy. Small intrapulmonary hemorrhage is relatively common after biopsy, but hemothorax and chylothorax are relatively rare after lung biopsy. Neuropathic pain is limited to instances where a nerve, usually an intercostal nerve, is violated during needle advancement and is rare. Pericardial laceration is extremely rare.

3. **c.** A peripheral noncalcified nodule is the most amenable lesion of those listed previously for CT-guided transcutaneous biopsy. Central nodules are more amenable to bronchoscopic biopsy. A calcified granuloma will likely prove stable in size on follow-up images and need not be biopsied. A "serpiginous mass" that enhances with contrast suggests an arteriovenous malformation that should absolutely not be biopsied.

CHAPTER 32: GASTROSTOMY TUBE PLACEMENT

1. **a.** INR should be less than 1.5. Platelet count should be greater than 50,000/μL. Plavix should be held for 5 days before the procedure, but aspirin can be continued.

2. **e.** All are absolute contraindications. A G-tube can be placed in a patient with SBO or gastric outlet obstruction for decompression; this is not so in the case of a patient with an esophageal mass.

3. **b.** Dysphagia, due to neurologic, neuromuscular, or obstructive causes, is the most common indication for G-tube placement. Weight loss is seen with esophageal cancer, but weight loss by itself is not an indication for G-tube placement. The placement of G-tubes has not been shown to increase patient survival rates.

CHAPTER 33: LYMPHANGIOGRAPHY AND THORACIC DUCT EMBOLIZATION

1. **b.** Thoracic surgery is the most common cause of chylothorax, which is the most common indication for thoracic duct embolization. Pneumothoraces and tracheoesophageal fistulas do not cause lymph leaks. Filariasis can cause lymphedema, but TDE is not the proper treatment.

2. **c.** Contraindications to TDE include uncorrectable coagulopathy, patient with intracardiac shunts (as there is a risk of cerebral embolism), and patient with decreased respiratory reserve, as Lipiodol can cause pulmonary embolism/pneumonitis.

3. **a.** Lipiodol can be the source of an embolus if it inadvertently gets into the internal jugular vein via the jugulovenous angle. In a normal patient, this can cause a PE. In a patient with an intracardiac shunt, this can lead to a cerebral embolism.

CHAPTER 34: PARACENTESIS

1. **b.** Disseminated intravascular coagulation (DIC) is the only absolute contraindication to paracentesis. The remaining choices are relative contraindications.

2. **b.** Spontaneous bacterial peritonitis (SBP) is defined by ascites with a PMN count of >250 cells/mm^3, which can be calculated by multiplying the WBC count by the neutrophil percentage. Choice *b*, with a PMN count of 360 cells/mm^3, is the only choice that meets criteria for SBP.

3. **d.** A portal pressure of approximately 12 mm Hg or greater is typically required for fluid retention, making choices *a* and *c* incorrect. Cirrhotic ascites is defined by a SAAG ≥1.1 g/dL, making choice *d* the correct answer.

CHAPTER 35: PERCUTANEOUS NEPHROSTOMY

1. **c.** Indications for percutaneous nephrostomy include obstructive uropathy, pyonephrosis, urinary diversion, and access for percutaneous interventions such as PCNL. Urinary incontinence is a lower urinary tract disorder, which would not be helped by percutaneous nephrostomy.

2. **b.** In general, accessing the renal collecting system via the mid/lower renal calyx avoids the complications of pleural transgression when accessing the upper poles or injury to the main renal artery/vein when accessing the renal pelvis or ureteropelvic junction.

3. **a.** The 0.035-inch guidewire provides a more stable platform for the nephrostomy catheter to be advanced over and through the extrarenal soft tissues and renal parenchyma, and minimizes damage to these tissues. Choices Guidewires, regardless of size, are easily seen under fluoroscopy. Guidewires are also not used to dilate the soft tissue tract (dilators are used for that purpose). A PCN catheter easily accommodates a 0.035-inch wire and therefore would also accommodate a thinner wire such as a 0.018-inch wire.

CHAPTER 36: THORACENTESIS

1. **b.** Thoracentesis is performed in the pleural space. It is not performed in the other listed options.
2. **c.** A thoracentesis is performed to drain fluid from the pleural space (pleural effusion). It would not be indicated for any of the other conditions listed.
3. **a.** An exudate is a protein-rich fluid, and to determine if an effusion is an exudative, Light's Criteria is used. Choices *b* and *d* describe transudative fluids and choice *c* is not part of Light's Criteria.
4. **d.** There are no absolute contraindications to thoracentesis.
5. **c.** CT provides far superior evaluation of bony structures, which appear as shadows on ultrasound. Ultrasound, on the other hand, is less expensive, does not expose the patient to ionizing radiation, and is portable.

INDEX

Note: Page numbers followed by *f* indicate figures, *t* indicate tables, and *b* indicate boxes.